Luc Lanthier, MD., MSc., FRCPC
General Internist
Head of the Internal Medicine Division
Centre Hospitalier Universitaire de Sherbrooke
Associate professor
Faculty of Medicine and Health Sciences
Université de Sherbrooke

PRACTICAL GUIDE TO INTERNAL MEDICINE

First Canadian Edition

September 2009

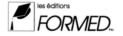

les éditions
FORMED inc.

Bibliothèque et Archives nationales du Québec and Library and Archives Canada cataloguing in publication

Lanthier, Luc, 1971-

Practical guide to internal medicine

1st Canadian ed.

Translation of: Guide pratique de médecine interne.
Includes bibliographical references and index.

ISBN 978-2-923026-15-2

1. Internal medicine - Handbooks, manuals, etc. 2. Diseases - Handbooks, manuals, etc.
3. Diseases - Causes and theories of causation - Handbooks, manuals, etc. 4. Diagnosis -
Handbooks, manuals, etc. 5. Therapeutics - Handbooks, manuals, etc. 6. Prognosis -
Handbooks, manuals, etc. I. Title.

RC55.L3613 2009   616   C2009-941842-8

First Canadian Edition, September 2009
Practical Guide to Internal Medicine

ISBN-13 : **978 – 2 – 923026 – 15 – 2**
Legal deposit- Quebec National Library, 2009
Legal deposit- National Library of Canada, 2009

"We would appreciate you notifying us of any suggestions in this edition. Simply inform us by sending an E-mail entitled "Practical Guide to Internal Medicine" to the following address: Luc.Lanthier@USherbrooke.ca"

© _Les Éditions Formed inc., September 2009, all rights reserved for all countries._
All partial or total reproduction of this guide is forbidden without a written consent from the Éditions Formed inc., 1871, rue Royale, Trois-Rivières, P.Q. G9A 4K7.
Internet : formed@videotron.ca
Tél. : (819) 371-9744 Fax : (819) 371-9744

Main Author:
Luc Lanthier MD, internist, CHUS, Sherbrooke.

Co-Authors:
Jean-Daniel Baillargeon MD, gastroenterologist, CHUS, Sherbrooke.
Frédéric Bernier, MD, endocrinologist, CHUS, Sherbrooke.
Simon Bérubé MD, cardiologist, specialist in hemodynamics, CHUS, Sherbrooke.
Nicole Bouchard MD, pneumologist, CHUS, Sherbrooke.
Charles Deacon MD, neurologist, CHUS, Sherbrooke.
Jean Dufresne MD, hemato-oncologist, CHUS, Sherbrooke.
Patrick Liang MD, rhumatologist, CHUS, Sherbrooke.
Mélanie Masse MD, MSc, nephrologist, CHUS, Sherbrooke.
Matthieu Touchette MD, internist, CHUS, Sherbrooke.
Louis Valiquette MD, MSc, microbiologist-infectious disease specialist, CHUS, Sherbrooke.

Collaborators:
Jean-Sébastien Aucoin MD, resident, Sherbrooke.
Annie Beaudoin MD, gastroenterologist, CHUS, Sherbrooke.
Damien Bélisle, MD, nephrologist, CSSS Chicoutimi.
Émilie Belley-Côté MD, resident, Sherbrooke.
Marco Bergevin MD, microbiologist-infectious disease specialist, Cité de la Santé, Laval.
Paul Bessette MD, gynecological oncologist, CHUS, Sherbrooke.
Mariane Breton-Thibodeau MD, nephrologist, CH La Sagamie, Chicoutimi.
Michel Carmel MD, urologist, CHUS, Sherbrooke.
Mariane Charron MD.
Anne-Marie Côté MD, nephrologist, CHUS.
Luc Cormier MD, resident, Sherbrooke.
Jean Desaulniers MD, family medicine, Trois-Rivières.
Véronique Duguay MD.
Donald Echenberg MD, internist, CHUS, Sherbrooke.
David Germain MD, pneumologist, CH Pierre-Boucher, Longueuil.
Mélanie Hamel MD, nephrologist, Cité De La Santé, Laval.
Noémie Juaire MD, resident, Sherbrooke.
Geneviève LeTemplier MD, internist, CHUS, Sherbrooke.
Vincent Masse MD, resident, Sherbrooke.
Michaël Mayette MD, resident, Sherbrooke.
Bruno Maynard MD, dermatologist, CHUS, Sherbrooke.

Collaborators: (to follow)

François Moreau MD, neurologist, CHUS, Sherbrooke.
Mohamed Nosair MD, resident, Sherbrooke.
Alain Piché MD, MSc, microbiologist-infectious disease specialist, CHUS, Sherbrooke.
John Robb MD, internist, CHUS, Sherbrooke.
Nadine Sauvé MD, internist, CHUS, Sherbrooke.
Jean Sétrakian MD, internist, CHUS, Sherbrooke.
Charles St-Arnaud MD, resident, Sherbrooke.
Catherine St-Pierre MD, internist and intensive care specialist, CHUS, Sherbrooke.
Marc-André Tremblay MD.
Daniel Viens MD, resident, Sherbrooke.
David Williamson, B. Pharm, MSc, Hôpital Sacré-Coeur de Montréal.
Philippe Yale MD, resident, Sherbrooke.
Matthias Ziller MD, resident, McGill University, Montreal.

With special thanks to Ms Sylvie Bruneau; and to Dr René Gagnon MD and Guy Tremblay MD, for SCORE Canada

Special regards to the following societies:

Association des médecins omnipraticiens de la Mauricie
Canadian Society of Internal Medicine
Faculty of medicine and Health Sciences, Université de Sherbrooke

FOREWORD

I have known Luc Lanthier since 1994 when he was a first year resident in internal medicine. I have had the opportunity to follow his career throughout his residency and during his years on staff at the *Centre Hospitalier Universitaire de Sherbrooke*.

Luc as a resident had an encyclopaedic knowledge of internal medicine and a remarkable ability to rapidly synthesize vast amounts of data. During his last years as a resident, while preparing for his final exams, he decided to attempt to make a synthesis of internal medicine in 100 tables. It was a pretty good attempt!!!

The result was so successful (both the work that he created and his exam results) that he decided to turn his work into a book entitled: *Guide Pratique de Médecine Interne*.

The first edition published in 1999 was an immediate success. It was a succinct summary of most of the problems encountered in an internal medicine practice but small and light enough to easily slip into and out of the pocket of a lab coat. It was based on the soundest principles of evidence-based medicine and included all of the relevant clinical practice guidelines. Each chapter and each table was reviewed and modified extensively by another member of our general internal medicine service. It rapidly became a must for residents in the core medical and general internal medical programs first in Sherbrooke and then all over Quebec. It was also used by many physicians in practice in general internal medicine (including the undersigned) and family doctors.

Luc's work is now in its fifth edition (first bilingual edition) with this latest edition undergoing the same extensive review as the first four. His book has sold an astounding 12 500 copies so far (quite amazing when you consider that it is intended mainly for internal medical and family practice residents in Quebec).

Luc and his publisher therefore decided to translate the book into English and make it available to a wider Canadian readership.

Do we need another book on internal medicine? Yes indeed, if it contributes to the ease of knowledge retrieval for the busy physician at the office, during hospital rounds and while on call at home. Yes, if it is a place where we can rapidly find the thousands of small diagnostic, preventive and therapeutic details that we need at a moment's notice. Yes if we know that we can rely on the information that it contains including the many clinical pearls that help to make up the knowledge base of the general internist.

A few years ago I came across a seminal article in the Annals of Internal Medicine (The Relation Between Clinical Experience and Quality of Health Care, Ann Intern Med 2005; 142: 260-73). This systematic review suggested that physician knowledge, adherence to clinical guidelines, and clinical outcomes do not necessarily improve with physician age or years of experience. In some cases the contrary might apply. In spite of remarkable advances in the art and science of medicine there is ample proof that the theory to practice gap is still as wide as ever. Amongst the solutions towards narrowing this gap: Continuing Professional Development (rather than traditional CME that is composed of discrete boluses of knowledge, often forgotten and never translated into practice), rapid diffusion of and easy access to the latest clinical guidelines available in the relevant practice setting and books such as the Practical Guide to Internal Medicine which offer rapid reference to relevant and reliable clinical information.

Whether you wish to rapidly review the differential diagnosis of coma, refresh your memory on the indications for colon cancer screening, or go over the treatment of various vasculitides the answer is in this book. If you cannot remember the dose and format of an inhaled bronchodilator, of a neuromuscular blocker, or of a specific anti-convulsive agent, check the appendices at the end of the book. If you cannot remember the half-lives of the various benzodiazepines, this is the place to look. There is even a table on drug interactions involving the Cytochrome P-450 system of enzymes.

Luc's book is proof that good things do indeed come in small packages. It will be of use to medical students, residents in family practice and internal medicine as well physicians in practice in these disciplines.

Therefore it is with great pleasure that I introduce the first Canadian edition of the Practical Guide to Internal Medicine.

Donald Echenberg, MD, FRCPC, FACP
Past President of the Canadian Society of Internal Medicine.

PREAMBLE

The majority of treatment and therapeutic in this volume reflect the current standards of internal medicine. Other treatment options may be effective and are not necessarily included in this collection.

The author, associated companies and publisher wish to caution, however, any physician to retain a critical and do not hesitate to consult an expert colleague for therapeutic or clinical situation where he feels uncomfortable.

We remind you that every physician is responsible for his acts and therefore should use this guide as an indication only.

To Catherine, for her great patience.
To Marie-Noël, Éloïse and Anaïs,
three lovers of books.

To medical students, clinical clerks and residents,
the sole *raison d'être* of this Guide.

TABLE OF CONTENT

Chapter 1

Cardiology

Bradyarrhythmias and Conduction Disturbances	
Sinus bradycardia	Definition: heart rate < 60 beats/min. Bradycardia as low as 30/min, or an asymptomatic pause up to 3 seconds or a 2nd degree AV block Mobitz I may occur in healthy individuals. Causes : – Intrinsic: idiopathic, physically active patient, ischemia-infarction, infiltrative diseases (sarcoidosis, amyloidosis, hemochromatosis), connective tissue disease, myotonic dystrophy, post valvular replacement, infections (Chagas disease, endocarditis), familial, etc. – Extrinsic: autonomic (neurocardiogenic syncope, hypersensitivity of the carotid sinus, situational), medication (digoxin, non-dihydropyridine calcium channel blockers, beta-blockers, clonidine, antiarrhythmics, etc), hypothermia, hypothyroidism, intracranial hypertension, hyperkalemia, sleep apnea, etc.
Sick sinus syndrome	Sinus node dysfunction is characterized by an abnormal rhythm: sinus pause or sino-auricular block or sinus bradycardia or supraventricular tachyarrhythmia (atrial fibrillation, flutter, reentry) ± bradycardia (tachycardia-bradycardia syndrome). Idiopathic or associated with diseases mentioned above or rarely CAD. Occurs mostly with older patients: most commonly asymptomatic or syncope, near syncope, faintness, dizziness, confusion, palpitations, angina, congestive heart failure, systemic embolism. With atrial fibrillation, pauses up to 5 seconds may be considered normal if asymptomatic. Diagnosis by cardiac monitoring (Holter). The relationship between rhythm and symptoms is important. External or internal loop recorder sometimes useful. Table tilt test if vagal etiology suspected. Electrophysiological studies are rarely needed. Stress test may show chronotropic incompetence where maximum heart rate is less than 85 % of predicted heart rate according to age (220 - age). Treatment: if symptomatic, DDD pacemaker (or AAI if normal conduction at the AV node level). Pindolol sometimes effective if atrial fibrillation alternates between fast and slow ventricular response.
Atrioventri-cular block (AV)	Definition : • 1st degree AV block: PR interval > 0.20 seconds. • 2nd degree AV block Mobitz I (Wenckebach): progressive ↑ PR interval followed by a non-conducted P wave: due to abnormal conduction in the AV node: may be associated with inferior wall infarction. Occurs sometimes in healthy, especially younger, patients. • 2nd degree AV block Mobitz II: P wave blocked suddenly with PR interval previously fixed or constant: due to abnormal conduction in His bundle (infranodal): may be associated with anterior wall infarction. QRS often widened. • 3rd degree AV block: No fixed relation between P wave and QRS. AV dissociation. Causes: idiopathic fibrosis, acute ischemia, iatrogenic ablation, calcified valvular disease, medication, infection (endocarditis, Lyme), inflammatory or infiltrative diseases, connective tissue disease, trauma, post cardiac surgery, etc. Diagnosis is as for sinus disease. Treatment: pacemaker if symptomatic or if 2nd AV block Mobitz II (especially with bi or trifascicular block or with wide QRS) or with persistent 3rd degree block (especially with ventricular response < 40/min [awake], pause > 3 s [awake], with certain neuromuscular diseases or with bi or trifascicular or certain congenital blocks) or post-op AV blocks.

Intraventricular conduction disturbances	After the His bundle, the conduction system splits into right and left bundle branches. The left bundle branch splits into anterior and posterior fascicles.
	Definition :
	- Right bundle branch block: QRS > 0.12 ms: RSR' in V_1 or V_2: S > 40 ms in I, V_6: ST-T changes in V_1-V_3.
	- Left bundle branch block: QRS > 0.12 ms; wide R wave in V_5-V_6 with notch or slow rise; absence of Q wave in V_5-V_6.
	- Left anterior fascicular block (LAFB): axis < -45 °: R/S < 1 in II, III, aVF: qR wave in I and rS in II, III: QRS < 0.12.
	- Left posterior fascicular block (LPFB): axis > + 90 °: rS wave in I and qR in II, III: QRS < 0.12.
	- Bifascicular block: if 2 of following: RBBB, LAFB, LPFB.
	- Trifascicular block:
	- RBBB + alternating fascicular block (LAFB, LPFB on different occasions).
	- Alternating RBBB and LBBB.
	- Bifascicular block with prolonged infranodal conduction (long His-ventricular interval in electrophysiological study).
	- Non-specific intraventricular conduction disturbance: QRS ≥ 0.12 ms without any bundle branch block morphology.
	Causes: can occur in normal person or associated with CAD, infiltrative, cardiomyopathy, postcardiotomy syndrome, inflammatory diseases, etc.
	Treatment: pacemaker indicated if symptomatic or if alternate bundle-branch block.
	Prognosis depends on the cause. Good prognosis if no organic disease.

Tachyarrhythmias

Supraventricular Tachyarrhythmias

Atrial Fibrillation

Irregularly irregular supraventricular rhythm.
Most frequent sustained cardiac arrhythmia, increasing in frequency with age (occurrence of 1 % at 50 years old, 11 % at 80 years old).

Symptoms: palpitations, chest pain, fatigue, dizziness, pre-syncope, syncope, congestive heart failure, decreased effort tolerance, tachycardia-induced cardiomyopathy, stroke, peripheral embolism; occasionally asymptomatic.
Risk factors: age, heart failure, smoking, diabetes, hypertension, male, LVH, MI, valvular heart disease.

Differential Diagnosis:
- Atrial Flutter (see below).
- Multifocal atrial tachycardia.
- Pre-excitation syndrome (Wolff-Parkinson-White): see below.

Clinical Classification of atrial fibrillation	- First-detected episode of atrial fibrillation: may be persistent or self-limited and symptomatic or not.
	- Recurrent atrial fibrillation: 2 or more episodes of atrial fibrillation lasting > 30 s.
	- Paroxysmal atrial fibrillation: recurrent atrial fibrillation terminating spontaneously (within 7 days).
	- Persistent atrial fibrillation: atrial fibrillation sustained beyond 7 days or requiring pharmacological therapy or electrical cardioversion for termination: may be a first episode or recurrent atrial fibrillation.
	- Permanent atrial fibrillation: Long term atrial fibrillation (> 1 year) or when cardioversion failed or has not been attempted.

Associated diseases	– Heart disease: valvular disease (more often mitral or tricuspid), CAD, cardiomyopathy, pericardial diseases, conduction system disease (sick sinus syndrome, pre-excitation), congenital heart disease, intracardiac or adjacent to left atrium tumor or metastasis, etc. – Post cardiothoracic or esophageal surgery. – Pulmonary disease (embolism, obstructive or interstitial disease). – Neurologic disease (stroke, subarachnoid haemorrhage, tumor). – Toxico-metabolic causes (hyperthyroidism, electrolytes imbalance, alcohol, coffee, pheochromocytoma, infections, anxiety, drugs, carbon monoxide, etc). – Neurogenic mediated causes: increased vagal or adrenergic tone. – Electrical injury. – Familial. – Idiopathic.
Risk of stroke with atrial fibrillation	**CHADS$_2$ score** in order to evaluate the risk of stroke per year for non-valvular atrial fibrillation (for patients not on anticoagulation nor aspirin): **C:** **C**ongestive heart failure: 1 point. **H:** **H**igh blood pressure: 1 point. **A:** **A**ge > 75: 1 point. **D:** **D**iabetes: 1 point. **S$_2$:** **S**troke history: 2 points. If score = 0 points, 1.9 % risk of stroke/year (adjusted). 1 point = 2.8 %, 2 points = 4 %, 3 points = 5.9 %, 4 points = 8.5 %, 5 points = 12.5 %, 6 points = 18.2 %.
Workup	CBC, INR, aPTT, electrolytes, creatinine, glucose, TSH. CK-troponin if ischemia is suspected. ECG. Chest X-ray. Echocardiography (valve evaluation, left and right atrial size, ventricular function, presence of thrombus). Holter or telemetry as needed. With infrequent episodes, external or internal loop recorder sometimes useful.
Acute Management	*If hemodynamically unstable* (angina, hypotension, heart failure) → immediate electrical cardioversion (with heparin or LMWH if no contraindication), followed by warfarin for at least 4 weeks if sinus rhythm persists. *If hemodynamically stable and duration < 48 h* → rapid cardioversion, with heparin or LMWH if not contraindicated: anticoagulation to be evaluated according to patient's risk of embolism. *If hemodynamically stable and duration > 48 h but < 1 year* → 2 options : 1- trans-esophageal echocardiography and rapid cardioversion if no thrombus (with heparin if not contraindicated) and anticoagulation for at least 4 weeks afterwards **or** 2- anticoagulation for a minimum of 3 weeks with a therapeutic INR before the planned cardioversion and anticoagulation at least 4 weeks afterwards. *If hemodynamically stable and duration > 1 year* → anticoagulation depending on CHADS$_2$ score and control ventricular rate (high failure rate for maintaining a sinus induced rhythm post cardioversion). *Rate control* with digoxin (less effective during exercise), beta-blockers, calcium channel blockers (non-dihydropyridine: verapamil or diltiazem). Electrical or pharmacological cardioversion (propafenone, flecainide, amiodarone, ibutilide, dofetilide). Spontaneous cardioversion often occurs.

Chronic Management	2 possible strategies, none being superior to the other (AFFIRM and AF-CHF trials): 1. Rate control and chronic anticoagulation (see next section for anticoagulation) (**Rate control strategy**): a strategy of rate control using beta-blockers or non-dihydropyridine calcium channel blockers if LVEF is normal **or** beta-blockers, digoxin (adequate at rest) or amiodarone if LVEF ↓; aim for heart rate between 60-80/min at rest, 90-115/min with moderate exertion. If failure to achieve: install a permanent pacemaker and adjust rate control with negative chronotropic drugs or concomitant AV node ablation. 2. Sinus rhythm control (**Rhythm control strategy**) : Give antiarrhythmic drug therapy after the 1st episode if hemodynamically unstable atrial fibrillation: otherwise start it at the 2nd episode. Choose anti-arrhythmic according to co-morbidities: - In the absence of heart disease: use flecainide or propafenone (combined with a negative chronotrope since there is a risk of 1:1 flutter with recurrence) or sotalol. If failure/recurrence, use amiodarone or dofetilide or pulmonary veins ablation or change strategy aiming for rate control. - If hypertension with LVH: use amiodarone: if failure/recurrence: pulmonary veins ablation or change strategy aiming for rate control. If hypertension without LVH, same treatment as for a patient without heart disease (above). - If CAD: use sotalol or dofetilide: if failure/recurrence use amiodarone or pulmonary veins ablation or change strategy and aim for rate control. - If heart failure: use amiodarone or dofetilide. If failure/recurrence, catheter ablation or change strategy aiming for rate control. Refractory AF > 100/min > 50 % of the time despite two medications = indication for ablation therapy via pulmonary veins ablation if rhythm control strategy or AV node ablation with concomitant pacemaker implantation if rate control strategy. Surgical ablation (Maze procedure) if patient is having cardiac surgery. Note: Start IC Class anti-arrhythmic and sotalol in hospital under cardiac monitoring except for sotalol if QTc < 460 ms, no structural heart disease, normal electrolytes and no pro-arrhythmic risk factor (renal failure, hypokalemia /hypomagnesemia...) and for IC class if lone atrial fibrillation without structural heart disease: then ambulatory treatment may be started. Stop anti-arrhythmic if QRS ↑ more than 50 %, except for amiodarone. Note: treatment of precipitating factors (hyperthyroid, pneumonia, CHF) must be achieved before cardioversion.
Anticoagulant treatment	In accordance with the 2006 ACC/AHA/ESC Guidelines: Each patient's individual risk of cardio-embolism is to be stratified and risk and benefits of anti-coagulant treatment must be evaluated: - High risk factors for stroke: prior stroke, TIA or systemic embolism, mitral stenosis, prosthetic heart valve. - Moderate risk factors: age > 75 y, hypertension, heart failure and/or left ventricle dysfunction with LVEF ≤ 35 % or diabetes. - Low risk factors (or less validated): age 65-74 y, woman, CAD, hyperthyroidism. For patient without any risk factor: **Aspirin (ASA) 81-325 mg/d.** For patient with one moderate-risk factor: **ASA 81-325 mg/d or warfarin, INR 2-3** (warfarin rather than aspirin suggested by ACCP 2008). For patient with any high-risk factors or with > one moderate-risk factor: **warfarin, INR 2-3.** ASA only if warfarin is contraindicated. In practice, if CHADS$_2$ score > 1, warfarin; if CHADS$_2$ = 1, ASA or warfarin; if CHADS$_2$ = 0, give ASA. Note: For paroxysmal AF, the risk of embolism is the same as for permanent AF and the same recommendations apply.

Atrial Flutter

Arrhythmia characterized by sawtooth flutter (F) waves with atrial rate 240-320/min. If normal conduction system AV ratio 2:1 conduction is usual, and the ventricular response is near 150 beats/min.
Higher AV block (3:1 or more) without medication slowing the AV node is suggestive of a disorder of conduction tissue.

Carotid massage slows the ventricular response and can be useful in establishing the diagnosis.

60 % of episodes are secondary to another acute process (acute exacerbation of COPD, post-op, myocardial infarction, etc).

Treatment:
Medication slowing AV node same as in atrial fibrillation (30-50 % success rate).
Radiofrequency ablation of re-entry pathway is very effective and highly recommended (> 90 % chance of success). Other options: AV node ablation and permanent pacemaker. Pharmacologic cardioversion can be attempted with propafenone, flecainide, procainamide or ibutilide.
No long term treatment when secondary to other disorders.

Note: Risk of embolism same as in AF; same anticoagulation strategy recommended.

Paroxysmal Supraventricular Tachycardia

The most frequent paroxysmal tachycardia. Often occurs in patients without structural heart disease. Regular rhythm 140-240/min. Occasionally secondary to digoxin intoxication.

Causes	#1 Nodal reentrant 60 %: typical 90%: p in QRS or right after (PR interval > RP).
	Atypical 10 %: inverted p before QRS (PR < RP).
	
	#2 Accessory pathway 30 %: orthodromic 90 %: narrow QRS (PR > RP).
	                                    Antidromic 10 %: wide QRS (See below pre-excitation syndrome).
	
	# 3 Other causes 10 %: sinoatrial nodal reentrant: p ⊕ before QRS.
	                               Unifocal or multifocal atrial tachycardia.

Treatment	Vagal stimulation: Valsalva, cough… carotid sinus massage.
	Pharmacological: adenosine 6 mg IV-12 mg IV rapid bolus. Side effects: hot flushes, chest pain, prolonged pause.
	    Calcium channel blockers (non-dihydropyridine): verapamil, diltiazem.
	    Other options (less recommended): beta-blockers: esmolol, metoprolol, etc.
	Electrical cardioversion: if hemodynamically unstable or drug failure (avoid if digoxin intoxication).

Prevention of recurrence	Radiofrequency ablation (effective in > 95 %). Alternatives to ablation (according to patient preference): verapamil, diltiazem, beta-blockers If no response; Class IC antiarrhythmic (if no structural cardiac disease and combined with a negative chronotropic) or class III antiarrhythmic.

Multifocal Atrial Tachycardia

Irregular rhythm characterized by P wave of different morphology (at least 3 on a lead II rhythm strip) and irregular PR interval.
Ventricular response between 100-140/min.
Associated with severe COPD, catecholamine excess, acid-base and electrolyte disturbances, rarely associated with digoxin intoxication.
Treatment: treat the underlying cause ± verapamil. No digoxin.

Pre-excitation Syndrome

Caused by conduction through an accessory pathway between the atrium and ventricle. Prevalence 1/500. 33 % of patients < 40 years old with pre-excitation are symptomatic.
Wolff-Parkinson-White (WPW) Syndrome: short PR (< 0.12 s.), delta wave, prolonged QRS (> 0.12 s.), ST-T changes discordant with the QRS, palpitations.
Lown-Ganong-Levine syndrome: short P-R, normal QRS, paroxysmal tachycardia.

Anterograde conduction thru AV node (orthodromic) with narrow QRS or thru an accessory pathway (antidromic) with wide QRS (see Paroxysmal Supraventricular Tachycardia).

Patients with WPW Syndrome may have a PSVT (70 %), AF (30 %) or atrial flutter. Risk of sudden death if symptomatic is 0.25-0.5% pt-year.

Treatment	If asymptomatic, observation alone (ablation can be done for patients with high-risk occupations).
	If PSVT: see PSVT treatment above.
	If AF or flutter: electrical cardioversion if hemodynamically unstable. If hemodynamically stable, procainamide IV. Avoid digoxin, verapamil and beta-blockers since it ↓ refractory period through accessory pathway. Risk of rapid AF with adenosine. Prophylaxis with procainamine, flecainide or ibutilide.
	Chronic: Radio-frequency ablation of accessory pathway.

Ventricular Tachyarrhythmias

Ventricular Tachycardia	– Wide complex tachycardia ≥ 100/minute (generally 160-240/min).
	– Asymptomatic or cerebral hypoperfusion (syncope).
	– **Non-sustained** if < 30 s vs **sustained** if > 30 s or < 30 s *and* hemodynamic instability.
	– Often associated with heart disease (ischemia, cardiomyopathy, myocarditis...).
	– Rare causes of malignant arrhythmia: congenital or acquired (drug related) long QT syndrome, Brugada syndrome (RBBB and ST elevation on V_1-V_3), RV outflow tract VT, idiopathic LV VT, arrhythmogenic right ventricular cardiomyopathy, tetralogy of Fallot, hypertrophic cardiomyopathy.
	
	Workup: echocardiography + coronary angiography, especially if sustained VT. Rule out electrolyte disorders (K^+, Mg^{++}).
	
	Treatment :
	Acute: – urgent electrical cardioversion if hemodynamically unstable.
	– Amiodarone IV.
	– Beta-blockers IV during acute MI for primary prevention.
	– If non-sustained: treatment controversial.
	
	Chronic: - Implantable cardioverter-defibrillator: consider for cardiac arrest with VF-VT without obvious reversible cause, post-syncope with inducible VT-VF, for CAD and LVEF 31-40 % and non-sustained and inducible VT at EPS or CAD with LVEF ≤ 30 % (measured > 1-3 months post-MI), for non-ischemic cardiomyopathy with LVEF ≤ 30 %, or for cardiac diseases at high risk of malignant arrhythmia (Brugada, hypertrophic cardiomyopathy...) in absence of contraindication.
	  - For long QT syndrome, beta-blockers, pacemaker, sympathectomy, implantable cardioverter-defibrillator. Family counseling necessary.
	  - Ablation of arrhythmogenic substrate sometimes possible (right ventricular outflow tract VT, idiopathic left septum VT) or if recurrence after implantable cardioverter-defibrillator.
	
	Note: if malignant arrhythmia within < 48 h after an MI, further investigation not necessarily and no antiarrhythmic treatment required (other than beta-blockers).

Ventricular Fibrillation	Caused by cardiac disorders or drugs. Management: as above. IV Amiodarone with VF refractory to defibrillation (ARREST study). Chronic treatment with implantable cardioverter-defibrillator.
Torsades de Pointes	Polymorphic tachycardia with $\uparrow$ QT, idiopathic or 2nd to drug that $\uparrow$ QT interval (e.g. : antiarrhythmics from Class IA, IC, III, tricyclic antidepressant), or 2nd to electrolyte disorders (hypokalemia) or bradycardia. Treatment: stop offending medication. IV Mg^{++}, isoproterenol. Temporary pacemaker if needed. IV beta-blockers + implantable cardioverter-defibrillator if congenital.

Distinguishing Supraventricular Tachycardia with Aberrancy from Ventricular Tachycardia :

– If regular: VT monomorphic vs PSVT with bundle branch block, aberrant conduction, accessory pathway or pacemaker.
– If irregular: VT polymorphic (normal QT) or torsades de pointes (prolonged QT) or atrial fibrillation or atrial flutter with bundle branch block, aberrant conduction, accessory pathway or pacemaker.

More likely VT if :
1. Positive or negative concordance of all derivations from V_1 to V_6.
2. Presence of fusion complexes or capture phenomenon.
3. Auriculoventricular dissociation.
4. QRS > 0.14 ms with RBBB pattern or > 0.16 with LBBB pattern.
5. RBBB QRS morphology with on V_1 qR or RSr' or Rs pattern.
6. LBBB QRS morphology with on V_6 qS or qR pattern.
7. RS interval in precordial > 100 ms.
8. Extreme axis.

More likely PSVT with aberrant conduction:
1. Carotid massage $\downarrow$ PSVT.

Note: 85 % of wide QRS tachycardia are of ventricular origin and up to 90-95 % among patients with CAD. **Never use** calcium channel blocker for wide QRS tachycardia, unless there is no doubt that it is of supra-ventricular origin.

Syncope

Sudden and transient loss of consciousness caused by cerebral hypoperfusion followed by spontaneous recovery.

Frequency: 3 % emergency visits, 5-6 % hospital admissions.

Look for a precipitating factor on history (pain, anxiety), prodrome, onset (effort, urinating, coughing, turning the head, orthostatic hypotension) residual symptoms, associated neurologic symptoms, history of cardiac or psychiatric disease, medications, family history of Wolff-Parkinson-White or sudden death.
On physical exam, look for orthostatic hypotension, do carotid massage with cardiac monitoring, do a cardiac and neurological exam.

Differential diagnosis: dizziness, vertigo, convulsions, drop attacks, metabolic disorders (hypoglycemia).

Causes	– Neurocardiogenic :
	  - vasovagal 18 % (prodrome of nausea, diaphoresis, pallor).
	  - situational 5 % (cough, micturition, defecation).
	  - psychiatric 2 %: frequent, no sequella.
	  - others 1 %: carotid sinus hypersensitivity (with neck pressure or head rotation
	  - 3 types of response: 35 % cardioinhibitory, 15 % vasodepressor, 60 % mixed).
	– Orthostatic 8 %: symptoms when rising. Idiopathic or 2^e to medication, autonomic insufficiency (diabetes, Parkinson, multisystem atrophy), hypovolemia hemorrhage, vasodilatators, etc: diagnostic 20 mmHg ↓ systolic BP or 10 mmHg diastolic after 3 minutes in a standing position.
	– Medication 3 %.
	– Neurological 10 %: subclavian steal syndrome.
	– Cardiac :
	  - Arrhythmias 14 %: bradyarrhythmia (sinus disease, 2-3rd degree AV block, pacemaker dysfunction, medication), tachyarrhythmia (VT, torsades de pointes - long QT syndrome, PSVT).
	  - Mechanical 4 %:
	    o Obstructive: pulmonary or aortic stenosis, hypertrophic cardiomyopathy, pulmonary embolism, pulmonary hypertension, myxoma.
	    o Autres : tamponade, aortic dissection.
	– Unknown cause: 34 %.

Diagnostic	See Figure of the *American College of Physicians 1997* (next page). Note: tilt table testing is occasionally indicated in certain situations where a neurocardiogenic cause is suspected (e.g.: high-risk work). Internal or external loop recorder sometimes useful.
Treatment	Indications for hospitalization : – *Indicated* if infarction, stroke, associated arrhythmia; history of CAD, CHF or ventricular arrhythmia; associated chest pain; significant valvular disease; focal neurologic deficit; ischemia; bundle branch block or ↑ QT interval on ECG. – *Often indicated if* syncope on exertion, frequent syncope, suspicion of CAD, arrhythmia, moderate to severe orthostatic hypotension, > 70 years old, or significant injury. Treatment according to cause or tilt-table test: – Neurocardiogenic syncope: Elastic stocking, salt supplement, fludrocortisone? Beta-blockers? Paroxetine? Midodrine? Electrophysiology consultation, if needed. – Carotid sinus hypersensitivity: if cardio-inhibitory response (pause > 3 s) = pacemaker. If vasodepressor response (↓ BP > 50 mmHg) = elastic stocking, anticholinergic. If mixed, combine treatment. – Orthostatism: stop associated medication, patient education, elastic stocking, salt

	supplementation, hydration, fludrocortisone, midodrine, other medications (clonidine, fluoxetine), and pacemaker if needed. – Malignant arrhythmia identified by electrophysiological study: implantable cardioverter-defibrillator, antiarrhythmic medication. See: Tachyarrhythmia table. Always evaluate possible contraindications to driving: If unexplained unique syncope (faint) or recurrent vagal syncope, wait one week (for private driving). If recurrent unexplained syncope, wait 3 months. For secondary syncope with avoidable trigger (e.g.: micturition, defecation), wait one week. No restriction for unique typical vagal syncope. See appropriate text for more details.
Prognosis	According to cause. If cardiac origin: mortality at one year 18-33 %. If unknown cause 6 %. Frequent recurrence if psychiatric cause. San Francisco Syncope Rule to predict patients with serious outcomes: **C**: **C**ongestive heart failure history. **H**: **H**ematocrit < 30 %. **E**: **E**CG abnormal: non-sinus rhythm or change from past ECG. **S**: **S**hortness of breath. **S**: **S**ystolic BP < 90 mmHg on arrival. 89-90 % sensibility and 42-56 % specificity to predict a serious outcome.

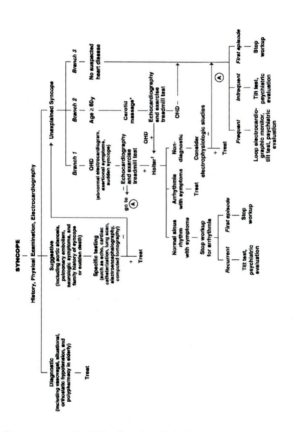

Carotid massage may be performed in the office setting only in the absence of bruits, ventricular tachycardia, recent stroke, or recent myocardial infarction. Carotid hypersensitivity should be diagnosed only if clinical history is suggestive and massage is diagnostically positive: asystole > 3 seconds, hypotension, or both. May be replaced by inpatient telemetry if there is concern about serious arrhythmia.
Echo: echocardiography. OHD: organic heart disease.

From: Linzer M et al. Ann Intern Med 1997 ; 127 : 76-86.

Unstable Angina and Non ST-Elevation MI

Chest Pain Causes	**Non ischemic:** costochondritis, skin disease (shingles), cervical or chest wall pain, muscle, esophagus or stomach (GERD, ulcer, esophageal spasm, Mallory-Weiss, nonulcer dyspepsia), abdominal (pancreatitis, biliary disease, etc), shoulder (arthritis, thoracic outlet syndrome, etc), lungs (pneumonia, pneumothorax, embolism, tumor, mediastinitis, aspiration, asthma, etc), aortic (dissection), cardiac (apical ballooning syndrome – "Takotsubo", mitral valve prolapse, pericarditis, postcardiotomy syndrome, Dressler's syndrome, myocarditis, valvular heart disease), psychogenic. **Ischemic:** CAD, endothelial dysfunction, vasospasm (variant angina, cocaine < 96 hours). Rarely: arteritis, embolism, dissection, congenital malformation, syndrome X, aortic stenosis or regurgitation, severe left ventricular hypertrophy, severe anemia, hypermetabolic state (hyperthyroidism), arrhythmia, vaso-occlusive crisis with sickle cell disease, fibromuscular dysplasia.
Clinical classification	Typical angina if : 1. Retrosternal discomfort with characteristic duration and quality. 2. Induced by physical effort or emotion. 3. Relieved by rest or nitroglycerin. Atypical angina (probable) if it meets 2 of the above criteria: Non-cardiac chest pain if it meets ≤ 1 of the above criteria. With history, physical exam, ECG, and cardiac biomarkers, chest pain may also be classified into one of 4 categories: non-cardiac chest pain, chronic stable angina, possible acute coronary syndrome or definite acute coronary syndrome.
Management	Workup according to clinical presentation (see below). During the acute phase, first determine if the patient has a life threatening pathology (acute ischemia, aortic dissection, pulmonary embolism). If not, investigate as an outpatient. Always consider cocaine consumption, amphetamine or recent use of phosphodiesterase type 5 (sildenafil, tadalafil, vardenafil). Note: A patient with chest pain has an 80% of chances of having an MI if there is new ST-segment elevation ≥ 1 mm, 20 % if there is ST-segment depression or new T wave inversion, 4 % if known CAD with no ECG changes, and 2 % if no history of CAD and no ECG change.
Stable Angina	Primary or secondary (anemia, hyperthyroidism, aortic stenosis, arrhythmia, etc).

Functional classification of angina	Canadian Cardiovascular Society Classification:
	  I: ordinary physical activity such as walking, climbing stairs does not cause angina. Angina occurs with strenuous, rapid or prolonged exertion.
	  II: Slight limitation of ordinary activity.
	  III: Marked limitation of ordinary physical activity.
	  IV: Inability to carry on any physical activity without discomfort - angina may be present at rest.

Workup	– CBC, glucose, lipids. – ECG. Chest X-ray as needed. – Exercise testing (diagnostic or prognostic: do not perform if pre-excitation syndrome, LBBB, pacemaker or > 1 mm of ST depression at rest, LVH, digoxin therapy). – Exercise or pharmacologic stress radionuclide myocardial perfusion imaging (if treadmill test is impossible or non diagnostic, or marked baseline ECG abnormalities). – Stress echocardiography or echo dobutamine (see above).

	– Coronary angiography (if angina is not controlled by medication, if high risk angina according to laboratory workup, if malignant arrhythmia-sudden death, if associated heart failure, if diagnosis is uncertain). – Ergonovine or acetylcholine test (if suspicion of vasospastic angina).

Treatment	Acute attack of angina: sublingual nitrate.
	 Preventive treatment :
	 – Treatment of precipitating factors: anemia, hypertension, arrhythmia, hyperthyroidism, etc.
	 – Beta-blockers (1st line), calcium channel blockers (but avoid non-dihydropyridine and nifedipine if LVEF ↓), topical-PO nitrate, alone or in combination.
	 – Antiplatelet agent (aspirin: if allergy, clopidogrel). With coronary stent, double antiplatelet therapy (aspirin + clopidogrel). Warfarin if antiplatelet agent contraindicated.
	 – ACE inhibitor or angiotensin II receptor blocker for most CAD patients (especially if diabetes or hypertension) unless contraindicated.
	 – Lipid lowering medication (See Dyslipidemia table).
	 – Revascularization:
	     - Coronary artery bypass (CABG) indicated for left main disease or three-vessel disease (Vx) (with ↓ LVEF or diabetes), 2 Vx with proximal left anterior descending (LAD) disease + ↓ LVEF and/or demonstrable ischemia.
	     - Percutaneous coronary intervention (PCI) indicated if 2-3 Vx with proximal left anterior descending and appropriate anatomy, normal LVEF without diabetes.
	     - CABG or PCI superior to medical treatment if 2-3 Vx, 1 Vx with moderate to severe ischemia, 1 Vx with proximal LAD disease or failure of medical treatment (2-3 anti-ischemic drugs).
	 – Risk factor management (smoking, obesity, diabetes, hypertension, stop hormone replacement therapy).
	 – Exercise: 30-60 minutes, almost every day (proven to ↓ mortality).
	 – Influenza and pneumococcal vaccinations.
	 – Other treatments (experimental): spinal stimulation, pluripotent stem cells, angiogenesis, etc.

Unstable Angina – non ST-Elevation Myocardial Infarction Definitions	**Unstable Angina** : 1. New angina (at least class III/IV within the last 2 months). 2. Crescendo angina (more frequent, more prolonged, more easily induced, i.e. functional class at least III/IV within the last 2 months). 3. Resting angina (usually > 20 min). Either primary or secondary. **Myocardial Infarction** (definition from ESC/ACCF/AHA/WHF 2007) : 1. Detection of rise and/or fall of cardiac biomarkers (CK, troponin*) with at least one of the following: a) Symptoms of ischemia. b) ECG changes indicative of new ischemia (new ST-T changes or new left bundle-branch block). c) Development of pathologic Q waves on ECG. d) Imaging evidence of new loss of viable myocardium or new regional wall motion abnormality. **or** 2. Pathological findings of an acute MI. * Biomarkers should be increased greater than 3 times normal post-angioplasty or 5 times normal post CABG to diagnosis MI in such circumstances. Non ST-elevation infarction cannot be clinically differentiated from unstable angina without cardiac markers (CK-MB elevation or troponin higher than a given threshold). We often use the term "acute coronary syndrome" to designate either angina or MI before a definitive diagnosis can be determined by laboratory testing.

Workup	- CBC, electrolytes, creatinine, INR, aPTT, CK every 8 h x 3, troponin STAT and every 6-12 hours x 1 (at least 9 hours after onset of chest pain), lipids (< 24 hours from acute event).
	- As needed: AST, LDH, TSH. Cocaine metabolite assay < 36 hours after symptom onset.
	- Standard 12-lead ECG ± "15-lead" ECG with right and posterior leads (V_4R, V_8, V_9) as needed. ECG if chest pain.
	- Cardiac monitoring.
	- As needed: echocardiography during chest pain.
	      Radionuclide myocardial perfusion imaging during pain.
	      Coronary angiography.

Management	Assess each patient's risk by evaluating CAD probability, ischemia severity, TIMI risk score (see below), age, ECG, biomarkers, LV dysfunction, etc.
	
	- Low risk (normal ECG and cardiac markers, no recurrence of retrosternal pain): emergency room treatment (short term) followed by discharge with:
	  - Aspirin (ASA).
	  - Beta-blockers or non-dihydropyridines CCB.
	  - ACE inhibitors or angiotensin II receptor blockers for most CAD patients (especially diabetes or hypertension).
	  - Hypolipidemic agents (see Dyslipidemia table).
	  - Revascularization should be considered according to the clinical course and stratification post-stabilization.
	
	- Intermediate: treatment in hospital:
	As indicated for low risk plus:
	  - Oxygen.
	  - Anticoagulant: IV heparin or enoxaparin or bivalirudin or fondaparinux s/c.
	    - early invasive strategy: consider IV heparin.
	    - conservative strategy: consider fondaparinux.
	  - Morphine as needed.
	  - Glycoprotein IIb/IIIa inhibitors (especially if recurrent ischemia, troponin ↑, ECG abnormalities or with moderate [3-4] or high [5-7] TIMI Risk Score: see below).
	  - Clopidogrel (combined with ASA) if ECG changes or cardiac biomarkers ↑ (CK-MB or troponin) and low risk of bleeding (CURE trial).
	  - Beta-blockers (or non-dihydropyridines calcium channel blockers 2nd line).
	  - Revascularization immediately or according to the clinical course and post-stabilization stratification.
	
	- If at high risk : treat in the intensive care unit with:
	As indicated for intermediate risk plus:
	  - Early coronary angiography if possible (TACTICS approach) with revascularization if needed (see below).
	  - Glycoprotein IIb/IIIa inhibitors to be highly considered (as indicated above).
	  - IV nitrates + beta-blockers ± calcium blockers ± intra-aortic balloon if refractory.
	
	⇒ in practice, use **GP IIb/IIIa inhibitors** in high risk acute coronary syndrome with chest pain within 24 hours, with ECG changes *__and/or__* elevated cardiac biomarkers in patients eligible for cardiac revascularization with no contraindication (e.g. : renal failure, ↓ Hb, ↑ INR, contraindication almost the same as for thrombolysis).
	Use **clopidogrel** in high risk coronary syndrome with chest pain < 24 hours, with ECG changes *__and/or__* elevated cardiac biomarkers with no contraindication. Combination of GP IIb/IIIa and clopidogrel possible.
	
	⇒ in practice, an early aggressive approach (i.e.: coronary angiography ± revascularization as needed) is suggested for patients without comorbidity when associated with a high risk acute coronary syndrome, i.e.: recurrent ischemia, troponin ↑, ST ↓, high risk stress test, FEVG < 40 %, hemodynamically unstable,

	sustained VT, PCI < 6 months, prior CABG.
	Otherwise, an aggressive or conservative approach (stabilization and stratification with stress test or radionuclide myocardial perfusion imaging and coronary angiography PRN if high risk) is acceptable.
	Choice of treatment must be individualized
	
	Note: Avoid nitrates with recent use of phosphodiesterase type 5 inhibitors (24 h except 48 h for tadalafil) since there is a risk of hypotension.
	
	- Management of cardiac risk factors (tobacco, lipids, obesity, diabetes, hypertension, stop hormone replacement therapy).
	- Influenza and pneumococcal vaccination.
	- Follow-up: lower risk patients or revascularized patient within 2-6 weeks and high risk patients within 1-2 weeks.
	- Patient education is essential.
	- Resumption of driving (private driving):
	  - In cases of unstable angina: car driving is permitted at 48 hours post-PCI or after 7 days if PCI is not performed during initial hospital stay.
	  - In case of non ST-elevation MI :
	    - With minor LV damage (in the absence of a new wall motion abnormality), no PCI done: wait 7 days.
	    - With minor LV damage, post-PCI: wait 48 hours after PCI.
	    - With significant LV damage (presence of a new wall motion abnormality): wait 1 month.

Prognosis	TIMI Risk Score for unstable angina and non ST-elevation MI : 1 point for each of the following criteria: age ≥ 65 years, 3 or more risk factors for CAD (family history of CAD, hypertension, dyslipidemia, diabetes, current smoking), significant coronary stenosis (prior coronary stenosis ≥ 50 %), ST deviation, severe angina symptoms (i.e.: ≥ 2 angina attacks in the last 24 h), use of aspirin in the last 7 days, elevated cardiac markers (CK-MB and/or troponin). Rate of all-cause mortality, MI or severe ischemia requiring urgent revascularization at 14 days: 4.7 % if 0/1 points: 8.3 % if 2: 13.2 % if 3: 19.9 % if 4: 26.2 % if 5: 40.9 % if 6/7 points.

ST-Elevation Myocardial Infarction	
Overview	Mostly secondary to a thrombosis of an atherosclerotic fissured plaque (> 70 % of infarctions occur on vulnerable plaque with coronary stenosis < 70 %). Rarely secondary to a vasospasm, hypotension, hypermetabolic state, embolism, vasculitis, coronary dissection, aortitis, cocaine. Prolonged chest pain symptoms > 30 minutes ± arrhythmia, hypotension, shock, CHF, etc. Occasionally asymptomatic, or presenting with syncope, symptoms of acute heart failure, shock, sudden death or cardiac embolism (stroke) or other. Always eliminate cocaine, amphetamines, or recent phosphodiesterase type 5 use (sildenafil or others) Note: 33-50 % of deaths due to MI occur before arrival at the hospital.

Definition of infarction (ESC/ACCF/AHA/WHF)	1. Detection of rise and/or fall of cardiac biomarkers (CK, troponin*) with at least one of the following:
	  a. Symptoms of ischemia.
	  b. ECG changes indicative of new ischemia (new ST-T changes or new left bundle-branch block).

	c. Development of pathologic Q waves in the ECG. d. Imaging evidence of new loss of viable myocardium or new regional wall motion abnormality. **or** 2. Pathological findings of an acute MI. * Biomarkers should be increased greater than 3 times normal post-angioplasty or 5 times normal post CABG to diagnose MI in such circumstances.

Risk stratification	Killip Classification:
	    I: No clinical signs of heart failure.
	    II: rales (up to < 50 % of lung fields), no S3.
	    IIb: rales (up to < 50 % of lung fields), S3 present.
	    III: pulmonary edema with rales > 50 % of lung fields.
	    IV: Cardiogenic shock.

Workup Acute phase	– Biochemistry : CBC, INR, aPTT, electrolytes, CK-MB every 8 hours x 3, troponin, as needed, glucose, creatinine, BUN, urinalysis, lipids (< 24 hours from acute event ideally), chest X-ray. – If needed: AST, ALT, TSH. Cocaine metabolite assay < 36 hours after symptom onset. – 12-lead ECG, to repeat every 5-10 minutes if not diagnostic at first. Repeat ECG at 24 hours, if chest pain recurs and on discharge. – "15-lead ECG" with right and posterior leads (V_4R, V_8, V_9) for inferior infarction or normal 12-lead ECG. – Vital signs, cardiac monitoring, etc. – As needed: echocardiography, diagnostic coronary angiography, pulmonary artery catheter (Swan-Ganz), arterial line, etc.
Treatment	
Initial stabilization	– Oxygen, venous access, etc. – IV morphine: pain control. If needed: Anxiolytic. – ICU until stable for 12-24 h, followed by transfer to floor with telemetry. – Bed rest maximum 12-24 h if stable, then progressive mobilization.
Reperfusion Therapy	– IV thrombolysis or percutaneous coronary intervention (PCI) as first-line treatment (primary PCI) or as a rescue (if failure of thrombolysis, especially if persistent ischemia, severe left heart failure, large territory in jeopardy or unstable hemodynamically/arrhythmia). – Reperfusion if symptoms < 12 hours, or between 12-24 hours in the following cases: when associated with persistent ischemia and ↑ ST - treat with thrombolysis or PCI - severe left heart failure or unstable hemodynamically/arrhythmia – treat with PCI. – See Thrombolysis table.

Thrombolysis is generally preferred if :	**Angioplasty is generally preferred if :**
– Early presentation (< 3 h from symptom onset and delay for angioplasty). – Angioplasty not possible (not available, vascular access difficulties) – Delay for angioplasty (door-to-balloon > 90 minutes or > 1 h longer than immediate lysis)	– Skilled PCI lab available in short delay (door-to-balloon < 90 minutes or < 1 hour longer than immediate lysis). – High risk MI (cardiogenic shock, Killip class ≥ 3). – Contraindications to thrombolysis including increased risk of bleeding (especially intracranial). – Late presentation (symptom onset > 3 h). – Diagnostic of STEMI is in doubt.

If presentation < 3 h and no delay for PCI, both strategies are acceptable.

Note: delay between patient arrival and thrombolysis should be < 30 minutes. Delay between patient arrival and PCI should be < 90 minutes.

Antiplatelet - antithrombin	– Aspirin: 160-325 mg chewable, then 75-162 mg daily. – Clopidogrel 300 mg STAT if ≤ 75 years of age, 75 mg if > 75 years of age followed by 75 mg/day for at least 28 days and ideally 1 year for any patient who did not undergo PCI. – Clopidogrel bolus of at least 300 mg for patient undergoing primary PCI, followed by 75 mg/day for ideally one year for any patient who has undergone PCI, minimal duration of treatment according to the type of stent used: bare metal stent : 4 weeks, drug-eluting stent : ≥ 12 months. – NSAIDs (COX- 2 selective and non-selective) must be stopped on admission. – Heparin (IV if PCI or if streptokinase, alteplase, tenecteplase, or reteplase used): low molecular weight heparin (enoxaparin) recommended with acute STEMI receiving thrombolysis with adequate renal function (creatinine < 220 μmol/L in males, < 175 μmol/L in females). Heparin 12 500 U s/c q 12h is an alternative with streptokinase. Give heparin IV ≥ 48 hours if thrombolysis is used. Heparin s/c or LMWH until mobilization for any MI patient not receiving warfarin. – Bivalirudin if heparin-induced thrombocytopenia. – Warfarin if AF or at high risk for systemic embolism (severe left ventricular dysfunction, congestive heart failure, mural thrombus, past thromboembolic event), or if contraindication to aspirin
Other pharmacological treatments	– PO beta-blockers to be started within 24 hours (except if heart failure, low cardiac output, risk of cardiogenic shock or contraindications). IV treatment reasonable in patients without contraindications (see above), especially if a tachyarrhythmia or hypertension is present. – IV nitroglycerin (recommended if continuous chest pain, left ventricular dysfunction, hypertension): avoid if hypotension, brady- or tachycardia, suspicion of a right ventricular infarction or recent use of phosphodiesterase type 5 inhibitors. – ACE inhibitors or angiotensin II receptor blockers for all patients. – Eplerenone with signs of heart failure and LVEF ≤ 40 % (and no contraindications). – Lipid lowering agent (see below). Avoid the routine use of: lidocaine, CCB, magnesium. Stop NSAIDs (COX -2 specific NSAIDs included).

Management before release	– Noninvasive evaluation:
	   1- Ejection fraction (by echocardiography or ventriculography).
	   2- If no coronary angiography done: early (≥ 4 days) stratification post-infarction by stress test (preferably), echo dobutamine or stress-echo, exercise or pharmacologic stress radionuclide myocardial perfusion imaging (except if spontaneous recurrent ischemia: see below).
	– Coronary angiography if spontaneous ischemia or if moderate-high risk after stratification: also if LVEF ≤ 40 %, congestive heart failure, diabetes, prior revascularization or serious ventricular arrhythmia: consider post-thrombolysis.
	– Medication on discharge: ASA 75-325 mg daily.
	   - Clopidogrel if ASA contraindicated or combined with ASA if stent.
	   - Warfarin if ASA contraindicated (alternative to clopidogrel) or if atrial fibrillation or mural thrombus or severe left ventricular dysfunction.
	   - ACE inhibitor or ARB ± eplerenone.
	   - Beta-blockers (if no contraindication).
	   - Lipid lowering agent: statin aiming for LDL< 2 mmol/L, CT/HDL ratio < 4.
	
	Avoid the routine use of: calcium channel blockers, antiarrhythmics.
	Patient education: life style changes, medication, action to be taken if cardiac symptoms recur.

Management after discharge	– Risk factor modification (smoking cessation, stop hormone replacement therapy). – Rehabilitation program recommended. – No work for 4-8 weeks, or until 16 weeks for complicated infarction (according to type of work). – No car driving for 1 month after discharge (private driving). – Return to normal sexual activity when negative stress test at 5 Mets. – Influenza and pneumococcal vaccinations.

Complications	– Post infarction ischemia: absolute indication for coronary angiography.
	– Arrhythmias: see Brady and Tachyarrhythmia tables.
	   - Bradycardia: temporary pacemaker if needed.
	   - Conduction defect: temporary pacemaker if needed.
	   - Supraventricular tachyarrhythmias (atrial fibrillation, sinus).
	   - Ventricular: aggressive intervention, especially if present > 48 hours after infarction.
	– Heart failure: see Heart Failure table.
	– Cardiogenic shock (if systolic BP < 90 mmHg for > 30 minutes without response to volume and with evidence of organ hypoperfusion): STAT coronary angiography. Rapid coronary revascularization if appropriate. Thrombolysis if not a candidate for invasive treatment. Intra-aortic balloon useful if shock does not resolve rapidly. Pulmonary artery catheterization (Swan-Ganz) if needed. Mortality ≈ 50-60 %.
	– Right ventricular infarction: present in 33 % of inferior infarction but clinically significant in half of them. Hypotension and jugular vein distension with clear lungs. Diagnosis if ↑ ST segment ≥ 1 mm in V_3R, V_4R or V_1. Treated with volume ± inotropes. Stop hypotensive medications. Early revascularization if available (but wait 4 weeks if possible for CABG). Manage bradycardia if present.
	– Papillary muscle rupture or ventricular septal rupture: 2-10 days post-anterior or inferior infarction. Pulmonary edema and new mitral murmur. Early surgical treatment. Intra-aortic balloon if needed ± nitroprusside ± inotropes. Poor prognosis.
	– Rupture of ventricular free wall: 2-14 days post-infarction, mostly anterior. Rapidly fatal. Pseudoaneurysm if incomplete rupture.
	– Left ventricular aneurysm: with an anterior infarction. To be suspected if persistent anterior ST ↑ > 4-8 weeks post-infarction. Possible embolic or arrhythmic source (warfarin to be considered). Surgical treatment possible.
	– Mural thrombus: more likely with anterior infarction. Anticoagulation ≥ 3 months if anterior infarction or if thrombus at echocardiography.
	– Pericarditis: 2-7 days post infarction. Avoid anticoagulation. Avoid ibuprofen with aspirin. Dressler's syndrome 1-12 weeks post-infarction also possible. See table of pericardial disorders.

Prognosis	TIMI Risk Score for ST-Elevation MI: Points according to the following criteria: age ≥ 75 (3 points) or 65-74 (2 points), diabetes, history of hypertension or history of angina (1 point), systolic BP < 100 mmHg (3 points), pulse > 100/min (2 points), Killip II-IV (2 points), weight < 67 kg (1 point) anterior infarction or left bundle branch (1 point), time from symptom onset to treatment > 4 hours (1 point). Risk of death within 30 days: 0.8 % if 0 points; 1.6 % if 1 point; 2.2 % if 2 points; 4.4 % if 3 points; 7.3 % if 4 points; 12 % if 5 points; 16 % if 6 points; 23 % if 7 points; 27 % if 8 points; 36 % if > 8 points.

Thrombolysis	
Indications	1. Ischemic cardiac pain ≥ 30 minutes **and** 2. At least 1 mm ST segment elevation in at least 2 adjacent limb leads or ≥ 1-2 mm ST segment elevation in at least 2 adjacent precordial leads, or complete LBBB. Possibilities of aortic dissection (more likely with inferior infarction) or acute pericarditis should always be considered.

Contra-indications	***Absolute :***
	  – Previous intracerebral hemorrhage.
	  – Known structural cerebral vascular lesion (arteriovenous malformation or aneurysm).
	  – Known malignant intracranial neoplasm (primary or metastatic).
	  – Ischemic stroke < 3 months.
	  – Suspected aortic dissection.
	  – Active internal bleeding or bleeding diathesis (excluding menstruation).
	  – Significant closed-head or facial trauma < 3 months.
	
	Relative :
	  – Poorly controlled or chronic sustained hypertension (Systolic BP > 180 and/or diastolic BP > 110 mmHg).
	  – Ischemic stroke > 3 months.
	  – Dementia or other intracranial pathology (except as above).
	  – Traumatic or prolonged cardiopulmonary resuscitation (> 10 min) or major surgery (< 3 weeks).
	  – Recent internal bleeding (< 2-4 weeks).
	  – Noncompressible vascular puncture.
	  – Active peptic ulcer.
	  – Pregnancy.
	  – Current use of anticoagulants.
	  – Streptokinase: prior exposure (> 5 days) or prior allergic reaction.

Doses	– Streptokinase: 1.5×10^6 U IV in 1 hour.
	  – Alteplase (Activase®): 15 mg IV bolus + 0.75 mg/kg in 30 min (max 50 mg) + 0.50 mg/kg in 60 min (max. 35 mg), maximum total = 100 mg.
	  – Reteplase (Retavase®): 10 MU in 2 doses 30 minutes apart.
	  – Tenecteplase (TNK-ase®): 30-50 mg IV (based on weight) bolus administration.

Options	- Use Alteplase, tenecteplase or reteplase if prior allergic or exposure to streptokinase.
	- Every patient who has received streptokinase must carry a card or wear a Medic-Alert bracelet indicating previous exposure to streptokinase.
	
	  – Thrombolytic treatment within the first 6 hours:
	       Choice of agent depends on many factors: alteplase or reteplase favored for patient < 75 years and/or retrosternal pain < 4 h and/or with anterior or bad prognostic inferior infarction (hemodynamic compromise, right ventricle, anterior ST depression).
	  – Thrombolytic treatment > 6 hours after occurrence of retrosternal pain:
	       Indicated for most patients between 6-12 hours, in selected between 13-24 hours.
	
	Use IV heparin for 48 hours or enoxaparin (1st choice) in patients with adequate renal function (creatinine < 220 µmol/L in males, < 175 µmol/L in females), continued up to 8 days.
	S/c heparin can also be used (12 500 U s/c q 12 hours) with streptokinase.

Side effects	– Bleeding: (major 5-6 %, intracranial 0.5 %): Treat with cryoprecipitate 10 U STAT and every 6 hours as required ± antifibrinolytic agents (tranexamic acid or aminocaproic acid) ± fresh frozen

	plasma ± protamine ± platelets. – Allergy/anaphylaxis with streptokinase (0.1-1.7 %). – Hypotension with streptokinase (2-10 %): if present, give volume and slow or stop streptokinase: do not modify alteplase.

Failure of thrombolysis	Definition: controversial: if chest pain or persistent ST elevation (< 50 % resolution of ST elevation 90 min post-treatment onset compared with the pretreatment ECG).
	    If hemodynamically unstable: STAT coronary angiography + rescue PCI.
	    Otherwise, evaluate the size of the affected territory :
	        - if significant and early presentation: consider PCI.
	        - otherwise: medical treatment (no benefit to repeat thrombolysis).

Heart Failure	
Overview	Heart failure may be systolic (decreased left ventricular ejection fraction) or diastolic (preserved left ventricular ejection fraction: an abnormality in ventricular filling during diastole, caused by left ventricular hypertrophy, ischemia, aortic or/and mitral valvular disorder, hypertension, infiltrative disease, constrictive pericarditis, tamponade, arrhythmia). 40-60 % of heart failure is diastolic in origin, more likely in older patients. Heart failure may be of low or high output (high output with severe anemia, hyperthyroidism, arteriovenous fistula, Paget, Beriberi). CHF is the number one reason for hospitalization for patients ≥ 65 years.
Clinical findings	Dyspnea, orthopnea, PND, supine cough, nocturia, jugular venous distension, abdominal jugular reflux, anorexia, nausea, edema, ascites, liver congestion, fatigue, hypotension, diaphoresis, abnormal cardiac exam (S3 present with systolic CHF or S4 if diastolic, displaced apex, parasternal lift, murmurs). "Flash pulmonary edema" can be a typical presentation of renovascular disease as well as ischemia or arrhythmia.
Stages of heart failure	According to *American College of Cardiology* : – Stage A: Patients at high risk for developing HF but with no identified structural or functional abnormalities of the heart and no symptoms or signs of HF. – Stage B: Patients with underlying structural heart disease who has always been asymptomatic. – Stage C: Patients who have current or prior symptoms of HF associated with underlying structural heart disease. – Stage D: Patient with advanced structural heart disease and marked symptoms of HF at rest despite medical therapy and who require specialized interventions.
Functional classification	*New York Heart Association* (NYHA) classification: – I: No limitation of activity. Asymptomatic on ordinary physical activity. – II: Slight limitation of physical activity; they are comfortable at rest or on mild exertion. Ordinary physical activity causes symptoms. – III: Marked limitation of physical activity; they are comfortable only at rest. Less than ordinary activity causes symptoms. – IV: Inability to carry out any physical activity. Symptoms may occur at rest.

Causes	– Ischemic* (50-70 %).
	– Valvular: stenosis, regurgitation, endocarditis*.
	– Hypertension*.
	– Pericardial disease: tamponade*, constrictive pericarditis (right-sided heart failure).
	– Congenital heart diseases or intracardiac shunt.
	– Pulmonary hypertension (right-sided heart failure).
	– Other nonischemic causes of cardiomyopathy:
	   - Inflammatory:
	     - infectious: viral myocarditis* (coxsackievirus, echovirus, adenovirus, influenza,
	      EBV, HIV, etc) : Rickettsia (Q fever) : Spirochetes (Lyme) : parasites
	      (Chagas), etc.
	     - noninfectious: connective tissue disease, vasculitis, hypereosinophilic,…
	   - Toxic: alcohol, cocaine, medication, chemotherapy (doxorubicine, trastuzumab,
	    cyclophosphamide, sunitinib), etc.
	   - Metabolic: hypo-hyperthyroidism, diabetes, uremia, pheochromocytoma,
	    acromegaly, etc.
	   - Infiltrative: sarcoidosis, amyloidosis, hemochromatosis, Whipple disease, Gaucher
	    disease, glycogen storage disease, etc.
	   - Idiopathic: dilated, restrictive, hypertrophic cardiomyopathy.
	   - Others: neuromuscular disease (Duchenne, Friedreich), endomyocardial
	    fibroelastosis, Löffler's syndrome, carcinoid syndrome, peripartum
	    cardiomyopathy, radiotherapy, tachycardia-induced cardiomyopathy, etc.
	
	* causes of acute heart failure.

Workup	According to diagnostic hypotheses. Ejection fraction *essential*: echocardiography and/or isotopic ventriculography. Repeat testing after 3-6 months sometimes useful. Routine testing: CBC, electrolytes (including Ca^{++}, PO_4^{3-}, Mg^{++}), creatinine, glucose, urinalysis, AST, ALT, lipid profile, TSH. ECG Chest X-ray. Usually required: coronary angiography in order to rule out underlying CAD if moderate-severe systolic dysfunction. Biochemistry as needed: B-type natriuretic peptide assay, if diagnosis uncertain. Ferritin, iron saturation, HIV, connective tissue disease workup, urinary catecholamines, etc. Cardiac workup as needed: exercise testing, exercise or pharmacologic imaging modality (echocardiography or radionuclide myocardial perfusion imaging), resting thallium or TEP scan (for myocardial viability), cardiac biopsy (rare). For idiopathic dilated cardiomyopathy, family screening of 1st degree parents with ECG and echocardiography. Follow weights regularly if right-sided heart failure or refractory heart failure.

Treatment of systolic dysfunction: Chronic phase	Treat reversible causes (ischemia, valvular disorder, etc) and precipitating factors. Control other cardiovascular risk factors.
	
	Non pharmacological: patient education, sodium restriction (2-3 g/d to 1-2 g/d if severe), fluid restriction (1.5-2 L/d if uncontrolled fluid retention), regular exercise if stable, limit alcohol intake, smoking cessation, weight loss, vaccinations (pneumococcus and influenza).
	
	Pharmacologic:
	– Vasodilatators:
	   - Angiotensin-converting enzyme inhibitors (ACEI): indispensable (reduce
	    mortality). Maximal tolerated dose.

- if contraindication/intolerance: Angiotensin II receptor blockers (ARB). An ARB could also be added to an ACEI if patient remains symptomatic despite optimal treatment.
- if contraindication/intolerance: hydralazine (up to 75 mg tid) combined with nitrates (but less effective than ACEI). Hydralazine + nitrates in addition to standard treatment should be considered among Afro-American patients.
- Beta-blockers: carvedilol, metoprolol and bisoprolol proven effective to reduce mortality. Effect in 2-4 months.
- Diuretics:
  - Furosemide 20-120 mg/day for symptomatic relief.
  - K^+ sparing diuretics (reduce mortality, but K^+ and creatinine must be followed closely, especially in patients with diabetes or CKD):
    - Spironolactone 25-50 mg daily if functional class IIIb-IV/IV **or**
    - Eplerenone 25-50 mg daily if post-MI heart failure and LVEF ≤ 40 % (and no contraindications, i.e: K^+ > 5 mmol/L, creatinine > 221 µmol/L or creatinine clearance < 50 mL/min).
  - Add hydrochlorothiazide or metolazone 2.5-5 mg daily if needed. Follow K^+ and Mg^{++} closely.
- Digoxin: for patients with functional classes II-IV symptomatic (↓ hospitalization in DIG study): aim for serum level 0.7-1 µg/L 8-12 hours post-dose.
- Calcium channel blockers: avoid except amlodipine and felodipine safe.
- Anticoagulants (warfarin): if atrial fibrillation, thrombus or prior embolism.

Surgical:
- Revascularization if ischemia.
- Left ventricular assist device ("mechanical pump") sometimes useful as a bridge to transplantation.
- Cardiac transplantation: if mortality estimated 25-50 % at 1 year without transplant. Evaluate VO_2 max: if < 15 mL/kg/min or < 55 % predicted → probably indicated.
- Ventricular resynchronization (if QRS ≥ 0.12 ms, LVEF < 35 % and FC 3-4/4 despite maximal treatment) with biventricular pacemaker.
- Implantable cardioverter-defibrillator indicated if LVEF ≤ 30 % (more controversial with LVEF 31-35 %) in absence of contraindications.

- If refractory: water restriction 1L/day, Na^+ 2 g/day, activity restriction, combination of diuretics or vasodilatators; bed time nitrates for nocturnal dyspnea. Intermittent dobutamine or milrinone if very severe (but no proven decrease in mortality).
Always consider noncompliance.
If there is deterioration, consult a heart failure specialist.

To summarize, heart failure patients should received an ACEI and a beta-blocker whether they experience symptoms or not, functional class I-IV/IV.
- If still symptomatic and functional class II-III/IV, consider adding ARBs ± digoxin ± nitrates.
- If still symptomatic and functional class IIIb-IV/IV give spironolactone or ↑/combine diuretics.

Diastolic Dysfunction: Chronic Treatment	Treat underlying cause (hypertension, ischemia, valvular disorder, etc). Slow heart rate: beta-blockers, non-dihydropyridines calcium-channel blockers. Use diuretics with caution, sometimes useful. Few studies available on diastolic dysfunction. Optimal treatment still uncertain.
Prognosis	According to etiology and symptoms. Prognosis better with diastolic than systolic heart failure. For post-hospitalization systolic heart failure, 1 year survival rate = 70%, but very variable. Readmission rate at 3 month = 20-30%.

Acute Heart Failure	
Overview	Most frequently associated with known chronic heart failure, exacerbated by one of the precipitating factor listed below. Can also be the mode of presentation of new onset congestive heart failure.
Clinical findings	Severe dyspnea, pink sputum, diaphoresis, cyanosis, chest pain, wheezing ("cardiac asthma"). Differential diagnosis: noncardiogenic pulmonary edema (see ARDS table), pulmonary embolism, sepsis, acute exacerbation of COPD, aspiration, pneumothorax, panic attack, severe anemia, acidosis, etc (see Dyspnea table).
Precipitating factors	Ischemia or infarction, arrhythmia, hypertension, noncompliance (medical therapy, salt intake), drugs (non-dihydropyridines calcium channel blockers, beta-blockers, NSAIDs, antiarrhythmics, thiazolidinediones, anagrelide, tricyclics antidepressants, antihistaminics, cocaine, amphetamines, etc), fluid intake, infection, pulmonary embolism, anemia, acute renal failure, hyperthyroidism, pregnancy, etc.
Management	**Urgent workup :** CBC, electrolytes, creatinine, BUN, glucose, urinalysis, CK and troponin, AST, ALT, INR, aPTT, ECG, chest X-ray. If needed: echocardiography, lipid workup, TSH, Ventilation/perfusion lung scan, viral serology, connective tissue disease workup, isotopic ventriculography, coronary angiography, etc, according to diagnostic hypothesis/ patient's condition/ laboratory results/clinical course. BNP (*B-type natriuretic peptide*) assay sometimes useful (if available) in order to determine if dyspnea is of cardiac origin (false $\oplus$ can occur with severe obesity, kidney disease, cancer). Investigation for etiology of heart failure should be done as discussed earlier. Note: Diastolic and systolic heart failure may be indistinguishable, however ejection fraction should *always* be evaluated. Urinary catheter could be inserted. Insert a Swan-Ganz catheter, as needed. **Emergency treatment of acute pulmonary edema:** According to precipitating factor and cause. Sodium + fluid restriction 1.2 L/day. Bed rest. Keep patient in a sitting position, oxygen therapy to obtain pO_2 > 60 mmHg. Furosemide 40-80 mg IV + morphine 2-5 mg s/c-IV (max. 8 mg) q 30-60 min as needed. Topical or sublingual or high dose IV Nitroglycerin (if BP > 100 mmHg) or positive inotropic (dopamine, dobutamine) according to severity of clinical presentation. Nesiritide for moderate to severe dyspnea persisting 2 hours after administration of Henle diuretics. Bronchodilators for bronchospasm as needed. Intra-aortic balloon pump as needed. Invasive or non-invasive assisted ventilation as needed. Coronary angiography ± angioplasty or CABG as needed according to the clinical course and test results. Chronic treatment of CHF as discussed previously. Note: pulmonary edema usually responds quickly to standard treatment; if not, an aggressive search for another etiology should be undertaken. Note: if severe post treatment hypotension, consider diastolic heart failure, especially hypertrophic cardiomyopathy.

Hypertrophic Cardiomyopathy

Overview	Definition: presence of myocardial hypertrophy in absence of an underlying cause such as hypertension, aortic stenosis or infiltrative disease. Prevalence: 1/500 adults. Mutation of a gene encoding the cardiac sarcomere present in 60 % of affected patients (but many other genetic abnormalities have been described), autosomal dominant transmission in most of families. Left ventricular outflow obstruction may occur in 25 % of patients during systole; this obstruction can be exacerbated by various factors which increase myocardial contractility (digoxin, extrasystoles, sympathetic stimulation) or decrease left ventricular filling (Valsalva, peripheral vasodilator, diuretics). Progression to a dilated cardiomyopathy = 1.5 %/year.
Clinical findings	Clinical manifestations: syncope, sudden death (mainly among young men), dyspnea, angina (in older patients), palpitations (ventricular or supra-ventricular arrhythmia). Often asymptomatic (incidental finding or during screening of affected relatives). Physical exam: abnormal if obstruction is present: Bifid carotid pulse, S4, systolic ejection murmur ↑ with Valsalva or in standing position and ↓ with squatting, apical holosystolic murmur.
Workup	ECG: left ventricular hypertrophy, left atrial dilation, repolarization abnormalities, arrhythmia. Echocardiography: myocardial hypertrophy (left ventricular thickness ≥ 15 mm in diastole) ± left ventricular outflow obstruction (if presence of a sub-aortic gradient ≥ 30 mmHg) ± diastolic dysfunction ± mitral regurgitation. Holter monitoring: 24-48 hours suggested for all patients. Exercise stress testing sometimes useful to evaluate symptoms, arrhythmia, and prognosis. Evaluate 1st degree relatives with ECG and echocardiography (each year between 12-18 years old and every five years thereafter). Genetic testing is not universally available. Other tests sometimes useful among adults: cardiac MRI, endomyocardial biopsy (rare), measurement of α-galactosidase A (to rule out Fabry disease), arterial blood gas on exertion (for mitochondrial disease).
Treatment	Symptomatic patients: - Avoid intense physical activity. - ↓ Contractility to ↓ left ventricular outflow obstruction with beta-blockers (1st choice), calcium channel blockers (verapamil or diltiazem: 2nd choice) ± disopyramide (if persistent symptoms despite maximum treatment with beta-blockers or CCB but side effects). - Avoid medication that ↓ preload and afterload. Be careful with diuretics. - Septal ablation (by alcohol ablation or surgical myectomy) for highly symptomatic patients despite maximum medical treatment (mortality risk: 1-5 %, risk of AV block, ventricular arrhythmia). - Implantable cardioverter-defibrillator after cardiac arrest or in presence of sudden death risk factors (sustained VT, family history with sudden death, unexplained syncope, massive LVH with wall thickness ≥ 30 mm). - Treatment of atrial fibrillation when present may improve symptoms. Patients with atrial fibrillation must be anticoagulated.

	Asymptomatic patients: treatment controversial. - Implantable cardioverter-defibrillator for patients at high risk of sudden death?
Prognosis	Prognosis variable. Risk of sudden death among adults: ≤ 1 % /year. Risk factors for sudden death: personal or family history of sudden death, unexplained syncope, abnormal BP response on exertion, non-sustained VT on Holter or severe LV hypertrophy (≥ 30 mm). In presence of several factors, risk of sudden death may be up to 3 %/year. Some mutations are more frequently associated with sudden death.

Valvular Heart Disease

Mitral Stenosis
Evaluation
	Causes: acute rheumatic fever in most cases. Other causes (rare): left atrial myxoma, thrombus, mucopolysaccharidosis, or severe annular calcification.
	Symptoms usually occur around 20 years after acute rheumatic fever.
	
	Left and right heart failure, fatigue, atrial fibrillation or systemic embolism.
	Rarely: hemoptysis, hoarse voice, dysphasia.
	
	Physical exam :
	   - ↑ S1.
	   - ↑ pulmonary S2.
	   - opening snap.
	   - low-pitched mid diastolic murmur, ↑ duration = ↑ severity.
	   - signs of pulmonary hypertension (jugular vein distension,
	           parasternal lift, ascites, leg edema).
	   - Graham-Steele diastolic murmur with severe pulmonary hypertension.
	
	Classification of severity:
	   - Normal valve area = 4-5 cm^2
	   - Minimal stenosis > 2.5 cm^2: no symptoms.
	   - **Mild** stenosis if valve area > 1.5 cm^2 or mean gradient < 5 mmHg or pulmonary artery systolic pressure < 30 mmHg: exertional dyspnea or dyspnea brought on by stress, infection, pregnancy or rapid atrial fibrillation.
	   - **Moderate** stenosis: valve area 1-1.5 cm^2 or mean gradient 5-10 mmHg or pulmonary artery systolic pressure 30-50 mmHg: exertional dyspnea, paroxysmal nocturnal dyspnea, orthopnea.
	   - **Severe** stenosis: < 1 cm^2 or mean gradient > 10 mmHg or pulmonary artery systolic pressure > 50 mmHg: symptoms at rest.
	
	Symptoms often brought on by new onset atrial fibrillation, infection, ↑ fluid or sodium intake, pregnancy, endocarditis …

Workup	− ECG: signs of pulmonary hypertension (right axis deviation, right atrial and ventricular hypertrophy), atrial fibrillation is common, left atrial hypertrophy. − Chest X-ray: valvular calcifications, left atrial dilation (double shadow on the right, quadruple shadow on the left). − Echocardiography-Doppler: to rule out myxoma and calculate a "mitral score": to be done for diagnosis and for asymptomatic patients after 3-5 year of follow-up for mild mitral stenosis (MS), after 1-2 year of follow-up for moderate MS or every year for severe or more often if there is a change in symptoms. − Stress-echocardiography or echo dobutamine as needed if discordance between symptoms and results of rest echocardiography. − Exercise stress testing if needed (to evaluate functional class [FC]). − Cardiac catheterization if above tests are inconclusive or are discordant.

Treatment	**Medical treatment :** – Avoid intense physical activity with moderate to severe stenosis. – Anticoagulation in presence of atrial fibrillation (even paroxysmal), prior embolism or mural thrombus. May be considered with severe MS, spontaneous contrast on echocardiography, or dilated left atrium (LA) ≥ 55 mm. – Negative chronotropic agent (beta-blockers or calcium channel blockers) for patients in sinus rhythm and symptomatic on exertion due to rapid heart rate. – Treatment of heart failure as needed. – Patients who have had rheumatic fever should receive prophylaxis for a minimum of 10 years post rheumatic fever or until age 40. **Treatment by percutaneous mitral balloon valvotomy:** - Recommended for patients with mitral stenosis ≤ 1.5 cm^2 symptomatic (FC 2-4/4) or with pulmonary hypertension (> 50 mmHg at rest, > 60 mmHg with exercise) and favorable morphology in absence of contraindications (left atrium thrombus or mitral regurgitation 3-4/4). - Reasonable for patients with MS ≤ 1.5 cm^2 symptomatic (FC 3-4/4) with nonpliable calcified valve but not candidates or at high risk for surgery. - May be considered for patients with MS ≤ 1.5 cm^2 asymptomatic who have new onset of atrial fibrillation (in absence of left atrial thrombus or mitral regurgitation 3-4/4) or for symptomatic patients with mild MS (FC 2-4/4) if there is evidence of hemodynamically significant MS (based on systolic pressure pulmonary artery > 60 mmHg, pulmonary artery wedge pressure ≥ 25 mmHg or mean mitral valve gradient > 15 mmHg during exercise). **Surgical treatment :** *Valvular repair* is recommended for patients with MS ≤ 1.5 cm^2 and FC 3-4/4 not candidates for valvotomy and who have valve morphology favorable for repair. May be considered if MS ≤ 1.5 cm^2 with recurrent embolic events while receiving adequate anticoagulation. *Valvular replacement* is recommended for patients with MS ≤ 1.5 cm^2 and FC 3-4/4 not candidates for valvotomy or valvular repair or if associated with moderate to severe mitral regurgitation: is reasonable for patients with MS < 1 cm^2 and severe pulmonary hypertension (systolic pulmonary artery pressure > 60 mmHg) and FC 1-2/4 not candidates for valvotomy or surgical mitral valve repair.
Mitral Regurgitation Evaluation	Causes : mitral prolapse (see below), acute rheumatic fever, endocarditis, connective tissue disease, papillary muscle or chordae tendineae dysfunction, ischemia, myxoma (rare), dilated or hypertrophic cardiomyopathy, drug induced (pergolide, cabergolide, dexfenfluramine before 1997). Clinical manifestations : Acute pulmonary edema if acute mitral regurgitation (MR). Exertional dyspnea and fatigue if chronic MR. Acute decompensation sometimes the result of new onset atrial fibrillation. Physical exam: high-pitched holosystolic murmur radiating to axilla or base, S3.
Workup	– ECG: left atrial enlargement and left ventricular hypertrophy. – Chest X-ray: left atrial dilation - left ventricular dilation if chronic. – Exercise testing if needed (e.g.: pre-op evaluation of functional class). – Isotopic ventriculography. – Echocardiography-Doppler: to be performed every year if asymptomatic moderate mitral regurgitation or every 6-12 months if severe. – Cardiac catheterization if above tests are inconclusive or are discordant.

Treatment	**Medical treatment:** – Vasodilatators? No proven benefit. Not indicated in absence of hypertension. **Surgical treatment:** - Recommended for symptomatic patients with acute severe mitral regurgitation (MR): for patients with chronic severe and symptomatic MR (FC 2-4/4), LVEF ≥ 30 % and LV end-systolic dimension ≤ 55 mm: for patients with asymptomatic MR and LVEF 30-60 % and/or LV end-systolic dimension ≥ 40 mm. - Is reasonable for asymptomatic patients with chronic severe MR with preserved LV function (EF > 60 % and end-systolic dimension < 40 mm) in whom the likelihood of successful repair without residual MR is greater than 90% or with new onset of atrial fibrillation, or with pulmonary hypertension (> 50 mmHg at rest, > 60 mmHg with exercise) or if severe MR is due to a primary abnormality of the mitral apparatus with FC 3-4/4 and severe LV dysfunction (LVEF < 30 % or LV end-systolic dimension ≥ 55 mm) in whom MV repair will very likely be successful. - May be considered for symptomatic patients with chronic severe MR due to severe LV dysfunction (LVEF < 30 %) FC 3-4/4 despite optimal therapy for heart failure, including biventricular pacing. Note: valvular repair preferable to valvular replacement if possible.
Mitral Valve Prolapse	Most frequent valvular heart disease. Displacement of the mitral valve leaflet into the left atrium during systole. Prevalence: 1-2.5 % of general population. Sometimes causes mitral regurgitation. Occasional family transmission. Tricuspid involvement: 40 %; pulmonary: 2-10 %, aortic: 2-10 %, ↑ incidence of atrial septal defect and left accessory pathway. ↑ endocarditis risk: controversial. ↑ risk of TIA. Sudden death: rare (< 2 %). Physical exam: midsystolic click ± followed by a late systolic murmur ↑ with maneuvers decreasing intracardiac volume (Valsalva, upright position). Diagnosis: echocardiography/Doppler. Family screening (1st degree) recommended. Treatment: no treatment if asymptomatic. Treatment of mitral regurgitation as indicated above. TIA-CVA treatment as among the general population except in case of infarction, thickening of leaflets at trans-thoracic echocardiography or recurrence on aspirin; anticoagulate.

Aortic Stenosis Evaluation	Causes: rheumatic fever (25 %; mitral valve always associated), bicuspid valve (< 70 years = 50 %, coarctation of the aorta associated in 10 %), degenerative or calcific aortic stenosis (> 70 years = 48 %).
	
	Differential diagnosis: supravalvular obstruction, idiopathic hypertrophic subaortic stenosis (IHSS).
	
	Symptoms :
	    Angina (CAD-related 50%) = 5 year prognosis.
	    Syncope (especially during exercise) = 3 year prognosis.
	    Heart failure = 2 year prognosis.
	Symptoms may be subtle (because of adaptation).
	↑ sudden death even without symptoms (rare < 1 %/year).
	
	Note: Prognosis for asymptomatic patients is identical to that of the general population.

	Physical exam: *pulsus parvus + tardus* (↓ volume and delayed carotid upstroke), ↓ A2, S3 ⊕ , S4 ⊕, midsystolic murmur at right second intercostal space, parasternal border or at apex radiating up to the neck (late peak). Note: Criteria of severity on examination: *pulsus parvus + tardus*, ↓ A2 or paradoxical S2, late peak, presence of a thrill. Classification of severity: - Normal valve area = 3-4 cm². - Mild stenosis if valve area > 1.5 cm², mean gradient < 25 mmHg or jet velocity < 3 m/s. - Moderate stenosis if valve area 1-1.5 cm², mean gradient 25-40 mmHg or jet velocity < 3-4 m/s. - Severe stenosis if valve area < 1 cm² (but relative to patient's size < 0.6 cm²/m²), mean gradient > 40 mmHg or jet velocity > 4 m/s. Under-estimation of gradient if LVEF↓. Stenosis usual progression is 0.1-0.3 cm²/year but individual variability exists.
Workup	– ECG: abnormal in 98 %, LVH, repolarization abnormality. – Chest X-ray: valve calcification. – Echocardiography-Doppler: if symptomatic or every 3-5 years if mild stenosis, every 1-2 years if moderate or every year if severe or more often if any change in symptoms. – Stress test may be done as needed if severe, asymptomatic aortic stenosis (AS) in order to evaluate potential exercise-induced symptoms or BP response to exercise. – If LVEF ↓: echo dobutamine in order to evaluate hemodynamic contribution of the AS. – Cardiac catheterization if above tests are inconclusive or are discordant.

Treatment	– Surgery is recommended in:
	  - Symptomatic patients with severe AS.
	  - Patients with severe AS undergoing CABG, surgery on the aorta or other heart valves.
	  - Patients with severe AS and LVEF < 50 %
	 – Surgery is reasonable in:
	  - Patients with moderate AS undergoing CABG, surgery on the aorta or other heart valves.
	 – Surgery may be considered in:
	  - Asymptomatic patients with severe AS and abnormal response to exercise.
	  - Adults with severe asymptomatic AS if there is a high likelihood of rapid progression (age, calcification, and CAD) or if surgery might be delayed at the time of symptom onset.
	  - Patients undergoing CABG who have mild AS when there is evidence that progression may be rapid (such as moderate to severe valve calcification).
	  - Asymptomatic patients with extremely severe AS (aortic valve area < 0,6 cm², mean gradient > 60 mm Hg, and jet velocity > 5 m/s) when the patient's expected operative mortality ≤1 %.
	
	 – Valvuloplasty = restenosis within 6-12 months for most of patients (indicated as a bridge to surgery in hemodynamically unstable patients, or in patients with severe comorbidity).
	 – Percutaneous aortic valvular replacement: under investigation.

Aortic Regurgitation Evaluation	Causes :
	– Rheumatic fever (mitral valve always involved).
	– Bicuspid aortic valve.
	– Endocarditis.
	– Arterial hypertension.
	– Aortic arch disease (dilation, idiopathic, Takayasu disease, temporal arteritis, Marfan, dissection of ascending aorta*, ankylosing spondylitis, Reiter, rheumatoid arthritis, syphilis).
	– Drug induced (pergolide, cabergolide, dexfenfluramine before 1997).
	– Others: trauma*, osteogenesis imperfecta, Ehlers-Danlos syndrome, mild subaortic stenosis.
	
	* most often: acute presentation.
	
	Symptoms :
	  - if acute: acute pulmonary edema.
	  - if chronic: exertional dyspnea, fatigue, chest pain.
	
	Physical examination :
	  - If acute = acute pulmonary edema. Absence of classic signs of aortic regurgitation.
	  - If chronic: ↑ pulse pressure, ↓ diastolic pressure, Hill's sign (difference in systolic BP > 60 mmHg between upper and lower limbs), Corrigan's pulse (pulse with rapid rise and fall), Duroziez's sign (murmur over a partially compressed peripheral artery, commonly the femoral), apical impulse forceful and displaced to left and downward, ↑ S2a, a high-pitched decrescendo diastolic murmur, ± a low-pitched mid diastolic murmur at apex (Austin Flint).
	
	Natural history:
	– For asymptomatic patient with normal LVEF: risk of progression towards symptoms and/or LV dysfunction < 6 %/year, risk of sudden death < 0.2 %/year.
	– For asymptomatic patient with ↓ LVEF: risk of progression towards symptoms > 25 %/year.
	– For symptomatic patient: risk of death > 10 %/year.

Workup	– ECG: LVH.
	– Chest X-ray: left ventricular enlargement.
	– Echocardiography-Doppler:
	  - At diagnosis or at onset of symptoms.
	  - After 2-3 months if the chronicity of the lesion is uncertain.
	  - Every 2-3 years if mild aortic regurgitation (AR), little or no LV dilation and normal LVEF.
	  - Every 6-12 months if severe AR and significant LV dilation (end-diastolic dimension > 60 mm); every 4-6 months if more advanced dilation (end-diastolic dimension > 70 mm or end-systolic dimension > 50 mm).
	– Treadmill testing for sedentary patients or with equivocal symptoms to evaluate functional capacity.
	– Ventriculography PRN if suboptimal echocardiography.
	– Cardiac catheterization if above tests are inconclusive or are discordant.

Treatment	Avoid isometric exercise.
	
	Medical treatment :
	– Vasodilatators (questionable benefit): nifedipine, ACEI.
	  - Recommended in patients with severe AR who have symptoms or LV dysfunction and who are non-operable.
	  - Reasonable for patients with severe heart failure symptoms and severe LV dysfunction before proceeding with valvular surgery.
	  - May be considered for asymptomatic patients with severe AR who have LV

dilation but normal LVEF.

– Beta -blockers for patients with a dilated aortic root (Marfan).
– Nitroprusside + dopamine or dobutamine for patients with acute AR waiting for surgery.

Surgical treatment:

Surgery is indicated for:
- Symptomatic severe AR (i.e.: NYHA FC 3-4/4 or angina FC ≥ 2/4 in a patient with normal LVEF or NYHA FC 2-4/4 for a patient with LVEF 25-50 %)
- Asymptomatic severe AR and LVEF ≤ 50 %.
- Severe AR in a patient undergoing CABG, surgery on the aorta or other heart valves.

Surgery is reasonable for:
- Asymptomatic patients with severe AR and normal LVEF but with severe LV dilation (end-diastolic dimension > 75 mm or end-systolic dimension > 55 mm)

Surgery may be considered for:
- Moderate AR undergoing CABG or surgery of the ascending aorta.
- Severe AR and normal LV systolic function at rest (LVEF > 50 %) with end-diastolic dimension > 70 mm or end-systolic dimension > 50 mm; when there is evidence of progressive LV dilation, declining exercise tolerance, or abnormal hemodynamic responses to exercise.

Note: If the patient has a functional class 4/4 and LVEF < 25 % or end-systolic dimension > 60 mm, the risk of the surgery is very high: medical treatment is usually preferred.

Concomitant surgery to repair the aortic root or replace the ascending aorta indicated if diameter of the aortic root or ascending aorta > 5 cm or if the rate of increase in diameter is 0.5 cm per year or more, or with bicuspid valves and diameter of the aortic root or ascending aorta > 4.5 cm.

Tricuspid Stenosis Evaluation	Causes: acute rheumatic fever (usually with mitral stenosis), carcinoid syndrome, atrial tumor. Physical exam: right-sided heart failure (pulsating liver), giant a wave, y descent ↓, ↑ S1, diastolic murmur along left sternal border = mitral stenosis, ↑ with inspiration. Severe if valvular area < 1 cm².
Workup	Chest X-ray: right atrium ↑. Echocardiography/Doppler. Right heart catheterization.
Treatment	Valvuloplasty or valvular replacement (rarely indicated).
Tricuspid Regurgitation Evaluation	Causes: left-sided heart failure, pulmonary hypertension, right ventricular infarction, endocarditis, carcinoid syndrome, SLE, tricuspid valve prolapse, congenital heart disease (such as Ebstein's anomaly), trauma. Physical exam: pansystolic murmur ↑ with inspiration along left sternal border, ↑ v wave, no x descent, ↑ y descent, S3 on inspiration.
Treatment	Valvuloplasty, valvular repair or replacement with a bioprosthesis (rarely indicated).

Pericardial Disorders

Acute Pericarditis	Chest pain ↑ with deep inspiration worse supine and with cough, frequently following a viral prodrome. Physical examination: evanescent pericardial rub (mono, bi or triphasic).

Causes	– *Idiopathic.*
	– *Infectious* :
	    - Viral (coxsackie, echovirus, adenovirus, influenza, mumps, hepatitis, VZV, EBV, HIV).
	    - Bacteria (streptococcus, staphylococcus, Gram negative rods, *Legionella*), mycoplasma, tuberculosis, histoplasmosis, Lyme disease, parasites, etc.
	– *Neoplasm*: metastases from lung, breast, thyroid, renal cancer; melanoma, lymphoma, acute leukemia, primary pericardial mesothelioma (rare).
	– *Immune/inflammatory* : rheumatoid arthritis, SLE, rheumatic fever, scleroderma, Wegener, polyarteritis nodosa, dermatomyositis, ankylosing spondylitis, Reiter, Behçet, Churg-Strauss, giant cell arteritis, inflammatory bowel disease, pancreatitis, Dressler's syndrome, etc.
	– *Metabolic disorders*: uremia, hypothyroidism, gout, Gaucher's disease.
	– *Iatrogenic*: post-radiotherapy, post-cardiotomy, drug-induced (procainamide, hydralazine, minoxidil, penicillin, etc).
	– *Traumatic.*
	– *Vascular*: post-infarction, post-coronary angioplasty.
	– *Contiguous structural disease*: aortic dissection, myocardial infarction, pneumonia, pulmonary embolism, empyema.
	
	Note: 90 % of acute pericarditis is idiopathic or post-viral.
	- Among young patients: trauma, myocarditis, SLE, purulent.
	- Among elderly patients: post-myocardial infarction, tuberculosis, neoplasm.

Workup	For most cases, the workup includes **CBC, electrolytes, creatinine, ESR, CK-MB, troponin, ECG, chest X-ray, echocardiography**. According to clinical findings : blood cultures, PPD, viral and fungal serology, ASO titres, cold agglutinins, heterophile antibodies, TSH, ANA, rheumatoid factor, complement, urinalysis, pericardial fluid analysis with culture + Gram + Ziehl + cytology + biochemical (glucose, LDH, protein), pericardial biopsy. Note: ECG: Diffuse concave ST elevation, PR depression, T wave abnormalities, and intermittent atrial arrhythmia in 5-10 %.

Treatment	According to cause.
	If idiopathic:
	    NSAIDs (e.g.: Aspirin 650 mg every 3-4 hours, ibuprofen 600-800 mg every 6 hours, etc). Duration: 2-6 weeks.
	    Addition of colchicine 0.6-1.2 mg/day for 3 months decreases risk of recurrence.
	    Prednisone if no response after a 7-10 days of treatment: 60-80 mg/day (but seems to increase risk of recurrence; bacterial infection and tuberculosis should be rule out first).
	    Narcotics if severe.
	    Duration of treatment = 2-6 weeks.
	    If recurrence: steroids, colchicine (1 mg/d), azathioprine, cyclophosphamide, pericardectomy.
	If post-infarction:
	    Avoid NSAIDs and steroids whenever possible (can extend area of infarct). ASA can be continued.
	    Simple analgesic (Acetaminophen).
	    Usually rapid response.
	
	Patients with pericarditis can be safely managed on an outpatient basis without a thorough diagnostic evaluation unless the patient has high risk features such as temperature > 38 °C, a subacute onset, immunodepression, a history of recent trauma,

	oral anticoagulant therapy, myopericarditis, a large pericardial effusion, and cardiac tamponade.
Prognosis	According to cause. 25 % recurrence: tamponade rare.
	Follow closely for heart failure if associated myocarditis (with ↑ cardiac markers).
	Complications: recurrence in 15-30 % of cases, tamponade (15 % if idiopathic, 60 % if neoplasm or tuberculosis), constrictive pericarditis (see below).
	Avoid strenuous activities for 3 to 6 months.
Constrictive Pericarditis	– Thickened fibrotic pericardium, limiting normal diastolic filling.
	– Symptoms of right heart congestion (ascites, hepatosplenomegaly, edema), dyspnea, fatigue, etc.
	– On physical examination: jugular distension or other signs of right ventricular failure, rapid y descent, Kussmaul's sign, pericardial knock, apical impulse often impalpable. Atrial fibrillation. Paradoxical pulse present in 1/3 of patients.
Causes	– Constrictive pericarditis is usually a long-term consequence of either acute or chronic pericarditis.
	– Most common: idiopathic, radiation, viral, post-PCI, cardiac trauma, recurrent pericarditis, renal failure, connective tissue disease, cancer. Tuberculosis and histoplasmosis rare.
	– May be difficult to distinguish from restrictive cardiomyopathy: hemodynamic workup and sometimes endomyocarditis biopsy may be required to differentiate between these entities.
Workup	– Liver enzymes elevations (↑ ALT, ↑ AST, ↑ LDH).
	– ECG non-specific: low voltage, T wave abnormalities, atrial fibrillation.
	– Chest X-ray: widening of cardiac silhouette, pericardial calcification, right atrial dilation.
	– Echocardiography: shows inspiratory changes in mitral ↓, and tricuspid inflow ↑ velocities; in pulmonary venous flow, and preserved myocardial relaxation index, ↑ pericardial thickness.
	– Pericardial CT: shows ↑ pericardial thickness: most useful test.
	– Hemodynamics: to confirm the diagnosis (characteristic square root sign).
Treatment	Prudent diuresis.
	Pericardectomy possible but significant morbidity.
Pericardial Effusion	– Accumulation of transudate, exudate or blood in the pericardial space. Asymptomatic if effusion accumulates slowly. Frequent symptoms include pain, dyspnea, and cough.
	– Causes: many of the same diseases causing pericarditis will generate an effusion (see above): very frequent after cardiac surgery: also associated with cardiac perforation post-intervention or post-infarction, aortic dissection, ruptured aortic aneurism, malignant tumor, trauma, myxœdema, amyloidosis, anticoagulants, HIV, idiopathic, etc.
Management	– Workup: ECG (low voltage, tachycardia), chest X-ray (widening of the cardiac silhouette), echocardiography (diagnostic).
	– Pericardiocentesis (with fluid analysis) if significant effusion (> 2 cm), tamponade, neoplasm, bacterial infection or tuberculosis or if recurrent or persistent > 3 months: possible complications of intervention = myocardial or coronary laceration, pneumothorax, acute right or left ventricular dysfunction: post-intervention: follow-up for 24 hours in the ICU.
Tamponade	– Caused by the accumulation of fluid in the pericardial space inducing an increase of ventricular and atrial diastolic pressures thereby impeding diastolic filling and causing a decrease in ejection volume and systolic BP.
	– Clinical features: variable: asymptomatic to severe retrosternal discomfort with dyspnea and hypotension.
	– On physical examination: elevated venous pressure, preserved x descent, absent y descent, pulsus paradoxicus. Beck's triad: hypotension, jugular venous distension, distant heart sound.

Workup	– ECG: low voltage, non-specific ST changes: electrical alternans (pathognomonic). – Echocardiography: diastolic right atrial and ventricular collapse and variation of tricuspid and mitral inflow velocities. – Swan-Ganz catheter or cardiac catheterization confirms ↑ right atrial diastolic pressure and ↑ pulmonary capillary pressure: absent y descent.
Management	– If life-threatening condition: increase volume and STAT pericardiocentesis: otherwise guided echocardiographic pericardiocentesis vs open surgical drainage (and fluid analysis). Inotropes if needed. – If recurrence: repeated pericardiocentesis, sclerotherapy, pericardial window, pericardectomy.

Aortic Disorders	

Aortic Dissection	Risk factors : arterial hypertension, aortic coarctation, iatrogenic, age, Marfan, Ehlers-Danlos, pregnancy, post-thoracic trauma, cocaine/crack intake, smoking, dyslipidemia, giant cell arteritis, Behçet, Takayasu, syphilis, bicuspid aortic valve.
	
	Stanford's classification :
	  – type A: dissection involving ascending aorta.
	  – type B: dissection distal to the brachiocephalic trunk (sparing the ascending aorta).
	Acute if diagnosis ≤ 14 days after symptom onset. Chronic thereafter.
	
	Symptoms: Acute severe chest pain maximal at onset. Sometimes tearing, radiating to the back, sometimes complicated by acute aortic regurgitation or tamponade. Occasionally upper and lower extremity, renal, myocardial, cerebral, mesenteric or spinal ischemia. Arterial hypertension common at presentation.
	
	Diagnosis: chest X-ray (mediastinal widening), transthoracic or transesophageal echocardiography, thoracic CT, thoracic MRI, arteriogram. ECG non-specific (but inferior infarction can occur). ↑ D-dimers.
	
	Treatment: surgery for type A aortic dissection: medical treatment for type B aortic dissection (with beta-blockers followed by nitroprusside to obtain the lowest tolerated BP): notable exceptions where surgery might be necessary; if aorta > 5 cm in diameter, progression of dissection on medical treatment, persistent pain, uncontrolled hypertension, ischemia or peripheral organ dysfunction, Marfan. Endovascular therapy to be considered for unstable descending aortic dissection or with hypoperfusion.
	
	Prognosis: mortality for an untreated type A dissection 50 % at 48 h vs type B 10 %. Intrahospital mortality < 30 %. Surgical mortality 10-25 %. Survival rate at 5 and 10 years for patients discharged from hospital = 80 and 40 %. Follow up with CT or MRI every 3 to 12 months for non-surgically treated dissection.

Coarctation of the Aorta	Stenosis usually distal to the origin of left subclavian, sometimes proximal to the left subclavian artery, rarely at the level of the abdominal aorta. Male predominance is 2:1. For women: the risk of dissection of the aorta is higher during pregnancy. ↑ frequency with Turner syndrome, bicuspid aortic valve (50 %) - aortic stenosis, ventricular septal defect, patent ductus arteriosus, mitral valvular disorder, aneurysm of the circle of Willis (3-5 %). Congenital causes, or acquired inflammatory disease (Takayasu) or rarely from atherosclerosis. Non-specific symptoms related to hypertension (headache, dizziness), claudication, heart failure, intracerebral hemorrhage.

	On physical exam, systolic BP in upper > lower extremities. ↑ S2. Sometimes BP in right arm > left. Rarely hypotension in 4 limbs. Delayed femoral pulse (radial-femoral delay). Thrill in the suprasternal notch. Systolic murmur may radiate to the back. Signs of bicuspid aortic valve. Workup: ECG (left or right ventricular hypertrophy), chest X-ray (posterior rib notching, "3" sign, cardiomegaly), echocardiography, thoracic CT, thoracic MRI, MR-Angio, arteriography, cerebral CT to screen for vascular abnormalities. Complications: hypertension, left ventricular failure (in 2/3 of patients > 40 years old), aortic dissection, early CAD, endocarditis, stroke (aneurysm rupture). Treatment: surgery if gradient > 30 mmHg. Alternative: angioplasty ± stent but complications to be considered. Surgical success depends on patient's age. Prognosis: if untreated, 75 % death rate before age of 50, 90 % before age of 60.
Abdominal Aortic Aneurysm (AAA)	Risk factors: smoking, age, male, atherosclerosis, family history of aneurysm, hypertension, COPD, etc. Prevalence: 5 % males > 65 years old. 3 males for 1 female. Men's rupture risk/year: 0 % if < 4 cm, 1 % if 4-4.9 cm, 11 % if 5-5.9, 25 % if > 6 cm. Rupture risk at a smaller diameter in women. Survival 10-15 % if rupture (a minority survive until hospital arrival): survival 50 % if emergency surgery. Physical Exam: most often asymptomatic. Frequent incidental finding at echography. Inflammatory AAA sometimes causes abdominal pain, back pain, claudication or ureteral obstruction. Treatment : - Surgery if AAA ≥ 5.5 cm in men (> 6 cm if significant comorbidity), ≥ 5 cm in women (?) or if symptomatic AAA: mortality at 30 days 3-5 %. - Endovascular therapy by inserting an endovascular stent sometimes possible if appropriate anatomy: mortality at 30 days 1%, endovascular leak 10-20 %. Optimal treatment (surgery vs stent) still undetermined. - Smoking cessation. Close follow up of AAA by echography every 24 months if 3-3.9 cm, every 12 months if AAA 4-4.9 cm, and every 6 months if ≥ 5 cm (in men) and at 12 months if AAA 3-4.4 cm, and at 6 months if 4.5-5 cm (in women). Serial CT scan follow-up post-stent insertion. Universal screening not recommended. Selective one-time screening by abdominal ultrasonography for men aged 65-75 who have ever smoked (2005 CCS Guidelines).

Congenital Heart Disease	
Acyanotic Conditions	
Atrial Septal Defect (ASD)	4 types of inter-atrial communication: - *ostium secundum* (75 % of cases). - sinus venosus (5-10 %). - *ostium primum* (15-20 %, also called partial atrioventricular canal. Associated with Down's syndrome). - coronary sinus (< 1 %) In presence of left-to-right shunt, there is risk of pulmonary hypertension which could lead to Eisenmenger syndrome (see below). **Clinical**: clinical manifestations depend on the extent of left-to-right shunt; if ratio of pulmonary/systemic flow (Qp/Qs) > 2, heart failure during childhood. If Qp/Qs 1.5-2: symptoms during adolescence and young adulthood (palpitations - atrial fibrillation -, dyspnea, heart failure). If Qp/Qs < 1.5; asymptomatic. Stroke due to paradoxical embolism can also occur. On cardiac examination, presence of wide and fixed split S2 and systolic murmur I-III/VI at pulmonary area. Left parasternal lift. **Workup**: ECG shows incomplete right bundle branch block + 1st degree AV block and either right axial deviation (with *ostium secundum*) or left axial deviation (with *ostium primum*). Chest X-ray shows prominent pulmonary arteries and enlargement of the right ventricle. Echocardiography diagnostic. Cardiac magnetic resonance sometimes useful for evaluating right heart chambers. **Treatment**: Indicated with dilation of right cavities (in absence of severe pulmonary hypertension), or cryptogenic TIA-stroke with bidirectional shunt. Closure of ASD by surgery or percutaneously.
Patent Foramen Ovale (PFO)	Caused by incomplete closure of the *septum secundum*, which produces a valve effect and provokes an intermittent right-to-left shunt. Opening persistent in 25 % of people after birth. Significant opening (≥ 0.5 cm) present in 6 % of autopsies. Potential cause of paradoxical embolism and cryptogenic stroke (45 % of patients with cryptogenic stroke under 55 years old have PFO). Treatment post-stroke is controversial.
Ventricular Septal Defect (VSD)	**Clinical**: depends on diameter of the defect; In adults, with restrictive VSD, asymptomatic with holosystolic murmur III-IV/VI. If moderately restrictive VSD, dyspnea, atrial fibrillation, pulmonary hypertension, possible murmur. If non-restrictive VSD, Eisenmenger syndrome. **Workup:** Diagnosis by echocardiography. Cardiac catheterization to evaluate pulmonary resistance. Cardiac magnetic resonance sometimes useful. **Treatment:** depends on diameter of the defect and symptoms. If significant shunt: treatment in order to prevent pulmonary hypertension or heart failure. Frequent spontaneous closure of shunt (40 %) before age 2, so delay surgery except if there are signs of pulmonary hypertension or heart failure. Treat significant VSD (Qp/QS > 1.5/1), if symptomatic, if LV dilation or dysfunction or if pulmonary artery pressure > 50 mmHg. Surgery is contraindicated if Eisenmenger syndrome. Percutaneous closure undergoing evaluation. No endocarditis prophylaxis.

Patent Ductus Arteriosus	Presence of a shunt between descending thoracic aorta and left pulmonary artery. Associated with maternal rubella. Prevalence: 1:2000-5000. Produces an arteriovenous fistula. **Clinical:** Often asymptomatic. Ventricular failure or pulmonary hypertension possible if significant. Systolo-diastolic murmur at 2nd left intercostal space. ↑ S2 and ↑ pulse pressure. **Workup:** Echocardiography. Cardiac catheterization as needed to evaluate pulmonary resistance and shunt severity. Arteriography as needed, cardiac magnetic resonance sometimes useful. **Treatment:** Could be considered for everyone due to the risk of infectious endarteritis; surgical ligature or through catheterization if available No endocarditis prophylaxis
Pulmonary Stenosis	**Clinical:** Often asymptomatic. If moderate to severe (maximum gradient > 50 mmHg), exertional dyspnea, angina, syncope, right-sided heart failure, arrhythmia. Systolic murmur, ↑ with inspiration and ↑ a wave. Parasternal lift. Systolic ejection click ↓ with inspiration. **Workup:** Echocardiography diagnostic. **Treatment:** Indicated if symptomatic (exertional dyspnea, angina or syncope) or if mean echographic gradient > 40 mmHg. Possibility of percutaneous valvuloplasty or valvular surgery.

Cyanotic Conditions

Eisenmenger Syndrome	Develops when a significant left-to-right shunt produces pulmonary hypertension and irreversible pulmonary vascular disease, causing the shunt to reverse, becoming a right-to-left shunt. This may complicate a ventricular septal defect, an atrial septal defect or a patent ductus arteriosus. **Clinical:** cyanosis with right-to-left shunt, exertional dyspnea, palpitations, hyper-viscosity, hemoptysis, bleeding, thrombosis, stroke, syncope, heart failure, sudden death. Risk of cerebral abscess. ↑ pulmonary S2, and pulmonary regurgitation murmur (Graham-Steel), central cyanosis. **Workup:** CBC (polycythemia), O_2 saturation (desaturation). Echocardiography to localize shunt. Cardiac catheterization to evaluate pulmonary vascular disease and quantify intra-cardiac shunt. **Treatment:** Avoid dehydration, intense exercise, altitude, systemic vasodilatation, pregnancy, and anesthesia. Pulmonary vasodilatators (epoprostenol, nitric oxide, etc) can be useful. Phlebotomy for symptoms of hyperviscosity with hematocrit > 65 %. Cardiopulmonary transplant or pulmonary transplant with repair of the cardiac defect possible if limited prognosis. Endocarditis prophylaxis.
Ebstein Anomaly	Congenital lesion in which tricuspid valve has migrated towards right ventricle, creating a smaller right ventricle. Tricuspid regurgitation frequent, occasional pulmonary stenosis. Frequently associated with atrial septal defect or patent foramen ovale (> 50 %) with 2nd right-to-left shunt. Pre-excitation syndrome in 25 % of cases. **Clinical:** cyanosis, dyspnea, fatigue, palpitations, syncope, heart failure, stroke, cerebral abscess. **Workup:** Echocardiography diagnostic. ECG: giant p wave and right bundle branch block ± delta wave. Electrophysiological study if arrhythmia. **Treatment:** Valvular repair or replacement with closure of atrial septal defect indicated if heart failure FC 3-4/4, paradoxical embolism, cyanosis (oxygen saturation < 90 %), right heart failure or PSVT. Ablation of accessory pathway if atrial arrhythmia. Endocarditis prophylaxis to be considered in cyanotic patient.

Chapter 1   Cardiology

Useful References: CARDIOLOGY

Abdominal Aorta Aneurysm: Lancet 2005; 365: 1577-89 (review article)
   … Endovascular Treatment: N Engl J Med 2008; 358: 494-501 (review article)
Acute Coronary Syndrome: JAMA 2005; 293: 349-357 (review article)
Acute Myocardial Infarction: Lancet 2008; 372: 570-84 (review article)
   - With ST Elevation: Circulation 2008; 117: 296-329 (American Guidelines)
        Treatment: J Am Coll Cardiol 2007; 50: 917-29 (review article)
        Primary PCI: N Engl J Med 2007; 356: 47-54 (review article)
   - Without ST Elevation: Circulation 2007; 116: 803-877 (American Guidelines)
   Complications: Mayo Clin Proc 1995: 70: 880- (review article)
Acute Pericarditis: N Engl J Med 2004; 351: 2195-2202 (review article)
   Eur Heart J 2004; 25: 587-610 (European Guidelines)
   Lancet 2004; 363: 717-27 (review article)
Amiodarone: JAMA 2007; 298: 1312-1322 (review article)
   … and Atrial fibrillation : N Engl J Med 2007; 356: 830-40 (review article)
Angina (Stable): N Engl J Med 2005; 352: 2524-33 (review article)
   Can J Cardiol 2000; 16: 1513-1536 (Canadian Guidelines)
   Circulation 2007; 116: 2762-2772 (ACC/AHA Guidelines)
Angina (Unstable): Circulation 2007; 116: 803-877 (American Guidelines)
   Mayo Clin Proc 2001; 76: 391-405 (review article on treatment)
Aortic Dissection: Lancet 2008; 372: 55-66 (review article)
   Circulation 2003: 108: 628-35 & 772-78 (review article)
Aortic Regurgitation: N Engl J Med 2004; 351: 1539-46 (review article)
   Circulation 2005; 112: 125-134 (review article)
Aortic Stenosis: Lancet 2009; 373: 956-66 (review article)
   J Am Coll Cardiol 2006; 47: 2141-51 (review article)
   … Asymptomatic Severe: J Am Coll Cardiol 2008; 52: 1279-92 (review article)
   Valvuloplasty: Circulation 2007; 115: 334-338 (review article)
Apical Ballooning Syndrome (Takotsubo): Circulation 2008; 118: 397-409 (review article)
   Circulation 2007; 115: 56-59 (review article)
Arrhythmogenic right ventricular cardiomyopathy: Lancet 2009; 373: 1289-1300 (review article)
Atrial Fibrillation: Circulation 2006; 114; 700-752 (ACC/AHA/ESC Guidelines)
   Can J Cardiol 2005; 21: 9B-73B (Canadian Guidelines)
   Mayo Clin Proc 2009; 84: 643-62 (review article)
   Lancet 2007; 370: 604-18 (review article)
   N Engl J Med 2004; 351: 2408-16 (review article)
   … After Cardiac Surgery: J Am Coll Cardiol 2008; 51: 793-801 (review article)
   … Ablation Treatment: Circulation 2007 ; 116 : 1515-23 (review article)
Atrial Septal Defect: Circulation 2006; 114; 1645-1653 (review article)
Bradycardia: N Engl J Med 2000; 342; 703-09 (review article)
CABG: Circulation 2004; 110: 1168-76 (American Guidelines)
Cardiac Rehabilitation: Mayo Clin Proc 2009; 84: 373-383 (review article)
   J Am Coll Cardiol 2008; 51: 1619-31 (review article)
Cardiac Resynchronisation: JAMA 2007; 297: 2502-2514 (review article)
   J Am Coll Cardiol 2005; 46: 2153-67 & 68-82 (review article)
Cardiogenic Shock: Circulation 2008; 117: 686-97 (review article)
Chest Pain evaluation: N Engl J Med 2000; 342: 1187-95 (review article)
Cocaine and Retrosternal Pain - Infarction: Circulation 2008; 117: 1897-1907 (review article)
Congenital heart disease in adults (aorta coarctation, etc):
   Circulation 2008; 118: 2395-2451 (ACC-AHA Guidelines)
   Circulation 2008; 117: 1090-99 & 1228-37 & 1340-50 (review article)
   Can J Cardiol 2001; 17: 940-59 & 1029-50 & 1137-58 (Canadian Guidelines)
   N Engl J Med 2000; 342: 256-63 & 334-42 (review article)
Coronary angiography: Circulation 1999; 99: 2345-57 (American Guidelines)
Eisenmenger syndrome: J Am Coll Cardiol 2009; 53: 733–40 (review article)
Fitness to drive and cardiovascular diseases: Can J Cardiol 2004; 20: 1313-34 (CCS Guidelines)
Heart Failure:
   Can J Cardiol 2006; 22: 23-45 & 2007; 23: 21-45 & 2008; 24: 21-40 & 2009; 25: 85-105 (Canadian
      Guidelines: updated)
   Circulation 2009; 119: 1977-2016 & 2005; 112: 1825-1852 (American Guidelines)
   Lancet 2009; 373: 941-55 (review article)
   Eur Heart J 2008; 29: 2388-2442 (ESC Guidelines)
   … Decompensated: CMAJ 2007; 176: 797-805 (review article)
      J Am Coll Cardiol 2009; 53: 557-73

... Diastolic: CMAJ 2009; 180: 520-527 (review article)
    J Am Coll Cardiol 2009; 53: 905-18 (review article)
Hypertrophic Cardiomyopathy: Lancet 2004; 363: 1881-91 (review article)
    J Am Coll Cardiol 2003; 42: 1687-1713 (ACC/AHA Guidelines)
Implantable Cardioverter-Defibrillators: J Am Coll Cardiol 2006; 47: 1507-17 (review article)
    ... After Myocardial Infarction: N Engl J Med 2008; 359: 2245-53 (review article)
Long QT syndrome: J Am Coll Cardiol 2008; 51: 2291-300 (review article)
    N Engl J Med 2008; 358: 169-76 (review article)
Mitral Regurgitation: Lancet 2009; 373: 1382-94 (review article)
    Treatment: J Am Coll Cardiol 2008; 52: 319-26 (review article)
Mitral Stenosis: Circulation 2005; 112: 432-37 (review article)
Mitral Valve Prolapse: Lancet 2005; 365: 507-18 (review article)
Myocarditis: N Engl J Med 2009; 360:1526-38 (review article)
Pacemaker: Circulation 2008; 117: 2820-40 (American Guidelines)
    Mayo Clin Proc 2008; 83: 1170-86 (review article)
Palpitations (evaluation): N Engl J Med 1998; 338: 1369-73 (review article)
Patent Ductus Arteriosus: Circulation 2006; 114: 1873-1882 (review article)
PCI: Circulation 2008; 117: 261-295 (American Guidelines)
Pericardial Disorders: Eur Heart J 2004; 25: 587-610 (European Guidelines)
    Circulation 2006; 113: 1622-32 (review article)
Pericardial Effusion: Heart 2001; 86: 235- (review article)
Pregnancy and Cardiovascular diseases: Eur Heart J 2003; 24: 761-781 (European Guidelines)
Pregnancy and Myocardial Infarction: J Am Coll Cardiol 2008; 52: 171-80 (review article)
PSVT: Mayo Clin Proc 2008; 83: 1400-11 (review article)
    N Engl J Med 2006; 354: 1039-51 (review article)
    Circulation 2003; 108: 1871-1909 (American Guidelines)
    ... Ablation: Circulation 2007; 116: 2465-2465 (review article)
Radionuclide Imaging: Circulation 2003; 108: 1404-18 (American Guidelines)
Right Ventricular Infarction: Lancet 2003; 362: 392-94 (review article)
    J Am Coll Cardiol 2002; 40: 841-53 (review article)
Stress Test: Circulation 2002; 106: 1883-92 (American Guidelines)
Sudden Cardiac Death: N Engl J Med 2001; 345: 1473-82 (review article)
    Can J Cardiol 2000; 16 (Suppl C)
Syncope: Circulation 2006; 113: 316-327 (American Guidelines)
    Eur Heart J 2004; 25: 2054-72 (European Guidelines)
    Mayo Clin Proc 2008; 83: 1280-93 (review article)
    ... Vasovagal: J Am Coll Cardiol 2008; 51: 599-606 (review article)
    ... Neurocardiogenic: N Engl J Med 2005; 352: 1004-1010 (review article)
    ... Treatment: J Am Coll Cardiol 2009; 53: 1741-51 (review article)
Tamponade: N Engl J Med 2003; 349: 684-90 (review article)
Thrombolysis: Can J Cardiol 1994; 10: 517- (Canadian Guidelines)
    Mayo Clin Proc 2000; 75: 1185-92 (review article)
Tricuspid Regurgitation: Circulation 2009; 119: 2718-25 (review article)
Troponins: CMAJ 2005; 173: 1191-202 (review article)
Valvular Heart Diseases: Circulation 2006; 114: 450-527 & 2008; 118: e523-e661 (American Guidelines)
    Eur Heart J 2007; 28: 230-268 (European Guidelines)
    ... and Pregnancy: J Am Coll Cardiol 2005 ; 46 : 223–30 & 403-10 (review article)
    N Engl J Med 2003; 349: 52-59 (review article)
Vasopressors: Circulation 2008; 118: 1047-56 (review article)
Ventricular Septal Defect: Circulation 2006; 114: 2190-2197 (review article)
Ventricular Arrhythmia and Sudden Cardiac Death: Circulation 2006; 114: 2190-2197 (review article)
    N Engl J Med 2001; 345: 1473-82 (review article)

Useful Web Site in Cardiology: Q-Tc Interval Prolongation by Drugs: www.qtdrugs.org

Chapter 2

Endocrinology

Dyslipidemias	

Classification	*Primary dyslipidemia*:
	- Familial hypercholesterolemia ($\uparrow$ LDL and often $\downarrow$ HDL).
	- Familial hypertriglyceridemia ($\uparrow$ TG and $\downarrow$ HDL).
	- Dysbetalipoproteinemia ($\uparrow$ TG and $\uparrow$ total cholesterol).
	- Familial combined hyperlipidemia ($\uparrow$ TG and $\uparrow$ LDL).
	- Familial hypoalphalipoproteinemia ($\downarrow$ HDL with normal LDL and TG).
	- Familial hyperchylomicronemia ($\uparrow$ TG and $\downarrow$ HDL).
	
	Secondary dyslipidemia:
	– LDL
	   - Hypothyroidism.
	   - Nephrotic syndrome.
	   - Chronic kidney disease.
	   - Bile duct obstruction.
	   - Medication: thiazides, ticlodipine, progesterone, cyclosporin, glucocorticoids, isotretinoin, protease inhibitors, etc.
	   - Rare: multiple myeloma, hypogonadism, primary biliary cirrhosis, acute intermittent porphyria, anorexia nervosa, sertraline.
	
	– $\uparrow$ triglycerides (TG)
	   - Diabetes (poorly controlled).
	   - Obesity.
	   - Alcoholism.
	   - Chronic kidney disease.
	   - Nephrotic syndrome.
	   - HIV infection.
	   - Medication: thiazides, non-ISA beta-blockers, oral estrogens, protease inhibitors, atypical antipsychotics, isotretinoin, glucocorticoids, etc.
	   - Rare: Cushing's syndrome, lipodystrophy, acromegaly, allopurinol, sertraline, hypothyroidism.
	
	– $\downarrow$ HDL
	   - Renal or liver failure.
	   - Diabetes.
	   - Hyperthyroidism.
	   - Nephrotic syndrome.
	   - Smoking.
	   - Acute or chronic inflammatory states.
	   - HIV infection.
	   - Medication: Non-ISA beta-blockers, anabolic steroids, isotretinoin, thiazides, benzodiazepines, etc.

Risk stratification	– Patients with atherosclerosis (coronary, carotid, peripheral: both symptomatic and asymptomatic), and most patients with diabetes or chronic kidney disease (< 30 mL/min/1.73 m^2) are in the "high risk" category. – For other patients, risk is determined using the Framingham Risk Charts (see below), combined with clinical judgment. – Also consider other risk factors: apolipoprotein B, Lp(a), $\uparrow$ homocysteine, $\uparrow$ hsCRP, positive family history (1st degree relatives), metabolic syndrome [present if $\geq$ 3 of the following risk factors: abdominal obesity (waist circumference > 102 cm in men or > 88 cm in women), triglycerides $\geq$ 1.7 mmol/L, HDL < 1.0 in men or < 1.3 mmol/L in women, BP $\geq$ 130/85 mmHg, fasting plasma glucose 5.6-7.0 mmol/L].

Targets		
Risk level	**10-year CAD risk**	**Recommendations (2006)**
High †	≥ 20 %	Treatment targets: Primary: LDL < 2 mmol/L. Secondary: TC/HDL < 4 mmol/L*.
Moderate #	11-19 %	Treat LDL ≥ 3.5 mmol/L **or** TC/HDL ≥ 5.
Low	≤ 10%	Treat LDL ≥ 5 mmol/L **or** TC/HDL ≥ 6

† Included: patients with CAD, PAD, cerebrovascular disease, and most patients with diabetes and chronic kidney disease.
* Apolipoprotein B can be used to evaluate risk of CAD and treatment benefits. Optimal level of apolipoprotein B is < 0.85 g/L in a high risk patient, < 1.05 g/L in a moderate risk patient, and < 1.2 g/L in a low risk patient.
# Treatment may be started at higher or lower values if a positive family history, the presence of metabolic syndrome, or other investigation results alter the risk level. Patients with genetic lipoproteins disorders (e.g.: familial hypercholesterolemia, dysbetalipoproteinemia) should be treated.

Screening	For: – All adults: men ≥ 40 y.o., women ≥ 50 y.o. or menopausal. – Adults with risk factors for CAD or diabetes. – Adults with family history of early CAD (1st degree relative < 55 y.o. men or a < 65 y.o. women relative). – Patients with atherosclerosis (cardiac, carotid or peripheral). – Patients with xanthomas or other physical signs of dyslipidemia. – Patients with retrosternal discomfort, dyspnea, erectile dysfunction, chronic kidney disease, SLE.
Treatment	Non-pharmacologic: Diet, exercise, limited alcohol intake, smoking cessation, weight loss (nevertheless, losing 5-10 % = beneficial effect), management of secondary causes + other risk factors. Pharmacologic: - LDL lowering: agents: Statin ± bile acid sequestrant or cholesterol absorption inhibitor. Aim for at least a 50 % ↓ in LDL in a high-risk patient and at least 40 % in a low- or moderate-risk patient. - TC/HDL ratio lowering agents: Statin ± niacin or fibrate or salmon oil supplementation (if TG increased). - TG lowering agents: Fibrate, niacin or salmon oil supplementation.

See the list of lipid-lowering drugs in the appendix.	
Comments	– LDL = Total cholesterol - HDL - (triglycerides/2.2): valid when TG < 4.5 mmol/L. – On physical exam, look for xanthelesma, signs of a primary dyslipidemia (eruptive xanthoma, tendon xanthomas, planar xanthoma, corneal arcus) and evidence of atherosclerosis (abdominal or carotid bruits, diminished peripheral pulses, ankle-brachial index < 0.9). – Take into account all the risk factors. – Avoid measuring lipids during periods of stress (assay valid if performed < 12 hours or > 6 weeks from the stress). – Measure lipids every 3-6 months. – Biochemical tests if using medication (hepatic enzymes [statin, fibrate, ezetimibe and niacin], CK [statin, fibrate], glycemia and uricemia [niacin], creatinine [fibrate], and CBC [fibrate]). – Beware of drug interactions (cytochrome P450). – Educate patients on side effects of medication (discontinue medication if weakness ± muscle pain). – Consultation in specialized lipid clinic as needed. – Pancreatitis risk increase when TG level > 10 mmol/L. – IV insulin perfusion may be used with fasting in the acute treatment of a high TG level (especially in presence of pancreatitis or chylomicronemia syndrome).

Estimation of 10-year risk of nonfatal myocardial infarction or coronary death in subjects without diabetes or evidence of cardiovascular disease according to *Framingham Heart Study* data.

Risk factor	Men Points					Risk factor	Women Points				
Age (yrs)						**Age (yrs)**					
20-34	-9					20-34	-7				
35-39	-4					35-39	-3				
40-44	0					40-44	0				
45-49	3					45-49	3				
50-54	6					50-54	6				
55-59	8					55-59	8				
60-64	10					60-64	10				
65-69	11					65-69	12				
70-74	12					70-74	14				
75-79	13					75-79	16				

Total cholesterol (mmol/L)	Age (yrs)					Total cholesterol (mmol/L)	Age (yrs)				
	20-39	40-49	50-59	60-69	70-79		20-39	40-49	50-59	60-69	70-79
< 4.14	0	0	0	0	0	< 4.14	0	0	0	0	0
4.15-5.19	4	3	2	1	0	4.15-5.19	4	3	2	1	1
5.20-6.19	7	5	3	1	0	5.20-6.19	8	6	4	2	1
6.20-7.20	9	6	4	2	1	6.20-7.20	11	8	5	3	2
> 7.21	11	8	5	3	1	> 7.21	13	10	7	4	2

Smoking						Smoking					
No	0	0	0	0	0	No	0	0	0	0	0
Yes	8	5	3	1	1	Yes	9	7	4	2	1

HDL (mmol/L)	Points	HDL (mmol/L)	Points
≥ 1.55	-1	≥ 1.55	-1
1.30-1.54	0	1.30-1.54	0
1.04-1.29	1	1.04-1.29	1
< 1.04	2	< 1.04	2

Systolic BP (mmHg)	Untreated	Treated	Systolic BP (mmHg)	Untreated	Treated
< 120	0	0	< 120	0	0
120-129	0	1	120-129	1	3
130-139	1	2	130-139	2	4
140-159	1	2	140-159	3	5
≥ 160	2	3	≥ 160	4	6

Points total	10-year risk (%)*	Points total	10-year risk (%)*
0	< 1	< 9	< 1
1-4	1	9-12	1
5-6	2	13-14	2
7	3	15	3
8	4	16	4
9	5	17	5
10	6	18	6
11	8	19	8
12	10	20	11
13	12	21	14
14	16	22	17
15	20	23	22
16	25	24	27
≥ 17	≥ 30	≥ 25	≥ 30

* Note: For patients with a family history of CAD (1st degree relative < 55 y.o. men, < 65 y.o. women), the calculated risk should be multiplied by a factor of 2.

Thyroid Disorders	
Hyperthyroidism	Palpitations, tremor, anxiety, weight loss despite a normal appetite, heat intolerance, excessive sweating, dyspnea, diarrhea or increased bowel movements, insomnia, menstrual disorders, irritability, emotional lability, gynecomastia (young men), atrial fibrillation, osteoporosis, high systolic BP, heart failure, proximal myopathy… With Graves disease: ophtalmopathy (eyelid retraction, exophthalmia, chemosis, diplopia, palpebral edema, optic nerve compression …), clubbing, pretibial myxedema. In elderly patients: weight loss, constipation, apathy, atrial fibrillation, heart failure, systemic embolism, osteoporosis ...
Causes	– Graves' disease: most frequent cause, especially in young adults and in women; autoimmune; positive family history; leads to specific infiltrative process (proptosis, myxedema). – Single toxic adenoma or toxic multinodular goiter (the latter more frequent in elderly patients). – Thyroiditis: subacute De Quervain thyroiditis (thyroid pain, fever, malaise, myalgia, odynophagia, sedimentation rate ↑) or silent (painless) thyroiditis; transient (2-3 months), often followed by a hypothyroidism state that is often temporary. May occur in post-partum period and be recurrent. – Medication: lithium, interferon, interleukin, amiodarone (type 1 = iodine-induced, type 2 = thyroiditis). – Secondary or tertiary hyperthyroidism: secondary to ↑ TSH or TRH secretion by tumor: rare. – Ectopic: struma ovarii, ectopic production of hCG (with molar, twin, and sometimes with normal pregnancy, choriocarcinoma or testicular cancer), metastasis from follicular carcinoma. – Exogenous causes: thyroid hormones, iodine (radiologic contrast agents, natural products, amiodarone [type 1], iodine disinfectants). Differential diagnosis of ↓ TSH with normal or low free T4 and T3 levels and clinical euthyroidism: steroids, dopamine, phenytoin, severe non-thyroid disease.
Workup	TSH, T3, free T4, thyroid scan (normal uptake = 10-25 %). As indicated: antibodies (TSH-receptor antibodies [TSI] or microsomal antibodies [anti-TPO]). If radioiodine uptake is low, the thyroglobulin level may be useful in differentiating exogenous hyperthyroidism (thyroglobulin ↓) from silent thyroiditis (thyroglobulin ↑). Pregnancy test for women of child-bearing age. Color-flow Doppler ultrasonography of the thyroid can be useful in amiodarone induced thyroiditis (↑ or normal in type 1 and ↓ in type 2). ⇒ When thyroid scan shows a homogenous increase in radioiodine uptake: Graves' disease vs secondary hyperthyroidism with ↑ TSH or hCG. ⇒ When thyroid scan shows hot areas or heterogenous radioiodine uptake: toxic adenoma or toxic multinodular goiter. ⇒ If thyroid scan has a decreased radioiodine uptake: thyroiditis vs exogenous thyroxine intake vs recent exposure to iodine (up to 6 months) vs secreting metastasis of a thyroid cancer vs struma ovarii.

Treatment	According to cause:
	– Graves' disease: radioactive iodine or antithyroid agent. In pregnancy: the antithyroid agent should be PTU, because of the possible teratogenic effects of methimazole. Rarely surgery.
	– Toxic adenoma: radioactive iodine or rarely surgery (if > 4 cm).
	– Toxic multinodular goiter: radioactive iodine ± temporary antithyroid agent, or rarely surgery.
	– Silent thyroiditis: symptomatic treatment (beta-blockers).
	– Subacute thyroiditis: symptomatic treatment (aspirin, NSAIDs) ± steroids (quick response to steroids, difficult to wean).
	– Secondary to tumor: surgery.
	Note: If severe hyperthyroidism: give antithyroid agent until euthyroid state, then radioactive iodine or surgery depending on the cause.
	Radioactive iodine: Side effects: secondary hypothyroidism (possibly transient [up to 6 months], up to 90% permanent depending on dosage): contraindicated during pregnancy, nursing, or with significant ophthalmopathy (risk of exacerbation: consider steroids as prophylaxis): consider restoring euthyroid state before radioactive iodine treatment (discontinue antithyroid agent 3-5 days prior to treatment): effective in 2-3 months: radiation-induced thyroiditis 7-10 days post-radiation (rare). Avoid pregnancy for ≥ 6 months post treatment.
	Antithyroid agents: Propylthiouracil (PTU) and methimazole. Prescribe for at least 1-2 years (aim for 1 year of a normal TSH before stopping). Remission is rare but possible in Graves' disease.
	Complete effect in 6-8 weeks. Recurrence of disease in more than 50 % at cessation of treatment. Recurrence less likely among women, in mild hyperthyroiditis or with a small goiter.
	Side effects: agranulocytosis, rash, fever, vasculitis, hepatitis, bone marrow aplasia, lupus-like syndrome. Follow free T4 + T3, liver profile and CBC (also obtain these tests prior to treatment).
	Surgery: for multinodular goiter with symptoms of compression or pregnant women with Graves' unresponsive to PTU: restore the euthyroid state pre-op with antithyroid agent and iodine for 7-10 days pre-op. Complications: recurrent laryngeal nerve or parathyroid injuries in 1-2 %.
	Inorganic iodine: transient inhibitor: indicated pre-op or if storm imminent.
	Beta-blockers: propranolol 40-340 mg/day: ↓ T4 conversion to T3. Adjuvant treatment (or as single agent in thyroiditis): control adrenergic symptoms.
	Steroids: for subacute thyroiditis, severe Graves ophthalmopathy, or amiodarone-induced thyroiditis (type 2): Prednisone 20-40 mg/day with rapid response. Treatment for 2-4 weeks (subacute thyroiditis), wean over 3 weeks or up to 3 months.
	Note: Treatment of subclinical hyperthyroidism (with ↓ TSH but normal free T4) is indicated if sustained for 8 weeks, especially in elderly patients … Look for atrial fibrillation, osteoporosis, menstrual disorders, infertility, etc.
"Thyroid storm"	Clinical: hyperthermia, changes in mental status (psychosis, anxiety, apathy, coma), tachycardia, tachypnea, nausea, vomiting, diarrhea, abdominal pain, arrhythmia, heart failure, shock … Significant mortality (10-75%).
	Thyroid disease + precipitating factors: infection, myocardial infarction or stroke, thyroid surgery, antithyroid agent withdrawal, radioactive iodine, iodine-based contrast agents, vigorous thyroid palpation, delivery…
	Treatment: ICU admission, hydrocortisone 100 mg IV every 6 hours + PTU 200-400 mg every 6-8 hrs (600 mg- loading dose) + Lugol 8 drops qid (1 hour post-PTU) + propranolol 80 mg every 6-8 hrs: esmolol if risk with beta-blocker. Add lithium 300 mg qid if storm uncontrolled (aim for serum lithium level of 1 mEq/L). Plasmapheresis as last resort. Treatment of precipitating factors and underlying cause. Avoid aspirin, use acetaminophen for fever.

Hypothyroidism	Psychomotor impairment, fatigue, cold dry skin, coarse hair, myxedema, cold intolerance, weight gain, constipation, prolonged relaxation phase of reflexes, ataxia, hoarseness, depression, dementia, carpal tunnel syndrome, bradycardia, high diastolic BP, respiratory depression, menstrual disorders, joint pain, myalgias, hypothermia, etc. Rarely: psychosis, deafness, cerebellar ataxia, hypoventilation, apnea, galactorrhea, pericardial effusions (if severe).
Causes	Primary hypothyroidism (> 90 % of cases) – Hashimoto's: autoimmune, positive family history. Goiter. Positive antimicrosomal antibody (TPO). – Post-ablation: surgical, radiotherapy, radioactive iodine, etc. – Thyroiditis: hypothyroid phase of silent or de Quervain's thyroiditis. – Iodine deficiency. – Medication: lithium, antithyroid agents, iodine, amiodarone, interleukin, interferon, etc. – Infiltrative diseases. Secondary hypothyroidism – Pituitary or hypothalamic malfunction: tumor, postpartum necrosis, etc. – Post-treatment phase of Graves' disease (TSH may be suppressed for up to 3-6 months even in the presence of post-treatment hypothyroidism): frequent. – Withdrawal from thyroid hormone therapy. May be a manifestation of a polyglandular autoimmune syndrome (with Addison's disease, type 1 diabetes, hypoparathyroidism, pernicious anemia, etc). Differential diagnosis of ↑ TSH with normal free T4 (may even be ↑ in some of these diseases): patients recovering from severe illness, acute adrenal insufficiency, lithium, amiodarone, phenytoin, heterophilic antibody interference in the TSH, TSH-secreting pituitary adenoma, thyroid hormones resistance syndrome, etc.
Workup	TSH, free T4, antimicrosomal antibodies. With ↑ TSH + normal T4 → subclinical hypothyroidism. With ↑ TSH + ↓ T4 → primary hypothyroidism. With normal or ↓ TSH + ↓ T4 → secondary hypothyroidism or severe illness. With ↑ TSH + ↑ T4 → assay interference problem (e.g.: with phenytoin, heterophilic antibodies…), TSH-secreting pituitary adenoma, thyroid hormones resistance syndrome. Normocytic or macrocytic anemia, ↓ Na⁺ (SIADH), hypercholesterolemia, ↑ CK (MM fraction), ↑ homocysteine, ↑ AST-ALT-LDH.
Treatment	Levothyroxine (L-T4) 1.6 µg/kg: check TSH 6-8 weeks after starting treatment (because T4 ½ life = 1 week). For elderly or CAD patient: begin with 0.025 mg daily with ↑ every 4 weeks. Target: normalize TSH in primary hypothyroidism (aim for TSH ≈ 1.0 mU/L) and free T4 in secondary hypothyroidism. Note: ↑ TSH despite adequate treatment may be secondary to lack of adherence, malabsorption (celiac disease or secondary to fiber, bile acid sequestrants, iron, sucralfate, antacids, calcium supplements, magnesium), ↑ clearance due to pregnancy (↑ 25-50 % dose during pregnancy), estrogens, phenytoin, or rifampicin. Adjust insulin and anticoagulants with treatment. Risk of cardiac disease deterioration, especially in elderly patients (but rare). In presence of concomitant untreated adrenal insufficiency, risk of adrenal shock with treatment. Subclinical hypothyroidism: 3-5 %/yr develop symptoms if untreated: treatment indicated if result confirmed on a second sample and a) TSH ≥ 10 mU/L or b) if TSH 3.5-10 mU/L, and ⊕ antithyroid antibody, goiter, history of irradiation for Graves' disease, male, fertility

	disorder, dyslipidemia, smoking, or vague symptoms, depression or bipolar disease, pregnancy (current or planned). Follow-up with regular TSH assays if untreated. Note: During pregnancy, aim for TSH < 2.
Myxedema coma	– Clinical findings: impaired consciousness, seizures, hypoventilation, hypothermia, bradycardia, hyponatremia, hypoglycemia… in patients with long-standing hypothyroidism left untreated (or undertreated). – Precipitating factors: infection, surgery, myocardial infarction, sedatives or opiates, stroke, cold exposure, deterioration of general health. – Treatment: ICU admission, L-T4 400 µg IV then 100 µg IV q 24h (PO when patient is able) ± L-T3 10 µg IV bid + hydrocortisone 100 mg then 25-50 mg every 8 hours (different regimes of T4 and T3 replacement exist and should be tailored to the patient). – Treatment of underlying infection. Mechanical ventilation, if needed. Passive warming of patient, if needed.
Thyroid Nodules	– 4-7% of the population have a palpable nodule: < 5 % malignant. – Risk factors for malignancy: age < 20 yrs or > 60 yrs, male, rapid growth, hoarseness, progressive dysphagia, dyspnea, history of radiation exposure to the head and neck, positive family history (including medullary carcinoma, MEN II), hard consistency, diameter > 4 cm, indurated and/or fixed lymphadenopathy, cold nodule found on thyroid scan. On ultrasound: solid or mixed texture, hypoechogenic, irregular margins, diffuse microcalcifications, irregular or absent halo, central vascularization on Doppler examination, round rather than oval shape.
Causes	Follicular adenoma, cyst, thyroid carcinoma, metastasis (kidney, breast, melanoma, lung), lymphoma, etc.
Management	Measure TSH: if low or suppressed = radioiodine uptake scan to rule out functional nodule. If positive family history of medullary cancer: measure CEA + calcitonin (and rule out pheochromocytoma before surgery if ⊕). Thyroid ultrasound useful in follow-up and in describing nodule characteristics. Fine needle aspiration biopsy for any nodule > 1 cm or if history of radiation exposure or family history of medullary neoplasia or echographic findings suggestive of cancer (see above) : → benign: follow-up with ultrasound examination every 6 months to 1 yr: if ↑ size, repeat needle biopsy, if material other than benign → surgery. → Malignant: surgery. → Suspected follicular or Hürthle cell tumor → obtain radioiodine scan: if hot, rule out hyperthyroidism, follow-up (or rarely, surgery): if cold, surgery. → Insufficient material: repeat needle biopsy under ultrasound guidance. Treatment of multi-nodular goiter: radioactive iodine vs surgery vs follow-up. Workup of any suspicious nodule in the multi-nodular goiter should be done before administration of a radioactive iodine treatment in the toxic multi-nodular goiter.

Pituitary Gland Disorders	
Physiology	Anterior pituitary gland secretes ACTH, FSH, LH, GH, TSH, prolactin. Posterior pituitary gland secretes ADH, oxytocin.
Diseases	***Secreting tumor***: hormonal effect and mass effect (headaches, cranial nerve paralysis, bitemporal hemianopsia, CSF rhinorrhea, temporal lobe epilepsy, hypopituitarism): **Prolactinoma**: most frequent tumor (40-50 %): symptoms of galactorrhea, amenorrhea, ↓ libido, infertility, erectile dysfunction ... Differential diagnosis of ↑ prolactin: tumor, medication, pregnancy, damage to pituitary stalk, chest wall disease, severe hypothyroidism, chronic kidney disease... Association with MEN I. Diagnosis: prolactin assay x 2-3: > 200 µg/L is diagnostic: if < 100 µg/L, rule out secondary causes → pregnancy, dopamine antagonist (neuroleptic, metoclopramide, antidepressants, verapamil, opiates, marijuana), chest wall irritation, chronic kidney disease, cirrhosis, severe hypothyroidism, compression of the pituitary stalk, nipple stimulation. Pregnancy test, TSH, MRI of the head, visual field examination. When prolactinoma established, rule out other pituitary deficit (free T4, 8 AM cortisol, IGF-1, free testosterone in males, menses history in women or FSH/H in post-menopausal women). Treatment: Bromocriptine (80% success rate), cabergoline (more effective than bromocriptine and better tolerated), quinagolide. High dose dopamine agonists have been associated with cardiac valvulopathies. Rarely surgery (if resistant or intolerant to medication or visual field defect not improved through medication) or radiotherapy. **Acromegaly**: 10-15 % of pituitary tumors. Clinical: Hand and feet growth, hyperhidrosis, oily skin, macroglossia, hyperpigmentation, ↑ soft tissues, osteoarthritis, cardiac involvement (left ventricular hypertrophy and dysfunction), stroke, headaches, compressive neuropathy (e.g.: carpal tunnel), sleep apnea, ↑ incidence of colon cancer, myopathy, hypogonadism, hypertension, glucose intolerance ... Association with MEN I. Increased cardiovascular mortality. Diagnosis: GH (fluctuant) and IGF-1 (more useful) assay: both ↑. Confirm with 75 g glucose tolerance test: if no suppression (suppression if nadir GH < 1 µg/L) = acromegaly. Pituitary MRI: if ∅ tumor: assay GHRH (because 1% is caused by ectopic tumor). Measure prolactin to rule out a mixed secreting tumor (prolactin and GH). Also rule out other pituitary deficit. Treatment: surgery (50-80% success rate). Primary treatment with somatostatin analogs could be considered in selected cases. Adjuvant treatment (may be started pre-op): octreotide (60-80 % effectiveness), cabergolin or bromocriptine (especially with mixed GH-prolactin tumor), pegvisomant (if octreotide ineffective or not tolerated: 90-100% effectiveness). Radiotherapy/gamma knife as needed. Screening for colon cancer (colonoscopy). **Gonadotropin-secreting tumor**: FSH and/or LH ↑. Rare. **TSH-secreting tumor**: see Thyroid diseases table: < 5 % of pituitary tumors. **Cushing's disease**: 10 - 15 % of pituitary tumors: see Adrenal diseases. ***Non-secreting tumor***: Frequent tumor (30-40 %). Mass effect, impaired vision, hypopituitarism ... Causes: adenoma, cysts, glioma ... ***Hypopituitarism***: sequence of hormonal deficiencies – GH, LH/FSH, TSH, ACTH, prolactin: acute or insidious (more frequent) symptoms. Causes: tumors (adenoma, craniopharyngioma, dysgerminoma, metastasis), radiotherapy, pituitary apoplexy, Sheehan's syndrome, lymphocytic hypophysitis, granulomatous disease (sarcoidosis, Langerhans cell histiocytosis), functional (stress, anorexia, chronic kidney disease, hormones, medication), post-operative. Clinical: symptoms according to deficiency; FSH/LH: in ♀, oligomenorrhea or amenorrhea, ↓ libido, vaginal dryness, dyspareunia: in ♂, ↓ libido, erectile dysfunction, testicular atrophy ± gynecomastia; ACTH: adrenal insufficiency; TSH: hypothyroidism;

	Prolactin: post-partum decreased lactation; GH: asymptomatic or fatigue, ↓ endurance to exercise, abdominal obesity, ↓ muscular mass. Diagnosis: pituitary MRI (or CT if MRI unavailable) and hormone evaluation: free T4, 8AM cortisol (± insulin-induced hypoglycemic test or ACTH stimulation test [depending on the suspected duration of the deficiency]), IGF-1 (± insulin-induced hypoglycemic test or arginine and GHRH stimulation test), free testosterone in males, menses history in women or FSH/LH in post-menopausal women, prolactin. Treatment: glucocorticoid replacement then thyroid and sex-hormone replacement (+ GH if a child and may be adequate for adults), Medic-Alert® bracelet. Diabetes insipidus: see Hypernatremia table.
Pituitary Incidentaloma	– Mass discovered incidentally by imaging procedure. Frequent = 10 % of CTs/MRIs. Sporadic or associated tumor with MEN 1. – So, do not screen for pituitary disease using imagery! – Hormone evaluation required: PRL, IGF-I, TSH, free T4, LH, FSH, testosterone/estradiol, plasma cortisol and urinary cortisol, midnight salivary cortisol or 1 mg dexamethasone suppression test: if ⊕, perform in-depth evaluation. Visual field evaluation if > 1 cm. – If hormone evaluation ⊖ and < 1 cm: MRI at 1-2-5 yrs: if no change, stop. If ↑ volume or symptoms = surgery (except if slowly ↑ volume without symptoms = functional evaluation every 1-2 years). – > 1 cm: MRI at 0.5-1-2-5 yrs: if no change, stop. If ↑ in volume or symptoms = surgery.

Diabetes	

Patho-physiology	Classification of Diabetes (2008 CDA Guidelines):
	Type 1: encompasses diabetes that is primarily a result of pancreatic beta cell destruction and is prone to ketoacidosis. This form includes cases due to an autoimmune process (including Latent Autoimmune Diabetes in Adult - *LADA* -, a form of autoimmune diabetes occurring in adults, treated differently from type 2 diabetes), and those for which the etiology of beta cell destruction is unknown.
	
	Type 2: may range from predominant insulin resistance with relative insulin deficiency to a predominant secretory defect with insulin resistance.
	
	Gestational diabetes: refers to glucose intolerance with onset or first recognition during pregnancy.
	
	Other specific types: include a wide variety of relatively uncommon conditions, primarily specific genetically defined forms of diabetes (genetic defects of β cell function, formerly known as Maturity-onset Diabetes of the Young - *MODY* - [up to 5% of diabetes in young patients], genetic defects in insulin action), drug use (atypical antipsychotics, beta-adrenergic agonists, cyclosporine, diazoxide, interferon, nicotinic acid, pentamidine, phenytoin, protease inhibitors, steroids, thiazides...), or diabetes associated with other diseases :
	    - Endocrinopathies: acromegaly, Cushing's, primary aldosteronism, glucagonoma, hyperthyroidism, pheochromocytoma, somatostatinoma.
	    - Diseases of the pancreas: cystic fibrosis, hemochromatosis, neoplasia, pancreatitis, etc.
	    - Other genetic syndromes sometimes associated with diabetes (myotonic dystrophy, Down's syndrome, Prader-Willi syndrome, etc).
	    - Infections (CMV, congenital rubella).
	    - Uncommon forms of immune-mediated diabetes.

Clinical findings	Symptoms: polyuria, polydipsia, polyphagia, weight loss, blurred vision, recurrent mucocutaneous fungal infections, recurrent urinary tract infections, fatigue, tingling, dysesthesia ... For type 1: ketoacidosis, age < 40 yrs (but not always), absence of obesity or insulin resistance, rapid progression (< 2 yrs) to insulin dependence. For type 2: usually a 4-7 yrs latency before diagnosis. Approx. 1/3 of diabetic patients are undiagnosed. 80% are obese. If not obese, suspect LADA. Family history often ⊕. Presence of complications of diabetes at diagnosis in up to 50% of cases.

Screening	Fasting blood glucose at age 40 then every 3 years if no other risk factors.
	Screen at a younger age and/or more frequently in patients with risk factors for diabetes (positive family history, member of high-risk ethnic group, history of impaired glucose tolerance or impaired fasting glucose, presence of complications associated with diabetes, vascular disease, history of gestational diabetes or delivery of a macrosomic infant, obesity, hypertension, dyslipidemia, schizophrenia, acanthosis nigricans, polycystic ovary syndrome ...)
	
	Measure fasting plasma glucose:
	    When plasma glucose is < 5.6 mmol/L: repeat tests every 3 yrs.
	    When plasma glucose is 5.6-6.0 with no other diabetes risk factors for diabetes: rescreen more often.
	    When plasma glucose is 5.6-6.0 with other risk factor for diabetes: consider a 75-g oral glucose tolerance test (OGTT).
	    When plasma glucose is 6.1-6.9: do an OGTT.
	    When plasma glucose ≥ 7.0: diabetes (confirmation needed).

Diagnostic criteria	1. Classic symptoms + plasma glucose ≥ 11.1 mmol/L at any time **or** 2. Fasting plasma glucose ≥ 7.0 mmol/L **or** 3. Plasma glucose ≥ 11.1 mmol/L (at 2 hrs) in a 75-g oral glucose tolerance test. *A confirmatory laboratory glucose test must be done in all cases on another day in the absence of unequivocal hyperglycemia accompanied by acute metabolic decompensation. However, individuals in whom type 1 is a possibility, to avoid rapid deterioration, confirmatory testing should not delay initiation of treatment.* Impaired glucose tolerance (IGT) when plasma glucose = 7.8 to 11.1 during glucose tolerance test (at 2 hrs). May be isolated (if fasting plasma glucose is < 6.1) or associated with impaired fasting glucose. Impaired fasting glucose (IFG) when fasting plasma glucose = 6.1-6.9. Can be isolated (if glucose tolerance test is normal: < 7.8) or associated with impaired glucose tolerance. The term "prediabetes" is a practical and convenient term for impaired fasting glucose and impaired glucose tolerance.
Targets	Recommended targets for glycemic control *† **(2008 CDA Guidelines)**

	HbA1c (%)	Fasting/pre-prandial glucose (mmol/L)	2-hour postprandial glucose (mmol/L)
Type 1 and type 2 diabetes	≤ 7	4.0-7.0	5.0-10.0 (5.0-8.0 if HbA1c targets not being met)

* Treatment goals and strategies must be tailored to the patient, with consideration given to individual risk factors and prognosis.
† Glycemic targets for children ≤12 years of age and pregnant women differ from these targets.
Note: A target HbA1c of 6.5% may be considered in some patients with type 2 diabetes to further lower the risk of nephropathy, but this must be balanced against the risk of hypoglycemia and increased mortality in patients who are at significantly elevated risk of cardiovascular disease.

Management	- Prescribe blood glucose meter, test strips, lancets, Medic-Alert® bracelet. Glucagon kit in patient treated with insulin or if significant risk of hypoglycemia.
	- Blood glucose meter readings should be compared to a laboratory plasma fasting glucose level at least once a year to check accuracy (difference < 20% acceptable).
	- Measure urinary ketones with reactive test strips in type 1 diabetes patient in presence of preprandial blood glucose > 14 mmol/L, during an acute disease or when there are symptoms of diabetic ketoacidosis (DKA).
	- Workup at first appointment: lipids, ECG, creatinine, electrolytes, TSH, urinalysis, ferritin, transferrin saturation (if suspicion of hemochromatosis), microalbuminuria (if urinalysis is normal), HbA1c or fructosamine (every 3 months), check diabetes logbook (capillary blood glucose). C-peptide levels sometimes useful to differentiate between type 1 and type 2 diabetes. Islet cell antibodies (ICA) and/or glutamic acid decarboxylase (GAD) antibodies if LADA suspected.
	- If morning hyperglycemia: rule out nocturnal hypoglycemia - Somogyi effect ($\rightarrow$ measure capillary blood glucose at night).
	- Immunization: influenza and pneumococcal vaccinations suggested.
	- Patient to be referred to a diabetes education clinic.
	- Patients with prediabetes should alter their lifestyle to reduce the risk of presenting type 2 diabetes: metformin, or acarbose, or rosiglitazone can be considered.
Complications	- Retinopathy: proliferative vs nonproliferative. Laser treatment, as needed (**$\rightarrow$ ophthalmologic examination necessary every year starting 5 years after diagnosis of type 1 diabetes in all individuals $\geq$ 15 y.o. and every year after diagnosis of type 2 diabetes**).
	- Nephropathy: progression from microalbuminuria $\rightarrow$ macroalbuminuria $\rightarrow$ chronic kidney failure. Acute disease may cause false $\oplus$. Always check for micro-albuminuria: to be confirmed with 2 out of 3 tests positive. Treatment: ACEI (for type 1 or type 2 and creatinine clearance > 60 mL/min) or ARB (for type 2), non-dihydropyridine calcium blockers, low protein diet, avoid nephrotoxic agents (**$\rightarrow$ check for microalbuminuria every year starting 5 yrs after diagnosis for type 1 diabetic patients, and every year after diagnosis for type 2 diabetic patients**).
	- Neuropathy: peripheral (glove and stocking anesthesia, focal, autonomic (orthostatic hypotension, gastroparesis, diarrhea, sexual dysfunction). Treatment: tricyclic antidepressants and/or anticonvulsants as needed.
	- Erectile dysfunction: screen at diagnosis and then periodically. Treatment: PDE5 inhibitors: consider referral to a specialist if unsuccessful or if treatment contraindicated.
	- Feet: examine at least once a year (vibration sense with 128-Hz tuning fork or 10-g monofilament on big toe and Achilles reflex). Patient is to perform daily self-examination of feet. Aggressive treatment of infection + look for PAD (arterial Doppler of the lower limbs as needed) (**$\rightarrow$ podiatrist as needed,** especially if deformations $\pm$ severe neuropathy $\pm$ history of plantar ulcer).
	- Cardiovascular: questionnaire on cardiovascular disease symptoms and a vascular examination. First cause of mortality among diabetic patients.
	Note: It has been proven that good control of diabetes lowers the risk of complications.
General treatment	- In people with type 1 diabetes: treat acute metabolic disorder and give multiple doses of insulin (qid). Intensive insulin therapy except if contraindicated (risk of severe hypoglycemia, poor life expectancy, intellectual, social or psychiatric disorder...).
	- In people with type 2 diabetes: Basic treatment is aggressive modification of lifestyle: balanced and slightly hypocaloric diet, physical exercise (walking or equivalent leisure activity for a minimum of 150 min/week).
	- For mild to moderate hyperglycemia (HbA1c < 9%): nonpharmacologic treatment for 2-3 months. If glycemic targets are not achieved, initiate antihyperglycemic

agent (metformin) (concomitant with lifestyle counselling):
- For marked hyperglycemia (HbA1c ≥ 9%): initiate pharmacotherapy immediately:
  - Consider initiating metformin concurrently with another agent from a different class; or
  - Initiate insulin.
- For patients with symptomatic hyperglycemia with metabolic decompensation : initiate insulin ± metformin:
- If not at target with above treatment: add an agent best suited to the individual based on the advantages/disadvantages of each drug class.
- If not at target with above treatment: add another drug from a different class; or add bedtime basal insulin to other agent(s); or intensify insulin regimen.

In the type 2 diabetes treated initially with insulin: if, with weight loss, insulin needs are < 20 U/day → treat with oral antihyperglycemic agents. If insulin needs are > 20 U/day → injection of intermediate-acting or long-acting HS insulin + oral antihyperglycemic agents. If needs are 60-80 U/day → divide into four injections (25% intermediate-acting HS insulin and 30% ultra-rapid-acting insulin AM, 20% noon and 25% supper). Alternatively, if non optimal control is tolerable (poor prognosis, compliance problems, lack of resources for injections in patients with loss of autonomy), divide into 2/3 AM -1/3 PM with pre-mixed insulins (30% rapid-acting and 70% intermediate-acting).

Specific treatment	Nonpharmacologic treatment = cornerstone of type 2 diabetes: - Exercise: aerobic exercise ≥ 150 min/wk. + resistance exercise 3x/wk. In sedentary patients with other vascular risk factor(s), consider exercise ECG testing before beginning an exercise program. - Diet (→ consultation and follow-up with nutritionist is ideal). Pharmacologic: see **appendix** of oral antihyperglycemic agents: - *Sulfonylureas*: e.g.: Glyburide (Diabeta®): ↑ insulin secretion. Side effects: hypoglycemia, weight gain. Gliclazide (Diamicron®) and glimeperid (Amaryl®) cause less hypoglycemia and are safe for CKD or elderly patients. - *Biguanides*: Metformin (Glucophage®): ↓ hepatic gluconeogenesis and ↓ insulin resistance: 250 mg bid up to 850 mg tid (1000 mg bid, has a similar efficiency to 850 mg tid). Side effects: gastrointestinal intolerance, risk of lactic acidosis with chronic kidney disease, hepatic or cardiac failure... but does not cause hypoglycemia. First-choice medication for type 2 patients. - *Alpha-glucosidase inhibitors*: Acarbose (Prandase®): ↓ absorption of carbohydrates (sucrose and starch): 50 mg tid with meals up to 100 mg tid. Side effects: diarrhea. - *Meglitinides*: repaglinide and nateglinide: ↑ insulin secretion modulated by the level of glycemia (less hypoglycemia than with sulfonylureas). Short ½ life. Take 15-30 minutes prior to meal. Side effects: hypoglycemia. Safer for patients with chronic kidney disease. - *Thiazolidinediones*: ↓ insulin resistance: Side effects: edema, resumption of ovulation in cases of polycystic ovary, fractures ... Contraindicated with heart failure, ALT > 2.5 x normal, pregnancy and nursing. Hepatotoxicity = extremely rare (measure ALT and AST 2-3 months after initiating treatment). Effective in 6-12 weeks. Rosiglitazone (Avandia®): 4-8 mg/day in 1 or 2 doses. Pioglitazone (Actos®): 15-45 mg daily. - *Incretines*: Sitagliptine (Januvia®): dipeptidyl peptidase-4 inhibitors (DPP-4); ↑ insulin secretion. Indicated in association with metformin. 100 mg daily (to be adjusted in case of renal failure). Less hypoglycemia than with sulfonylurea. - *Weight loss agent* (Orlistat or sibutramine): See Obesity Table. - *Insulin*: Ultra-rapid-acting (60-90 minute spike) or regular-acting (2-3 hour spike), intermediate-acting (N or NPH) (5-8 hour spike), analogue to slow action, premixed insulins... 　　　Initiating insulin treatment with antihyperglycemic agent; start at 0.25 U/kg HS,

to increase as needed.

Alone: 0.5 U/kg divided as follows: 40-50 % HS and 20-25 % at meals to increase as needed; or 60% AM (2/3 N, 1/3 R) + 40% PM (½ N, ½ R) if optimal control not deemed important.

Insulin Lispro or aspart (Humalog® or NovoRapid®): fast-acting.

Basal insulin: insulin glargine or detemir: low spike of action with a 24-hour lasting action, may help in decreasing nocturnal hypoglycemia while improving blood sugar control.

Insulin pump available (indicated in type 1 diabetes with inability to maintain adequate control of HbA1c without incurring severe and/or frequent hypoglycemic episodes despite adherence and rigorous self-control, or pregnant diabetic uncontrolled by other insulin injection methods). Reimbursed by many health insurance plans but not by the *Régie d'Assurance Maladie du Québec*.

Intensive insulin therapy (basal + meal boluses [based on glucose ingestion]) for type 1 diabetes (DCCT study).

Pancreas ± kidney transplant for very labile type 1 with severe hypoglycemic episodes or in combination with kidney transplant if nephropathy.

Islets of Langerhans cell transplant.

Management of the other risk factors: stop smoking, aim for BP < 130/80 mmHg, aim for LDL < 2 mmol/L and TC/HDL < 4 for diabetic patients considered at high risk of a vascular event (≥ 45 y.o. men, ≥ 50 y.o. women, or younger men and women with ≥ 1 of the following: macrovascular disease, microvascular disease, multiple additional risk factors, extreme level of a single risk factor, duration of diabetes > 15 years with age > 30 years). Clinical judgement should be used to decide whether additional LDL lowering is required for individuals with a LDL of 2.0-2.5 mmol/L on treatment. Statins should also be considered in diabetic patients > 40 y.o. even if their LDL ≤ 2.5 mmol/L (HPS and CARDS studies).

Add aspirin in diabetic patients with vascular disease (coronary or cerebrovascular or peripheral), and to consider for patients at high risk of a vascular event (see above). Add ACEI or ARB in diabetic patients with vascular disease (coronary or cerebrovascular or peripheral), or at high risk of a vascular event, or if microalbuminuria is present.

Emergencies	Causes of hyperglycemic emergencies: infection (30-40%), insulin omission (15-20%), idiopathic (20-25%), myocardial infarction, new diagnosis of diabetes, pregnancy, medication (steroids, thiazides, sympathomimetics, atypical antipsychotics, pentamidine, protease inhibitors, niacin,…), total parenteral nutrition, stroke, alcohol intake, pancreatitis, trauma, drugs, psychological disorder, burns, hypothermia, renal failure… Mortality from diabetic ketoacidosis = 0.65-3.3 %, especially due to precipitant factors. Mortality from hyperosmolar coma = 50 % (historically, probably less today).
Criteria	**Diabetic ketoacidosis (DKA):** blood glucose > 13.8 mmol/L (except with pregnancy): pH < 7.3: HCO_3 < 15 mmol/L: anion gap > 10-12: ketonuria, ketonemia. False ⊕: HCO_3, fasting, aspirin, captopril. False ⊖: lactate, alcohol, aspirin, hypoxia. **Hyperosmolar hyperglycemic state (HHS):** blood glucose > 33 mmol/L: osmolality > 320 mmol/kg: pH > 7.3: HCO_3 > 15 mmol/L: no ketonuria: anion gap < 12. **Differential diagnosis**: fasting or alcoholic ketoacidosis, lactic acidosis, drug ingestion (salicylates…), alcohol ingestion (methanol, ethylene glycol…), chronic kidney disease.

Management	For a 70 kg man: water loss = 100-200 mL/kg (5-7 L): Na^+ = 5-13 mEq/kg (300-400 mEq): K^+ = 2-6 mEq/kg (200-400 mEq): Ca^{++} = 1000-1500 mg: PO_4^{3-} = 75-150 mmol.

Workup: CBC, glucose, creatinine, BUN, electrolytes (Na, K, Cl), osmolality, plasma and urinary ketones (by dipstick), urinalysis, arterial blood gas, HbA1c, ECG, CXR: urine and throat culture, blood culture as needed if clinical suspicion. Amylase, lipase as needed.

Always search for the cause (do cardiac workup, infectious workup...). If stupor or coma with plasma osmolality < 320 mOsm/kg, search for another cause of stupor.

Treatment:
1 - Hydrate:
- For severe deficit (shock), give NaCl 0.9% 1-2 L for the 1st hour to correct hypotension, then NaCl 0.9% 500 mL/h x 4 h, then 250 mL/h x 4 h.
- For mild to moderate deficit, NaCl 0.9% 500 mL/h x 4 h, then 250 mL/h x 4 h.
- Once euvolemic, switch to NaCl 0.45% if corrected plasma Na^+ is normal or ↑; and rate of fall of effective plasma osmolality is < 3 mmol/kg/h. If not, continue with NaCl 0.9 %.
- Once glucose < 14 mmol/L, add D5W or D10W to IV fluids to maintain glucose of 12-14 mmol/L.
Note: For persons with a HHS, IV fluid administration should be individualized based on the patient's needs.

2 - Insulin: 0.1 U/kg (10 U) R insulin IV bolus; then 0.1 U/kg/h. Target: ↓ blood glucose by 2-4 mmol/h. Measure capillary blood glucose every 2 hours. If K^+ < 3.3 mmol/L, correct hypokalemia before starting insulin.

The insulin infusion rate should be maintained until the resolution of ketosis as measured by the normalization of the plasma anion gap.

If acidosis does not correct itself despite correction of blood glucose, consider increasing glucose in the IV in order to maintain a higher insulin drip rate.

3 - KCl if normal or ↓ K^+: e.g.: 20 mEq in 1st litre:
Monitor K^+ every 2 h then every 4 h.
  - if < 3.3 mmol/L: discontinue insulin - give 40 mEq/h KCl (max 40 mmol/h) - monitor every hour.
  - if 3.3-5.5: give 10-40mEq/h KCl (max 40 mmol/h).
  - if > 5.5: 0.

4 - Phosphate supplement as needed if < 0.3 mmol/L or if heart failure, respiratory depression or anemia.

5 - $NaHCO_3$ as needed but *controversial*: if pH < 7.0: give $NaHCO_3$ 1 vial/h until pH > 7.0. Avoid hypokalemia.

Complications: hypo- or hyperglycemia, hypokalemia, hyperchloremic acidosis, hypoxemia, pulmonary edema, aspiration, ARDS, DVT, PE, cerebral edema, stroke, acute renal failure, hypocalcemia (if phosphate given).

Note: hospitalization not necessary for patient in good general condition and able to eat, pH ≥ 7.3 and HCO_3^- > 15, and if blood glucose rapidly ↓ to normal and precipitating event identified is corrected.

Pre-Existing Diabetes and Pregnancy	Among pregnant women who are known to have diabetes, 35% have type 1, 65% have type 2 diabetes.
	Maternal consequences: exacerbation of retinopathy and nephropathy (hypertension, proteinuria $\uparrow$, GFR $\downarrow$ - temporary or permanent), CAD known or unknown, infections, hypoglycemia. Polyhydramnios.
	Fetal and neonatal consequences: congenital malformations (13% vs normally 2%: proportional to HbA1c pre-conception/ 1st trimester), spontaneous abortion (proportional to HbA1c), macrosomia, intrauterine growth retardation, death in utero. If ketosis: possible neuro-developmental disorder. $\uparrow$ preeclampsia (mainly with renal disease, HBP or vasculopathy). Neonatal metabolic disorders.
	Pre-conception care essential (since organogenesis occurs at 0-7 weeks) = aim for HbA1c < 7% pre-conception and during pregnancy.
	Folic acid 5 mg/day during pre-conception up to 12 weeks.
	Capillary blood glucose: ≤ 5.3 fasting and ≤ 6.7 2 hours PC.
Management	Pre-conception evaluation is essential: assessment of glycemic control, evaluation and investigation of end organ damage, evaluation of and explanation concerning maternal and fetal risks.
	In type 2 diabetes, discontinue oral agents and start insulin as soon as the pregnancy is diagnosed or pre-conception if poor control. Use of glyburide and metformin has not been approved during pregnancy and is not recommended by CDA guidelines (2008), but these medications have not been associated with an increase in malformations. Discontinue ACEI, ARB and antihyperlipidemic agents ideally in the pre-conception period. Exception: renal disease or significant heart disease, if discontinuation of these medications while waiting for conception may have undesirable long term consequences. Then, discontinue as soon as conception takes place. Aspirin 75-100 mg/daily to be kept, decreased or started early for preeclampsia prevention.
	Frequent HbA1c. Initial basic preeclampsia workup and, as needed, immediately upon suspecting preeclampsia.
	Regular testing for proteinuria. Ophthalmologic examination every trimester if pre-proliferative or proliferative retinopathy present. Monitor ketonuria and renal function as needed.
	Baby monitoring begins at 26-28th week (growth, well-being).
	Peri-partum: blood glucose every 1-2 hours: s/c insulin during latent phase, insulin infusion pump during active phase. D5W at delivery of placenta and stop insulin in the pump - resume according to blood glucose levels.
	Breast-feeding: Resume intake of metformin (safe, < 1 % secreted into breast milk). Otherwise, keep on insulin therapy. Small doses of glyburide may be added if necessary (5-10 mg/day), 1.5 % secreted through breast milk. Other anti-hyperglycemic medications not recommended. TSH should be checked at 6 weeks in type 1 diabetes patient as they are at risk of post-partum thyroiditis.

Gestational Diabetes

Definition: diabetes diagnosed during pregnancy (undiagnosed pregestational diabetes possible).
Incidence: ~ 4 % (higher in high-risk ethnic population).

Pregnancy-induced change in hormones increases resistance to insulin causing hyperglycemia, especially post-prandial.

Fetal/neonatal* consequences:
- Macrosomia (17-29 %), shoulder dystocia, clavicular fracture, brachial plexus lesion, hypoglycemia, hypocalcemia, polycythemia, hyperbilirubinemia can occur. ↑ admission to neonatoalogy unit. ↑ perinatal mortality? Congenital abnormalities only if pregestational diabetes.
- Childhood obesity, early adult-onset diabetes, neuropsychological disorders?

Maternal consequences*: ↑ caesarean rate, instrumental delivery, ↑ preeclampsia? (bias ++).

* Stronger association in women with higher glycemia (> 11.1 mmol/L at 2 hours post 75 g).

Diagnosis	Gestational diabetes: diagnosis established if fasting plasma glucose ≥ 7.0 or random ≥ 11.1 mmol /L on two separate occasions.
	Screening : optimal screening still debated:
	– All women should be screened between 24 and 28 weeks.
	– To be done during 1st trimester depending of the risk factors: age > 35 y.o., high-risk ethnic group (Hispanic, African, South Asian, Asian, Aboriginal), obesity, personal past history of gestational diabetes, PCOS, acanthosis nigricans, family history of diabetes, steroid use, persistent glycosuria.
	Screening ± confirmation vs confirmation alone :
	– Screening test (O'Sullivan's test): 50 g glucose (at random): if glucose 1 h PC is between 7.8 and 10.2 mmol/L, do a confirmation test. If ≥ 10.3, diagnostic of gestational diabetes.
	– Confirmation test (fasting):
	– **75 g glucose** (CDA Guidelines): glycemia at 0-1-2 h; abnormal if fasting glucose ≥ 5.3: 1 h ≥ 10.6: 2 h ≥ 8.9: if 1/3 values ⊕ = impaired glucose tolerance; if ≥ 2/3 values ⊕ = gestational diabetes.
	– Multiple daily glycemia measures: diagnostic if > 5.5 mmol/L fasting or > 7.0 mmol/L postprandial (not an official diagnostic test, less well validated, not in CDA Guidelines).
	If impaired glucose tolerance: follow with self monitoring of blood glucose.

Management	– Diabetic diet, moderate exercise (if not contraindicated).
	– Ketosis monitoring to rule out starvation ketosis (with low calorie diet).
	– Workup: self-monitoring blood glucose ≥ 4 x/d (AM and 1 or 2 h PC x 3): HbA1c: serial fetal growth ultrasound (early 3rd trimester abdominal circumference ≥ 70th percentile better predictor of macrosomia).
	– Insulin therapy if target not reached after 2 weeks of diet.
	– Benefit of insulin therapy = ACHOIS sudy (still controversial):
	- ↓ shoulder dystocia >>> perinatal mortality, fracture, neurological lesions (combined 4 % to 1 %); ↓ macrosomia.
	- ↑ labor induction but number of caesareans identical, ↑ admission to neonatalogy unit but severe metabolic complications identical, ↓ post-partum depression, ↑ health-related quality of life.
	– Target: fasting glucose 3.8-5.2: 1 h PC 5.5-7.7: 2 h PC 5.0-6.6. Avoid hypoglycemia.
	– Insulin dose to be adjusted according to the needs of the patient.
	– Many insulin regimens possible: e.g.: insulin N HS + R or Lispro AC as needed, insulin N and R AM and PM. No data for Glargine.
	– Alternative during 2nd or 3rd trimester: glyburide (similar perinatal outcomes).
	– Other oral hypoglycemics: metformin used during 1st trimester/any pregnancy in order to prevent fetal loss in woman with polycystic ovaries without harmful effects. ↓ gestational diabetes. All other oral hypoglycemics are contraindicated in the absence of data. Use of metformin or glyburide during pregnancy is not an approved indication in Canada. Such use is considered off-label and thus appropriate discussions are required with the patient.
	– In intra and peripartum: perfusion D5W; glycemia every 1-2 h: insulin perfusion if glycemia > 6.0 mmol/L: monitoring of the baby.
Prognosis	Risk of gestational diabetes recurrence = 50 % in subsequent pregnancies. **Risk of acquiring type 2 diabetes = 30-60 % at 20 years,** especially during first 5 years, especially if insulin is necessary during pregnancy. Do a 75 g glucose tolerance test or fasting glycemia between 6 weeks and 6 months postpartum in order to screen for diabetes. 15-20 % will be ↑. Follow-up every year if impaired fasting glucose or impaired glucose tolerance, every 3 years if normal. Lifestyle and risk factor modification.

Hypoglycemia

Causes	Postprandial hypoglycemia (symptomatic 1-6 hours postprandial): idiopathic (rare), "diabetic" (with prediabetes), "alimentary" (post-gastrectomy, jejunostomy, sudden withdrawal of total parenteral nutrition ...), medication (insulin, oral antihyperglycemic agents, quinine, pentamidine, disopyramide, MAO Inhibitors).
	Fasting hypoglycemia: hepatic (severe hepatic failure), endocrine (insulinoma, insulin, oral hypoglycemic agents - sulfonylurea and meglitinide, hypopituitarism, adrenal insufficiency), auto-immune with anti-insulin antibodies, alcohol, severe medical illness (sepsis, malaria), tumors (mesenchymal, hepatocellular carcinoma, adrenal, gastro-intestinal, pancreatic), severe malnutrition (anorexia), intense exercise (e.g.: marathon), medications and drugs (beta-blockers, salicylates, chloroquine, "magic mushrooms"...). Chronic kidney disease patients more at risk to experience hypoglycemia. Any cause of fasting hypoglycemia may also cause post-prandial hypoglycemia.
	Pseudo-hypoglycemia with leukemia, leukemoid reaction and *polycythaemia vera* (normal real glycemia but low measured blood glucose 2nd to glucose consumption by leukocytes or erythrocytes in test tube before measuring).
Clinical findings	2 groups of symptoms: neuroglycopenic (impaired cognitive function, weakness, drowsiness, visual disturbances, difficulty speaking, confusion, headaches, dizziness, convulsion, coma) and hyperadrenergic (palpitations, sweating, tremors, anxiety, hunger, nausea, tingling).
	If mild: adrenergic symptoms. If moderate: neuroglycopenic ± adrenergic symptoms. If severe: loss of consciousness or when patient unable to reverse the episode himself. Symptoms usually reversible unless they are prolonged.
	Whipple's triad: typical symptoms during hypoglycemia episodes reversed by glucose administration.
Diagnosis	*Controversial* definition: blood glucose < 2.5 mmol/L associated with symptoms.
	Always: 1- Document hypoglycemia. 　　　　2- Demonstrate that the symptoms are due to hypoglycemia. 　　　　3 - Find the cause.
	Measure glucose, insulin, and C-peptide levels during hypoglycemia:
	- If insulin ↑ (insulin > 35 pmol/L when plasma glucose ↓): secondary to exogenous insulin administration (↓ C-peptide), oral hypoglycemic agents (can be measured in urine), insulinoma (72 hour fasting test with insulin assay + C-peptide [reference test] or glucagon test, pro-insulin/insulin ratio > 20%, localization through MRI, CT of the abdomen, angiography or intra-operative ultrasound if not seen at CT/MRI). - If insulin ↓: alcohol, mesenchymal or adrenal neoplasm, glucocorticoid or GH deficiency, hepatic failure, malnutrition, severe chronic kidney disease with malnutrition.
Treatment	According to cause. Adjust dosage if insulin or oral hypoglycemic agents are the cause. Education (diet), etc. Glucagon Kit 1 mg IM, as needed. Surgery for insulinoma: diazoxide if refusal of surgery.

Adrenal disorders	
Hypercorticism (Cushing's Syndrome)	Central obesity, plethoric moon facies, fragile skin, ecchymosis, muscular atrophy, proximal weakness, acne, hirsutism, headaches, amenorrhea, arterial hypertension, purple striae, leukocytosis, glucose intolerance, supraclavicular fat pads, buffalo hump, osteoporosis ...
Causes	1. ACTH-dependent: Cushing's disease (60 % of cases: pituitary tumor: hyperpigmentation), ectopic ACTH (15 % of cases, associated with neoplasm: lung, carcinoid, thymus, pancreas and bronchial adenoma: muscular atrophy, hypokalemia, weight loss, ++ hyperpigmentation, arterial hypertension), ectopic CRH (rare) ... 2. ACTH-independent: iatrogenic, adrenal tumor (25 % of cases: adenoma, carcinoma, or, rarely, hyperplasia) ... Pseudo-Cushing's with depression, obesity, stress, hospitalization, chronic alcoholism ...
Workup	1- 24-hour urinary cortisol on 2-3 occasions: diagnostic if > 250 nmol/L + variation in urinary creatinine < 10% or dexamethasone suppression test, low dose (1 mg at 11 PM, plasma cortisol the next day at 8 AM); normal if < 50 nmol/L, abnormal if > 138 nmol/L or an elevated salivary cortisol at midnight at home can help make the diagnosis (when available). If pseudo-Cushing's suspected, 2-day low-dose dexamethasone suppression test with IV CRH may be helpful. 2- ACTH on 2-3 occasions ($\uparrow$ if > 4.4 pmol/L or $\downarrow$ if < 1.1 pmol/L). Also valuable for diagnosis: cortisol $\uparrow$ with loss of diurnal variation, glucose, Na^+, K^+, chest X-ray... $\rightarrow$ If ACTH $\downarrow$: abdominal CT. $\rightarrow$ If ACTH normal or $\uparrow$: Pituitary MRI (but normal in 50 % of patients with Cushing's disease), CRH test and « high dose » dexamethasone suppression test (8 mg at 11 PM and serum cortisol at 8 AM with a > 50 % reduction suggestive of Cushing's disease but low yield): if non diagnostic, measure ACTH by petrosal sinus catheterization during CRH administration: if central to peripheral gradient > 2 pre-CRH and > 3 post-CRH, compatible with Cushing's disease. Note: Total cortisol may be increased because of increased binding proteins (with estrogen, for example) while free cortisol is normal. Cortisol level should always be assessed when performing lab tests to ensure it is elevated at that time (some patients have a cyclic variant of Cushing's syndrome).
Treatment	Cushing's disease: transsphenoidal surgery (80 % long-term success rate): radiotherapy, bilateral adrenalectomy (side effect: Nelson's syndrome), octreotide, dopamine agonists, enzyme inhibitor (ketoconazole, mitotane, metyrapone), radio-surgery ... Adrenal tumor: surgery. If impossible: mitotane, enzyme inhibitor... Ectopic ACTH: surgery: enzyme inhibition, adrenalectomy.
Hypoadreno-corticism	- Presentation is often insidious: fatigue, muscular weakness, lethargy, weight loss, dizziness, orthostatic hypotension, anorexia, nausea, vomiting, diarrhea, headaches, apathy and non specific complaints. - If primary: "salt-cravings", hyperpigmentation, hyponatremia and hyperkalemia. - If secondary: possible visual field defect, possible hyponatremia but normokalemia. - Acute: abdominal pain, diarrhea, vomiting, fever, hypoglycemia, shock.
Causes	- Primary (or Addison's disease) : - Autoimmune: rule out autoimmune polyglandular syndrome: type I (in children, mucocutaneous candidiasis, hypoparathyroidism), type II (in adult with type 1

	diabetes, hypothyroidism). - Non-autoimmune: tuberculous or fungal adrenalitis, bilateral adrenal hemorrhage (with anticoagulants, DIC, trauma, antiphospholipid syndrome, sepsis [Waterhouse-Friderichsen syndrome]), surgery, medication (spironolactone, etomidate, ketoconazole, rifampicin, TMP), metastasis, infiltrative process (sarcoidosis, amyloidosis, hemochromatosis), congenital, adrenoleukodystrophy (in boys or young men), AIDS – with cytomegalovirus infections, *Mycobacterium avium intracellulare* ... - Secondary (with ACTH deficiency): medication (IV, PO or inhaled steroid), hypopituitarism (adenoma, tumor, infarction, granuloma, infiltrative process, lymphocytic hypophisitis), hypothalamic disease, congenital.
Workup	- 8 AM plasma cortisol (< 100 nmol/L is diagnostic; > 525 → ruled out) + plasma ACTH (on ice). - Stress-related plasma cortisol (< 550 nmol/L is diagnostic; > 700 → ruled out). - 250 µg IV ACTH (Cortrosyn) stimulation test if primary adrenal insufficiency or secondary of > 3 months duration: measure cortisol at 0-30-60 min: if peak > 500-550 → ruled out; if 360-500 → repeat x 1, if needed. - If suspicion of secondary adrenal insufficiency, insulin-induced hypoglycemic test = gold standard (hypoglycemia < 2.2 and cortisol > 550). 1 µg ACTH IV test is an acceptable alternative. - If workup suggests hypoadrenocorticism, proceed with electrolytes, CBC (normochromic normocytic anemia, eosinophilia ...). As indicated: serum glucose, tests of coagulation, septic workup, hypopituitarism workup, serum very long-chain fatty acids (if boy or young man, especially if there is presence of neurologic or neuro-psychiatric manifestations). - Imaging depending on the results of biochemical investigation: CT of the abdomen or pituitary MRI.
Treatment	- Steroids: begin with Cortef 25 mg/day (15 mg AM +10 mg PM) to be reduced to 20 mg/day ± fludrocortisone 50-200 µg (if signs of hypoaldosteronism). DHEA supplements remain controversial. - Medic Alert® bracelet. Injectable 4 mg dexamethasone, as needed if patient unable to take oral medication. - Educate patient: has to increase doses (↑ dose of steroids x 2-3) with infection (stress). - In **acute adrenal crisis**: classically volume- + pressor-resistant shock. When suspected: give dexamethasone 8 mg IV STAT then quickly perform an ACTH test ± adrenal imaging then hydrocortisone 50-100 mg IV every 8 hours until stabilization then gradual weaning until maintenance dose.
Prevention	Perioperative supplementation (or with medical stress) required if patient received > 5 mg Prednisone or its equivalent for 1 month *or* ≥ 20 mg/day for 5 days *in the past year*. If any doubt, measure cortisol or do ACTH test. 1. For minor medical or surgical stress (e.g.: inguinal hernia repair, gastroenteritis, mild febrile illness ...): need is equivalent to 25 mg hydrocortisone for one day. e.g.: administer Prednisone 5 mg on day of procedure only. 2. For moderate medical or surgical stress (e.g.: open cholecystectomy, hemicolectomy, pneumonia, severe gastroenteritis ...): 50-75 mg/day of hydrocortisone is needed for 1-2 days. e.g.: administer 10 mg Prednisone pre-op, then SoluCortef® 50mg IV per-op, then 20 mg IV every 8 hrs on day #1 then usual dose on day #2. 3. For major medical or surgical stress (e.g.: cardiac, Whipple's procedure, pancreatitis...): 100-150 mg/day of hydrocortisone is needed for 2-3 days. e.g.: administer SoluCortef® 50mg IV every 8 hours for 48-72 hrs. 4. For seriously ill patients (intensive care, septic shock): hydrocortisone 50-100 mg every 6-8 hours or 0.18 mg/kg/hr as a continuous infusion until shock resolved (may take days to weeks): then gradually taper.

Primary hyperaldosteronism	Underlying cause of 1-5 % of cases of hypertension. Rarely causes severe hypertension. To be considered in the following situations: hypertension with spontaneous hypokalemia (< 3.5 mmol/L) or marked diuretic-induced hypokalemia (< 3 mmol/L), hypertension in a young patient, hypertension refractory to ≥ 3 medications, or hypertension with an incidental adrenal adenoma. Note: 30 % of patients with primary hyperaldosteronism have a normal serum K^+.
Clinical findings	Most cases are asymptomatic. Weakness/muscular cramps may be present (sometimes with paralysis similar to periodic hypokalemic paralysis), tingling, polyuria, nocturia, polydipsia, headaches, palpitations, Trousseau's sign or Chvostek's sign (rare) …
Causes	Primary hyperaldosteronism: unilateral aldosterone-producing adrenal adenoma (aldosteronoma or Conn's syndrome), bilateral adrenal hyperplasia, adrenal carcinoma (rare); glucocorticoid-remediable aldosteronism (autosomal dominant, occurring at young age: rare). Secondary hyperaldosteronism: renovascular disease, renin-secreting juxtaglomerular tumor, malignant hypertension, volume depletion, ovarian tumor (rare). Differential diagnosis of hypertension with hypokalemia (but without hyperaldosteronism): diuretics, Cushing's syndrome, Liddle's syndrome, hyperthyroidism, 17 α-hydroxylase deficiency, 11 ß-hydroxylase deficiency, cortisol-secreting tumor, 11 beta-hydroxysteroid dehydrogenase deficiency (idiopathic or secondary to chewing tobacco, black licorice), glucocorticoid resistance (receptor anomaly)…
Workup	Screening by assessment of plasma aldosterone/plasma renin activity (pmol/L + ng/L) ratio (after 15 minutes in sitting position): if aldosterone/plasma renin ratio > 140, compatible with primary hyperaldosteronism, especially if aldosterone > 416 pmol/L. Medications can cause false ⊕ and false ⊖ results. Stop aldosterone antagonists, angiotensin-II receptor blockers, clonidine and beta-blockers if possible. If ↑ aldosterone and renin: secondary hyperaldosteronism. If screening for primary hyperaldosteronism is positive, confirm autonomous hypersecretion of aldosterone with: saline loading tests (2 L of NaCl 0.9 % in 4 hours) or suppression test with Captopril or fludrocortisone: measuring aldosterone before and after: if aldosterone remains ↑, compatible with primary hyperaldosteronism. Some medications must be stopped with these tests. If confirmation test ⊕, obtain localization test with: adrenal CT or MRI, selective adrenal venous sampling: if adenoma ⊕, especially with lateralization of aldosterone/cortisol secretion (ratio > 4), compatible with aldosteronoma. Without lateralization of aldosterone hypersecretion, bilateral hyperplasia probable (or glucocorticoid-remediable aldosteronism). Iodocholesterol scan may sometimes be useful for localization. Postural tests also useful to differentiate causes of hyperaldosteronism (but lower sensitivity / specificity). Genetic testing for glucocorticoid-remediable aldosteronism.
Treatment	With aldosteronoma, adrenalectomy by laparoscopy or medical treatment with spironolactone. Hypertension reversible in 66 % of cases, especially if mild or of recent onset. Pre-operative response to spironolactone is a good predictor of the BP response to surgery. With bilateral adrenal hyperplasia: medical treatment with spironolactone. Also useful: amiloride or triamterene. Other anti-hypertensive drugs as needed. Restriction of salt intake. Dexamethasone for glucocorticoid-remediable aldosteronism.

Pheochromocytoma	Rare cause of HBP (< 0.3 %). Adrenal medullary tumor or tumor of the sympathetic chain (paraganglioma), rarely in other sites (thorax, bladder, brain). To be suspected in the following situations: paroxysmal/severe hypertension refractory to standard treatment; presence of multiple symptoms suggestive of catecholamine excess (eg, headaches, palpitations, sweating, panic attack or pallor); hypertension triggered by beta-blockers, MAOI, micturition or changes in abdominal pressure; presence of incidentally discovered adrenal adenoma: a family history of pheochromocytoma; hypertension and type 1 neuro-fibromatosis, or von Hippel-Lindau disease, or multiple endocrine neoplasia type 2A or 2B. Ten percent Rule (10 % are extra-adrenal, 10 % malignant, 10 % familial, 10 % bilateral, 10 % multiple, 10 % in children, 10 % normotensive). Familial pheochromocytoma is often bilateral, sometimes with multiple endocrine neoplasia type 2, neurofibromatosis, or pancreatic islet cell tumors (rare). Differential diagnosis: pseudo-pheochromocytoma (typical symptoms but normal workup), hyperthyroidism, anxiety, drugs, autonomic dysfunction, etc.
Clinical findings	20 % have sustained HBP, 50 % sustained HBP with paroxysms, 25 % have paroxysmal HBP only. Orthostatic hypotension sometimes associated. Triad of headaches (80 %), diaphoresis (70%), palpitations (60 %): pallor, tremor, anxiety, weight loss, weakness, thoraco-abdominal pain, orthostatic dizziness. Symptoms sometimes triggered by: tumor manipulation, exercise, fever, surgery, tyramine-containing food (cheeses, wines, chocolate) medications (contrast agents, glucagon, anaesthetics, MAOI, beta-blockers, metoclopramide, nicotine), renal artery stenosis secondary to compression.
Workup	Urinary metanephrines + catecholamines or plasma catecholamines (especially with paroxysm) (often > x 2 normal). Be careful with medication-test interactions (e.g.: labetalol, levodopa, tricyclics, methyldopa, MAOI, pressors), food (bananas, coffee, black pepper) or some specific medical situations with ↑ catecholamines (systemic diseases, myocardial infarction, amyotrophic lateral sclerosis, heart failure, sleep apnea). As needed: clonidine suppression test (rarely necessary). MRI localisation (T2 hyperintense signal) or CT abdomen and/or MIBG scan. PET scan rarely useful. Hypercalcemia, polycythemia, hyperglycemia also associated. Genetic testing if suspicion of hereditary syndrome (age < 21, bilateral, family history or multiple paraganglioma), with family genetic screening, as needed. These patients must be referred to a specialist.
Treatment	Surgical treatment: Pre-op preparation to be conducted with volume repletion (± transfusions) and medical treatment: phenoxybenzamine (beginning with 10 mg bid to be increased by 10 to 20 mg increments every 2 or 3 days until control of symptoms is reached); prazosin, doxazosin, terazosin PO ± calcium-channel blocker ± metyrosine ± phentolamine IV as needed: beta-blockers after alpha blockade as needed if tachycardia or residual HBP. Begin pre-op preparation 14 days prior to surgery. Aim to normal BP sitting but > 90 mmHg systolic standing pre-op. Be careful with post operative hypotension and hypoglycemia. Operative mortality risk < 3 %. Chemotherapy available if metastatic or non operable. Possible recurrence with familial pheochromocytoma.

	Urinary catecholamines to be done in post-operative period (> 2 weeks) and every 6 to 12 months for 5 years in order to ensure absence of multiple tumors or recurrence.
Adrenal incidentaloma	Prevalence: 0.2 % at age 20 to 29 and 7 % at age > 70. Etiologies: non-secreting adrenal adenoma (# 1), metastasis (lung, breast, kidney, colon, pancreas, liver, esophagus and stomach), adrenal carcinoma, nodular hyperplasia, pheochromocytoma, lipoma, cyst, secreting adenoma (aldosterone, cortisol, androgen). Workup: 1 - Screening tests for pheochromocytoma (urinary catecholamines and metanephrines) and for Cushing's syndrome (see Cushing syndrome above). 2 - Screening test for hyperaldosteronism if arterial hypertension (measure potassium and aldosterone/renin ratio). Stop spironolactone and amiloride for test. 3 - Assessment of tissue attenuation on unenhanced CT (adenoma suggested if homogenous and ≤ 10 Hounsfield units); if tumor > 10 HU, assess further (with percentage of CT contrast-medium washout at 10 minutes, MRI, PET scan or fine-needle aspiration biopsy …). 4 - DHEAS assay if there is hirsutism or virilization. – If secreting tumor (cortisol or pheochromocytoma) or non-secreting and > 6 cm diameter or suspicion of adrenal carcinoma at imaging = surgery. – If metastasis, management according to stage or type of cancer. – If aldosteronoma, surgery or medical treatment. – If non-secreting tumor of < 4 cm diameter: repeat CT at 6 or 12 months ± 24 months. Repeat biochemical workup every year for 4 years: if no growth and non-secreting = no follow-up necessary. If growth = surgery. – If non-secreting and 4-6 cm diameter: close follow-up or surgery. Note: Biopsy to differentiate between metastasis and adrenal tissue (benign or malignant). Always rule out pheochromocytoma before biopsy. MRI can help distinguish causes.

Steroid Equivalence Table

	Glucocorticoid effect	Mineralocorticoid effect
Short action		
Cortisol (Solu-Cortef®, Cortef®)	1	1
Cortisone (Cortate®)	0.8	0.8
Intermediate action		
Prednisone	4	0.25
Prednisolone	4	0.25
Methylprednisone (Solu-Medrol®)	5	< 0.01
Triamcilonone	5	< 0.01
Long action		
Paramethasone	10	< 0.01
Betamethasone	25	< 0.01
Dexamethasone (Decadron®)	30-40	< 0.01

Hirsutism	
Overview	**Hirsutism**: androgen-induced growth of terminal hair following a male-pattern (side burns, torso, upper lip, chin, etc) in women. Differential diagnosis: hypertrichosis (generally increased hair growth, usually in areas that are normally hairy in woman). **Virilization**: a decrease in women's secondary sexual characteristics (breast volume) and the appearance of masculine sexual characteristics (deep voice, growing muscle mass, clitoromegaly) (thus always associated with hirsutism). Reflecting a more serious case of hyperandrogenism.

Causes	- Endogenous :
	    - Ovarian origin (LH-dependent vs secondary to insulin resistance): polycystic ovary syndrome (PCOS: most frequent cause), benign and malignant tumors, acromegaly (insulin resistance).
	    - Adrenal origin: congenital adrenal hyperplasia, Cushing's syndrome, androgen-secreting adrenal cancer.
	- Exogenous: exposure to androgens, anabolic steroids, and some other medication …
	- Idiopathic (hyperactivity of 5 α-reductase).

Clinical findings	Acne, menstrual and ovulatory disorders, temporal alopecia, virilization and often among overweight or obese patients. Patients with PCOS may have *acanthosis nigricans*. On history, look for age of onset, progression and severity of hirsutism: appearance at puberty, with slow progression suggests a benign pathology. Rapid progression as well as presence of virilization suggests a malignant process. Occasionally: positive family history of familial hirsutism, polycystic ovary syndrome or congenital adrenal hyperplasia.
Workup	Total and free testosterone, DHEA-S, FSH, LH, androstenedione and 17-OH progesterone. Tests must be obtained ideally within the first 10 days of the menstrual cycle. Do a 24-hour urinary cortisol or « low dose » dexamethasone test if Cushing's suspected; assay prolactin if menstrual irregularity or galactorrhea. If congenital adrenal hyperplasia suspected, assay 17-hydroxyprogesterone with stimulation using ACTH 250 µg. Assay IGF-1 if signs of acromegaly. If DHEA-S > 19 µmol/L: adrenal tumor or congenital adrenal hyperplasia. If DHEA-S < 19 µmol/L and if total testosterone > 6.9 nmol/L: ovarian tumor to be ruled out. If tumor is suspected, obtain an adrenal CT, a pelvic ultrasound or pelvic MRI. A young woman with mild hirsutism appearing at puberty, of Mediterranean descent and with normal menses without signs of virilization and other endocrinopathies, does not require additional tests. If PCOS is diagnosed, a dyslipidemia and glucose intolerance screening (preferably with OGTT 75g) is required.
Treatment	According to cause. May take between 6 and 12 months to get complete response. Weight loss for overweight or obese PCOS. Oral contraceptives for idiopathic hirsutism, polycystic ovary syndrome or adrenal hyperplasia without ↓ cortisol. Glucocorticoids for more severe congenital adrenal hyperplasia. Metformin and thiazolidinediones also used for polycystic ovary syndrome. Other treatments (reliable contraception required): androgen receptor blockers (spironolactone, flutamide, cyproterone) or 5α-reductase inhibitor (finasteride). Contraceptive method necessary. Other treatments: local 5α-reductase inhibitor (eflornithine), aesthetic methods (waxing, electrolysis, laser).

Amenorrhea	
Overview	**Primary** amenorrhea is present if menarche has not occurred at age 15, in the presence of normal secondary sexual characteristics, or at age 14 in the absence of secondary sexual characteristics or within 5 years from breast development if this occurs before age 10. **Secondary** amenorrhea is present if a woman with prior menses does not menstruate for the equivalent of 3 of her usual menstrual cycles, or for a duration of 6 months (whichever occurs first).

Causes	Amenorrhea may be physiologic (pregnancy, menopause).
	 It may be secondary to a hypothalamic, pituitary, ovarian, uterine or vaginal disorder.
	
	 Causes of primary amenorrhea:
	 - Ovarian disorders (gonadal dysgenesis 45 % of cases).
	 - Anatomic anomalies: Imperforate hymen, müllerian agenesis (10 %), (Mayer-Rokitansky-Kuster-Hauser syndrome; rule out urinary anomalies), complete androgen insensitivity syndrome, transverse vaginal septum, vaginal/cervical agenesis (rare).
	 - Hypogonadotropic hypogonadism: Functional suppression of the hypothalamic-pituitary-ovarian axis by a nutritional or psychiatric disorder, prolonged heavy exercise, systemic illness, hyperprolactinemia, or thyroid or adrenal disorders: Organic hypothalamic or pituitary disease (rare - e.g.: craniopharyngioma), constitutional delay of puberty (20 %), Kallmann syndrome (anosmia).
	
	 Causes of secondary amenorrhea:
	 - Hypogonadotropic hypogonadism (WHO class 1)
	     - Hypothalamic disease (40 % - e.g.: functional hypogonadism with situational stress, weigh loss, diet, anorexia, exercise or systemic disease - hyperthyroidism, Cushing's -, tumor, hypothalamic infiltration or infection).
	     - Pituitary disease (20 % - e.g.: tumor, pituitary gland infiltration or infection, postpartum pituitary necrosis).
	 - Eugonadotropic hypogonadism (WHO class 2)
	     - Polycystic ovary syndrome (30 % - diagnosis in presence of 2/3 of following criteria: clinical or biological hyperandrogenism, oligo/amenorrhea, polycystic ovarian morphology (ultrasound - Rotterdam criteria).
	 - Hypergonadotropic hypogonadism (WHO class 3)
	     - Ovarian failure (10 % - e.g.: premature ovarian failure (< 40 y.o.) – autoimmune oophoritis, post-radiotherapy, post-chemotherapy - cyclophosphamide, vincristine).
	 - Others: androgen secreting ovarian tumor, intrauterine synechiae (Asherman's syndrome: – post-partum endometritis, intra-uterine adhesions post-dilation and curettage - rare), adrenal tumor: rare.

Workup	For secondary amenorrhea:
	 - 1st step: pregnancy test.
	 - 2nd step: measurement of prolactin TSH, FSH and LH.
	     - If FSH ↑ = ovarian failure: without evident cause (chemotherapy), probable autoimmune cause (search for other autoimmune disease). If < 35 y.o., karyotype (turner syndrome), screening for fragile X permutation.
	     - If FSH, LH normal or ↓ = hypothalamo-pituitary cause or PCOS: proceed with appropriate workup (see pituitary gland chart and step 3).
	 - 3rd step: if acne or hirsutism, measure testosterone and DHEA-S (in order to rule out adrenal or ovarian tumor) ± 17-hydroxyprogesterone if congenital adrenal hyperplasia is suspected ± test for Cushing's disease.
	    Polycystic ovary syndrome remains the most frequent diagnosis for women with acne and hirsutism.
	 - 4th step: In a woman with a history of gynecologic manipulation, normal FSH and prolactin, do a progestin challenge test (Provera 5 mg each day x 7 days). If no withdrawal bleeding, rule out Asherman's syndrome (gynecologic consultation).
	
	 For primary amenorrhea:
	 - If patient's appearance is normal and no pregnancy, proceed with gynecologic

	examination:
	    - If normal, workup as secondary amenorrhea.
	    - If abnormal or impossible to do a pelvic examination, ultrasound or MRI to evaluate internal genital organs.
	    - In absence of uterus, measure testosterone: if normal, suggestive of müllerian agenesis: if ↑, suggestive of androgenic insensitivity syndrome (testicular feminization): obtain a karyotype.
	- If sexual infantilism, measure FSH and LH:
	    - If FSH ↑, primary ovarian failure; obtain a karyotype (Turner's syndrome), rule out X fragile permutation, rule out ovarian enzyme deficiency (17 α-hydroxylase), rule out galactosemia.
	    - If FSH normal or ↓, suggestive of hypogonadotropic hypogonadism or delayed puberty. Rule out anosmia (with Kallmann's syndrome).

Treatment	According to cause. For hypogonadic women, hormone replacement therapy or oral contraceptives and bone protection with calcium and vitamin D. In polycystic ovary syndrome, oral contraceptives or cyclic progesterone therapy, androgen receptor blockers or 5α-reductase, metformin or thiazolidinediones. Clomiphene when fertility is desired.

Useful References: ENDOCRINOLOGY

Acromegaly: N Engl J Med 2006; 355: 2558-73 (review article)
    Clin Invest Med 2006; 29: 29-39 (Canadian guidelines)
    J Clin Endocrinol Metab 2009; 94: 1509-17 (Guidelines)
Addison's Disease: J Clin Endocrinol Metab 2001; 86: 2909-22 (review article)
Adrenal Insufficiency: Lancet 2003; 361: 1881-93 (review article)
    Diagnosis: Ann Intern Med 2003; 139: 194-204 (review article)
    Treatment: JAMA 2002; 287: 236-40 (review article)
Adrenal Incidentaloma: N Engl J Med 2007; 356: 601-10 (review article)
    Ann Intern Med 2003; 138: 424-29 (review article)
    Endocr Rev 2004; 25: 309-340 (review article)
Adrenal Tumor: Ann Intern Med 1999; 130: 759-71 (review article)
Adrogen Deficiency Syndromes: J Clin Endocrinol Metab 2006; 91: 1995-2010 (Guidelines)
Amenorrhea: Fertil Steril 2006; 86: S148-55 (Guidelines)
Androgen Deficiency: J Clin Endocrinol Metab 2006; 91: 1995-2010 (Guidelines)
Autoimmune Polyglandular Syndrome: N Engl J Med 2004; 350: 2068-79 (review article)
Cushing's Syndrome: Ann Intern Med 2003; 138: 980-91 (review article)
    J Clin Endocrinol Metab 2008; 93: 1526-40 (Guidelines)
    Lancet 2001; 357: 783-91 (review article)
    … Diagnosis: J Clin Endocrinol Metab 2008; 93: 1526-40 (Guidelines)
    … ACTH-dependant Cushing Syndrome - Treatment: J Clin endocrinol Metab 2007; 93: 2454-2462 (Guidelines)
Diabetes:
    Can J Diabetes 2008; 32 (suppl 1): S1-S201 or http://www.diabetes.ca/files/cpg2008/cpg-2008.pdf (Canadian Guidelines)
    Diabetes Care 2009; 32 (suppl 1): S1-S97 (American Guidelines)
    Intra-Hospital Hyperglycemia: N Engl J Med 2006; 355: 1903-11 (review article)
    Diabetic Neuropathy: Diabetes Care 2005; 28: 956-62 (Guidelines)
    Diabetic Foot: JAMA 2005; 293: 217-228 (review article)
        Treatment: Lancet 2005; 366: 1725-35 (review article)
    Type 1: Lancet 2006; 367: 847-58 (review article)
    Oral antihyperglycemic agents: CMAJ 2005; 172: 213-26 (review article)
    Hyperglycemia: Diabetes Care 2009; 32: 193-203 (ADA-EASD Guidelines)
    Hyperglycemic crisis: CMAJ 2003; 168: 859-66 (review article)
        Diabetes Care 2009; 32: 1335-43 (American Guidelines)
    Diabetic retinopathy: N Engl J Med 2004; 350: 48-58 (review article)
    Thiazolidinediones: N Engl J Med 2004; 351: 1106-1118 (review article)
Dyslipidemia:
    Can J Cardio 2006; 22: 913-27 (Canadian Guidelines)
    JAMA 2001; 285: 2486-2497 (American Guidelines)
    Circulation 2004; 110: 227-239 (American Guidelines - update)
    Drug Treatment: N Engl J Med 1999; 341: 498-511 (review article)

HDL: JAMA 2007; 298: 786-798 (review article)
Hirsutism: N Engl J Med 2005; 353: 2578-2588 (review article)
Graves' Disease: N Engl J Med 2008; 358: 2594-605 (review article)
     CMAJ 2003; 168: 575-86 (review article)
Graves' Ophtalmopathy: N Engl J Med 2009; 360: 994-1001 (review article)
Growth Hormone Deficiency: J Clin Endocrinol Metab 2006; 91: 1621-34 (Guidelines)
Hirtsutism: J Clin Endocrinol Metab 2008; 93: 1105-20 (Guidelines)
HDL: JAMA 2007; 298: 786-798 (review article)
Hirsutism: N Engl J Med 2005; 353: 2578-2588 (review article)
Hyperparathyroidism: Lancet 2009; 374: 14-58 (review article)
Hyperthyroidism: Lancet 2003; 362: 459-68 (review article)
     Subclinical Hyperthyroidism: N Engl J Med 2001; 345: 512-6 (review article)
         JAMA 2004; 291: 228-238 (American Guidelines)
Hypertriglyceridemia: N Engl J Med 2007; 357: 1009-17 (review article)
     CMAJ 2007; 176: 1113-20 (review article)
Hypoglycemia: J Clin Endocrinol Metab 2009; 94: 709-28 (Guidelines)
     ... in Diabetic Patients: Diabetes Care 2003; 26: 1902-12 (review article)
Hypoparathyroidism: N Engl J Med 2008; 359: 391-403 (review article)
Hypopituitarism: Lancet 2007; 369: 1461-70 (review article)
Hypothyroidism: Lancet 2004; 363: 793-803 (review article)
     Subclinical: JAMA 2004; 291: 228-238 (American Guidelines)
         Mayo Clin Proc 2009; 84: 65-71 (review article)
Incretins: J Clin Endocrinol Metab 2008; 93: 3703-16 (review article)
Insulin (analogs): N Engl J Med 2005; 352: 174-83 (review article)
Pheochromocytoma: Endocr Rev 2003; 24: 539-553 (review article)
     Ann Intern Med 2001; 134: 315-29 (review article)
     Pre-op: J Clin Endocrinol Metab 2007; 92: 4069-79 (review article)
Pituitary Incidentaloma: Cleve Clin J Med 2008; 75: 793-801 (review article)
     Endocrinol Metab Clin North Am 2008; 37: 151-171 (review article)
Pituitary Tumor: J Clin Endocrinol Metab 1999; 84: 3859-66 (review article)
     Ann Intern Med 1998; 129: 472-83 (review article)
Polycystic Ovary Syndrome: Lancet 2007; 370: 685-97 (review article)
     Am J Med 2007; 120: 128-32 (review article)
Prediabetes: J Clin Endocrinol Metab 2008; 93: 3259-65 (review article)
Primary Hyperaldosteronism: J Clin Endocrinol Metab 2008; 93: 3266-81 (Guidelines)
     Endocrinology 2003; 144: 2208-13 (review article)
Primary Ovarian Insufficiency: N Engl J Med 2009; 360: 606-14 (review article)
Prolactinoma: N Engl J Med 2003; 349: 2035-41 (review article)
Thyroiditis: N Engl J Med 2003; 348: 2646-55 (review article)
     Post-Partum Thyroiditis: J Clin Endocrinol Metab 2002; 87: 4042-4047 (review article)
Thyroid nodules: N Eng J Med 2004; 351: 1764-71 (review article)
     Endocr Pract 2006; 12: 63-102 (American Guidelines)
     Treatment: N Engl J Med 1998; 338: 1438-47 (review article)

Chapter 3

Gastroenterology

Gastrointestinal Bleeding	
Upper GI Bleeding	Presentation: hematemesis, "coffee ground" vomitus, melena (> 50-100 mL of blood) or hematochezia (> 1000 mL of blood), syncope, dizziness, weakness, etc.
Causes	1- Peptic ulcer 50%. 2- Portal hypertension (esophageal or gastric varices) 10-20%. 3- Erosive gastritis or duodenitis (NSAIDs, alcohol) 20%. 4- Mallory-Weiss syndrome 7%. 5- Esophagitis 2%. 6- Neoplasms. 7- Vascular lesions: Telangiectasia (Osler-Weber-Rendu, CREST), Dieulafoy. 8- Aortoenteric fistula. 9- Hemobilia. 10- Hemosuccus pancreaticus (pancreas). ⇒ **Differential diagnosis: epistaxis, hemoptysis. "Pseudo-melena"** with iron, Pepto-Bismol, black pudding, spinach, beets, blueberries, charcoal, licorice.
Management	– **Volume repletion:** 2 intravenous accesses, NaCl 0.9 % or Lactate Ringer bolus, blood: typed and cross-matched, 4-6 red blood cells units banked, transfusion to keep Hb > 90-100 g/L, hemodynamic monitoring (blood pressure, pulse, urinary output ± central line as needed). – **Important history:** Upper digestive symptoms (epigastric pain or burning, vomiting effort), peptic ulcer disease, cirrhosis, aortic replacement, anemia, coagulopathy, alcohol consumption, medication (NSAIDs, ASA, anticoagulants), rule out pseudo-melena (iron, Pepto-Bismol, black pudding), cardio-pulmonary-neurologic effects of bleeding. – **Physical examination:** Vital signs, orthostatic hypotension, skin and mucous membranes (telangiectasia, petechia), signs of chronic liver disease, abdomen (liver, spleen, ascites, pain, tumor), rectal exam. – **Workup:** CBC, INR, aPTT, BUN, creatinine, AST, ALT, alkaline phosphatase, bilirubin, ECG, nasogastric tube if needed. – **Correct coagulopathy** if present: Fresh frozen plasma, protamine, etc. – **Gastroenterology consultation:** Esophagogastroduodenoscopy (EGD). Note: 80% of upper GI bleeding cases stop spontaneously.
Treatment	**Peptic ulcer**: treatment is based on ulcer's appearance at EGD: – Clean base (3-5 % rebleeding) or nonprotuberant pigmented dot (10% rebleeding): No endoscopic treatment required. Early PO feeding and oral PPI. Same-day release if patient is young, no comorbidity, no hemodynamic instability and hemoglobin OK. Otherwise, observation 24-48 hours on the ward. – Adherent clot (22 % rebleeding), visible vessel (50 % rebleeding) or active bleeding (90% rebleeding): Endoscopic treatment (injection + cauterization or clip) and I.V. PPI. Intensive care observation for 24 hours then on the ward (observation time of 3 days minimum). – If rebleeding occurs after 1st treatment: Second endoscopic treatment attempt to consider vs immediate surgery if massive hemorrhage or large posterior duodenal ulcer. In the event of rebleeding after 2 endoscopic treatments: surgery (vs arterial embolization). **Varices**: (See Cirrhosis table, complications). **Erosive gastritis**: Stop causal factor. PPI. **Mallory-Weiss**: Good prognosis (< 2 % rebleed). Oral PPI. Endoscopic injection if active bleeding or rebleeding. **Aortoenteric fistula**: Abdominal CT vs STAT arteriography, emergent surgery.

Lower GI Bleeding	Presentation: Hematochezia, melena. Non massive lower GI bleeding: typically, blood streaks on stool, in water, on toilet paper.
Causes	1- Diverticulosis 30-40% (acute painless bleeding). 2- Angiodysplasia 3-10% (acute painless bleeding). 3- Colitis: (bleeding associated with diarrhea and abdominal pain): ischemic (elderly patient and/or atherosclerotic disease, vasculitis), infectious (*Campylobacter, Salmonella, Shigella, E. coli* O157H7, Yersinia, *Entamoeba*, CMV), inflammatory (ulcerative colitis, Crohn's), radiation-induced. 4- Tumor: benign (rare: polyp, adenoma) or malignant (more occult bleeding). 5- Small bowel 3-5%: Angiodysplasia, Meckel's diverticulum (young patient), neoplasms, enteritis, intussusception (pain), aortoenteric fistula, etc. 6- Esophagus-stomach-duodenum (See above): 10% of lower gastrointestinal bleeding cases are secondary to an upper GI bleed! 7- Anorectal: Generally non massive. Hemorrhoids, rectal varices, fissures, etc.
Management	– **Volume repletion:** see Upper gastrointestinal bleeding. – **Important history:** Lower digestive symptoms (diarrhea, abdominal pain), upper digestive symptoms (epigastric pain, hematemesis), history of peptic ulcer, cirrhosis, aortic replacement, atherosclerotic disease, radiotherapy, coagulopathy, weight loss, medication (NSAIDs, ASA, anticoagulants), cardio-pulmonary-neurologic effects of bleeding. – **Physical examination:** Vital signs, orthostatic hypotension, skin and mucous membranes (telangiectasia, petechia), signs of chronic liver disease, abdomen (pain, mass, liver, spleen, ascites), rectal examination (hemorrhoids, fissures, tumor, stool color). – **Workup:** CBC, INR, aPTT, BUN, creatinine, AST, ALT, alkaline phosphatase, bilirubin, ECG. Nasogastric tube if upper GI bleed suspected (massive hematochezia, hemodynamic instability). Stool culture + research of parasites if associated diarrhea. – **Correct coagulopathy** if present: Fresh frozen plasma, protamine, etc. – **Gastroenterology consultation:** Esophagogastroduodenoscopy if upper GI bleed suspected. Total colonoscopy with preparation within 24 hours. – **Persistent hemorrhage:** Angiography and/or surgery (vs arterial embolization). – **If no source of bleeding is identified:** Technetium scan (Meckel's scan) in young patients. Tagged red blood cells scan (bleeding > 0.1 mL/min; rarely useful). Angiography only if bleeding active (> 0.5-1 mL/min). Enteroscopy ± enteroscan ± capsule endoscopy if available. Small bowel follow through ± enteroclysis (not in acute setting, because of barium). Note: 80% of lower GI bleed cases stop spontaneously.
Treatment	**Diverticulosis:** Observation alone. Surgery or embolization if bleeding persists or 2nd episode. **Angiodysplasia:** Laser, argon. Hemicolectomy or embolization if persistent or recurrent. **Colitis:** Watchful waiting if infectious or ischemic. Treatment of underlying illness if inflammatory. **Hemorrhoids, fissures:** Reassurance, local treatment.

Abdominal Pain	
Causes	**Digestive causes of abdominal pain:** – **Bile ducts**: Cholelithiasis, choledocholithiasis, cholecystitis, sphincter of Oddi dyskinesia. – **Liver**: Hepatitis, metastasis, hepatocellular carcinoma, abscess, etc. – **Stomach**: Ulcer, GERD, cancer, functional dyspepsia, NSAIDs, volvulus, etc. – **Pancreas**: Acute or chronic pancreatitis, cancer, etc. – **Small bowel**: Obstruction, ischemia (Henoch-Schönlein), inflammation (Crohn's, infection), cancer, etc. – **Ileum**: Crohn's, infection (*Yersinia*, tuberculosis, etc), Meckel's diverticulum, etc. – **Appendix**: Appendicitis. – **Colon**: Diverticulitis, colitis (infectious, inflammatory, ischemic), cancer, obstruction, volvulus, constipation, irritable bowel syndrome, etc. **Non-digestive causes of abdominal pain:** – **Heart**: Infarction, angina, pericarditis, etc. – **Aorta**: Abdominal aortic aneurysm dissection. – **Lung**: Pneumonia, pulmonary embolism, empyema, pleuritis, pneumothorax … – **Spleen**: Splenomegaly, infarction, abscess, etc. – **Urinary**: Lithiasis, pyelonephritis, neoplasm, distended bladder, cystitis, etc. – **Gynecological**: Pregnancy, ectopic pregnancy, ovarian torsion, ruptured ovarian cyst, pelvic inflammatory disease, endometritis, sexually transmitted disease (STD), etc. – **Abdominal wall**: Lumbar strain, disc herniation, neuropathy, herpes zoster, abdominal wall hernia, muscle strain, spontaneous hematoma or secondary to coagulopathy, etc. – **Metabolic**: Porphyria, sickle-cell anemia, hemolysis, diabetic ketoacidosis, uremia, adrenal insufficiency, lead poisoning, etc.

Management	1. **Determine the location and radiation of the pain.**
	
	2. **Establish potential organs based on location:**
	   Right upper quadrant: Digestive (bile ducts, liver, stomach, pancreas), lung, abdominal wall.
	   Epigastrium: Digestive (stomach, bile ducts, liver, pancreas, small intestine), heart, aorta, lung, abdominal wall, metabolic.
	   Left upper quadrant: Digestive (pancreas, stomach, colon), heart, lung, spleen, abdominal wall.
	   Right flank: Digestive (appendix, colon, bile ducts, liver), urinary, gynecological, abdominal wall.
	   Peri-umbilical: Digestive (stomach, bile ducts, pancreas, small intestine, appendix, colon), aorta, urinary, gynecological, abdominal wall, metabolic.
	   Left flank: Digestive (colon, pancreas), spleen, urinary, gynecological, abdominal wall.
	   Right iliac fossa: Digestive (appendix, ileum, colon), urinary, gynecological, abdominal wall.
	   Left iliac fossa: Digestive (colon), urinary, gynecological, abdominal wall.
	   Hypogastrium: Digestive (colon, ileum, appendix, small intestine), urinary, gynecological, aorta, abdominal wall.
	
	3. **For each potential organ, look for pertinent associated symptoms:**
	   E.g.: **Digestive**: Vomiting, hematemesis, dysphagia, diarrhea, hematochezia, Constipation, etc.
	      Lung: Cough, expectoration, hemoptysis, dyspnea, pleuritic pain.
	      Heart: Retrosternal pain, dyspnea, heart disease risk factors.
	      Urinary: Dysuria, urinary frequency, hematuria.
	      Gynecological: Last menstrual period, vaginal discharge, meno-metrorrhagia, STD, risk factors.

Abdominal wall: Low back pain, arthritis, osteoarthrosis, musculoskeletal disease, coagulopathy.

4. **Assess pain modifying factors based on potential organs activity:**
   E.g.: **Digestive**: Pain changes with meals? Defecation?
   Lung: Pain changes with deep breathing? Coughing?
   Heart: Pain changes with exercise? Deep breathing?
   Urinary: Pain changes with urination?
   Gynecological: Pain changes with menstrual cycle? With sexual intercourse?
   Abdominal wall: Pain changes with position? Movements?

5. **Physical examination: Specify location of pain. Look for associated signs:**
   E.g.: **Digestive**: Murphy sign, McBurney sign, rebound tenderness, psoas sign, rectal examination.
   Heart: S3, S4, murmur, friction rub.
   Lung: Rales, effusion, pleural rub, bronchial breath sounds.
   Urinary: Costovertebral angle tenderness, kidney palpation, bladder distension.
   Gynecological: Vaginal and gynecologic examination.
   Abdominal wall: Hernia, lumbar pain, cellulalgia. Assess mobilization and muscular contraction, Carnett's sign (palpation of the painful area with muscles contracted). If pain ↓: Carnett negative = visceral pain. If pain = or ↑: Carnett ⊕: parietal pain).

6. **Workup based on pathological organs and/or entities selected:**
   E.g.: **Digestive**: Liver enzymes, pancreatic enzymes, plain film of the abdomen, ultrasonography, CT, gastroscopy, colonoscopy, blood gases and lactate level (if ischemia suspected).
   Lung: Chest X-ray, D-dimers, arterial blood gas, ventilation-perfusion scan, etc.
   Heart: CK, troponins, ECG.
   Urinary: Urinalysis, urine culture, ultrasonography, CT, etc.
   Gynecological: β-hCG, pelvic ultrasonography.
   Aorta: abdominal ultrasonography, CT.
   Abdominal wall: spinal X-ray, rib views.
   Metabolic: CBC, LDH, creatinine, glycemia, venous gases, cortisol, porphyrins, etc.

Esophageal Disorders	
Dysphagia	Difficulty swallowing.

Causes	– **Oropharyngeal**: difficulty to initiate deglutition. Associated with coughing, nasal regurgitation, choking, nasal voice and/or aspiration.
	  - Motor: stroke, Parkinson's, multiple sclerosis, amyotrophic lateral sclerosis, muscular dystrophy, myasthenia gravis, polymyositis, oculopharyngeal syndrome, etc.
	  - Mechanical: Zenker's diverticulum, cricopharyngeal hypertonia, osteophytes, thyromegaly, ENT cancer, foreign body, etc.
	– **Esophageal**: blockage of food bolus after deglutition.
	  - Motor: Dysphagia with solids and liquids.
	    • Intermittent: Esophageal spasm.
	    • Progressive: Achalasia, scleroderma, Chagas disease (South America).
	  - Mechanical: Dysphagia with solids > liquids.
	    • Intermittent: Schatzki ring, eosinophilic esophagitis.
	    • Slowly progressive: Benign stricture (peptic, caustic).
	    • Rapidly progressive: Cancer.

Workup	Depending on cause: – Oropharyngeal: look for systemic neuromuscular disease ± head CT. Oropharyngeal endoscopy ± videofluoroscopic swallowing ± manometry if mechanical cause not excluded. – Esophageal: esophagoscopy (barium swallow sometimes done before esophagoscopy). If normal, consider esophageal manometry.
Treatment	Depending on cause: – Oropharyngeal: treatment of the underlying disease if motor problem. Speech therapy, occupational therapy, sometimes gastrostomy. Surgery if mechanical. – Esophageal: stricture = dilation: Schatzki = PPI or dilation: eosinophilic esophagitis = PPI or fluticasone: Achalasia = pneumatic dilation, myotomy or botulinum toxin injection: spasms = nitrates, calcium channel blockers: Scleroderma = PPI.
Gastro-Esophageal Reflux Disease (GERD)	– Prevalence: 20 % have GERD ≥ once/week. 60 % have GERD ≥ once/month. – Mainly 2nd to ↑ of physiological transient relaxation of lower esophageal sphincter. Sometimes 2nd to hypotonia of the lower esophageal sphincter, or ↓ esophageal clearance. – **Typical symptoms**: Pyrosis, regurgitation. – **Atypical symptoms**: Non-coronary retrosternal pain, asthma, hoarseness, chronic cough, dental erosions, posterior laryngitis, aspiration and recurrent pneumonia. – Worsened by recumbent position, fatty foods, chocolate, alcohol, coffee, onions, garlic, mint, tomatoes, citrus juice, medication (anticholinergics, sedatives, theophylline, progesterone, nitrates, calcium channel blockers, beta-blockers). Improved by antacids.
Management	– Look for red flags suggesting cancer (dysphagia, weight loss, anemia, bleeding). If present: gastroscopy. – Typical symptoms and no warning sign: empirical treatment. ***Treatment*** – Lifestyle modifications: elevate the head of the bed 15 cm, low-fat diet, avoid lying down within 3 hours after meals, weight loss if overweight, stop smoking, avoid worsening food and medication (see above). – **Mild symptoms** (≤ twice/week): Antacids + H2-receptors antagonists (H2-RA) as needed. If symptoms persist, see severe symptoms, below. – **Severe symptoms** (> twice/week): Proton pump inhibitors (PPI) once a day for 4-

	8 weeks. If symptoms persist, increase PPI bid dose. Stop after 4-8 weeks.
	– If symptoms persist despite PPI bid: Reconsider diagnosis. Gastroscopy ± esophageal pH testing-esophageal manometry.
	
	Maintenance
	– 80% of GERD comes back after stopping treatment: Consider long-term treatment (H2-RA or PPI depending on initial response).
	– Consider gastroscopy "once in a lifetime" if significant GERD for > 5 years.
	– Surgery useful for patients who respond to medical treatment but don't want long-term medication. Same effectiveness as medical treatment.
	
	Complications
	– Strictures: treat with PPI ± dilation.
	– Barrett's esophagus (occurs in 10-15 % of chronic GERD cases):
	    - Treatment with PPI.
	    - Monitoring with gastroscopy + biopsies every 2-5 years.
	    - If mild dysplasia: gastroscopy every 6-12 months; If severe dysplasia: consider esophagectomy or photodynamic therapy.
	    - Monitoring not recommended if patient is not a surgical candidate (esophagectomy).
	– Esophageal adenocarcinoma.

Odynophagia	Pain on swallowing. Differential diagnosis: esophagitis 2nd to radiotherapy, infection (HSV, CMV, *Candida*), medication (tetracycline, doxycycline, quinidine, NSAIDs, potassium, iron, bisphosphonates), caustic esophagitis, rarely GERD or neoplasm. Treatment depending on cause.

Gastric Disorders	
Dyspepsia	Refers to acute, chronic, or recurrent pain or discomfort centered in the upper abdomen and related to digestion (nausea, vomiting, early satiety...). Prevalence: 29 % of Canadian adults. - Uninvestigated dyspepsia: dyspepsia in a patient who has never undergone an investigation. - Non-ulcerous dyspepsia: dyspepsia in a patient for whom gastroduodenal investigation showed nothing. Descriptive term, not a diagnostic entity. - Functional dyspepsia: diagnostic entity: dyspepsia without underlying organic cause.

Uninvestigated Dyspepsia	
Causes	– **Esophagus-stomach-duodenum**: ulcer, GERD, malignancy, gastroparesis, etc. – **Liver and bile ducts**: metastasis, lithiasis, sphincter of Oddi dysfunction, etc. – **Pancreas**: malignancy, chronic pancreatitis, etc. – **Small intestine**: mesenteric ischemia, sprue, lactose intolerance, etc. – **Heart**: angina pectoris, etc. – **Abdominal wall**. – **Medication**: NSAIDs, aspirin, etc. – **Functional**.

Workup	1. Rule out non-gastric causes for symptoms (heart, bile ducts, medication, diet).
	2. If new dyspepsia and > 50 years **or** red flags suggesting cancer (vomiting, anemia/bleeding, abdominal mass/weight loss, dysphagia) → gastroscopy in order to rule out gastric cancer.
	3. If NSAIDs or regular ASA used → stop medication if possible. Without improvement, go to step 4. If impossible to stop ASA-NSAIDs, add PPI and/or change for a COX 2 inhibitor. If no improvement: endoscopy.
	4. If dominant symptoms are pyrosis or reflux → PPI or H2-receptors antagonists (H2-RA) (see Esophageal disorders table - GERD).
	5. otherwise, look for *H. pylori* through serology:
	    → If *H. pylori* ⊕: eradicate with antibiotic therapy (see below).
	        If no improvement, confirm eradication with breath test.
	        If still ⊕, retreat. If ⊖: treatment as above.
	    → If *H. pylori* ⊖: PPI for 4 weeks, then stop.
	        If resistant to PPI or relapse after stopping: gastroscopy.
	Other treatments: stop alcohol, caffeine, exacerbating medication.
	Document symptoms with diet.

Peptic Ulcer	
Causes	1. *Helicobacter pylori*. 2. NSAIDs-Aspirin. 3. Other: acid hypersecretion (Zollinger-Ellison), Crohn's, viral infection, cocaine, etc.
Workup	– Gastroscopy + antral biopsy for *H. pylori* (+ biopsy of ulcer if gastric ulcer) **or** – Barium meal + *H. pylori* serology (+ gastroscopy and biopsy of ulcer if gastric ulcer with suspicious appearance).
Treatment and follow-up	1- Discontinue NSAIDs-ASA. Stop tobacco and alcohol abuse. 2- If *H. pylori* ⊕: PPI bid + Clarithromycin 500 mg bid + (Amoxicillin 1000 mg bid or Metronidazole 500 mg bid) for 7 days. If *H. pylori* ⊖: H2-RA for 8 weeks or PPI for 6-8 weeks. Gastric ulcer: Gastroscopy + biopsy of the ulcer every 6-8 weeks until fully healed. Consider surgery if ulcer persists after 12 weeks. Duodenal ulcer: No follow-up necessary if asymptomatic since there is no risk of cancer.

Complications	<ul><li>Obstruction: aggressive medical treatment with PPI. Surgery if persistent.</li><li>Perforation: surgical treatment.</li><li>Hemorrhage: (see Gastrointestinal bleeding table).</li></ul>
Refractory Peptic Ulcer	No endoscopic healing of the ulcer after 8 to 12 weeks of treatment. (≠ persistence of symptoms without persistent ulcer identified).
Causes	<table><tr><td>• Persistence of *H. pylori*.</td><td>• Slow-healing giant ulcer.</td></tr><tr><td>• NSAIDs or ASA, acknowledged or not.</td><td>• Hypersecretory condition.</td></tr><tr><td>• Noncompliance with treatment.</td><td>• Malignancy.</td></tr><tr><td>• Heavy smoking.</td><td>• Infection, Crohn's, etc.</td></tr></table>
Workup	1- Re-evaluate medication and compliance to treatments. 2- Gastroscopy + antral biopsy for *H. pylori* + biopsy of ulcer. 3- Measure serum gastrin (Zollinger-Ellison).
Gastritis	<ul><li>Erosive: Alcohol, NSAIDs, "stress" (trauma, burns, central nervous system disease).</li><li>Non erosive: type A = autoimmune (pernicious anemia) vs type B = *H. pylori*.</li><li>Specific: bacterial, viral, granulomatous, Ménétrier, eosinophilic.</li></ul>
Helicobacter pylori	Gram-negative bacillus. Prevalence: 30 % of the Canadian population. Only 15 % will have complications (especially ulcers).
Clinical findings	<ul><li>Active chronic gastritis (100 %). Asymptomatic.</li><li>Gastric or duodenal peptic ulcer (15 %).</li><li>Maltoma (rare).</li><li>Gastric adenocarcinoma (rare).</li></ul>
Diagnosis	<ul><li>Non invasive: serology (1st choice for a person never treated), Breath test (to confirm eradication).</li><li>Invasive: antral biopsy by gastroscopy (only when gastroscopy needed).</li></ul> - **Test** for *H. pylori* if ulcer (gastric or duodenal) identified, maltoma or uninvestigated dyspepsia (see non investigated dyspepsia section). - **Not recommended** to test for *H. pylori* in functional dyspepsia, GERD or asymptomatic individual. Treat *H. pylori* if test is positive.
Treatment	1st line: Clarithromycin 500 mg bid + amoxicillin 1000 mg bid + PPI bid for 7 days **or** Clarithromycin 500 mg bid + metronidazole 500 mg bid + PPI bid for 7 days. 2nd line: Bismuth 2 co qid + PPI bid + tetracycline 500 mg qid + metronidazole 250 mg qid for 14 days.
Follow-up	<ul><li>Not necessary to control eradication if asymptomatic.</li><li>Exception: complicated ulcer (hemorrhage, perforation, obstruction).</li><li>To confirm eradication: Breath test or gastroscopy (only if indicated).</li></ul>

Intestinal Disorders

Crohn's Disease	Can involve the GI tract anywhere from the esophagus to the anus. 40-50% ileocolitis, 30-40% ileitis alone, 20% colitis alone. Characterized by transmural inflammation, with granuloma, strictures, fistulas and abscesses.
Clinical findings	Diarrhea, abdominal pain, bleeding, weight loss, fever… Sometimes intestinal obstruction, fistula, abscess, perianal disease, fulminating colitis. Extra-intestinal manifestations: Oral ulcers, erythema nodosum, pyoderma gangrenosum, episcleritis, arthritis, nephrolithiasis, cholelithiasis.
Workup	CBC, C-reactive protein, albumin, AST, ALT, bilirubin, alkaline phosphatase, nutritional workup as needed. Bone densitometry. Exclude infection: Stool culture, seek parasites and *C. difficile* cytoxin. Staging: Colonoscopy, barium meal with small bowel follow through ± enteroclysis ± entero-CT ± entero-MRI. Capsule endoscopy if persisting doubt and negative small bowels imaging. Fistula in ano and/or perianal illness: Pelvic IRM ± endoanal ultrasound.
Treatment	**Active intestinal disease**: Low fiber diet during the symptomatic period. Maximize nutritional status. Enteral vs parenteral feeding as needed. Stop tobacco (tobacco ↑ recurrence). 1. **5-ASA**: For mild to moderate symptoms: Salazopyrine (treats colon), Asacol® (ileum and colon), Pentasa® (duodenum, ileum, colon). Moderate effectiveness. Note: If only left colon affected, 5-ASA enema (± 5-ASA per os) can be used. 2. **Corticosteroids**: For moderate to severe symptoms, or refractory to 5-ASA: Prednisone 40 mg/d to be tapered slowly. Budesonide per os if ileo-caecal illness and intolerance to conventional steroids. Note: If only left colon affected, steroid or budesonide enema (± prednisone per os) can be used. IV steroids if very severe symptoms or refractory to steroids per os and/or enema. 3. **Antibiotics** (metronidazole + ciprofloxacin): Sometimes used for slight colon damage (associated with 5-ASA or not) or for severe colon inflammation in association with steroids. 4. **Anti-TNF-α antibodies** (infliximab, adalimumab): For significant illness, refractory to previous treatments. To compare with surgery. 5. **Surgery**: When illness resistant to medical treatment, abscess, perforation and/or toxic megacolon. **Maintenance therapy**: Stop tobacco (tobacco ↑ recurrence). 1. **5-ASA** (PO or IR): Moderate effectiveness. Useful for maintenance of a less severe illness. 2. **Immunosuppressive drugs** (Azathioprine, 6-mercaptopurine, methotrexate): Very effective. Useful for maintenance of a problematic illness, i.e. corticodependence, corticoresistance, frequent recurrences (> once/year), severe recurrences, multiple past or extensive surgeries, fistula … Takes 3-6 months to be effective. 3. **Anti-TNF-α antibodies**: For patients who are intolerant or refractory to immunosuppressive drugs and for whom surgery is not considered. **Fistula in ano and/or perianal illness**: 1. **Surgery consultation** for adequate examination and drainage of abscesses and fistulas. 2. **Antibiotics** (metronidazole + ciprofloxacin): Especially with perianal illness and/or abscess. 3. **Immunosuppressive drugs** (Azathioprine, 6-mercaptopurine). Take 3-6 months to be effective. Long-term treatment. 4. **Anti-TNF-α antibodies**: If resistant to immunosuppressive drugs or if cannot wait 3-6 months. Rule out abscesses before using anti-TNF. To compare with surgery.

	5. **Stomy**: When resistant to previous treatments. Monitoring of colon cancer if colic disease (after 7 years if pancolitis or after 14 years if left colitis). Colonoscopy and biopsy every 1-2 years.
Ulcerative Colitis	Affects only the mucous membrane of the colon. Rectum always affected with variable proximal extension: 50% rectosigmoid, 30% up to the splenic angle, 20% pancolic.
Clinical findings	Diarrhea with bleeding, abdominal pain, emergency and tenesmus: severity = – **mild** if < 4 stools/d, pulse < 90/min, Hct N, weight stable, temperature N, sedimentation rate (SR) < 20, albumin N. – **moderate** if 4-6 stools/d, pulse 90-100, Hct 30-40 %, weight ↓ 1-10%, temperature 37.3-37.7°C, VS 20-30, albumin 30-35 g/L. – **severe** if > 6 stools/d, pulse > 100, Hct < 30 %, ↓ weight > 10%, temperature > 37.8°C, VS > 30, albumin < 30 g/L. Toxic megacolon if patient toxic, colon dilation > 6 cm or cæcum dilation >12 cm (risk of perforation). Extra-intestinal manifestations: erythema nodosum, pyoderma gangrenosum, episcleritis, arthritis, sclerosing cholangitis (cholangiocarcinoma).
Workup	CBC, albumin, AST, ALT, bilirubin, alkaline phosphatase, nutritional workup as needed. Rule out infection: Stool culture, look for parasites and *C. difficile* cytotoxin. Rule out Crohn's and assess extent: Colonoscopy + ileoscopy, barium meal with small bowel follow through.

Treatment	**Active illness:**
	Low fiber diet during the asymptomatic period. Maximize nutritional condition. Enteral vs parenteral feeding as needed.
	1. **5-ASA**: For mild to moderate symptoms: Salazopyrin, Asacol®, Salofalk®. Very effective.
	   NB: If only left colon affected, 5-ASA enema (± 5-ASA per os) may be used.
	2. **Corticosteroids**: For moderate to severe symptoms, or refractory to 5-ASA: Prednisone 40 mg/d with slow tapering**.**
	   Note: If only left colon affected resistant to topical 5-ASA, steroid or budesonide enema (± prednisone per os) can be used. IV steroids if symptoms very severe or refractory to steroids per os and/or enema.
	3. **Anti-TNF-□ Antibodies**: when resistant to IV steroids (> 7 days). Alternative to colectomy.
	4. **Cyclosporine**: alternative to anti-TNF-α antibodies in trying to avoid a colectomy.
	5. **Surgery**: Colectomy if refractory to previous treatments or toxic megacolon not improving in 48-72 hours.
	
	Maintenance therapy:
	1. **5-ASA** (PO or IR): Good effectiveness. 1st choice.
	2. **Immunosuppressive drugs** (Azathioprine, 6-mercaptopurine): Good effectiveness. Useful for corticodependent illness, severe recurrences or frequent recurrences despite optimal 5-ASA. Takes 3-6 months to be effective.
	3. **Surgery**: When severe or frequent recurrences despite previous treatments.
	4. **Anti-TNF-□ antibodies**: for non-tolerant patients or patients resistant to immuno-suppressors; and for whom surgery is not considered.
	5. **Cyclosporine PO**: For patients who had cyclosporine and responded to it. Ideally, convert to azathioprine or 6-MP.
	
	Monitor for colon cancer (after 7 years if pancolitis, after 14 years if left colitis). Colonoscopy and biopsy every 1-2 years.

Celiac disease	**Synonyms:** non-tropical sprue, gluten-sensitive enteropathy. Inflammation of the small intestine triggered by gluten intake. May be associated with autoimmune disorders (type 1 diabetes, thyroid disease, primary biliary cirrhosis), dermatitis herpetiformis, IgA deficiency, Howell-Jolly bodies (splenic atrophy). **Clinical findings:** diarrhea, weight loss, malabsorption, anemia, hypocalcemia, osteoporosis… May be slightly or not at all symptomatic. Increases the risk of lymphoma of the small intestine + other malignancies (adenocarcinoma of the esophagus, oropharyngeal, small intestine) if not treated. **Screening:** anti-transglutaminase antibody. Note: possible false negative with IgA deficiency. Family screening (1st degree relatives). **Diagnosis:** small bowel biopsy confirms diagnosis. Absence of HLA DQ2 or DQ8 haplotypes virtually rules out celiac disease. **Workup:** bone densitometry. CBC. Nutritional workup. **Treatment:** nutritionist consultation for diet without gluten (in wheat, barley and rye; oats to a lesser degree). Avoid lactose, initially. Iron supplement and vitamins as needed. **Note: Tropical sprue:** 2-3 months after travel in tropical area. Antibiotic treatment.
Whipple disease	Intestinal and/or systemic infection to *Tropheryma whippelli.* **Clinical findings:** diarrhea, malabsorption, heart, articular, renal, system nervous central involvement, lymphadenopathy, hyperpigmentation. **Diagnosis:** duodenal biopsy: accumulation of macrophages PAS ⊕ . **Treatment:** Ceftriaxone 2 g IV daily for 1 month followed by TMP/SMX DS 1 co bid for 1 year.
Bacterial Overgrowth	Bacterial overgrowth in the small intestine. Causes deconjugation of bile salts and malabsorption. Caused by structural abnormalities of the small bowel (e.g.: blind loop syndrome, small intestine diverticulum), motility disorders (e.g.: scleroderma, diabetes), achlorhydria, age, altered immunity. **Clinical findings:** chronic diarrhea, malabsorption, vitamin B12 deficiency. **Diagnosis:** therapeutic antibiotic trial. Jejunum culture >10^5 bacteria/mL or breath test if antibiotic test inconclusive. **Treatment:** Antibiotics (tetracycline, ciprofloxacin, TMP/SMX, amoxicillin/ clavulanic acid …). Treat 1 week per month for chronic cases. If possible, correct anatomic anomaly.
Colic Diverticulosis	Very prevalent (66 % at 80 years). Especially in sigmoid. Can be pancolic. Connective tissue diseases increases risk (scleroderma, Marfan, etc).
Clinical findings	**Diverticulosis:** 80 % asymptomatic. Sometimes chronic constipation, abdominal pain (controversial). **Diverticulitis:** Acute abdominal pain, change in intestinal habits, fever, leukocytosis. Sometimes abscess, fistula, peritonitis, obstruction. Recurrence in 1/3. **Diverticular bleeding:** see Gastrointestinal bleeding table.
Workup	**Diverticulitis:** CBC, plain film of the abdomen (rule out perforation). *Typical clinical presentation*: presumptive diagnosis and immediate treatment. *Doubtful diagnosis*: ultrasonography and/or abdominal CT. Colonoscopy if suspicion of cancer.

Treatment	**Diverticulitis:**
	– **Mild symptoms** and reliable home support: Ambulatory treatment. Fiber-free diet, ciprofloxacin 500 mg bid + metronidazole 500 mg tid PO for 7-10 days.
	– **Severe symptoms, elderly patient, immunosuppression or comorbidity ++:** Hospitalization, keep "nil per mouth", IV antibiotics. Then progressive diet and PO antibiotics based on progress.
	Note: Perform CT of the abdomen if fever persists after 2-3 days of antibiotics. Colonoscopy or barium enema after 6-8 weeks to confirm diverticulosis and rule out malignancy. Long term: high fiber diet.
	Surgery: if abscess > 5 cm, fistula, peritonitis, infection refractory to IV antibiotics, obstruction, ≥ 2 documented episodes of diverticulitis (or ≥ 1 episode in individual < 40 years or immunosuppressed).
Irritable Bowel Syndrome	Functional disorder of the digestive tract. Affects 15-20% of the population. Essentially a viscerosensitivity disorder. Motility abnormality probably secondary. Psychological disorders change the patient's perception of symptoms.
Clinical findings	Abdominal pain is the cardinal symptom. Associated with diarrhea, constipation (or alternation of both), bloating, mucus in stools. Associations: Non-ulcerous dyspepsia, dysmenorrhea, interstitial cystitis, dyspareunia, migraine, fibromyalgia, chronic fatigue, sleep disorders.
Diagnosis	Rome III Criteria: 1. At least 3 months, with onset at least 6 months previously of recurrent abdominal pain or discomfort associated with 2 or more of the following: – Improvement with defecation. – Onset associated with a change in frequency of stool. – Onset associated with a change in form (appearance) of stool. 2. Absence of structural or metabolic illness to explain symptoms.
Treatment	– Reassurance. – Fiber rich diet ± fiber supplement. Avoid food that ↑ symptoms. – Find and treat causes of stress, psychological or psychiatric disorders. – Medication if needed and depending on symptoms: • Diarrhea: fiber supplements, loperamide, lomotil, cholestyramine. • Constipation: fiber supplements, stool softeners, osmotic laxative (milk of magnesia). • Abdominal pain: fiber supplements, antispasmodics, amitriptyline.

Diarrhea	
Increase in frequency of bowel movements or decrease in consistency of stools. Objectively: weight of stools > 200 g/day. To be distinguished from fecal incontinence.	
Acute Diarrhea	Duration < 2 weeks. Infectious in > 90 % of cases.

Causes	1. Gastro-intestinal infections (see below) or other infections with diarrhea as non specific manifestation (ex.: acute pyelonephritis, malaria ...).
	 2. Medication: laxatives, antacids, colchicine, prokinetics, natural products ...
	 3. Food: dairy products, alcohol, coffee, sorbitol, food additives ...
	 4. Ischemic colitis.
	
	 Infectious agents causing diarrhea:
	 C. difficile: History of antibiotic intake in 99 % (up to 3 months after stopping). Most frequent cause of nosocomial diarrhea. Fever, occasional extreme leukocytosis, risk of ileus, sepsis, toxic megacolon.
	 Treatment: If possible, stop causal antibiotic. Hydrate. Avoid antimobility agents and opiates. Enteric isolation until 3 days without diarrhea.
	 If mild: metronidazole 500 mg PO tid.
	 If moderate: vancomycine 125-500 mg PO qid.
	 If severe (sepsis, paralytic ileus, megacolon): vancomycine 500 mg PO + intrarectal + IV metronidazole + surgery consultation.
	 Treat for 10 days. Frequent relapse (20 %).
	 Campylobacter jejuni: With chicken, contaminated water or non pasteurized milk: summer-fall. Treatment: Erythromycin or quinolone for severe illness.
	 Non-typhi Salmonella: With chicken, turtle, cheese. Severe diarrhea (bloody or not): septicemia with AIDS. Reiter's can occur. Treat if blood cultures ⊕, severe diarrhea, > 50 years, severe CAD, valvular heart disease, prosthesis, cancer, uremia or immunosuppression. Treatment: TMP/SMX, quinolone, etc.
	 Shigella: With food or water consumed outside. Bloody diarrhea + fever, bacteremia. Treatment TMP/SMX, quinolone, etc.
	 E. coli O157:H7: With improperly cooked beef, contaminated water, non-pasteurized milk. Enterohemorragic: cramps, toxic, fever (rarer than other entero-invasive pathogens); hemolytic uremic syndrome can occur. To be considered if bloody diarrhea. No specific treatment: (possible adverse effect of antibiotics and anti-motility agents).
	 Enterotoxigenic E. coli: "traveller's diarrhea". Treatment: TMP/SMX or quinolone.
	 Yersinia enterolitica: Rare in Canada. With pork. Enterocolitis syndrome (hemorrhagic in 25%), mesenteric adenitis, pseudo-appendicitis, bacteremia (with alcohol, cirrhosis), polyarthritis, erythema nodosum, Reiter's can occur. Treatment if bacteremia, if severe or immunosuppression (with doxycycline, aminoglycoside antibiotics, TMP/SMX, quinolone).
	 Staph. aureus: With salad, seafood: vomiting + + and cramps. No treatment.
	 Clostridium perfringens: With meat, chicken: diarrhea + +. No specific treatment.
	 Aeromonas/Plesiomonas: Rarely pathogenic. Mild diarrhea, sometimes bloody or chronic. Contact with oysters and contaminated water. Treatment: TMP/SMX, quinolone.
	 Vibrio parahemolyticus: With shellfish, cruises. Explosive aqueous diarrhea + fever. No specific treatment.
	 Bacillus cereus: With rice. 2 syndromes: vomiting or limited severe diarrhea. No treatment.
	 Vibrio cholera: With shellfish (toxins). Treatment: fluid + doxycycline or tetracycline or quinolone.
	 Vibrio vulnificus: With oysters: gastroenteritis, bacteremia, cellulitis (with cirrhosis). Treatment: tetracycline.
	
	 Virus:
	     Rotavirus: winter infection, child < 2 YO. No specific treatment.
	     Norwalk: Outbreak in close circle (cruise, hospital). No specific treatment.

	Parasites:
	    Giardiasis: Contact with contaminated water. Associated with IgA deficiency.
	    Treatment: metronidazole.
	    Entamoeba histolytica: Exposure in tropical regions or among immigrants.
	    Homosexual contact. May also cause liver abscess. Treatment: metronidazole
	    combined with iodoquinol or paromomycine. ↑ complications with steroids.
	    Cryptosporidium, Isospora, Cyclospora…
	
	For AIDS patient: Salmonella, cryptosporidiasis, *Microsporidia, Cyclospora, Isospora belli*, CMV, *Mycobacterium avium intracellulare*, etc.

Workup	Stool cultures only if systemic symptoms, fever or bloody diarrhea. Parasite examination if risk factors. Presence of leukocytes in stools supports inflammatory diarrhea. *C. difficile* cytotoxine if history of antibiotic intake. Possible endoscopy if needed for fast *C. difficile* diagnosis. HIV test if risk factors.
Treatment	Hydration + supportive treatment: At home if general condition is good. Hospitalization and intravenous hydration if severely dehydrated or unable to drink. Anti-motility agents must be avoided if bleeding or inflammatory diarrhea. Empirical antibiotics for patients with severe inflammatory diarrhea (but who aren't suspected to have *E.Coli* 0157:H7) while waiting for stool cultures is acceptable. Treatment of specific germs: see above.
Chronic Diarrhea	Duration > 4 weeks.
Causes	– **Infectious**: Amebiasis, giardia, *C. difficile*, opportunistic (HIV), etc. – **Inflammatory**: Crohn's, ulcerative colitis, collagenous colitis, lymphocytic, GVHD, etc. – **Malabsorption**: Bile salt deficiency, pancreatic insufficiency, small bowel diseases (sprue, Whipple's, short bowel, bacterial proliferation, lymphoma). – **Diet:** Caffeine, alcohol, diet food (sorbitol), dairy products, etc. – **Medication:** Antacids, laxatives, antibiotics, colchicine, antihypertensive drugs, diuretics, theophylline, prokinetics, chemotherapy, etc. – **Previous surgeries:** Gastrectomy, vagotomy, cholecystectomy, intestinal resection, etc. – **Obstructive:** Neoplasia, fecal impaction, etc. – **Ischemic:** Ischemic colitis, mesenteric ischemia. – **Radiation-induced:** Radiation-induced colitis, radiation-induced enteritis. – **Endocrine:** Hyperthyroidism, Addison, diabetes, carcinoid, gastrinoma, medullary carcinoma of the thyroid, VIPoma, etc. – **Functional**: irritable bowel syndrome, functional diarrhea.
Assessment	**Step I:** **History:** Describe stools (consistency, frequency, nocturnal stools, bleeding, steatorrhea, constipation), associated symptoms (abdominal pain, fever, weight loss), infectious risk factors (travel, antibiotics, contacts, suspicious food), diet (milk, coffee, alcohol, carbonated beverages, fruit juice, diet products), medication (including antacids, natural products), past surgeries, and associated diseases (diabetes, thyroid, scleroderma, etc). Distinguish between diarrhea and incontinence. **Physical exam:** Assess hydration and nutritional condition. Examine thyroid, abdomen and anorectum. Look for skin lesions, oral ulcers, lymphadenopathy and arthritis. **Basic workup:** CBC, sedimentation rate, electrolytes, creatinine, glycemia, albumin, calcium, TSH. Malabsorption workup according to clinical findings (See below). **Stool analysis:** Bacterial culture, parasite examination and *C. difficile* toxin.

Step II: If step I unrevealing:

Therapeutic tests: Stop dairy products. Fiber if functional cause suspected.
Metronidazole if parasites suspected despite negative examination.
Anti-transglutaminase antibody + immunoglobulin A levels. False negatives for
celiac disease with IgA deficiency.
Colonoscopy + biopsies: Short if age < 50 years. Total if age > 50 years.

Step III: If step II unrevealing **and** organic cause suspected (nocturnal diarrhea, recent onset, weight loss, anemia, blood in stool, hypoalbuminemia…)

Total colonoscopy + staged biopsies.
Gastroscopy + biopsies and aspiration of the small intestine.
Small bowel follow through.
CT of the abdomen.

Step IV: If step III unrevealing **and** organic cause suspected **or** patient very uncomfortable.

Hospitalization + stool collection: Measure fecal volume, calculate osmolar gap, fecal fat measurement, look for laxatives.
Osmolar gap: [Plasma Osm] - [(Na$^+$ + K$^+$ in stools) x 2] =
If < 40: Secretory diarrhea.
If > 40: Osmotic diarrhea.

Diagnostic approach based on physiopathological mechanisms:

Physiopathological mechanisms of diarrhea:
1. **Secretory:** Endocrine tumor (VIPoma, carcinoid, gastrinoma, medullary carcinoma of the thyroid, systemic mastocytosis), laxatives, bile salts malabsorption, enteropathy (infectious toxins, villous adenoma, lymphocytic colitis, collagenous colitis, GVHD, etc).
2. **Osmotic:** Lactase deficiency, sorbitol, antacids, laxatives, malabsorption.
3. **Motility disorders:** Short bowel syndrome, hyperthyroidism, visceral neuropathy (diabetes), scleroderma, amyloidosis, etc.
4. **Inflammatory:** inflammatory bowel disease, acute radiation-induced colitis, enteroinvasive infection (*Shigella, Yersinia, E. coli* O157H7, amoebae…)
5. **Mixed.**
6. **Functional.**

Malabsorption workup: if steatorrhea, weight loss, malnutrition, fecal fat > 7g/day:
1. D-xylose absorption test ± small bowel biopsy ± small bowel follow through.
2. If abnormal: Malabsorption secondary to small bowel illness (sprue, bacterial overgrowth…).
3. If normal: Suspect pancreatic insufficiency: Try pancreatic enzyme therapy ± plain film of the abdomen ± abdominal CT ± pancreatic-MRI ± endoscopic ultrasound ± ERCP.

Treatment based on cause.

Hepatic Disorders (excluding cirrhosis)

Icterus	Clinically apparent if bilirubin > 51.3 µmol/L.
	Differential diagnosis: hypercarotenemia (present in hypothyroidism).
	
	Causes:
	1. **Nonconjugated hyperbilirubinemia**:
	    – ↑ production: Hemolysis, hematoma, transfusion.
	    – ↓ capture and/or ↓ conjugation: Gilbert's, medication, Crigler-Najjar.
	2. **Conjugated hyperbilirubinemia**:
	    – Hepatocellular dysfunction: Hepatitis, cirrhosis, malignant infiltration, etc.
	    – Intrahepatic cholestasis: primary biliary cirrhosis, medication, total parenteral nutrition, sepsis, viral or alcoholic hepatitis, cancer, cholestasis of pregnancy, amyloidosis, sarcoidosis, mycobacteria, etc.
	    – Extrahepatic cholestasis: Choledocholithiasis, stricture, sclerosing cholangitis, cholangiocarcinoma, compression (pancreas cancer, pancreatitis, lymphadenopathy), etc.
	    – Hereditary cholestatic syndromes: Dubin-Johnson, Rotor's.

Disturbance of Liver Enzymes	**Determine predominance:** 1. If ↑ ALT >> ↑ alkaline phosphatase = hepatocellular damage (see below). 2. If ↑ alkaline phosphatase >> ↑ ALT = cholestatic disease (see below). 3. If ↑ ALT ≈ ↑ alkaline phosphatase = mixed illness, non specific.

Hepatocellular Damage

Causes	- Alcohol - Hemochromatosis - Medication - Wilson's disease - Viral hepatitis (A, B, C, D, E, HSV, CMV ...) - α1-antitrypsin deficit - Autoimmune hepatitis - Right-sided heart failure - Nonalcoholic fatty liver disease - Budd-Chiari syndrome - Acute fatty liver of pregnancy - Ischemic hepatitis - Acute biliary obstruction, cholecystitis (1st 24-48 hours). Non-hepatic causes of ↑ AST-ALT: celiac disease, muscle disease, intense exercise, hyperthyroidism, adrenal insufficiency, Stauffer's syndrome (with renal adenocarcinoma), sepsis ...
Workup	– Hepatitis A, B, C serologies – Anti-smooth muscle antibody, antinuclear factor antibodies – Serum iron, ferritin, transferrin saturation – Antimitochondrial antibodies – Ceruloplasmin – Protein electrophoresis – Abdominal ultrasonography Consider liver biopsy if enzymes ↑ > 2 x normal for > 3 month and above workup negative.

Cholestatic Disease

Causes	1. With bile ducts dilation:
	    - Intrabiliary obstruction: Choledocholithiasis, biliary strictures, sphincter of Oddi dysfunction, cholangiocarcinoma, recurrent pyogenic cholangitis ...
	    - Extrabiliary compression: Pancreatic cancer, chronic pancreatitis, lymphadenopathy, Mirizzi's syndrome ...
	2. Without bile ducts dilation:
	    - Extrahepatic: Sclerosing cholangitis (see below).
	    - Intrahepatic: Primary biliary cirrhosis (see below), medication, sepsis, total parenteral nutrition, viral or alcoholic hepatitis, malignant infiltration, granulomatous disease, amyloidosis, autoimmune cholangitis, secondary syphilis ...
	3. Non hepatic: Bone disease, pregnancy, renal failure, GVHD.

Workup	– GGT and/or alkaline phosphatase isoenzyme if doubt on hepatic origin.
	– Abdominal ultrasonography:
	  - With bile ducts dilation: CT, MRCP ± ERCP.
	  - Without bile ducts dilation: Antimitochondrial antibodies, viral serologies, CT.
	    If ⊖, cholangio-MRI ± ERCP ± liver biopsy.

Hepatitis A	Fecal-oral transmission. Incubation 15-45 days. Contagious for 2 weeks before and up to 7 days after the appearance of the icterus. No chronicity. Rare fulminant hepatitis (generally with preexisting liver disease or > 40 years). **Risk factors:** Contact with infected individual, travel to endemic country, childcare work. **Diagnosis:** Serology: IgG and IgM anti-HAV. **Treatment:** Symptomatic. Prednisone 30 mg OD x 2 weeks if extended cholestasis. **Prevention:** Hygienic measures. Immunoglobulins for contacts and travellers to high-risk countries. Anti-HAV vaccine recommended for homosexuals, IV drug users, travellers to endemic countries, healthcare workers, patients with chronic liver disease.
Hepatitis B	Blood-related, sexual or perinatal transmission. Incubation 1-6 months. Chronicity (HBsAg ⊕ > 6 months): adults: 5%; children 95%. Fulminant hepatitis < 1%. Sometimes complicated with arthritis, rash, glomerulonephritis, polyarteritis nodosa, serum sickness. **Risk factors:** IV drug users, high-risk sexual behavior, transfusions, tattoos, immigrant or aboriginal. Risk of transmission via needle 30%; mother-fetus 90%. **Diagnosis:** Serology:

	HBsAg	Anti-HBs	Anti-HBc
Acute hepatitis B	+ (< 6 months)	–	+ (IgM)
Chronic hepatitis B	+ (≥ 6 months)	–	+ (IgG)
Recovery from hepatitis B	–	+	+
Vaccination	–	+	–

Treatment:
Acute hepatitis B: Hepatic enzymes and serial INR. Symptomatic treatment: ambulatory treatment if patient looks well with normal INR. Otherwise: hospitalization. HIV and HCV testing.
Serology at 6 month: HBsAg - and AntiHBs +: recovery from hepatitis B.
                                   HBsAg + and Anti HBs - : chronic hepatitis B.

Chronic hepatitis B:
Workup: CBC, ALT, AST, Alk. P, bilirubin, INR, albumin, creatinine, AFP.
            HBsAg, Anti HBs, HBeAg, Anti-HBe, HBV-DNA, ± genotype.
            Anti-HCV, Anti-HIV ± Anti-HDV.
            Abdominal ultrasound.

Types:	HBsAg	HBeAg	Anti-HBe	HBV-DNA (IU/mL)	ALT
Immunotolerance	+	+	–	≥ 20 000	N
Active hepatitis HBeAg +	+	+	–	≥ 20 000	↑
Active hepatitis HBeAg -	+	–	+	≥ 20 000	↑
Inactive infection	+	–	+	< 20 000	N

Therapeutic recommendations: Treatment must be conducted by an expert in this field. Stop alcohol. Anti-HAV vaccine.

HBeAg + and HBV-DNA < 20 000 IU/mL **or**
HBeAg - and HBV-DNA < 2 000 IU/mL:
- Normal ALT: No treatment. Follow ALT and HBV-DNA every 3 months.
- High ALT: Search for other causes of hepatitis.

	HBeAg + and HBV-DNA ≥ 20 000 IU/mL **or** HBeAg - and HBV-DNA ≥ 2 000 IU/mL:<ul><li>Normal ALT: Consider liver biopsy (if > 35 y.o.) and treatment if inflammation and/or significant fibrosis. Otherwise, follow ALT every 3 months. Hepatocellular carcinoma screening every 6 months.</li><li>High ALT: to be treated.</li></ul>Medication: PEG-interferon-α2a (24-48 weeks based on HBe status. Side effects ++). Adefovir. Entecavir. Tenofovir (duration of treatment undefined. Well tolerated. Less development of resistance on the long term). 30-40 % seroconversion to HBe - after 3 years with oral medication. 32 % after 1 year with PEG-interferon. **Chronic cirrhotic hepatitis B**: Compensated cirrhosis and HBV-DNA < 2 000 IU/mL: Observe if ALT normal. If not, treat with long term Adefovir or Entecavir. Decompensated cirrhosis: Lamivudine (or telbivudine) + Adefovir (or entecavir) and consider liver transplant. **HIV and HBV co-infection:** HAART including Tenofovir and Lamivudine or Emtricitabine, combined with non-nucleosidic reverse transcriptase inhibitors or protease inhibitors. **HBV and HCV co-infection**: Measure HBV-DNA and HCV-RNA. Treat predominant virus. **Prevention**: Immunoglobulins for newborn, needle prick injury or sexual intercourse exposed to HBV. Anti-HBV vaccine for patients with high-risk sexual behavior, IV drug users, surrogate mother newborns, healthcare workers, travellers to endemic countries (> 6 months), patients with chronic liver disease. In Québec, vaccination of all school-age children.
Hepatitis C	Blood-related transmission. Sexual and perinatal rare. Incubation 6-7 weeks. Acute symptomatic hepatitis rare. Chronicity (HCV-RNA ⊕ > 6 months) = 85%. Cirrhosis = 20%: accelerated by alcohol intake and HIV coinfection. Hepatocellular carcinoma = 1-5%. May be complicated by cryoglobulinemia, glomerulonephritis, porphyria. **Risk factors:** IV drug users, transfusions. Transmission risk via needle prick injury < 5%, mother-fetus 0-3%. **Diagnosis:** Anti-HCV-ELISA and anti-HCV RIBA (= presence of antibodies). HCV-RNA (= presence of virus) may be useful to confirm diagnosis. Also look for HIV and HBV. **Treatment**: By specialist. Stop alcohol. Give anti-HAV and anti-HBV vaccines. ***Acute hepatitis C:*** (recent acquisition of HCV-RNA: < 6 months)<ul><li>Icteric: Observe and treat if HCV-RNA is still positive after 12 weeks.</li><li>Non-icteric: Treat as soon as known diagnosis. Treatment: PEG-interferon-α 12 weeks if genotype 2 or 3. 24 weeks if genotype 1.</li></ul>***Chronic hepatitis C:*** (HCV-RNA ⊕ > 6 months) Workup: HCV genotype, viral load, hepatic biopsy recommended. Recommendations: Genotype 1, 4, 5 and 6: PEG-Interferon-α + Ribavirin (dose based on weight) for ± 48 weeks according to viral response. 42-46 % of sustained viral response (HCV-RNA ⊖ 6 months after stopping treatment). Genotype 2 and 3: PEG-interferon-α+ Ribavirin for ± 24 weeks according to viral response. 72-80 % of sustained viral response (HVC-RNA ⊖ 6 months after stopping treatment). ***Cirrhotic chronic hepatitis C:*** PEG-interferon + Ribavirin not tolerated with decompensated cirrhosis. Contemplate liver transplantation. **Prevention**: No vaccine. Prevent risk factors.

Hepatitis D	Blood-related transmission. Coinfection or superinfection with HBV. Follows the pattern of hepatitis B (unsustained in the absence of HBV). Sometimes fulminant hepatitis when superinfection. **Diagnosis:** Anti-HDV ± HDV-RNA. **Treatment:** By expert in specialized centre: PEG-interferon for 48 weeks. Treat hepatitis B. **Prevention:** prevent risk factors.
Hepatitis E	Fecal/oral transmission. Infection in India, Pakistan, Southeast Asia. Symptoms similar to hepatitis A. Risk of fulminant hepatitis in pregnant women (mortality 10-20%). **Diagnosis:** HVE-RNA or Anti-HVE IGM. **Treatment:** Symptomatic. **Prevention:** Hygienic measures when visiting endemic countries.
Other Types of Viral Hepatitis	**Hepatitis G:** New virus: clinical significance uncertain. No evidence of chronic illness. **EBV, CMV, HSV, etc:** ↑ alkaline phosphatase + atypical lymphocytes.
Autoimmune Hepatitis	Most often affects young women. Acute ± fulminant hepatitis or chronic hepatitis or cirrhosis. Sometimes associated with other autoimmune manifestations. **Diagnosis:** Hypergammaglobulinemia (80%), ANA, antismooth muscle antibodies, anti-LKM antibodies and liver biopsy. Frequent false ⊕ for anti-HCV. **Treatment:** HAV and HBV vaccination. Screening for hepatocellular carcinoma every 6 months if cirrhosis. Treat hepatitis if transaminases ≥ 10 times normal; or transaminases ≥ 5 times normal and γ-globulins ≥ twice normal; or transaminases < 5 times normal but symptomatic patient; or necrosis with « *bridging* » or multi-acinous necrosis on liver biopsy; or pediatric patient. *If no treatment indicated:* Frequent follow-up of enzymes and hepatic biopsy after 2 years. *If treatment indicated:* Prednisone ± azathioprine. Remission if transaminases < twice times normal, bilirubin and normal γ-globulines, histologic resolution and asymptomatic patient. 80 % of remission after 3 years. Cyclosporine for refractory cases. Liver transplantation if liver failure or advanced cirrhosis. For patients in state of remission, weaning may be tried. Frequent recurrences: 60-90 % will require long term treatment.
Alcoholic Hepatitis	Generally secondary to > 80 g/day alcohol consumption for more than 15 years. Fever, jaundice, hepatomegaly, and sometimes liver failure (ascites, variceal bleeding, encephalopathy). Frequent leukocytosis. AST/ALT ↑ but less than 10 times normal. AST/ALT ratio > 2, GGT ↑, INR ↑. **Treatment:** Stop alcohol. Septic workup and peritoneal tap if fever. Nutritional support, hydration, thiamine, folic acid, and other vitamin supplements. Phosphate, magnesium and vitamin K as needed. Prednisone if 4,6 x [PT (s) – control (s)] + 1,7 x bilirubin > 32 and/or hepatic encephalopathy. Not recommended with pancreatitis, GI hemorrhage, renal failure or active infection.
Non Alcoholic Fatty Liver Disease	Metabolic disease consisting of steatosis, steatohepatitis and nonalcoholic steatonecrosis. Asymptomatic. Sometimes hepatomegaly. 20 % will evolve into cirrhosis. **Risk factors:** Obesity, diabetes, dyslipidemia, medication (steroids, amiodarone), malnutrition, total parenteral nutrition, post-op of bariatric surgery. 40% have no risk factors. **Diagnosis:** Suggestive: elevation of AST-ALT < 4 x normal, absence of alcohol (< 40 g/d) and liver workup negative. Steatosis at liver biopsy + absence of alcohol + HBV and HCV serology negative. **Treatment:** Lose weight, control of diabetes and dyslipidemia, stop causative medication. Metformin, pioglitazone, and rosiglitazone could be promising treatments.

Wilson's Disease	Autosomal recessive hereditary disease. ↓ Copper excretion in bile with accumulation in liver, brain, kidney and cornea. Mainly in men < 40 years. Acute hepatitis, chronic hepatitis or cirrhosis. May be associated with neuropsychiatric syndrome, hemolysis, Fanconi. **Diagnosis**: ↓ ceruloplasmin, ↑ 24 h urinary copper. In presence of Kayser-Fleischer rings (K-F) and ceruloplasmin < 200 mg/L = Diagnosis. If K-F rings and normal ceruloplasmin, proceed with biopsy and hepatic copper assay. If ceruloplasmin < 50 mg/L or 24 h urinary cooper > 40 µg and absence of K-F rings, proceed with biopsy and hepatic copper assay. **Treatment**: Copper-deficient diet. Trientine (1st choice) or penicillamine induction to normalize copper parameters. Oral zinc, trientine or penicillamine in maintenance treatment, for life. Measure 24 h urinary copper annually. Cerebral MRI if neurologic findings. Liver transplantation if advanced cirrhosis or fulminant hepatitis. **Prevention**: family screening.

Hemochromatosis	Autosomal recessive hereditary disease. HFE gene mutation (chromosome 6) causing ↑ iron absorption and accumulation in liver, pancreas, pituitary gland, heart, gonads, articulations. Prevalence of genotype = 1/200. 5 men for 1 woman.
	 95 % of hemochromatoses have mutation C282Y/C282Y, 4 % have C282Y/H63D and 1 % has H63D/H63D.
	 Clinical findings: Fatigue, arthralgias/arthritis, ↓ libido, erectile dysfunction, diabetes, amenorrhea, heart failure, arrhythmia, ↑ liver enzymes, hepato-splenomegaly, cirrhosis, hepatocellular carcinoma, dilated cardiomyopathy, hyperpigmentation, testicular atrophy, hypogonadism, hypothyroidism.
	 Diagnosis: Measure transferrin saturation: If < 45 %: no hemochromatosis. If ≥ 45 %: proceed to genotyping :
	 • C282Y/C282Y: = diagnostic for hemochromatosis:
	    o If age < 40 years, ferritin < 1000 µg/L and normal AST/ALT: Biopsy not needed. Proceed right away with phlebotomy.
	    o If ferritin > 1000 µg/L or AST/ALT ↑ and/or age > 40 years: liver biopsy to evaluate fibrosis severity. Start phlebotomy.
	 • C282Y/H63D or H63D/H63D: rule out other hepatic or hematologic disease. Liver biopsy and calculate hepatic iron index (HII) which can be useful if needed. HII (Intra-hepatic iron (µmol/g)/age) > 1.9 confirms diagnosis. Phlebotomy if diagnosis of hemochromatosis or if doubt persists.
	 Treatment: Weekly phlebotomy (500 mL) (to start if ferritin ≥ 200 µg/L in non pregnant women or ≥ 300 µg/L in men), until saturation < 45 % and ferritin < 50 µg/L.
	 Phlebotomies 3-4 times/year subsequently for life in order to maintain ferritin < 50 µg/L. Avoid alcohol and vitamin C supplements. Screen for hepatocellular carcinoma every 6 months if cirrhosis.
	 Prevention: family screening: Transferrin saturation and HFE genotyping when older than 18 years old.

α 1-antitrypsin Deficiency	Autosomal recessive genetic disease. Prevalence 1/1500. Accumulation of α 1-antitrypsin in the liver. Causes cirrhosis ± hepatocellular carcinoma and emphysema. **Diagnosis**: Absence of α protein electrophoresis peak. A α 1-antitrypsine < 11 µmol/L and genetic mutation confirm diagnosis. **Treatment**: HBV and HAV vaccination. Alcohol abstinence. Transplantation for advanced cirrhosis. Enzyme supplement for lung disease.

Drug-Induced Hepatotoxicity	Hepatitis (cytolytic predominance with $\uparrow$ ALT > $\uparrow$ alkaline phosphatase) – Acute: Acetaminophen, statins, valproic acid, azathioprine, 6-mercaptopurine, antiretroviral drugs, isoniazid, nitrofurantoin, minocycline, ketoconazole, troglitazone, sulfonamides, phenytoin, barbiturates, halothane, niacin, methyldopa, sulfasalazine, aspirin, NSAIDs, trazodone, ACEI, herbs, cocaine, MDMA (*"ecstasy"*), phencyclidine (PCP), glue and solvents, etc. – Granulomatous: Allopurinol, carbamazepine, hydralazine, quinine, quinidine, etc. Cholestasis (cholestatic predominance with $\uparrow$ alkaline phosphatase > $\uparrow$ ALT) – Estrogen, androgen, oral contraceptives, chlorpromazine, tricyclic antidepressants, trimethoprim-sulfamethoxazole, erythromycin, amoxicillin/clavulanic acid, ceftriaxone, etc. Cirrhosis: Methotrexate, amiodarone, vitamin A, etc. Treatment: Stop all hepatotoxic medication. N-acetylcysteine if acetaminophen intoxication. Transplantation for fulminant hepatitis or advanced cirrhosis.
Acute Liver Failure	Hepatocellular dysfunction (INR $\geq$ 1.5) and encephalopathy occurring < 8 weeks after onset of liver disease. Fulminant if < 2 weeks. Subfulminant if > 2 weeks. Causes: Viral (mainly HBV, HAV), medication (mainly acetaminophen) or drugs, auto-immune, shock, hyper-hypothermia, Budd-Chiari, metastatic cancer (lung, melanoma, breast, lymphoma), Wilson's, Reye's, acute fatty liver of pregnancy, some fungi, etc. 15% of causes undetermined. Workup: CBC, electrolytes, creatinine, glycemia, PO_4^{3-}, Mg^{++}, arterial blood gas, plasma acetaminophen level, hepatitis A and B serology, ANA and anti-smooth muscle antibody, tests for Wilson's, serum ammoniac and ß-hCG. If needed: hepatic biopsy. Treatment: Supportive treatment: hydration; Follow and correct metabolic abnormalities (acidosis, glycemia, K^+, Mg^{++}, PO_4^{3-}, etc); Gastro-prophylaxis with H2-RA; repeated septic workup ± prophylactic antibiotic; Correct coagulopathy only if bleeding. If encephalopathy, intensive care admission. • Grade I or II (lethargy): Lactulose, avoid sedatives. • Grade III (stupor) or IV (coma): Idem + endotracheal intubation + keep bed's head up 30°. Dilantin + benzodiazepine if convulsion. Invasive monitoring of intra-cranial pressure (ICP) controversial. Mannitol + hyperventilation if intracranial pressure $\uparrow$. Specific treatment according to cause. E.g.: N-acetylcysteine with confirmed or suspected acetaminophen intoxication, steroids if auto-immune hepatitis, etc. Transplantation need based on King's College criteria: • Acetaminophen intoxication: pH < 7.3 **or** PT > 100 s + creatinine > 300 μmol/L + grade III or IV encephalopathy. • Other causes: PT > 100 s **or** 3 of the following criteria: age < 10 or > 40 y.o., non A/non B hepatitis, halothane hepatitis or idiosyncratic drug reactions, duration of jaundice of more than 7 days before onset of encephalopathy, PT > 50 s, bilirubin > 300 μmol/L. Note: Early transfer to transplant center, even before getting above criteria. Occurrence of encephalopathy in itself justifies transfer.

Cholelithiasis	2 types of gallstones: pure or mixed cholesterol stones (90 % in Canada) and pigment stones.
	Risk factors: Woman, old age, obesity or rapid weight loss, family history, hypertriglyceridemia, diabetes, cirrhosis, pregnancy, hemolytic anemia, terminal ileum disease, medication (octreotide, hormone replacement therapy, ceftriaxone), total parenteral nutrition.
	Clinical findings: Frequently asymptomatic. Biliary colic (epigastric or RUQ pain or discomfort, quite sudden, lasting 1-4 hours) in 10-25 %, complications (e.g. acute cholecystitis) in 3 % at 10 years. Biliary ileus (obstruction of small intestine secondary to lithiasis) rare. Frequent recurrence following a first biliary colic.
	Treatment: Cholecystectomy (by laparoscopy) if symptomatic. Ursodeoxycholic acid to be considered if surgery refusal (may be useful for small non calcified gallstones < 1.5 cm with functional gallbladder) but 50 % recurrence 5 years after stopping treatment. Enterolithotomy if biliary ileus. Prophylactic cholecystectomy for asymptomatic patients to be considered with calcified gallbladder (porcelain), lithiasis > 3 cm in diameter or heart transplantation candidate. Not indicated for diabetes.
Acute Cholecystitis	90-95 % associated with gallstones. Occurs when a stone enters cystic duct and inflammation develops upstream of obstruction. An acalculus cholecystitis may appear 2-4 weeks post-op of major surgery or in ICU with prolonged fasting. May also be secondary to *Salmonella* infection. May also be secondary to infection (CMV, cryptosporidiosis, microsporidiosis) in AIDS patients.
	Clinical findings: Epigastric or RUQ sudden pain, prolonged, lasting 12-18 hours, with fever, nausea, vomiting, anorexia, RUQ sensibility (± Murphy's sign), jaundice (in 25 %).
	Diagnosis: leukocytosis. Rarely: ↑ AST, ↑ alkaline phosphatase, hyperbilirubinemia. Plain abdominal film shows radio-opaque gallstones in 15 %. Abdominal ultrasound is the best initial test. Some characteristics are suggestive (thickened of gallbladder wall, pericholecystic liquid, echographic Murphy's sign). HIDA scan ⊕ in general (most sensitive test). Abdominal CT useful for doubtful cases.
	Complications: Gangrene (if symptoms persist for 24-48 hours), perforation, abscess, emphysemetous cholecystitis, empyema, or cholecystoenteric fistula (possible biliary ileus).
	Treatment: Keep fasting with nasogastric tube as needed. IV hydration. Analgesia. Antibiotics if sepsis (such as piperacilline-tazobactam). Urgent cholecystectomy (in 2-3 days, or immediately if perforation/gangrene). Pre-operative ERCP if bilirubin > 85 μmol/L, bile duct dilation > 7 mm or choledocholithiasis on imaging. If surgery is too risky, percutaneous cholecystotomy or needle aspiration of gallbladder, with cholecystectomy later if acceptable risk.
Choledocho-lithiasis and Cholangitis	15-20 % of patients with gallstone have choledocholithiasis. ↑ with age or among Asians. 5 % of choledocholithiasis are formed *de novo* in bile duct, 95 % being stones that have migrated from gallbladder.
	Clinical findings: Patients with choledocholithiasis can be asymptomatic, or suffer from biliary colic or other complications like cholangitis, pancreatitis, obstructive jaundice or secondary biliary cirrhosis. Charcot's triad (pain, fever, jaundice) and Reynold's pentad (Charcot's triad + hypotension and altered mental status) are typical manifestations of cholangitis. Hepatomegaly can occur.

	Diagnosis: ↑ AST/ALT, hyperbilirubinemia, ↑ alkaline phosphatase. ↑ amylase with associated pancreatitis. Leukocytosis with cholangitis. Imaging studies: EUS or magnetic resonance cholangiopancreatography (MRCP) if low suspicion of persisting choledocolithiasis. ERCP if EUS or MRCP unavailable or high suspicion of persisting choledocolithiasis, for diagnosis and therapy. If ERCP is not available, percutaneous transhepatic cholangiography possible. Abdominal ultrasound, CT of the bile ducts, or HIDA scan also useful for diagnosis in certain circumstances. **Treatment**: Endoscopic sphincterotomy with stone extraction followed by elective cholecystectomy when stable (if acceptable risk).
Primary Biliary Cirrhosis (PBC)	Autoimmune granulomatosis destruction of intrahepatic bile ducts. Especially in middle-aged women. Asymptomatic at onset. Subsequently: fatigue, pruritus. Icterus and cirrhosis at end. Often associated with hypo-hyperthyroidism, Sjögren, celiac disease … **Complications:** Steatorrhea and malnutrition, osteoporosis, hyperlipidemia (xanthoma). **Diagnosis:** Alkaline phosphate (alk. P) ↑ and antimitochondrial antibodies (AAM) ≥ 1:40 (95% sensitivity) = diagnosis. If AAM ↑ and Alk P. normal: PBC?: Follow Alk P. If Alk P. ↑ and AAM normal; rule out other causes of choletasis. Liver biopsy if doubt persists. **Treatment:** Ursodiol, lifelong treatment (13-15 mg/kg). Colchicine ± methotrexate for refractory cases (controversial). Cholestyramine for pruritus. Prevention and treatment of complications: EGD every 3 years (rule out varices), bone densitometry every 2 years (rule out osteoporosis). Measure TSH periodically. ADEK vitamin supplements if hyperbilirubinemia. Liver transplantation when advanced cirrhosis: hyperbilirubinaemia or Mayo risk score elevation: R = 0.871 x log$_e$ (bilirubin/17) + -2.53 x log$_e$ (albumin) + 0.039 x age + 0.881 x log$_e$ (INR) + 0.859 x (edema score : 0, 0.5 or 1). Easy calculation on the WEB. http://depts.washington.edu/uwahep/calculations/rscoreoriginal.htm **Prognosis:** 15-20 years of survival on average. Survival ↓ if bilirubin increases.
Primary Sclerosing Cholangitis (PSC)	Inflammatory obliteration of intra and extrahepatic bile ducts. Especially in young men. Often associated with inflammatory bowel disease. Asymptomatic (90%) or recurring episodes of cholangitis (abdominal pain, icterus, fever, pruritus). Can progress to cirrhosis. **Complications:** Steatorrhea and malnutrition, intra-hepatic lithiasis, cirrhosis, cholangitis, cholangiocarcinoma, colon cancer. **Diagnosis:** MRCP ± ERCP. **Treatment:** Ursodiol: lifelong treatment (20-30 mg/kg) but effectiveness not proven. Cholestyramine for pruritus. Prevention and treatment of complications. ERCP and cytology ± dilation if dominant stricture. Liver transplantation when advanced cirrhosis. **Prognosis:** mean survival = 12 years.
Liver Disease in Pregnancy	**Cholestasis of pregnancy:** Onset during 3rd trimester. Icterus and ↑ alkaline phosphatase. Can have an impact on the fetus. Treatment: ursodiol ± cholestyramine for pruritus. Fetal monitoring. Induction when baby shows enough maturity. **HELLP Syndrome:** Associated with preeclampsia. Onset after 20th week. Diagnosis: Hypertension, abdominal pain, hemolysis, elevated liver enzymes and thrombocytopenia. Risk of hematoma, infarct, hepatic rupture. Treatment = same as for preeclampsia. Deliver as soon as possible based on mother's condition. **Acute fatty liver of pregnancy:** Hepatocellular dysfunction with coagulopathy and encephalopathy in the 3nd trimester. Diagnosis: ↑ INR, ↓ fibrinogen. ↓ glycemia and ↑ ammonia can occur. Treatment: deliver as soon as possible based on mother's condition.

Cirrhosis

Symptoms: generally asymptomatic. Otherwise, anorexia, nausea, vomiting, abdominal pain, dysmenorrhea, erectile dysfunction, hematemesis.
Signs: spider nevi, palmar erythema, parotid hypertrophy, testicular atrophy, Dupuytren's contracture, gynecomastia, glossitis, icterus, ascites, lower limb edema, ecchymosis, asterixis, hepatosplenomegaly, Terry's nails, muscular atrophy, caput medusa.

Causes	– Toxins: Alcohol 45% (micronodular). – Infections: Hepatitis B, C, D (macronodular). – Medication: Methotrexate, methyldopa, isoniazid, amiodarone. – Metabolic: Non alcoholic fatty liver disease, hemochromatosis, Wilson's disease, α-1 antitrypsin deficiency. – Autoimmune: Primary biliary cirrhosis, autoimmune hepatitis. – Cardiovascular: right-sided heart failure, constrictive pericarditis, Budd-Chiari, veno-occlusive disease. – Biliary: Primary sclerosing cholangitis, biliary strictures, chronic pancreatitis, cystic fibrosis. – Cryptogenic.
Workup	**Etiology**: – AST, ALT, alkaline phosphatase, bilirubin; hepatitis B and C serology; ferritin, transferrin saturation (hemochromatosis); ANA, anti-smooth muscle antibodies, anti-LKM antibodies (autoimmune hepatitis); antimitochondrial (PBC); protein electrophoresis (α-1 antitrypsin deficiency, ↑ IgG); ceruloplasmin (Wilson's); abdominal ultrasonography. – Liver biopsy to be considered if etiology still undetermined. **Hepatic function** (severity): – INR, albumin, bilirubin. – When in doubt: Liver-spleen scan. **Complications**: – CBC (hypersplenism); electrolytes, creatinine; abdominal ultrasonography and portal vein Doppler (ascites, thrombosis, hepatocellular carcinoma); α-fetoprotein (hepatocellular carcinoma); gastroscopy (varices).
Severity	**Child-Pugh criteria** *(see table below)*

Points	1	2	3
Bilirubin (μmol/L)	< 35	35-50	> 50
Serum albumin (g/L)	> 35	28-35	< 28
PT extended by (s)	< 4	4-6	> 6
or INR	< 1.7	1.7-23	> 2.3
Encephalopathy (grade)	Absent	1-2	3-4
Ascites	Absent	Mild/moderate	Severe/refractory

5-6 points: Child A.
7-9 points: Child B.
10-15 points: Child C.

MELD score (*Model for End-stage Liver Disease*):
R = 3.8 log$_e$ (bilirubin/17) + 11.2 x log$_e$ (INR) + 9.6 x log$_e$ (creatinine/88.4) + 6.4.

Easy calculation on the WEB:
Http://depts.washington.edu/uwhep/calculations/meldscore.htm

Management	1. Treat causal factor when possible
	2. Treat complications (ascites, encephalopathy, etc): see below.
	3. Prevent or screen complications:
	– Beta-blockers with esophageal and/or gastric varices (see Variceal hemorrhage).
	– α-fetoprotein and abdominal ultrasonography every 6 months (screen hepatocellular carcinoma) if candidate.
	– Hepatitis A and B vaccination.
	4. Liver transplantation based on MELD score or with Child C cirrhosis or complication refractory to medical treatment. Must be < 65 years and abstinent from alcohol for > 6 months.
Complications	Secondary to hepatocellular dysfunction, systemic shunt or portal hypertension.
Ascites	Every new or decompensated ascites must be tapped for diagnosis (unless ovarian cancer suspected).

(continuation of Ascites cell)

Workup on ascites:
- **Albumin**: Calculate **S**erum-**A**scites **A**lbumin **G**radient (SAAG) (= serum albumin - ascitic fluid albumin):
  - ≥ 11g/L = portal hypertension: cirrhosis, hepatitis, heart failure, acute liver failure, Budd-Chiari, venoocclusive disease, portal vein thrombosis, etc.
  - < 11g/L: carcinomatosis, tuberculosis, pancreatitis, nephrotic syndrome, etc.
    Note: 4% have "mixed" ascites with gradient of ≥ 11g/L.
- **Amylase, triglycerides**: pancreatic, chylous ascites.
- **White cell count with differential**: if > 0.250 polymorphonuclear x 10^9/L = spontaneous bacterial peritonitis (see below).
- **Cultures**: in blood cultures bottles (aerobes and anaerobes).
- **Cytology**.

Treatment:
1. Evacuating paracentesis if ascites voluminous or under strain. IV albumin when ≥ 5 L ascites is withdrawn (benefits not formally proven).
2. Na^+ restriction (90 mmol/d). Fluid restriction if Na^+ < 126 mEq/L (up to 1 L/d).
3. Stop or avoid NSAIDs.
4. Diuretic: Start a combination of spironolactone 100 mg/furosemide 40 mg daily. Target 0.5-1.0 kg/d weight loss. If weight loss less than optimal, double diuretics as needed up to a maximum of spironolactone 400 mg/furosemide 160 mg. Amiloride if painful gynecomastia with spironolactone. Watch for dehydration (hepatorenal syndrome).

Refractory ascites: If no response to maximum dose of diuretics or increasing creatinine with diuretics:
1. Verify compliance to diuretics and sodium restriction. Na/K ratio on urine or Na^+ urinary measure on 24 h urine collection can be useful.
2. Repeated paracentesis vs TIPS (transjugular intrahepatic portosystemic shunts).
3. Consider liver transplantation if candidate.

Prognosis: 50 % survival at 2 years.

Spontaneous Bacterial Peritonitis	Occurs in 10-20 % of cirrhotic patients. Mortality = 20 %. Patient at risk if proteins in ascites < 10 g/L. Symptoms of abdominal pain, fever, ↑ volume of ascites, progressive encephalopathy, general condition worsening. Sometimes only subtle symptoms. **Diagnosis:** Paracentesis: > 0.250 polymorphonuclears (PMN) x 10^9/L is diagnostic. Culture ⊕ 90 % (E. coli, pneumococcus more frequent: 1 single germ as a rule). Blood cultures ⊕ in 50 %. **Treatment:** 1. Cefotaxime or ceftriaxone for at least 5 days. 2. Albumin 1.5 g/kg on day 1 and 1 g/kg on day 3. 3. Control paracentesis in 48 h if evolution less than optimal. If ↓ PMN < 50 %, reevaluate antibiotics and consider secondary peritonitis. 4. Secondary prevention with norfloxacin, ciprofloxacin or trimethoprim/sulfamethoxazole. Start once IV antibiotics are stopped.
Encephalopathy	Secondary to ammonia ± hypersensitivity to GABA or ↑ endogenous benzodiazepines. Asterixis, altered level of consciousness: ↑ ammonia level (but not sensitive): typical EEG abnormalities. **Precipitating factors:** Dehydration (diuretics, paracentesis, uremia, etc) alkalosis, hypokalemia, hypoxemia, infection, ↑ protein intake (gastro-intestinal bleeding, transfusion, constipation, etc), narcotics, hypnotics, sedatives, deteriorating liver function (alcohol, hepatitis, progressive liver disease, etc), hepatocellular carcinoma, portosystemic shunt (TIPS, surgical, spontaneous), etc. **Grade:** 0: normal; 1: personality changes, decreased attention, abnormal sleep; 2: lethargy, moderate confusion; 3: somnolent, marked confusion; 4: coma. **Treatment:** 1. Look for precipitating factors and treat them. 2. Look for other causes of depressed level of consciousness (alcohol, intoxication, subdural hematoma, etc). 3. Restrict protein 0.8-1 g/kg. 4. Avoid sedatives, narcotics, tranquilizers. 5. Lactulose 30 mL tid-qid PO or IR for 2-4 stools/day. 6. Antibiotic therapy (neomycin, metronidazole) if resistant to above treatment. Sodium benzoate (3 g tid), ornithine aspartate ? 7. Liver transplantation if indicated for chronic and refractory cases.

Variceal Hemorrhage	Massive GI bleeding. Causes 50% of upper GI bleeding episodes in cirrhotic patients.
	
	Primary prophylaxis:
	Gastroscopy for all cirrhotic patients at diagnosis.
	– When no varices: repeat gastroscopy every 2-3 years.
	– When varices present, assess risk of rupture (criteria: varices ≥ II/IV, Child B or C, red wale marks on the varices):
	  - No criteria: no treatment. Repeat gastroscopy every 1-2 years.
	  - ≥ 1 criterion: non-selective beta-blockers for ↓ pulse of 25 %.
	  - Endoscopic variceal ligation if intolerant to beta-blockers or very high risk of rupture.

	Treatment:
	1. Ventilatory and hemodynamic support treatment (A-B-C).
	2. Correct coagulopathy as needed (fresh frozen plasma).
	3. IV octreotide perfusion for 5 days (bolus of 50 μg and perfusion of 50 μg/h).
	4. Gastroscopy for diagnosis and treatment: Variceal ligation (sometimes sclerotherapy). Blakemore Tube if bleeding persists despite ligation.
	5. Treat and prevent complications:
	   - Avoid excessive hydration (keep Hb 90-100 g/L).
	   - Lactulose to prevent hepatic encephalopathy.
	   - Peritoneal tap. Norfloxacin (or IV ceftriaxone) for 7 days (spontaneous bacterial peritonitis).
	   - Thiamine, multivitamins (vitamin deficiency).
	   - Watch for alcohol withdrawal.
	6. Think of secondary prevention (see below).
	
	If recurrence after a 1st endoscopic treatment: Try a 2nd ligation session.
	If recurrence after a 2nd endoscopic treatment:
	– Child A: Surgical shunt or TIPS.
	– Child B or C: TIPS and/or liver transplantation if candidate.
	
	Secondary prophylaxis:
	– Ideally, completely eradicate varices through several endoscopic ligation sessions. Then annual gastroscopy and ligations as needed, if varices recur.
	– Add beta-blockers ± nitrates if not already received as part of primary prevention.
	– Evaluation for liver transplantation is recommended for Child B or C cirrhosis after a variceal hemorrhage.
	If recurrence despite optimal secondary prophylaxis:
	– Child A: Surgical shunt or TIPS.
	– Child B or C: TIPS and/or liver transplantation if candidate.
	
	Prognosis: 8% immediate mortality, 50 % mortality at 6 weeks, 60 % mortality at 2 years.

Hepatorenal Syndrome	Functional kidney failure caused by a hepatocellular dysfunction.
	Precipitating factor: excessive diuresis, paracentesis, and spontaneous bacterial peritonitis.
	
	Criteria:
	– Cirrhosis with ascites.
	– Serum creatinine > 133 μmol/L.
	– No improvement after 2 days of
	    o Diuretic withdrawal
	    o Volume expansion with albumin (1g/kg/d)
	– Absence of shock or nephrotoxic medication.
	– Absence of proteinuria (< 500 mg/d) or hematuria (< 50 RBC/field).
	– Normal kidney ultrasound.
	
	Treatment:
	1. Arterial vasoconstrictors (midodrine 10 mg PO tid) + octreotide (200 μg s/c tid) + albumin (1 g/kg day 1 then 50 g daily) for 5-15 days. Effective in 2/3 of cases.
	2. Liver transplantation if candidate ± TIPS.
	3. Hemodialysis only when candidate for transplantation.

| Hepatocellular Carcinoma | Usually with cirrhosis due to HBV, HCV, hemochromatosis, alcohol, α1-antitrypsin deficiency.
Metastases to lymph nodes, lungs, bones, and brain.
Paraneoplasic syndromes: Hypercalcemia, polycythemia, hypoglycemia, clubbing, gynecomastia.
Screen with α-fetoprotein (AFP) and abdominal ultrasound every 6-12 months for the cirrhotic patients (benefit not proven). AFP ↑ in only 50 % of hepatocellular carcinoma.

Treatment:
Surgery possible if tumor < 5 cm or ≤ 3 nodules of < 3 cm.
– Child A: partial hepatectomy if tumor limited to only one lobe. Otherwise, transplantation.
– Child B or C: liver transplantation.

Palliative treatment if tumor has an extrahepatic extension or patient not candidate for surgery or transplantation: intra-tumoral alcohol injection, radio-frequency ablation, embolization ± chemoembolization, chemotherapy. |
| Other Complications | Portal vein thrombosis, hepatopulmonary or hepatorenal syndrome, anemia, hemorrhagic or infectious tendency, hydrothorax, malnutrition, gonad dysfunction, etc. |

Acute Pancreatitis	
Overview	Pathophysiology: "auto-digestion" of pancreas. Pancreatitis can be interstitial (85 % of cases) or necrotizing (15 % of cases).
Clinical findings	Prolonged upper abdominal pain (± dorsal irradiation), nausea, vomiting, ± fever. Icterus if choledocholithiasis (rarely because of compression secondary to edema). Shock, Cullen's or Grey Turner's sign if severe.
Causes	1. **Lithiasis** 45 %. 2. **Alcohol** 35 %. 3. **Metabolic**: Hypertriglyceridemia (> 11 mmol/L), hypercalcemia, methanol intoxication, etc. 4. **Traumatic**: Post-ERCP, post-surgery, post-trauma. 5. **Medication**: Ergotamine, tetracycline, L-asparaginase, azathioprine, 6-mercaptopurine, sulphonamides, 5-ASA, metronidazole, furosemide, methyldopa, pentamidine, didanosine, valproic acid, estrogen, thiazides, nitrofurantoin, etc. 6. **Obstructive**: Pancreas divisum, cancer, Wirsung's stenosis, sphincter of Oddi dyskinesia. 7. **Infectious**: Mumps, coxsackies, HIV. 8. **Genetic**: Hereditary pancreatitis, cystic fibrosis of the pancreas, mutation of CFTR gene, SPINK gene. 9. **Ischemic**: SLE, vasculitis, shock, cholesterol embolism, post cardiopulmonary bypass, etc. 10. **Idiopathic:** 10-15%.
Diagnosis	**Diagnostic criteria:** 1- Amylase and/or lipase > 3 x normal without any other evident cause. 2- Typical abdominal pain of an acute pancreatitis. 3- Characteristic abnormalities on CT. If ≥ 2 criteria present = acute pancreatitis. If < 2 criteria: May be acute pancreatitis but assess for other potential diagnoses.

	Differential diagnosis:
	– ***Hyper-amylasemia***: Pancreas (neoplasia, pseudocyst, chronic pancreatitis), intestine (perforation, ischemia, Crohn's), gastro-duodenal ulcer, esophageal rupture, bile ducts (cholecystitis, choledocholithiases), ovarian or fallopian tube disease, opiates, vomiting, salivary glands, diabetic ketoacidosis, renal failure, macroamylasemia.
	– ***Hyperlipasemia***: Pancreas (neoplasia, pseudocyst, chronic pancreatitis), intestine (perforation, ischemia, Crohn's), gastro-duodenal ulcer, esophageal rupture, bile ducts (cholecystitis, choledocholithiases), opiates, vomiting, salivary glands, renal failure, macrolipasemia.
Workup	– Lipase and/or amylase.
	– CBC, electrolytes, BUN, creatinine, glycemia, AST, ALT, alkaline phosphatase, bilirubin, LDH, ionized calcium, triglycerides, C-reactive protein at 72 h.
	– Plain abdominal film (ileus), abdominal ultrasonography (bile ducts).
	– Dynamic abdominal CT at 48-72 hours if severity criteria or Ranson $\geq$ 3 or APACHE II $\geq$ 8 (to assess if interstitial vs necrotizing pancreatitis and local complications).
	Balthazar-Ranson CT Grading Scale:
	Grade A: Normal pancreas.
	Grade B: Pancreatic enlargement.
	Grade C: Inflammation involving pancreas and peripancreatic fat.
	Grade D: Single fluid collection or phlegmon.
	Grade E: Two or more fluid collections or phlegmons.
	Necrosis probable if grade D or E
Severity criteria	**Organ failure:** Shock (BP systolic < 90 mmHg), renal failure (creatinine > 200 μmol/L), respiratory failure (PaO_2 < 60 mmHg) or GI hemorrhage (> 500 mL/24 h) **and/or**
	Local complication: Pancreatic necrosis, pancreatic abscess or pseudocyst.

Criteria predictive of severity

$\Rightarrow$ **Ranson's criteria:**

	Lithiasic pancreatitis	Non-lithiasic pancreatitis
Upon admission:		
– Age	> 70 yrs	> 55 yrs
– Leukocytes	> 18 000/μL	> 16 000/μL
– Glycemia	> 12.2 mmol/L	> 11.1 mmol/L
– LDH	> 400 U/L	> 350 U/L
– AST	> 250 U/L	> 250 U/L

$\Rightarrow$ **Ranson's criteria:**

	Lithiasic pancreatitis	Non-lithiasic pancreatitis
After 48 hours:		
– $\downarrow$ Hct	> 10%	> 10%
– $\uparrow$ BUN	> 0.7 mmol/L	> 1.8 mmol/L
– Calcemia	< 2 mmol/L	< 2 mmol/L
– PaO_2		< 60 mmHg
– Base deficit	> 5 mEq/L	> 4 mEq/L
– Fluid sequestration	> 4 L	> 6 L

Mortality: < 3 criteria: 1-5%; 3-5 criteria: 10%; > 5 criteria: > 50%

$\Rightarrow$ **APACHE II score**: if $\geq$ 8, severe, or if $\uparrow$ within first 48 hours.

$\Rightarrow$ **Hematocrit:** If Hct $\geq$ 44-47 % upon admission and/or absence of $\downarrow$ Hct after 24 hrs = 50 % risk of necrosis. Otherwise, very low risk of necrosis.

Treatment	**Mild pancreatitis** (usually interstitial):
	– Treat cause.
	– Nil by mouth, IV ranitidine, nasogastric tube if nausea, IV fluids 150-200 mL/h, analgesia.
	– Resume feeding after 24 h without pain (and no analgesia).
	
	Severe pancreatitis (often necrotizing):
	– Treat cause.
	– Intensive care with oximetry, cardiac, urinary ± pulmonary monitoring.
	– Hydration 250-300 mL/h (adjust with central line as needed).
	– Oxygen.
	– Nil by mouth, IV ranitidine, nasogastric tube, analgesia.
	– Jejunal feeding (if impossible, total parenteral nutrition).
	– Prophylactic antibiotic (imipenem) with necrotizing pancreatitis documented generally not recommended (controversial). Could be acceptable in a necrotizing pancreatitis associated with fever, leukocytosis and/or target organ failure while waiting for culture results.
	– Gastroenterology + surgical consultation.
	– Early ERCP (< 72 hours) if severe lithiasic pancreatitis and associated biliary obstruction (hyperbilirubinemia).
	– After 7 days, if worsening state, repeat CT with needle aspiration of necrosis.
	   o Continue with medical treatment if sterile necrosis.
	   o Surgical debridement of infected necrosis (in 33% of necrotizing pancreatitis). Surgery to be performed according to patient's condition. Ideally, as late as possible.
	   o Surgical treatment of sterile necrosis can be indicated if patient's condition worsens and becomes critical despite optimal medical treatment **or** target organ failure that persists after 4 weeks **or** painful re-feeding with persistence after 4 weeks.

Complications	– **Local:** Acute fluid collections, pancreatic necrosis, abscess, biliary obstruction, intestinal or splenic necrosis, gastro-intestinal bleeding, splenic vein thrombosis. – **Systemic:** Organ failure (kidney ± lung ± heart ± encephalopathy). – **Delayed:** Pseudocyst (10-20 %): Treatment by internal drainage (surgical or endoscopic) if symptomatic.
Prognosis	Average mortality = 5 %. If interstitial pancreatitis, mortality of 3 %; necrotizing pancreatitis 17 %. If sterile necrosis 12 %, infected necrosis 30 %.

Chronic Pancreatitis

History	– Abdominal pain, constant or recurring (10-20 % without pain). – Weight loss secondary to ↓ uptake, malabsorption, diabetes, etc. – Endocrine and exocrine insufficiency (80-90 % destruction necessary).
Causes	– **Toxic-metabolic:** Alcohol (70-80 %), medication, hypertriglyceridemia, hypercalcemia, chronic kidney disease. – **Idiopathic** 10-20 %. – **Genetic:** Hereditary pancreatitis, CFTR gene, SPINK gene mutation. – **Autoimmune:** Autoimmune pancreatitis, Sjögren, inflammatory bowel disease, etc. – **Recurrent** (pancreatitis): Multiple episodes of acute pancreatitis or severe pancreatitis. – **Obstructive:** Wirsung's stenosis, pancreas divisum, tumor, sphincter of Oddi dyskinesia, etc.

Workup	– Imaging studies (more accessible and more commonly used):
	    Abdominal X-ray (calcifications). Abdominal CT.
	    Magnetic Resonance Pancreatography (MRP) vs endoscopic ultrasonography vs ERCP when previous tests non-diagnostic.
	– Functional tests (less used because less accessible):
	    Secretin or cholecystokinin stimulation test (gold standard).
	    Bentiromide test (less sensitive).
	    Fecal elastase, serum trypsinogen level.
	    Measure fecal fat (non specific).

Treatment	1. Stop alcohol + smoking.
	2. If malabsorption: Pancreatic enzymes (e.g.: Cotazym ECS-20® 1-3 co with meals and 1 with snacks).
	3. If diabetes: Insulin.
	4. If pain:
	  - Analgesia: Non-narcotic. Consider narcotics if pain refractory.
	  - Proton pump inhibitors (↓ pancreatic secretion).
	  - Try non-coated pancreatic enzymes (Viokase-16 tablets: 4 tablets with meals and 2 with snacks).
	  - Trial of anti-oxydant (Selenium, vitamin A, E, C, methionine).
	  - Surgery if refractory pain and dilated Wirsung's duct (Puestow procedure).
	  - If refractory pain and normal Wirsung's duct: Celiac block vs octreotide vs endoscopic drainage vs resection surgery vs long-term narcotics.

Complications	– Exocrine insufficiency (malabsorption). – Endocrine insufficiency (diabetes). – Drug addiction. – Pseudocysts (25%): Surgical drainage vs endoscopic if symptomatic (pain). – Duodenal ulcer: Caused by ↓ HCO_3 secretion in duodenum. Treatment: PPI. – Increased risk of pancreatic malignancy. – Other: Splenic vein thrombosis, duodenum or bile ducts obstruction, stenosis of the small intestine or colon, pancreatic ascites, pleural effusion, pseudoaneurysm, etc.

Chapter 3   Gastroenterology

Useful References: GASTROENTEROLOGY

Achalasia: Am J Gastroenterol 1999; 94: 3406-12 (ACG Guidelines)
Acute Abdominal Pain: Med Clin N Am 2006; 90: 481-503 (review article)
Acute Abdominal Vascular Disorders: Med Clin N Am 2008; 92: 627-47 (review article)
Acute Cholecystitis with Lithiasis: N Engl J Med 2008; 358: 2804-11 (review article)
Acute Liver Failure: Med Clin N Am 2008; 92: 761-94 (review article)
        Hepatology 2005; 41: 1179-97 (Guidelines)
Ascites: N Engl J Med 2004; 350: 1639-45 (review article)
        Hepatology 2009; 49: 2086-2107 (AASLD Guidelines)
        Gut 2006; 55 (Suppl 6): vi1-vi12 (Guidelines)
Barrett's Esophagus: Am J Gastroenterol 2008; 103: 788-797 (ACG Guidelines)
        Lancet 2009; 373: 850-61 (review article)
        Gastroenterology 2004; 127: 310-30 (review article)
Budd-Chiari Syndrome: N Engl J Med 2004; 350: 578-85 (review article)
Celiac Disease: Lancet 2009; 373: 1480-93 (review article)
        N Engl J Med 2007; 357: 1731-43 (review article)
        Gastroenterology 2006; 131: 1977-80 (AGA Guidelines)
Choledocolithiasis, Cholangitis, Biliary Pancreatitis: Med Clin N Am 2008; 92: 925-60 (review article)
Cholestasis: Am J Gastroenterol 2000; 95: 1130-38 (review article)
C. difficile Colitis:
        Cleve Clin J Med 2006; 73: 187-197 (review article)
        … Recurrent: Gastroenterology 2006; 130: 1311-16 (review article)
        … Fulminant Infection: Am J Gastroenterol 2008; 103: 3195-3203 (review article)
Cirrhosis: Lancet 2008; 371: 838-51 (review article)
        Med Clin N Am 2008; 92: 839-60 (review article)
Colorectal Polyps: N Engl J Med 2006; 355: 2551-7 (review article)
        Am J Gastroenterol 2000; 95: 3053-63 (Guidelines)
Constipation: N Engl J Med 2003; 349: 1360-68 (review article)
        Can J Gastroenterol 2007; 21: suppl B (Canadian Guidelines)
Crohn's Disease: Am J Gastroenterol 2009; 104: 465-83 (American Guidelines)
Diabetic Gastroparesis: N Engl J Med 2007; 356: 820-9 (review article)
Diarrhea:
        Acute: Am J Med 1999; 106: 670-76 (review article)
        Chronic: Gut 2003; 52 (suppl V) (Guidelines)
                Gastroenterology 1999; 116: 1461-86 (American Guidelines)
        Infectious: N Engl J Med 2004; 350: 38-47 (review article)
                Clin Infect Dis 2001; 32: 331-50 (American Guidelines)
Diverticular Disease of the colon: Lancet 2004; 363: 631-39 (review article)
        Am J Gastroenterol 1999; 94: 3110-21 (Guidelines)
Diverticulitis: N Engl J Med 2007; 357: 2057-66 (review article)
Diverticulosis - Diverticulitis: Am J Gastroenterol 2008; 103: 1550-56 (review article)
Drug-Related Hepatotoxicity: N Engl J Med 2006; 354: 731-9 (review article)
Dyspepsia: Gastroenterology 2003; 125: 1219-26 (review article)
        CMAJ 2000; 162 (Suppl 12): S3-23 (Canadian Guidelines)
        Gastroenterology 2005; 129: 1753-1755 (AGA Guidelines)
Dysphagia: Can J Gastroenterol 1998; 12: 409-13 (review article)
        … Oropharyngeal: Gastroenterology 1999; 116: 452-54 (Guidelines)
        … Esophageal: Gastroenterology 1999; 117: 229-232 (Guidelines)
Esophageal Motility Disorders: Lancet 2001; 358: 823-8 (review article)
Esophageal Spasms: Am J Gastroenterol 2008; 103: 450-457 (review article)
Esophageal Varices: Am J Gastroenterol 2007; 102: 2086-2102 (ACG Guidelines)
        Hepatology 2007; 46: 922-38 (AASLD Guidelines)
        Gastroenterology 2004; 126: 1860-67 (review article)
        N Engl J Med 2001; 345: 669-681 (review article)
Fecal Incontinence: N Engl J Med 2007; 356: 1648-55 (review article)
Functional Dyspepsia: Gastroenterology 2004; 127: 1239-55 (review article)
Gastrointestinal Perforation and Acute Abdomen:
        Med Clin N Am 2008; 92: 599-625 (review article)
Gastroesophageal Reflux Disease: N Engl J Med 2008; 359: 1700-7 (review article)
        Gastroenterology 2008; 135: 1383-91 (AGA Guidelines)
        Am J Gastroenterol 2005; 100: 190-200 (ACG Guidelines)
        Can J Gastroenterol 2005; 19:15-35 (Canadian Guidelines)

Gastrointestinal Bleeding:
    Lower, acute: Can J Gastroenterol 2001; 15: 509-521 (review article)
    Upper, nonvariceal: Med Clin N Am 2008; 92: 511-50 (review article)
        Can J Gastroenterol 2004; 18: 605-9 (Canadian Guidelines)
    Occult: N Engl J Med 1999; 341: 38-46 (review article)
        Gastroenterology 2000; 118: 197-200 (American Guidelines)
Helicobacter pylori: N Engl J Med 2002; 347: 1175-86 (review article)
    Am J Gastroenterol 2007; 102: 1808-1825 (ACG Guidelines)
    Can J Gastroenterol 1999; 13: 213-7 (Canadian Guidelines)
Hemochromatosis: Lancet 2007; 370: 1855-60 (review article)
    N Engl J Med 2004; 350: 2383-97 (review article)
    Hepatology 2001; 33: 1321-28 (Guidelines)
Hemorrhoids: Gastroenterology 2004; 126: 1461-2 (Guidelines)
Hepatic Encephalopathy: Am J Gastroenterol 2001; 96: 1968-76 (American Guidelines)
    Med Clin N Am 2008; 92: 795-812 (review article)
Hepatitis:
    Alcoholic: N Engl J Med 2009; 360: 2758-69 (review article)
    Autoimmune: N Engl J Med 2006; 354: 54-66 (review article)
        Hepatology 2002; 36: 479-97 (Guidelines)
    A: Lancet 1998; 351: 1643-49 (review article)
    B: Lancet 2009; 373: 582-92 (review article)
        Can J Gastroenterol 2007; 21: 5C-24C (Canadian Guidelines)
        … Management: Ann Intern Med 2009; 150: 104-110 (NIH Guidelines)
        … Treatment: N Engl J Med 2008; 359: 1486-500 (review article)
            Ann Intern Med 2009; 150: 111-124 (NIH Guidelines)
    C: CMAJ 2006; 174: 649-59 (review article)
        Gastroenterology 2004; 126: 1409-15 (review article)
        Can J Gastroenterol 2007; 21: 25C-34C (Canadian Guidelines)
        Hepatology 2009; 49: 1335-1374 (AASLD Guidelines)
        … Acute: Lancet 2008; 372: 321-32 (review article)
        … and HIV : Clin Infect Dis 2008 ; 47 : 94-101 (review article)
    Viral Hepatitis and HIV: N Engl J Med 2007; 356: 1445-54 (review article)
Hepatocellular Carcinoma: Am J Med 2007; 120: 194-202 (review article)
    Lancet 2003; 362: 1907-17 (review article)
Hepatopulmonary Syndrome and Portopulmonary Hypertension:
    N Engl J Med 2008; 358: 2378-87 (review article)
    Lancet 2004; 363: 1461-68 (review article)
Hepatorenal Syndrome: N Engl J Med 2008; 358: 2378-87 (review article)
    Gut 2007; 56: 1310-18 (review article)
Inflammatory Bowel Disease: Gut 2004; 53 (suppl V) (Guidelines)
        N Engl J Med 2002; 347: 417-29 (review article)
    Diagnosis: Gastroenterology 2007; 133: 1670-89 (review article)
    Treatment: Gastroenterology 2006; 130: 935-9 (review article)
    Infliximab: Can J Gastroenterol 2004; 18: 503-8 (Guidelines)
    … and Pregnancy: Gut 2006; 55: 1198-1206 (review article)
Irritable Bowel Disease: N Engl J Med 2008; 358: 1692-9 (review article)
        Am J Gastroenterol 2009; 104: S1-S35 (ACG Guidelines)
    Treatment: N Engl J Med 2003; 349: 2136-46 (review article)
Liver and Pregnancy: Am J Gastro 1999; 94: 1728-32 (review article)
Liver Biopsy: Hepatology 2009; 49: 1017-44 (AASLD Guidelines)
    N Engl J Med 2001; 344: 495-500 (review article)
Liver Enzyme Alteration: CMAJ 2005; 172: 367-79 (review article)
    Gastroenterology 2002; 123: 1364-66 (review article)
    N Engl J Med 2000; 342: 1266-71 (review article)
Liver Transplantation: Med Clin N Am 2008; 92: 861-88 (review article)
Nausea and Vomiting: Gastroenterology 2003; 125: 586-90 (review article)
Nonalcoholic Fatty Liver Disease: Clev Clin J Med 2008; 75: 721-8 (review article)
    CMAJ 2005; 172: 899-905 (review article)
Noncardiac Chest Pain: Am J Gastroenterol 2001; 96: 958-68 (review article)
    Can J Gastroenterol 1998; 12: 401-7 (review article)
NSAID-Related Ulcer - Prevention: Am J Gastroenterol 2009; 104: 728-38 (ACG Guidelines)
Pancreatitis:
    … Acute: Am J Gastroenterol 2006 ; 101 : 2379-2400 (ACG Guidelines)
        Gastroenterology 2007; 132: 2019-21 & 2022-44 (AGA Guidelines)
        Lancet 2008; 371: 143-52 (review article)
        N Engl J Med 2006; 354: 2142-50 (review article)
    … Acute Necroziting: N Engl J Med 1999; 340: 1412-17 (review article)

... Auto-immune: N Engl J Med 2006; 355: 2670-6 (review article)
... Biliary: Gastroenterology 2003; 125: 229-35 (review article)
... Chronic: Gastroenterology 2007; 132: 1557-1573 (review article)
         Lancet 1997; 350: 1379-85 (review article)
... Recurrent: Am J Gastroenterol 2001; 96: 2540-55 (review article)
Peptic-Ulcer Disease: Lancet 2002; 360: 933-41 (review article)
         Am J Gastroenterol 2002; 97: 2950-61 (review article)
... Bleeding Peptic Ulcer-Management: N Engl J Med 2008; 359: 928-37 (review article)
Portal Hypertension: CMAJ 2006; 174: 1433-43 (review article)
Primary Biliary Cirrhosis: N Engl J Med 2005; 353: 1261-73 (review article)
         Hepatology 2009; 50: 291-308 (AASLD Guidelines)
Primary Sclerosing Cholangitis: Am J Gastroenterol 2002; 97: 528-34 (Guidelines)
Small Bowel and Colon Obstruction: Med Clin N Am 2008; 92: 575-97 (review article)
Spontaneous Bacterial Peritonitis: Clin Infect Dis 1998; 27: 669-76 (review article)
         J Hepatol 2000; 32: 142-153 (review article)
Toxic Megacolon: Am J Gastroenterol 2003; 98: 2363-71 (review article)
Ulcerative Colitis: Inflamm Bowel Dis 2006; 12: 972-78 (Guidelines)
         Am J Gastroenterol 2004; 99: 1371-85 (ACG Guidelines)
Vascular disorders of the liver: Hepatology 2009; 49: 1729-64 (AASLD Guidelines)
Whipple's Disease: N Engl J Med 2007; 356: 55-66 (review article)
         Hepatology 2003; 37: 1475-92 (Guidelines)
Wilson's Disease: Hepatology 2008; 47: 2089-2111 (AASLD Guidelines)
         Lancet 2007; 369: 397-408 (review article)

Chapter 4

General Internal Medicine

Shock	
\multicolumn{2}{l}{State of tissue hypoperfusion leading to cellular dysfunction and multisystem failure.}	
Clinical findings	Markers of shock : • Hypotension: Mean BP < 65 mmHg if acute or ↓ of mean BP > 40 mmHg if prior hypertension. • Oliguria. • Encephalopathy. • Tachycardia. • Metabolic acidosis.

Classification	**C**ardiogenic:
	  Arrhythmia, cardiomyopathy, acute valvular disease, septal/ventricular rupture.
	Hypovolemic:
	  Hemorrhagic, capillary leak, dehydration, third space.
	Obstructive:
	  Tension pneumothorax, pericardial disorders (cardiac tamponade, constriction), myxoma, mural thrombus, valvular stenosis, pulmonary circulatory disorders (embolism, pulmonary hypertension).
	Distributive:
	  Septic, adrenal, anaphylactic, neurogenic, toxic, vasodilator medication, systemic mastocytosis.

Workup	CBC, INR, aPTT, electrolytes, glucose, creatinine, lactate, arterial or venous blood gas, CK-MB, troponin, blood cultures, urinalysis, ECG, chest X-ray. If needed: AST, ALT, toxicologic screening, TSH, Ca^{++}, albumin, DIC workup, cortisol, ACTH stimulation test, echocardiography… according to clinical findings.

Hemodynamic workup	Resistance ↓ Cardiac index↑	Mixed	Resistance ↑ Cardiac index ↓
	Septic Anaphylactic Neurogenic Toxic Adrenal Drugs		Cardiogenic (CVP ↑ Wedge ↑) Hypovolemic (CVP ↓ Wedge ↓) Obstructive

Management	Liberal fluid administration: 20 cc/kg bolus if hypotension and noncardiogenic cause. Oxygen 100%. Mechanical ventilation if needed. Urinary catheter. Arterial line. Cardiac monitoring. Levine tube as needed, if gastric bleeding suspected. Central access (± catheterization of the pulmonary artery - Swan-Ganz, especially for cardiogenic shock or etiology?) for optimization of filling pressure with crystalloids and/or colloids. Treatment according to cause : – If cardiogenic shock due to ischemia: coronary angiography STAT, especially if < 75 years old. Early coronary revascularisation appropriate if possible. Thrombolysis if not candidate for invasive treatment. Intra-aortic balloon pump useful if shock does not respond quickly. – If cardiogenic shock due to bradyarrhythmia: pacemaker. – If cardiogenic shock due to pulmonary embolism: consider thrombolysis or surgery. – If septic shock: see Sepsis table. – If distributive shock of adrenal origin: steroids. – If anaphylactic shock: see Anaphylaxis table. – If toxic shock: supportive, drainage if needed and antistaphylococcus or streptococcus antibiotics.

	Vasopressors (see appendix). $NaHCO_3$ if needed (role?). Mitigated response to vasopressors in severe acidosis. Avoid hypotensive medication. Prophylaxis: antithrombotic, anti-stress ulcer, bed 30-45 ° if intubated … Note: if no response to amines, suspect relative adrenal failure, measure cortisol ± ACTH stimulation test and give steroids (especially in a context of septic shock).

Anaphylaxis

Immunological reaction induced by the release of mediators of mastocytes or basophils after exposure to a specific allergen.

Reaction said to be "anaphylactic" if IgE-mediated or "anaphylactoid" if not IgE-mediated (but clinically undistinguishable)

Clinical findings	Generalized reaction occurring within minutes following the exposure (but sometimes up to 1 hour post-exposure) with multisystem manifestations: - Cutaneous: diaphoresis, erythema, pruritus, urticaria, angioedema, maculopapular eruption... - Cardiovascular: tachycardia, hypotension, arrhythmia, ischemia, cardiac arrest. - Upper and lower respiratory tract: congestion, stridor, laryngeal edema, cough, obstruction, dyspnea, bronchospasm, cyanosis, respiratory arrest. - Neurological: weakness, dizziness, syncope, seizure (rare). - Ocular: pruritus, conjunctival erythema, tearing. - Gastrointestinal: nausea, vomiting, abdominal pain, diarrhea. Typically 2 phases: an initial phase, followed by a second phase in 20% 1-8 hours later, sometimes even more severe than the initial phase. Can even occur up to 72 hours later. Steroids minimize this second phase.
Causes	– Foods: eggs, milk, nuts, fish, shellfish and molluscs … Cause 1/3 of cases. – Venoms and saliva: hymenoptera, ants – Antibiotics: penicillin, cephalosporins, vancomycin, ciprofloxacin – Aspirin and NSAIDs. – Other drugs: iron, mannitol, methylprednisolone, opiates, protamine, ACEI, streptokinase, succinylcholine, vaccines – Latex (occasional cross reactions with kiwis, bananas, pineapples… More frequent in patient with spina bifida). – Contrast media (1/100 000 fatal). – Blood products or seminal fluid. – Physical factors (cold, heat, exercise). – Idiopathic: most frequent cause.
Differential diagnosis	– Loss of consciousness: vasovagal reaction, seizure, myocardial infarction/arrhythmia… – Acute respiratory failure with asthma, aspiration, embolism… – Disorders resembling anaphylaxis: systemic mastocytosis, carcinoid syndrome, use of monosodium glutamate or with certain fish, pheochromocytoma, hereditary angioedema, hereditary or acquired C1 esterase inhibitor deficiency. – Nonorganic diseases: hyperventilation, panic attack, Münchausen, vocal cord dysfunction.
Management	– Intramuscular adrenalin 0.3-0.5 mL diluted 1:1000 every 5-15 min until improvement (s/c or endotracheal possible, IV 1:10 000 if severe hypotension, under cardiac monitoring). – Stabilisation of *Airway, Breathing, Circulation* as usual. Oxygen. Open an intravenous access + liberal fluid administration (1-2 L rapidly). Trendelenburg's position as

| | needed.
– Other treatments: diphenhydramine (Benadryl®) 25-50 mg IV every 4-6 hours as needed + ranitidine 50 mg IV every 8 hours, as needed.
– Methylprednisolone 125 mg IV or Prednisone 50 mg PO (to ↓ recurrence) and every 6 hours as needed.
– Continue diphenhydramine + Prednisone regular for 4 days after the discharge.
– Bronchodilators as needed if bronchospasm. Vaponefrine® (0.5-0.75 mL) if laryngeal edema.
– Other vasopressors (dopamine, noradrenalin) if refractory to adrenalin.
– If use of beta-blockers: give glucagon (1 mg IV slowly, then 1-5 mg/h: nausea + vomiting occasional).
– Tourniquet or injection of adrenalin at the site if needle, insect sting or drug.

Observation for 24 hours in hospital ideally before discharge.
Warn the patient that he must be observed closely for 72 hours post-anaphylaxis and to come back to hospital quickly if recurrent symptoms.

Prescribe Twinject®, Epipen® or Anakit® and Medic-Alert bracelet at discharge.

Referral to an allergist on an outpatient basis (for identification of causative agent with allergy test ± possible desensitization with penicillin or hymenoptera).

Avoid if possible use of beta-blockers, ACEI, ARB, monoamine oxidase inhibitor and tricyclic antidepressants.

If allergy to iodine and radiological examination necessary: prophylactic treatment with Prednisone 50 mg 13h, 7h and 1h before + diphenhydramine 50 mg 7h and 1h before + ranitidine 150 mg 13h and 1h before the exam. |

Fatigue

Accounts for 1 to 3 % of GP consultations.
Organic cause responsible for 10 % of cases seen in primary care.

Can be classified as recent if < 1 month, persistent if > 1 month, chronic if > 6 months.

To be distinguished from muscular weakness (of neurological origin).

| Causes | - Nonorganic: depression, fibromyalgia, panic attack, anxiety disorder, somatoform disorder, eating disorder, bipolar disease, psychosis ...

- Organic:
    - Inflammatory: polymyalgia rheumatica, vasculitis (temporal arteritis...), connective tissue disease (Rheumatoid arthritis, inflammatory myositis...).
    - Toxicological: medications (β-blockers, sedatives, antihistamines...), alcohol or drugs, heavy metal intoxication.
    - Endocrinological: hypo-hyperthyroidism, diabetes, adrenal failure, Cushing's disease, menopause, andropause, panhypopituitarism...
    - Metabolic: hypo-hypercalcemia, hypo-hyperphosphemia, anemia, acute or chronic renal failure, hepatic insufficiency...
    - Neoplastic.
    - Cardiopulmonary: heart failure, COPD ...
    - Degenerative: dementia, amyotrophic lateral sclerosis, multiple sclerosis, myasthenia gravis, Parkinson's disease...
    - Infectious: endocarditis, tuberculosis, infectious mononucleosis, CMV, HIV, hepatitis, Lyme disease...
    - Sleeping disorder: apnea, insomnia, narcolepsy, nocturnal asthma ...
    - Orthostatic hypotension.

- Idiopathic: chronic fatigue syndrome (see below), idiopathic chronic fatigue. |

Workup	Primary importance of the history and physical exam to search for other more specific symptoms/signs in order to guide the workup; isolated fatigue reduces the probability of a specific etiology.
	In the absence of other specific symptoms/signs, do: CBC, electrolytes, glucose, creatinine, CK, TSH, liver enzymes, Ca^{++}, PO_4^{3-}, total protein, albumin, urinalysis, sedimentation rate or C-reactive protein, appropriate screening test for age and sex (e.g.: mammography).
	If needed, according to clinical evaluation: Monotest, cortisol, protein electrophoresis, rheumatoid factor, ANA, HIV, PPD, blood cultures, serology for Lyme disease, testosterone (if sexual dysfunction), chest X-ray, abdominal ultrasound ...
	Psychiatric evaluation, if needed.

Chronic Fatigue Syndrome

Unknown cause.
Prevalence 0.3-1 %. More frequently women, mainly between 30-40 years old, of all ethnic groups.
Frequent association with fibromyalgia, irritable bowel syndrome, chronic anxiety, migraine.

Diagnostic criteria	Criteria from *Centers for Disease Control* (1994) :
	
	- Persistent fatigue, unexplained, not relieved by rest and leading to a reduction of professional, social or personal activity for at least 6 months.
	and
	- Presence of at least 4 of the symptoms listed below for at least 6 months, the appearance of which did not precede the fatigue:
	   – Impaired memory or concentration sufficiently important to provoke a marked reduction of the usual activities of the patient.
	   – Sore throat.
	   – Tender cervical or axillary lymph nodes.
	   – Muscle pain.
	   – Pain in several joints without synovitis.
	   – New headache.
	   – Unrefreshing sleep.
	   – Post-exertional malaise lasting ≥ 24 hours.
	
	Exclusion criteria: medical condition causing fatigue, bipolar disorder, major depressive disorder, psychosis, dementia, anorexia or bulimia, alcoholism, or substance abuse, severe obesity (BMI ≥ 45).
	
	The chronic fatigue syndrome is a diagnosis of exclusion.
	If the chronic fatigue does not fulfill the criteria of the syndrome, use the term "idiopathic chronic fatigue".

Workup	Bio-psycho-social evaluation and mental exam. Search for prior depression or relationship disorders, trigger events, course over time, medications, and occupational history. Workup: CBC, electrolytes, sedimentation rate, glucose, creatinine, BUN, ALT, alkaline phosphatase, Ca^{++}, PO_4^{3-}, proteins, albumin, TSH, urinalysis. The remaining: as needed, according to clinical evaluation. The workup serves to eliminate an organic cause. No test is diagnostic.
Treatment	Reassure and inform (educate) the patient. Regular physical activity. Maintain healthy sleeping habits. Keep working (limit sick leave to ≤ 1 month if possible). Close follow-up by a primary care physician. If needed: consultation with psychologist or psychiatrist.

	Psychotherapy (behavior therapy) as needed. To consider, especially if other treatments fail. Medication according to symptoms: try drug for at least 4-8 weeks. – If muscular pain: tricyclic antidepressants (amitriptyline), clonazepam (if muscular spasm), cyclobenzaprine or carisoprodol (maximum 3 weeks) ... – If sleeping disorder: improve sleeping habits. Medication if non pharmacologic treatment ineffective; trazodone, tricyclic antidepressants (amitriptyline, nortriptyline). – If affective symptoms: antidepressants (tricyclic or SSRI). Consider antidepressants even in absence of symptoms.

Arterial Hypertension

Risk factor for coronary heart disease, heart failure, stroke, peripheral arterial disease, renal failure, dementia, and atrial fibrillation.

Affects 27 % of Canadians 35-64 years old, and more than 50 % of patients > 65 y.o.
Isolated systolic hypertension affects mainly patients who are ≥ 50 y.o.

Causes	**Essential (≥ 95 %):** typically after 30 years old, exacerbated by obesity, alcohol, tobacco, NSAIDs, polycythemia.
	
	Secondary causes:
	Renovascular disease:
	  - Suspect in patients with: sudden onset or worsening of hypertension in patient < 30 years old or > 55 years old, presence of abdominal bruit, hypertension resistant to ≥ 3 drugs, rise in serum creatinine level associated with use of ACEI/ARB or in patient with other atherosclerotic vascular disease or recurrent pulmonary edema associated with hypertensive surges.
	  - Young woman = fibromuscular dysplasia; elderly patient = atherosclerosis, cholesterol embolism, arterial dissection.
	  - Diagnosis: captopril-enhanced radioisotope renal scan (but less useful in patients with chronic renal failure), Doppler ultrasound, MRI/CT-angiography, renal angiography (gold standard): Measure of creatinine clearance and of proteinuria useful.
	  - Treatment:
	    - Medical: equivalent to angioplasty for control of the BP in atherosclerotic stenosis?
	    - Percutaneous angioplasty if stenosis > 50-70 % and kidney > 8 cm: especially useful for fibromuscular dysplasia, or if need of ≥ 3 antihypertensive agents to control hypertension, if ↑ creatinine or if loss of renal function on renal scan or history of "flash pulmonary edema": prognosis postangioplasty: 50-60 % have BP lowering, 1/6 have acute renal failure. Especially useful if index of resistance < 0.8 on renal Doppler (controversial).
	    - Surgery: bypass rarely done. Nephrectomy if severe hypertension not controlled by drugs and kidney < 8 cm.
	    - Treatment of atherosclerosis risk factors + ASA.
	Renal disease: secondary to parenchymal diseases, polycystic kidneys, post-transplantation (cyclosporine), etc.
	Primary hyperaldosteronism: see Adrenal disorders table.
	Secondary hyperaldosteronism: Secondary to hypercortisolism, renal artery stenosis, severe hypertension.
	Cushing disease - ectopic ACTH: See Adrenal disorders Table.
	Pheochromocytoma: See Adrenal disorders table.
	Coarctation of the aorta: See Aortic disorders table.
	Pregnancy
	Hypercalcemia
	Hypo-hyperthyroidism
	Intracranial hypertension
	Sleep apnea
	Drugs: Oral contraceptive, NSAIDs (including COX-2 specific), alcohol,

	sympathomimetics (anti-cold drugs), sibutramine, steroids, cocaine, amphetamines, ecstasy, phencyclidine, erythropoietine, cyclosporine, tacrolimus, bevacizumab, midodrine, bromocriptine, venlafaxine, MAOI + tyramine, secondary to drug withdrawal (beta-blockers, clonidine), natural products (sea salt, licorice, Ma Huang, ephedra, etc)
	
	Rule out "white-coat" hypertension (hypertension noted at the office but not ambulatory). Rule out pseudo-hypertension (uncommon: secondary to arterial calcification: on elderly patient: Osler maneuver (sometimes present).
	"Masked" hypertension: with ambulatory hypertension and normal blood pressure in general practitioner's office; risk seems to be identical to sustained hypertension.
	
	Causes of **severe** arterial hypertension:
	   - Essential 50 %.
	   - Central nervous system disease (subarachnoid hemorrhage, intracranial hemorrhage, stroke, trauma).
	   - Cardiac disease (ischemia, aortic dissection, post-CABG).
	   - Acute renal failure.
	   - Others: eclampsia, epistaxis, post-op, catecholamine excess (pheochromocytoma, MAOI, intoxication), serotoninergic syndrome, drug withdrawal (beta-blockers, clonidine).

Classification	American (JNC 7) :
	   - Normal: SBP < 120 and DBP < 80 mmHg.
	   - "Prehypertension": SBP 120-139 or DBP 80-89 mmHg.
	   - Hypertension:
	       - grade 1 : SBP ≥ 140-159 or DBP ≥ 90-99 mmHg.
	       - grade 2 : SBP ≥ 160 or DBP ≥ 100 mmHg.
	
	– Malignant hypertension = grade 4 retinopathy (papilledema).
	– Hypertensive emergency: target organ dysfunction (encephalopathy, nephropathy, infarction, angina, dissection, intracranial hemorrhage, preeclampsia): immediate treatment for urgent BP lowering.
	– Hypertensive urgency: no target organ dysfunction: rapid treatment for BP lowering over a few hours (see below) …

Diagnosis	A diagnosis of arterial hypertension is made: – After a first consultation if features of hypertensive emergency. – After a second visit in presence of target organ damage, chronic renal failure, diabetes or if BP is ≥ 180/100 mmHg or – On third visit if BP is between 160-179/100-109 mmHg*. – Otherwise, wait for 5 visits with BP ≥ 140/90 mmHg before making a diagnosis of hypertension. * Various methods can be used to establish the diagnosis: Office BP, home BP (if BP ≥ 135/85 mmHg) or with an ambulatory blood pressure monitoring (ABPM) (if BP ≥ 135/85 mmHg during day time or ≥ 130/80 mmHg over a 24 hour period), assuming that equipment and technique are reliable.
Target organ damage	- Atherosclerotic coronary disease. - Left ventricular hypertrophy. - Heart failure. - Stroke, including transient cerebral ischemia and vascular dementia. - Peripheral arterial disease. - Hypertensive nephropathy. - Hypertensive retinopathy. - Other asymptomatic atherosclerotic diseases.

Workup	To screen for secondary causes, evaluate target organ damage and other cardiovascular risk factors:
	- Basic workup: Na^+, K^+, creatinine, glucose, lipids, urinalysis, ECG.
	- As needed, according to clinical evaluation: CBC, renal ultrasound, microalbuminuria, chest X-ray, echocardiography, calcium, uric acid, TSH, etc.
	Note: If hypertension and ↓ K^+ with diuretics: consider secondary hyperaldosteronism (severe hypertension, Cushing, ectopic ACTH, exogenous steroids, renovascular disease...), primary hyperaldosteronism, licorice...
Management	- Oriented physical exam: measure bilateral BP and sitting/standing BP, peripheral pulses (coarctation) - Osler's sign - fundi - heart - vascular (bruits, pulses...) - lungs, summary neurological exam.
	- Evaluate urgency.
	- Identify the other cardiovascular risk factors in order to evaluate patient's global cardiovascular risk.
	- Assess for secondary cause if history or physical exam is suggestive, if poor response to treatment, systolic BP > 180 mmHg and/or diastolic > 110 mmHg or sudden worsening of hypertension.
	- Assess for target organ damage.
	- Ambulatory BP monitoring as needed (especially if suspicion of white-coat effect).
	- Home BP Monitoring by the patient as needed (especially if non-adherence, diabetes, chronic renal failure, white-coat effect or masked hypertension): use valid apparatus: target BP < 135/85 mmHg.
Treatment	Canadian consensus (2009) :
	Targets values for blood pressure: SBP < 140 mmHg and DBP < 90 mmHg.
	For patients with diabetes or CKD, target BP < 130/80 mmHg.
	Treat if average SBP > 160 or DBP > 100 mmHg.
	Strongly consider treatment if SBP ≥ 140 mmHg or DBP ≥ 90 mmHg, especially with target organ damage or other risk factors. If diabetes, start treatment if SBP ≥ 130 or DBP ≥ 80 mmHg.
	Nonpharmacological treatment:
	– ↓ alcohol (≤ 14 standard drinks per week for men; ≤ 9 standard drinks per week for women: one standard drink = 13.6 g ethanol = 45 mL spirits (40%), 150 mL 12% wine, 360 mL 5% beer).
	– ↓ weight (aim for a body mass index between 18.5-25 kg/m^2).
	– Physical exercise (moderately intense 30-60 minutes 4-7 times a week).
	– Sodium restriction (limited to 65-100 mmol/day).
	– "Healthy" diet based on fruits, vegetables, low in fat and cholesterol (type *Dietary Approaches to Stop Hypertension - DASH*).
	– Control stress management.
	Pharmacological treatment:
	Class of antihypertensive agents to be individualized according to associated conditions:
	- **Systolo-diastolic** hypertension without compelling indications: thiazide diuretics, beta-blockers (except for patient ≥ 60 years old), long-acting calcium channel blockers, ACEI (except for black patients), ARB.
	- **Isolated systolic** hypertension without compelling indications: thiazide diuretics, long-acting dihydropyridine calcium channel blockers, ARB.
	- With angina: Beta-blockers. ACEI (except in low-risk patient). Long action calcium channel blockers also useful.
	- With prior myocardial infarction: beta-blockers + ACEI, ARB if ACEI-intolerant.
	- With systolic heart failure: ACEI + beta-blockers. Spironolactone in patient with NYHA class III-IV/IV. Other diuretics if needed. ARB if ACEI-intolerant or combined with ACEI if BP not controlled.
	- With left ventricular hypertrophy: does not affect initial treatment recommendations. Avoid hydralazine/minoxidil.

	- Past stroke or TIA: ACEI/diuretic combinations.
	- With diabetes :
	    - And microalbuminuria/proteinuria : ACEI or ARB
	    - Without microalbuminuria: ACEI, ARB, dihydropyridine calcium channel blocker
	      or thiazide diuretics.
	- With nondiabetic chronic kidney disease with proteinuria: ACEI (ARB if ACEI-intolerant).
	  Diuretics as additive therapy (if CKD and fluid overload, use aldosterone blocker
	  diuretic).
	- With renovascular disease: be careful with ACEI and ARB (risk with bilateral or
	  unilateral disease with solitary kidney).
	
	Note: it seems that the efficacy of the antihypertension treatment depends more on the magnitude of pressure lowering rather than on the class used.
	
	- Combination treatment often necessary in hypertension: combine thiazide diuretics or
	  calcium channel blockers with beta-blocker, ACEI or ARB. A combination treatment
	  may be considered if BP is > 20/10 mmHg above treatment target but caution should
	  be exercised.
	- If not controlled by different combinations, add alpha-blocker, centrally acting agents or
	  other classes if needed.
	
	- A statin is recommended for a hypertensive patient with evidence of atherosclerotic
	  disease or if > 40 years old with ≥ 3 of the following cardiovascular risk factors: male, ≥
	  55 years old, LVH, abnormal ECG, peripheral arterial disease, past TIA/stroke,
	  microalbuminuria/proteinuria, diabetes, tobacco, familial history of early CAD, ratio
	  total cholesterol/HDL ≥ 6.
	
	- Consider low dose of aspirin for primary prevention in a hypertensive patient (especially
	  if > 50 years old) with controlled blood pressure.
	
	Treatment of hypertensive crisis:
	    IV treatment favored if hypertensive emergency or malignant hypertension:
	    PO treatment for hypertensive urgency with:
	        Nitroprusside IV, Nitroglycerine IV, Enalaprilat: IV, Clonidine PO, Nifedipine PA
	        PO, Captopril PO, Hydralazine IV or PO …

Follow-up	Ideally, the patient undergoing nonpharmacological treatment should be seen every 3-6 months or more frequently if needed. The patient submitted to pharmacological treatment should be re-examined every 1-2 months or more frequently as needed, until the BP is normal on 2 consecutive visits then every 3-6 months. Consultation with a specialist is to be considered for resistant hypertension (not controlled by 3 antihypertensive agents of which one is a diuretic) or if hypertension remains uncontrolled with target organ damage or comorbidity.

Arterial Hypertension and Pregnancy	
Definition	Diastolic BP (DBP) ≥ 90 mmHg, on at least two measurements (Korotkoff phase V). If systolic BP (SBP) ≥ 140 mmHg, follow closely for development of diastolic hypertension. Severe hypertension if SBP ≥ 160 or DBP ≥ 110 mmHg (confirmed after 15 minutes). BP taken in the sitting position, with manual device (most of automated BP machines underestimate BP, especially in presence of preeclampsia).
Classification	1. Pre-existing hypertension: hypertension before pregnancy or diagnosed before 20 weeks' gestation. - Essential. - Secondary: hyperthyroidism, substance abuse, pheochromocytoma, renal artery stenosis or renal disease, coarctation of the aorta, etc. - With comorbid conditions: diabetes, nephropathy, vascular or cerebrovascular disease, or an indication for antihypertensive therapy outside pregnancy. - With preeclampsia: if resistant hypertension (≥ 3 antihypertensive agents), new or worsening proteinuria, or ≥ 1 other adverse conditions (see below). 2. Gestational hypertension: hypertension diagnosed after 20 weeks' gestation. - With comorbid conditions. - With pre-eclampsia: With ≥ 1 other adverse conditions: maternal symptoms (persistent or new/unusual headache, visual disturbances, persistent abdominal or right upper quadrant pain, severe nausea or vomiting, chest pain or dyspnea), maternal signs of end-organ dysfunction (eclampsia, severe hypertension, pulmonary edema, or suspected placental abruption), abnormal maternal laboratory testing (elevated serum creatinine; elevated AST, ALT or LDH with symptoms; platelet count <100 x 10^9/L; or serum albumin < 20 g/L), or fetal morbidity (oligohydramnios, intrauterine growth restriction, absent or reversed end-diastolic flow in the umbilical artery by Doppler velocimetry, or intrauterine fetal death). and/or New-onset proteinuria ≥ 0.3 g/d. Severe preeclampsia with onset before 34 weeks' gestation, with heavy proteinuria (3-5 g/d according to other international guidelines), or with one or more adverse conditions. Note: Preeclampsia before 20 weeks of gestation can occur with molar pregnancy or antiphospholipid syndrome.
Differential diagnosis	SLE, TTP, HUS, primary nephropathy, catastrophic antiphospholipid syndrome, acute fatty liver of pregnancy, etc.
Epidemiology	- Pre-existing hypertension: 1 % of all pregnancies. - Gestational hypertension: 5-6 % of all pregnancies. If before 34 weeks, 35 % risk of developing preeclampsia. - Preeclampsia: 1-2 % of all pregnancies. Preeclampsia: among the 3 main causes of maternal mortality and first cause of peri-natal mortality; can occur post-partum (usually up to 7-10 days, theorically up to 6 weeks).
Clinical findings Preeclampsia	Clinical manifestations: see adverse conditions (above) + edema, important especially upper limb and face, retinal arteriolar vasospasm, clonus. Maternal complications: eclampsia (convulsion: 10 % without hypertension and without proteinuria, 10 % with isolated proteinuria), hemorrhagic or ischemic stroke, acute renal failure with oligoanuria, hepatic failure, hepatic hematoma or rupture, pulmonary edema, heart failure, HELLP syndrome. Fetal complications: prematurity, IUGR, oligohydramnios, placental abruption, in-utero

	death.
	Risk factors: MAJOR: primiparity or ≥ 10 years between pregnancies, age ≥ 40 years, past history (especially if early) or family history of preeclampsia, pre-existing hypertension (15-20% risk of preeclampsia), renal disease, diabetes (type 1 > 2 >> gestational diabetes), BMI ≥ 35, antiphospholipid syndrome, multiple pregnancy. MINOR: Other thrombophilia, fetal abnormalities, SLE, black race, non-smoker, triglycerides ↑, early CAD family history, < 2 year interval between pregnancies, reproductive technics, primipaternity, cocaine/amphetamine use, trophoblastic disease, excessive weight gain during pregnancy.

Workup	Workup necessary for pre-existing hypertension: creatinine, potassium, urinanalysis.
	
	Workup necessary to rule out preeclampsia.
	- **CBC**: hemoconcentration supports preeclampsia. Hemolysis with schistocytes = HELLP. Thrombopenia. Neutrophilic leukocytosis.
	- INR, aPTT, D-Dimer, fibrinogen (search for DIC if thrombopenia or placental abruption).
	- **AST + ALT**; LDH: if HELLP suspected. Bilirubin ↑ if hemolysis or hepatic dysfunction.
	- **Proteinuria**:
	   • **Urinalysis**: Sensitivity of 50 %, especially with low level of proteinuria. Unreliable for diagnosis, screening only in low risk population. High suspicion if ≥ 2 +.
	   • **Proteinuria 24 h**: diagnostic (≥ 0.3 g/d).
	   • **Urine spot** for proteins/creatinin ratio: diagnostic ≥ 30 mg/mmol. Quantification less reliable.
	- **Uric acid**: abnormal > 300 µmol/L. Can increase early, could be prognostic.
	- **Creatinine**: abnormal > 70 µmol/L.
	- **Albumine**: < 20 g/L is an adverse condition (see above).
	- **Glucose**: for differential diagnosis of acute fatty liver of pregnancy.
	- **Fetal monitoring:** (non-stress test, biophysical profile, fetal movements, Doppler of umbilical arteries, measuring of amniotic fluid, fetal growth)

Management	Indications for hospitalization: severe hypertension or severe preeclampsia.
	Consider hospitalization or hospital day unit/ home care management (for non-severe cases) in order to make a diagnosis (serial BP, blood and urinary workup), evaluate severity, exclude associated diseases, evaluate fetal well-being.
	Transfer to a tertiary center to be considered if severe and/or prematurity.
	
	For gestational hypertension or preeclampsia:
	- Hospitalization with BP every 15 minutes to 4 hours, daily weight. Rest + evaluation of symptoms and serial lab (from every day to every 6 hours, according to severity).
	- Ambulatory management possible after initial intrahospital evaluation if hypertension or preeclampsia ARE NOT SEVERE, if patient reliable and lives nearby. Restricted activity. Measure BP. Daily fetal movement counts, report new symptoms immediately, medical evaluation ≥ 1x/week, daily verbal contact, fetal monitoring and serial workups.
	
	Preeclampsia:
	The only cure = delivery (vaginal not necessarily contraindicated, according to emergency or obstetrical indications).
	- Fetus at term (> 37 weeks) or non-viable (< 23 weeks) = consider immediate delivery.
	- If > 34 weeks and severe = delivery.
	- If 34-36 weeks and non-severe = assess maternal-fetal risk vs fetal benefit.
	- If < 34 weeks and non-severe = expectant management in perinatal centres.
	- If < 34 weeks and severe = ≥ 24 h with MgSO₄, antihypertensive treatment, steroids for acceleration of fetal pulmonary maturity; consider delivery if:
	   • Uncontrolled severe hypertension development of a severe adverse condition, premature labor, rupture of membranes, fetal distress (variable decelerations or repeated late decelerations, bio-physical profile ≤ 4).
	   • Neonatal benefit demonstrated: 2 weeks gain in utero (but without ↓ neonatal mortality), without any maternal risk of ↑ eclampsia.

Antihypertensive treatment for non-severe hypertension	**Pre-existing hypertension**: If on antihypertensive agents pre-conception, 3 options: 1) Replace medication before conception with medication known to be safe during pregnancy (Continuation of ACEI/ARB may sometimes be considered until conception if nephropathy is progressing despite good BP control). 2) Continuation of on-going medication as long as not contraindicated. 3) Stop medication during first trimester and follow BP closely. Normal physiology of pregnancy causes ↓ 10-15 mmHg during 2nd trimester: thus, medication can often be stopped during pregnancy. **Treatment threshold/targets:** controversial. - For non-severe hypertension: Early treatment prevents only the progression toward severe hypertension (but not to preeclampsia nor abruptio placentae). - In short and long term, there is no increased risk of cardiovascular events if BP is less well controlled during the 9 months of pregnancy. Possible ↑ risk of low birth weight infant with lower BP targets. - Treatment threshold: always treat if ≥ 160/110 mmHg, certainly treat if > 155/105, or if > 140/90 and comorbidity. - Target BP: 130-155/80-105. If comorbidity: 130-139/80-89 mmHg. **Agents**: - Most commonly used: Methyldopa, labetalol (becoming the 1st choice since it is better tolerated and is more effective than methyldopa), nifedipine, other beta-blockers (pindolol, metoprolol, acebutolol, propranolol). - Other choices: thiazide, verapamil, clonidine, hydralazine + beta-blocker. - Note: ACEI and ARB contraindicated due to teratogenicity. Avoid atenolol and prazocin.
Antihypertensive treatment for severe hypertension	Confirm after 15 minutes: target < 160/110 mmHg, to avoid maternal cerebral complications; LOWER BP CAREFULLY to avoid the risks of placenta hypoperfusion and fetal distress. All agents can cause abrupt hypotension, use smaller doses since there is a state of severe hemoconcentration and vasoconstriction in preeclampsia. Fetal monitoring continued until stable BP. Transient fall in BP 30 minutes post-bolus of $MgSO_4$. Agents: - Labetalol: 10 mg IV initially up to 80 mg every 10-30 minutes (300 mg maximum): can be given as a perfusion 0.5-2 mg/min. Caution if asthma or heart failure. - Nifedipine: capsule 5-10 mg PO initial then every 30 minutes or PA 10 mg every 45 minutes, maximum 80 mg/day. Side effects: headaches, neuromuscular block if given with $MgSO_4$ (< 1 %, antidote 10 g of calcium gluconate). - IV Hydralazine 2.5 mg initially, then 5-10 mg every 30 minutes or 0.5-10 mg/hour (up to 20 mg maximum). Side effects: tachycardia, flushing, headache. If insufficient: - Diazoxide: 30 mg every 5 minutes. - IV Nitroprussiate if life-threatening hypertension: 0.25 µg/kg/min for a short period of time. Side effect: cyanide fetal toxicity.

Eclampsia treatment	Magnesium sulphate: Well documented indications: 1. Primary prevention of eclampsia in patients with severe preeclampsia: more effective than in non-severe preeclampsia (during delivery or 1st 24 hours if subsequent observation). 2. Secondary prevention if seizure and to prevent recurrence (for ≥ 24 hours) until improvement of clinical (including abundant diuresis) and laboratory parameters. $MgSO_4$ 4-6 g/50 mL D5W over 20-30 minutes, followed by 1-3 g/h. Side effects: hypotension, hyporeflexia, muscle weakness, respiratory depression. Close clinical follow-up with Mg^{++} level only if side effects vs serial Mg^{++} level: target Mg^{++} 2-3.5 mmol/L.
HELLP (*Hemolysis, elevated liver enzymes, low platelets*)	Corticosteroids (Dexamethasone or methylprednisolone) ↑ platelets and, thus, ↑ possibility of peridural anesthesia but no benefit for maternal and fetal issues. Consider platelets transfusion if < 20 x 10^9/L for vaginal delivery and < 20-50 x 10^9/L for caesarean.
Volume considerations	In severe preeclampsia: close fluid balance monitoring, minimal fluids because high risk of pulmonary edema (endothelial dysfunction, hypoalbuminaemia, $MgSO_4$, hypertension with systolo-diastolic cardiac dysfunction, etc). If oliguria and no sign of dehydration: use IV fluid with caution, no diuretics (unless pulmonary edema) and wait for reestablishment of diuresis; ↓ $MgSO_4$ or check Mg^{++} levels.
Anaesthetic considerations	Regional anesthesia: risk of fetal distress if BP drops with vasodilatation. Avoid fixed bolus fluids: phenylephrine or ephedrine as needed. Not contraindicated if on ASA. To consider if platelets > 75 x 10^9/L except in presence of coagulopathy, rapid drop in platelets, ASA or concomitant heparin. General anesthesia: higher risk of difficult/failed intubation and sudden BP increase during intubation.
Post-partum	Close BP follow-up necessary because BP peaks on days 3-6 post-partum, especially after early and severe preeclampsia. If new-onset post-partum hypertension: treat if severe (≥ 160/110) or symptoms. Consider treatment in mild-moderate hypertension. Close follow-up of maternal adverse conditions: repeat labs when necessary. Avoid NSAIDs in resistant hypertension, acute renal failure, oliguria, thrombocytopenia < 50 x 10^9/L. Consider thromboprophylaxis especially if bedrest > 4 days antepartum or caesarean. Resolution of hypertension and proteinuria usually occurs by 6 weeks but can occasionally take up to 6 months. Always make sure that the BP and laboratory data have returned to normal > 6 weeks post-partum. Evaluate for pre-existing hypertension, nephropathy, thrombophilia as needed. Breastfeeding: Best choices are: labetalol, nifedipine, methyldopa, captopril/enalapril (but ACEI to avoid if premature baby or with renal failure). Short duration of action preferable because dose adjustment easier in short and medium term (or if pre-existing hypertension: use the same treatment as before pregnancy if compatible with breastfeeding). Weekly follow-up often necessary since BP is very unpredictable.

Preeclampsia prevention	Close antenatal follow-up is the best method to early identify complications. Laboratory workup and measure of proteinuria as soon as clinical suspicion arises. Calcium 1 g/day if poor intake (< 600 mg daily/ < 2 portions of dairy products). Aspirin (75-100 mg HS) early (pre-conception, as soon as possible, at least < 16 weeks) if high risk. Consider rest at home during third trimester, reduced work duties and stress: strict bed rest harmful. Avoid weight gain between pregnancies.
Prognosis	Pre-existing hypertension: – Good prognosis in 90 % of cases. – Risk depends on the severity of hypertension, target organ dysfunction, nonobservance of the antenatal follow-ups, and especially on the presence of preeclampsia. – Perinatal mortality risk (RR 3.4), preeclampsia (15-20 % if mild hypertension, 50 % if severe hypertension), prematurity, IUGR, abruptio placentae (5-10 % if severe), renal or heart failure, stroke. Gestational hypertension and preeclampsia: – Global risk of recurrence in subsequent pregnancy: 18 % – If severe and early (< 27 weeks) preeclampsia: risk of recurrence up to 66 % of which 21 % before 27 weeks. – More frequent if underlying disease: nephropathy, thrombophilia. – Preeclampsia increases long term risk of hypertension, nephropathy, cardiac/ cerebrovascular disease, and thromboembolic events. – Counselling on healthy life style changes. Early screening for other CV risk factors?
Medications	ACEI and angiotensin receptor blockers are contraindicated because of teratogenicity. Atenolol to be avoided (could cause growth retardation). Prazocin to be avoided ($\uparrow$ stillbirths).

Name	Dose	Side effects
Methyldopa	125 mg qid $\rightarrow$ up to 2-3 g/d in 4 doses.	Headache, weakness, depression
Labetalol	100-200 mg bid up to 1200 mg/day.	Neonatal bradycardia.
Beta-blockers (pindolol > metoprolol).		Neonatal bradycardia and hypoglycemia.
Nifedipine	PA 10-20 mg PO bid-tid (max. 80 mg/day) or XL up to 120 mg.	
Hydralazine	25-50 mg PO qid	Maternal intolerance (tachycardia) if used alone, Neonatal thrombocytopenia rare.

Weight Loss	
Body weight is determined by intake, absorptive capacity, metabolism and energy expenditure. Weight loss is clinically significative if > 4.5 kg or > 5 % on a period of 6-12 months. Determine if the weight loss is voluntary (diet) or involuntary. If voluntary, is it appropriate or not (psychiatric cause).	

Causes	With appetite ↑ :
	– Hyperthyroidism.
	– Diabetes mellitus.
	– Gastrointestinal loss: malabsorption, inflammatory bowel disease …
	– Pheochromocytoma.
	– ↑ physical activity.
	
	With appetite ↓ :
	– Nonneoplasic organic causes: ≈ 40-50 %
	    • Gastrointestinal disorders: the most frequent (30-50 %) : malabsorption, obstruction, pancreatic insufficiency, peptic ulcer, gastric motility disorder or of swallowing, mesenteric or gastric ischemia, etc.
	    • Chronic disorders: cardiac, pulmonary, renal or rheumatologic.
	    • Endocrine disorders: diabetes, hyper-hypothyroidism, hypocorticism, panhypopituitarism, hyperparathyroidism, etc.
	    • Infection (chronic): endocarditis, tuberculosis, HIV, AIDS, etc.
	    • Medications and drugs : digoxin, metformin, levodopa, selective serotonin reuptake inhibitors, laxative abuse, medication side effects, alcohol, drugs (cocaine), etc.
	    • ENT disorders: dentition problems, candidiasis, loss of taste, sense of smell, etc.
	    • Neurological disorders: stroke, Parkinson, dementia, etc.
	
	– Neoplastic ≈ 20-30 %: in general, the weight loss is not isolated: 30 % digestive (colon, stomach, pancreas, hepatobiliary), lung, hematologic, breast, genito-urinary, ovarian, ENT, prostate, unknown primary, etc.
	– Psychiatric ≈ 10-20 %: depression (frequent), anorexia, anxiety, alcoholism, functional…
	– Socio-economic causes (isolation).
	– Idiopathic ≈ 5-25 %.
	
	Note: sometimes there is more than one cause, especially in elderly patient.
	
	In > 80 %, the cause is obvious after the initial clinical and laboratory evaluation.

Workup	– Document the weight loss as accurately as possible because of frequent overestimation or underestimation. – "1st line" workup: CBC, electrolytes, creatinine, liver enzymes, glucose, sedimentation rate, C-reactive protein, calcium, phosphorus, protein electrophoresis, albumin, TSH, stool for occult blood, urinalysis, chest X-ray, abdominal ultrasound, ECG. Cancer screening appropriate for age/sex (PSA, Pap test, mammography …). – "2nd line" workup to do if needed according to signs/symptoms and 1st line workup results: upper and lower GI endoscopy, malabsorption workup, fecal fat if diarrhea, blood culture, HIV, rheumatoid factor, ANA, CT thorax, abdomen … If workup negative, serious organic disease unlikely: see again in 3-6 months for follow-up. In general, if in presence of an organic cause, il will be evident within the next 6 months. – Psychology or psychiatry evaluation as needed.

Treatment	According to cause. Dietary education. Parenteral nutrition rarely useful. Drugs to increase appetite rarely useful (limited benefits).
Prognosis	Mortality at 18 months 25-30 %, in general secondary to cancer and other terminal diseases. The prognosis is good for the majority of nonneoplasic causes, including the idiopathic category, most patients having a stable weight after 30 months.

Obesity	
Overview	Body mass index (BMI) = $\dfrac{\text{weight (kg)}}{\text{height}^2\ (\text{m}^2)}$ Prevalence in Canada (2004): BMI $\geq$ 25 in 59 %, obesity in 23 %. Second risk factor responsible for the highest number of deaths after tobacco.
Causes	Complex and multifactorial: Genetics (polygenic: responsible for 40-70 %), family history, environment (diet, exercise ...), drugs (steroids, sulfonylurea, resistance to insulin, antidepressants, valproic acid, propranolol, clonidine, prazocin, progesterone, lithium, phenothiazine, clozapine, olanzapine ...), stress, metabolic and endocrine disease (hypothyroidism, insulinoma, Cushing, hypogonadism, hypothalamic damage, menopause...: cause < 1 % obesity).
Associated complications	– Cardiac: atherosclerosis, arterial hypertension, left ventricular hypertrophy, heart failure (*adipositas cordis*), valvular disease (if prior use of certain anti-obesity drugs). – Dermatologic: venous stasis, *acanthosis nigricans*. – Endocrino-metabolic: resistance to insulin, diabetes, dyslipidemia, gout, growth hormone hyposecretion, polycystic ovarian syndrome. – Gastro-enterologic: cholelithiases, nonalcoholic steatohepatitis, gastroesophageal reflux disease, "intraabdominal" syndrome. – Locomotor: osteoarthritis. – Neurological: Stroke, pseudotumor cerebri, *adiposis dolorosa*. – Oncological: breast, endometrium, ovary, esophagus, prostate, kidney, colon, pancreas, gall blader, lymphoma, leukaemia, etc. – Pulmonary: restrictive syndrome, obesity-hypoventilation syndrome, pulmonary hypertension, sleep apnea, asthma. – Other: altered immunity, dysmenorrhea, urinary incontinence, post-surgical complications, venous insufficiency, psycho-social disorders (depression).
Stages of severity	Criteria of the World Health Organisation (not applicable if patient < 18 years old or in pregnant or breast feeding women): BMI < 18.5 kg/m^2: underweight. BMI 18.5-24.9 kg/m^2: normal. BMI 25-29.9 kg/m^2: overweight. BMI 30-34.9 kg/m^2: class 1 obesity. BMI 35-39.9 kg/m^2: class 2 obesity. BMI > 40 kg/m^2: class 3 obesity (morbid obesity). For patients $\geq$ 65 years old, a normal BMI can extend to a slightly higher value than 18.5 up to a value situated in the overweight range.

Workup	Measure blood pressure. Measure waist if BMI 25-35 (among europoid man, ↑ of the risk of complications linked to obesity if ≥ 94 cm, ↑↑ of risk if ≥ 102 cm : among europoid woman ↑ of risk if ≥ 80 cm, ↑↑ of risk if ≥ 88 cm) and waist-hip ratio (↑ of risk if > 1.0 for men and > 0.8 for women). Measure lipids, glucose. According to clinic findings: TSH, urinary cortisol, hirsutism workup, FSH, LH, AST, ALT, polysomnography …

Treatment	– Aggressivity of treatment depends on severity and on associated risk.
	– Diet: evaluation by a dietitian (↓ intake by 500-1000 kcal/day).
	– Activity level: physical exercise 30 minutes 3-5 times/week …
	– Pharmacotherapy : indicated if BMI ≥ 30 or if BMI ≥ 27 with risk factors linked to obesity or comorbid conditions associated with obesity:
	  o Orlistat (Xenical®): intestinal lipase inhibitor. 120 mg tid with meals. Give lipid soluble multivitamins concomitantly. Side effects: flatulence, abdominal pain, fecal incontinence, fatty stools, especially with fat ingestion. Efficacy: ↓ weight 8-10 % after 2 years. Maximal length of the studies = 2 years.
	  o Sibutramine (Meridia®): serotonin-norepinephrine reuptake inhibitor. 10-15 mg daily. Side effects: xerostomia, headache, constipation, dizziness, insomnia, tachycardia, hypertension … Contraindicated if CAD, TIA/stroke, heart failure, arrhythmia, uncontrolled arterial hypertension, anorexia and bulimia. Efficacy comparable to orlistat. Maximal length of the studies = 2 years.
	  o Other medications under investigation: topiramate, bupropion, metformin, recombinant human leptine.
	– Bariatric surgery: if failure of medical treatment and BMI ≥ 35 with severe co-morbidities or a BMI ≥ 40. Most effective treatment currently. Complications: peri-op mortality 0.5 % depending on type of surgery, dumping syndrome, vitamin, iron, and calcium deficit, wound dehiscence, incisional hernia, infection...
	– Control of the other cardiovascular risk factors (stop tobacco, control diabetes, dyslipidemia, arterial hypertension …)
	
	Note: Maintain realistic treatment goals (5-10 % weight loss), because even such a modest weight loss is associated with risk factor benefits.

Prognosis	Morbidity and mortality are proportional to the BMI. 280 000 to 325 000 deaths/year attributable to obesity in the USA.

Intoxications	Poison Control Centre 1-800-463-5060 (Québec)
Overview	Of vital importance in the care of the overdose patient is to rapidly initiate supportive care and to recognize the toxic agents that require specific therapy (elimination, antidote). Review patient's history in order to determine which drug was taken, at what time, in what quantity ... from patient, family, friend or paramedic according to case. Don't forget over-the-counter drugs or alcohol. On physical exam: vital signs, mental status, odor, neurological exam, cardiopulmonary exam, bowel sounds … Special attention to pupils and skin in order to identify "toxidromes".

"Toxidrome"	Pupils	Skin	Other clinical findings	Toxic agents
Sympathomimetic	Dilated	Moist	Hypertension, tachycardia, fever, anxiety	Amphetamines, cocaine, phencyclidine (PCP) ...
Anticholinergic	Dilated	Dry	Tachycardia, hypertension, fever, vomiting, agitation, ↓ peristalsis, urinary retention	Atropine, antihistamines, tricyclics ...
Cholinergic	Small	Moist	Bradycardia, diaphoresis, ↑ peristalsis, ↑ salivation, wheezing, ↑ tearing.	Organophosphates
Sympatholytic	Small	Dry	Hypotension, bradycardia, hypothermia, ↓ peristalsis, respiratory depression	Sedative, narcotics, benzodiazepines, alcohol ...
Workup	Basic workup: CBC, electrolytes, glycemia, creatinine, BUN, serum osmolality, liver enzymes, CK, calcium, phosphate, urinalysis, INR, aPTT, arterial blood gas, ethanol level, acetaminophen and salicytates levels, ECG, chest X-ray. If needed: urinary toxicologic screening, plain abdominal X-ray, specific serum drug levels. Pregnancy test for woman of child-bearing age. Calculation of 3 gaps as needed: anionic-gap, osmolar gap, oxygen saturation gap.			
Treatment	Stabilisation of *Airway, Breathing, Circulation* as usual. General approach: 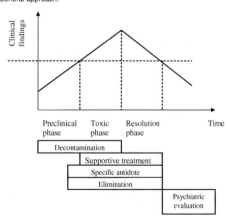 **Decontamination:** Activated charcoal: adsorbs the toxic agent and can prevent its absorption by the body. Maximum effect < 2 hours post-ingestion. Certain substances are poorly adsorbed (lithium, alcohol, magnesium). Contraindicated if peritonitis, intestinal obstruction, ileus. Initial dose: 1 g/kg (max 100 g) (ideally in water, with only 1 dose of sorbitol for the taste if taken PO). Repeated doses possible according to toxic agent (up to 3 doses every 2-4 hours).			

	– Gastric lavage: limited indications: potentially severe intoxication, with ingestion < 1 hour, substance not adsorbable by activated charcoal. Need protection of the respiratory tract. Contraindicated if risk of seizure or use of corrosive.
	– Intestinal irrigation: mechanical cleaning of the gastrointestinal tract with Golytely®. Give Golytely® 2L/hour for adult via nasogastric tube until clear rectal liquid (4-6 hours). Not a routine intervention !
	– Potential indications: ingestion of high doses of toxic substances, late presentation, use of prolonged liberation pills, agents not adsorbed by activated charcoal (lithium, iron, lead, body packing with cocaine, heroin). If vomiting, stop for 30 minutes and start over at half dose.

Supportive treatment:
– Intravenous access. Large volume fluid administration (unless contraindicated).
– Dextrose 50 % 50 mL if needed (according to capillary glycemia).
– Atropine if bradycardia of any cause.
– Noradrenaline if hypotension refractory to fluid administration, because most often distributive shock occurs.
– Thiamine 100 mg IV if alcoholism.

Specific antidotes:
– No automatic cocktail.
– Naloxone (Narcan®): antidote for opiates. Use selectively: altered mental status and 1 of the 3 following criteria: respiratory rate < 12/min, miosis, suspicion of opiates. 0.1- 2 mg IV. Caution if chronic use: risk of acute withdrawal. If pCO_2 ↑↑, risk of pulmonary edema. Short ½ life.
– Flumazenil (Anexate®): benzodiazepine antidote. Selective use: altered mental status and suspicion of use of benzodiazepines and absence of contraindications (epilepsy, use of tricyclic antidepressants or anticonvulsants, convulsive risk, head trauma). 0.2 mg IV every 30 seconds up to 5 mg. Quick action in 1-3 minutes, peak 6-10 minutes, duration of action 1 hour. Risk of recurring sedation if use of long-acting benzodiazepine.
– Other antidotes according to specific toxin (see individual agents below).

Elimination:
– According to specific toxin (urinary alkalinization, hemodialysis, hemoperfusion): (see individual agents below).

Suicide risk evaluation (psychiatric consultation if needed). Constant supervision sometimes necessary while waiting for psychiatric evaluation.

Call **Poison Control Center** (1-800-463-5060 in Québec) if needed.

Most frequent agents (in alphabetical order)	
Acetaminophen	Clinical features:
	Stage 1: (30 min - 24 h): nausea, vomiting, anorexia, sweating.
	Stage 2: (24-48 h): hepatic tenderness, jaundice, renal failure, ↑ bilirubin, INR, then AST, ALT.
	Stage 3: (48-96 h): hepatic failure, encephalopathy, coagulopathy, hypoglycemia, renal failure.
	Stage 4: (96 h - 2 weeks.): recuperation.
	Toxic dose ≥ 150 mg/kg (less if use of alcohol, isoniazide, anticonvulsants, anorexia, chronic treatment).
	See Rumack-Matthew nomogram (next page). Nomogram less reliable if time of ingestion unknown, dosage < 4 hours post-ingestion, chronic ingestion, high risk population (alcoholic, malnutrition, on P450 cytochrome inducer, glutathione deficiency).

Plasma Acetaminophen Concentration Table

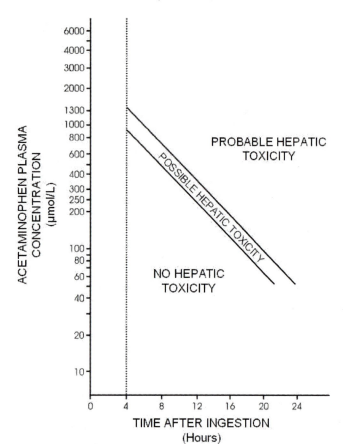

Adaptation of the Rumack and Matthew Nomogram.
(Rumack, B & H. Matthew: Acetaminophen poisoning
and toxicity. Pediatrics 55:871, 1975.)

	Follow liver function tests, INR, glycemia, creatinine. Tx: Activated charcoal (1 dose only). - IV N-acetylcysteine: o Indications: If plasma concentration > hepatotoxicity threshold: plasma level higher than 1000 µmol/L after 4 h or 200 µmol/L after 12 h (or higher than 700 µmol/L after 4 h if use of alcohol, isoniazide, anticonvulsant, anorexia, malnutrition, chronic treatment). If ingestion > 150 mg/kg and plasma concentration not available before 8 hours. If ingestion time unknown and dosage > 32 µmol/L. If evidence of hepatotoxicity and history of intoxication. o Early protocol if ingestion < 10 hours: 150 mg/kg over 45 min then 50 mg/kg over 4 hours and 100 mg/kg over 16 hours. o Late protocol if ingestion > 10 hours or if severe (> 2500 µmol/L at any time): 140 mg/kg over 60 minutes and 70 mg/kg over 60 minutes every 4 hours for 12 doses. Repeat plasma level at the end of the treatment: if still ⊕, continue treatment every 4 hours until ⊖ or restart 16 hours perfusion protocol until ⊖. If severe intoxication and hepatotoxicity: continue doses every 4 hours until diminution of liver enzymes and improvement > 20 % of INR. - Consider transfer to a liver transplantation center if APACHE II ≥ 15 (because risk of mortality ↑).
Anticholinergic - Tricyclic Antidepressants (Elavil®, Norpramine®, Sinequan®, Tofranyl®, Aventyl®, Desyrel®, Surmontil®,...) Datura. Amanita …	Toxidrome: tachycardia, dry skin, visual disorder, mydriasis, delirium, confusion, coma, hypotension. ECG: QRS > 0.10-0.12 sec, QT ↑, PR ↑, atrio-ventricular and intra-ventricular block (Bundle-branch block). Lethal dose 10-30 mg/kg. Period of observation if asymptomatic = 6 hours. Do ECG every 4 h + cardiac monitoring (until return to sinus rhythm, normal QRS and normal level of consciousness for > 24 hours). Tx: aggressive because very toxic and extracorporeal elimination inefficient (high distribution volume and significant protein binding). Delayed absorption due to anticholinergic effects: gastric lavage useful up to 12 hours post-ingestion. Entero-hepatic circulation and long half-life: give repeated doses of activated charcoal. - Cardiotoxicity via inhibition of sodium channels: - If QRS > 0.10 sec or coma: NaHCO₃ 2 ampoule/1L D5W for pH ≥ 7.5. - If ventricular arrhythmia: NaHCO₃ 1-2 mEq/kg IV → Lidocaine IV. Do not give any antiarrhythmic agents from class Ia and Ic. - If block: temporary pacemaker. - If seizures: diazepam, lorazepam, phenobarbital, propofol. NaHCO₃ IV. - If hypotension: fluids ± noradrenaline. Extracorporeal circulation if needed. - If pure anticholinergic intoxication: physostigmine.
Benzodiazepines	Toxidrome: Central nervous system depression. Tx: Gastric lavage if indicated. Activated charcoal. Supportive treatment. Flumazenil: if altered mental status and suspicion of use of benzodiazepines and absence of contraindications (epilepsy, use of tricyclic antidepressants or anticonvulsants, risk of convulsion, head trauma). 0.2 mg IV every 30 seconds up to 5 mg. Quick action: within 1-3 minutes, peak 6-10 minutes, duration of action 1 hour. Risk of recurrence of sedation if use of long-acting benzodiazepine.
Beta-blockers	Toxidrome: bradycardia, hypotension, block, bronchospasm, hypoglycemia, hyperkalemia, seizure, coma, torsades de pointe. Tx: Decontamination - Activated charcoal (multiple doses) (not useful for propranolol). Glucagon: if hypotension caused by bradycardia, cardiac depression or conduction disturbances. 2-5 mg IV over 1 min. If no effect, 5-10 mg IV over 1 minute and perfusion if needed 2-10 mg/h diluted in D5W for 5-12 hours. - If block: atropine - temporary pacemaker.

	- If hypotension: fluids.
	    Noradrenaline, adrenalin, milrinone.
	    Calcium chloride + insulin 0.1-1 u/kg/h + D5W 1 g/kg/h (check capillary
	    glycemia every 30-60 minutes).
	    If refractory hypotension: invasive monitoring + amines at very high doses.
	- If torsades de pointe: MgSO$_4$ IV.
	Caution with dopamine, adrenalin, isoproterenol.
	Hemodialysis if hydrosoluble agent (atenolol, nadolol, sotalol).
	Intra-aortic balloon pump or extracorporeal circulation as needed.

Calcium Channel Blockers	Toxidrome: hypotension, nausea, vomiting, hyperglycemia, confusion, coma, atrioventricular block. Tx: gastric lavage if indicated - charcoal - Golytely®. Fluids. - Ca^{++} gluconate 10 % (30 mL) IV or Ca^{++} chloride 10 % (10 mL) over 5 minutes, can be repeated every 15-20 min x 4 doses as needed if hypotension, bradycardia, block. Monitor serum Ca^{++}. Do not give calcium if co-intoxication with digoxin: risk of asystole. - Atropine for severe bradycardia (but ineffective if severe intoxication). - Glucagon if hypotension, block (same dose as for beta-blockers). - Adrenalin, milrinone, intra-aortic balloon pump as needed. - Insulin 0.1-1 u/kg/h + D5W 1 g/kg/h (check capillary glucose) - Hemoperfusion if use of verapamil and hepatic failure. - Temporary pacemaker if needed (not very effective)
Carbon Monoxide	Clinical findings: headache, dizziness, weakness, nausea, dyspnea, seizures, myocardial ischemia, ventricular arrhythmia, pulmonary edema, lactic acidosis, coma (according to severity of exposure). Fetus much more susceptible. Delayed neuropsychiatric sequela (3 days-6 months) post-intoxication possible, but usually reversible. Diagnosis: carboxyhemoglobin level (but does not always correlate with clinical findings). Tx: Oxygen 100 % until carboxyhemoglobin normalized. Oxygen in hyperbaric chamber if coma, if history of loss of consciousness, carboxyhemoglobin > 40 % (or > 15 % in a pregnant woman), if cardiac ischemia or arrhythmia, known CAD and carboxyhemoglobin > 20 %, if persistent symptoms after 4-6 h of normobaric oxygen, recurring symptoms for 3 weeks. Reduce neuropsychiatric sequela (still controversial).
Cocaine	Toxidrome: euphoria, anxiety, delirium, psychosis, mydriasis, tachypnea, tachycardia, chest pain, hypertension, hyperthermia, hallucinations, vomiting, chronic perforation of the nasal septum. Complications: seizure, cardiac or cerebral ischemia, arrhythmias, aortic dissection, rhabdomyolysis, DIC, renal or hepatic failure, bronchospasm, pulmonary edema, barotrauma ... Cardiac monitoring - Follow CK, INR, aPTT, liver enzymes. Tx: Charcoal. Total intestinal irrigation (Golytely®) if body packers. Treat hyperthermia if needed. - Diazepam or lorazepam. Liberal fluid administration if significant rhabdomyolysis (CK > 10 000 IU/L). - If infarction: aspirin, benzodiazepines, nitrates, heparin (beta-blockers contraindicated), calcium channel blockers. - If ventricular arrhythmia: benzodiazepines, lidocaine, defibrillation...
Digoxin	Toxidrome: GI symptoms, headaches, arrhythmia, block, ↑ K$^+$. Digoxin level can be in the therapeutic range due to slow redistribution. Tx: gastric lavage if indicated, charcoal (repeated doses because active metabolites eliminiated by biliary tract). - Antibodies (Digibind®) indicated if severe intoxication (i.e.: ingestion of > 10 mg, blood level > 6.5 nmol/L 6-8 hours post-ingestion, K$^+$ > 5.5 mmol/L, ventricular arrhythmias, bradycardia refractory to atropine, progression of cardiac or digestive

	symptoms).

	- Dose for acute intox. : 1 vial (38 mg) per 0.6 mg absorbed digoxin (= total dose ingested x 0.8).
	   If unknown quantity: give 10-20 vials over 15-30 minutes or in bolus if cardiac arrest.
	   If digoxinemia available or chronic intoxication: # vials = digoxin level (nmol/L) x weight (kg) x 0.0073.
	
	Note: Digibind® can falsely ↑ digoxin level. Can also cause hypokalemia.
	- If block: atropine - temporary pacemaker - antibodies (Digibind®).
	- If ventricular tachyarrhythmia: phenytoin, lidocaine (while waiting for Digibind®).

Ethanol	Tx: supportive.
Ethylene Glycol (antifreeze, windshield washer)	Toxidrome: State of intoxication, ataxia, seizures, cerebral edema → Heart failure, pulmonary edema → acute renal failure (oxalate crystals). Symptoms can be delayed and elevated osmolar gap present with normal anionic gap if concomitant use of alcohol. Crystalluria (Wood lamp ⊕ for oxalate crystals, but low sensitivity). Hypocalcemia. Acidosis with ↑ anionic and osmolar gap. Toxic dose: 2 mL/kg. Tx: Same as methanol except no folinic or folic acid. - Fomepizole (Antizol®) (indicated if ethylene glycol > 3.0 mmol/L or suspicion of ethylene glycol ingestion and either osmolar gap > 10 mOsm/L or metabolic acidosis or oxaluria) *or* ethanol (indicated if ethylene glycol > 3.0 mmol/L) until ethylene glycol < 1.6 mmol/L. Follow ethanol blood concentration every 8 h. - Hemodialysis if ethylene glycol > 8 mmol/L, if refractory acidosis or target organ damage or significant hypernatremia secondary to NaHCO₃, until ethylene glycol undetectable and acidosis resolved. - Thiamine 100 mg IV + pyridoxine 100 mg IV every 6 h for 24 hours until ethylene glycol level = 0 and acidosis corrected. - Treat hypocalcemia, hypoglycemia as needed. Bicarbonate as needed.
Isopropyl Alcohol (rubbing alcohol, after-shave)	Toxidrome: isopropyl alcohol induces an alteration of consciousness, including coma and cardiac depression with hypotension. Metabolized in the liver via alcohol dehydrogenase to nontoxic metabolites (acetone) eliminated by the kidney > lungs. Characteristic odor (acetone). Ketonuria, Ketonemia without metabolic acidosis. Osmolar gap ↑, euglycemia. Tx: supportive. Hemodialysis if refractory hypotension, coma or isopropanol level > 67 mmol/L or preexistent hepatic or renal failure.
Lithium	Toxidrome: tremor, ataxia, nystagmus, agitation, confusion, nausea, vomiting, diarrhea, seizure, coma, bradycardia, hypotension, nephrogenic diabetes insipidus. ECG: QT ↑. Anionic gap can be decreased. Follow lithium level, serial Na⁺ and creatinine. Tx: Total intestinal irrigation (Golytely®) 1-2 L/h (see above in overview). - Gastric lavage if indicated - charcoal ineffective. - Fluid: bolus 1-2 L NaCl 0.9 % over 2-3 hours: for volume repletion (hypovolemia is frequent). Follow electrolytes closely. - Hemodialysis if lithium level > 3.5 (with **acute** intoxication), > 2.5 mmol/L (with **chronic** intoxication), or if < 2.5 mmol/l but severe symptoms or if renal failure or significant intoxication where an increase of the plasma level is anticipated. Repeat hemodialysis until lithium level < 1 mmol/L. Caution: rebound phenomenon after stopping hemodialysis.

Methanol (wood alcohol, antifreeze, windshield washer, adulterated alcohol)	Toxidrome: State of intoxication, ataxia, confusion, headache. Visual disturbances (re: formic acid) . Occasional pancreatitis. Symptoms can be delayed and elevated osmolar gap present with normal anionic gap if concomitant use of alcohol. Acidosis with ↑ anionic and osmolar gap. Toxic dose 0.4 mL/kg. Tx:
	- Hemodialysis if methanol blood concentration > 15.6 mmol/L, if hemodynamic instability, if anionic gap > 10, severe refractory acidosis (pH < 7.1), acute or chronic renal failure, visual or mental symptoms (by doubling ethanol per-dialysis) until methanol blood concentration < 6.0 mmol/L and correction of the acidosis.
	- fomepizole (Antizol®): indicated if methanol blood concentration > 6.0 mmol/L or suspicion of ingestion with methanol and either osmolar gap > 10 mOsm/L or metabolic acidosis or HCO_3^- < 20 mmol/L until methanolia < 6.0 mmol/L.
	  or ethanol if acidosis or methanol blood concentration > 6.0 mmol/L (aiming for ethanol blood concentration 22-43 mmol/L) to stop when methanol blood concentration < 5.0 mmol/L, no acidosis, normal anion gap and no neurological symptoms.
	   - loading dose : 0.6 g/kg of ethanol solution 10 % IV :
	   - infusion : ethanol 10 % IV (mL/kg/h) :
	      for non alcoholic patients = 66 mg/kg/h : for alcoholic = 154 mg/kg/h (and double per-dialysis).
	   Follow ethanol blood concentration every 8 hours.
	- Folinic acid 1 mg/kg (max. 50 mg) IV (if symptomatic) followed by folic acid 1 mg/kg IV for everybody (max. 50 mg) every 4 h x 6 doses.
	- Bicarbonates as needed.

Narcotic - Opiates	Toxidrome: lethargy, respiratory depression, coma, adult respiratory distress syndrome, aspiration pneumonia, hypothermia, seizure, bradycardia, miosis. Tx: Gastric lavage if indicated – activated charcoal. Supportive treatment. Give naloxone 0.2-0.4 mg IV, repeat every 2-3 min. If no response and no chronic use of opiates, give 1-2 mg IV, up to 20 mg IV. - If seizure: diazepam, lorazepam.
Salicylates	Present in lots of over-the-counter products (Percodan®, Pepto-Bismol®, forest tea ...). Toxidrome : hyperventilation, tinnitus, confusion, fever, vomiting, GI hemorrhage, diarrhea, lethargy, seizure, coma, shock, adult respiratory distress syndrome , hypokalemia, renal or hepatic insufficiency, ↑ INR, hypoglycemia, respiratory alkalosis, metabolic acidosis or both. Toxic dose: < 150 mg/kg = mild intox.: 150-300 = moderate ; 300-500 mg/kg = severe. If salicylatemia = 5 mmol/L = severe intoxication. If > 7.2 mmol/L = very severe intoxication. Salicylate level every 2 hours until stable or in ↓ x 2 (erratic absorption in intoxication due to pylorospasm). Do arterial blood gas every 2 hours. Tx: gastric lavage if indicated (even if > 1 h) – activated charcoal (multiple doses) - Golytely® if coated medication. - Urinary alkalinization if salicylate level > 2.9 mmol/L: with bolus $NaHCO_3$ 1-2 mmol/kg then perfusion 3 ampoules $NaHCO_3$ /1 L D5W at 100-200 mL/h (or up to 10-15 mL/kg/h if hypovolemic) + KCl 20-30 mEq/L → target = aim for plasma pH 7.45-7.5 and urinary pH 7.5-8. Stop when blood salicylate concentration < 2 mmol/L. Avoid hypokalemia because interferes with urinary alkalinization. - Hemodialysis if salicylate level > 8.7 mmol/L initially or > 6.5 mmol/L 6h post-ingestion or if refractory acidosis, coma, seizure, fluid overload, pulmonary edema or renal failure with acute intoxication or if > 4.3 mmol/L and symptomatic with **chronic** intoxication. - Vitamin K if INR elevated. - Glucose if alteration of state of consciousness even if normal glycemia. - If intubation is inevitable, hyperventilate + +. Do not intubate in order to "avoid fatigue".

Selective Serotonin Reuptake Inhibitors (SSRIs)	Toxidrome: nausea, vomiting, dizziness, blurred vision, fever. Rarely central nervous system depression and tachycardia. Serotoninergic syndrome possible: altered consciousness, myoclonus, hyperreflexia, diaphoresis, tremor, fever, nausea, diarrhea, seizure, coma, DIC, rhabdomyolysis, hyponatremia, SIADH. More frequent if combined with MAOI or medication interacting with cytochrome P450. Also possible with MDMA ("ecstasy"), dextromethorphan, meperidine. Tx: supportive mainly + decontamination. Serotoninergic syndrome: benzodiazepines, cyproheptadine, chlorpromazine, methysergide, propranolol.
Stimulants (amphetamines, phencyclidine-PCP, ecstasy, "ice", etc)	Toxidrome: confusion, agitation, tremor, anxiety, mydriasis, tachyarrhythmia, hypertension, myocardial ischemia, hyperthermia, rhabdomyolysis, seizure, coagulopathy, renal or hepatic failure. Tx: supportive. Treat hyperthermia as needed. Adequate hydration. - If severe arterial hypertension: phentolamine 2-5 mg IV every 5-10 min - nitroprusside IV. - If tachyarrhythmia: beta-blockers (esmolol IV). - If agitation: benzodiazepine, phenothiazines, haloperidol.
Other Agents	**Barbiturates**: Alteration of consciousness, hypothermia, hypotension, cardio-respiratory depression, adult respiratory distress syndrome, coma. Tx: supportive. Urinary alkalinization with phenobarbital only. Hemoperfusion useful if coma/hypotension refractory or renal failure (controversial) **Corrosives**: Gastroscopy. Tx: water, milk as needed. **Cyanide**: venous O_2 saturation > 90 %. Severe lactic acidosis. Tx: gastric lavage - charcoal - Oxygen 100 %. Na^+ nitrite 300 mg IV in 3 min. Na^+ thiosulfate 12.5 g IV over 10 minutes. - Hydroxycobalamine 4-5 g IV. **γ-hydroxybutyrate (GHB)**: euphoria, hypothermia, hypotension, lethargy or coma with respiratory depression. Seizures or occasional muscular contractions. Quick recovery (usually < 5 hours). Detection of GHB by specialized laboratory. Tx: activated charcoal. Supportive. Physostigmine? (controversial). **Iron**: Tx: total intestinal irrigation (Golytely®). Chelation (deferoxamine) if severe: coma, shock, hemorrhage, serum level > 63 μmol/L with symptoms or > 90 μmol/L asymptomatic → start slowly to reach 15 mg/kg/h (side effects: hypotension, ARDS). Stop chelation when 3 conditions fulfilled: serum level < 32 μmol/L and normal urine, decontamination finished, and patient asymptomatic. **Isoniazide (INH)**: lactic acidosis, seizures. Tx: activated charcoal - Diazepam as needed - Pyridoxine if > 3-5 g INH (give gram = ingested gram; 5-10 g IV over 10 minutes). **Lead**: total intestinal irrigation (Golytely®) - chelation (if lead level > 2.42 μmol/L). **Methemoglobinemia**: Side effect of certain drugs (dapsone, pyridium, sulfonamides, nitrates) or hereditary, dietetic or idiopathic causes: cyanosis with normal O_2 saturation, "chocolate" blood. Tx: if symptomatic → methylene blue 1-2 mg/kg IV within 5 minutes, repeatable as needed. Contraindicated if G6PD deficiency or with renal failure. **Organophosphates**: cholinergic toxidrome. Measure acetylcholinesterase and pseudocholinesterase. Tx: atropine 2-5 mg IV over 1-2 min repeatable every 10-30 min as needed - pralidoxime 1-2 g IV, then 3-4 mg/kg/h until resolution - Hemoperfusion (for parathion). **Theophylline**: vomiting, tremors, tachycardia, arrhythmias, seizures, metabolic disorders. Serum level every 2-3 hours. Tx: gastric lavage -activated charcoal (multiple doses) - total intestinal irrigation (Golytely®) if prolonged release medication. Beta-blocker (if not bronchospastic) or nondihydropyridine calcium channel blocker or lidocaine if arrhythmia. Benzodiazepine for seizures. Hemoperfusion if seizures, refractory hypotension or refractory arrhythmia or if theophylline level > 550 μmol/L 2 h post-ingestion, if > 275 (with chronic intox.) or if > 193 (for clinically unstable patient or at higher risk of complications : > 60 years old or with hepatic or heart failure).

Thromboembolic Disease

Deep Vein Thrombosis (DVT)

Annual incidence of thromboembolic disease: about 0.1 %/year.

Risk factors (see Hypercoagulability table):
- Inherited: Protein C, Protein S or antithrombin III deficiency, resistance to activated protein C (factor V Leiden), factor II 20210A mutation, ↑ factor VIII, ↑ homocysteinemia …
- Acquired: cancer, chemotherapy, immobilization, surgery, travel, estrogen, pregnancy, nephrotic syndrome, antiphospholipid syndrome, DIC, heparin-induced thrombocytopenia, myeloproliferative syndromes, inflammatory bowel diseases, foreign body (catheter) …

Clinical findings	Pain, edema, superficial vein distension, fever. *Phlegmasia caerulea dolens* if severe venous obstruction, pain, edema and cyanosis. *Phlegmasia alba dolens* if arterial obstruction, pain, palour and edema. May-Thurner syndrome: secondary to compression of left common iliac vein by right common iliac artery and the vertebral body: DVT sometimes extensive, poorly responding to treatment or recurring. More frequent in women 20-50 years old. Paget-Schroetter syndrome: upper limb DVT, often secondary to anatomic abnormality at thoracic level, associated with repeated trauma or with upper limb exercises, occurring more frequently in a young (male/female) patient. Differential diagnosis: muscle streching or contusion, cellulitis, lymphatic or arterial obstruction, rupture of Baker cyst, reflex sympathetic dystrophy Complications: pulmonary embolism, postphlebitic syndrome (chronic venous insufficiency if thrombophlebitis above knee). Wells' criteria: for predicting pretest probability of deep-vein thrombosis: 1. Active cancer (treatment ongoing, administered within previous 6 mo or palliative): 1 point. 2. Paralysis, paresis or recent plaster immobilization of the lower extremities: 1 point. 3. Recently bedridden > 3 d and/or major surgery within previous 12 wk requiring general or regional anesthesia: 1 point. 4. Localized tenderness along the distribution of the deep venous system: 1 point. 5. Swelling of entire leg: 1 point. 6. Calf swelling > 3 cm larger than asymptomatic side (measured 10 cm below tibial tuberosity): 1 point. 7. Pitting edema confined to the symptomatic leg: 1 point. 8. Collateral superficial veins (nonvaricose): 1 point. 9. Previous documented DVT: 1 point. 10. Alternative diagnosis at least as likely as DVT: -2 points. Calculate the score: level of probability of DVT: low risk (6 %) if ≤ 1 point, high (28 %) if ≥ 2 points.
Workup	– Basic workup: CBC, electrolytes, INR, aPTT, creatinine, hepatic workup, urinalysis, chest X-ray. – D-Dimer: very sensitive but not very specific: to do if low clinical probability, in an outpatient. Could also be useful if high clinical probability and ⊖ Doppler, to exclude DVT in such cases (without proceeding to a repeat Doppler: see below). – Hypercoagulability workup as needed: indicated if idiopathic DVT and family history or age < 50 years old or DVT at an unusual site or recurrent DVT (but controversial). – Malignancy workup according to age (mammography, prostate, colonoscopy …). No proven benefit for extensive workup, but prevalence of undiagnosed cancer in unprovoked DVT is around 10 %. – Venous Doppler ultrasound: sensitivity and specificity > 95 % for proximal DVT, but less for isolated calf DVT. If test ⊖ and high clinical probability and ⊕ D-dimer, repeat Doppler in 5-7 days. – Impedance plethysmography as needed (rarely available). – Venography if uncertain diagnosis and high clinical probability or Doppler ⊕ and low

	clinical probability (rarely done).
	– MRI: sensitive and specific: could be done instead of venography.
	– If suspicion of embolism: see below.
	– If recurrence of DVT suspected: repeat Doppler → if ⊕ and previously ⊖ = diagnostic: if ⊕ and previously ⊕ → do venography: diagnosis if new filling defect: if → repeat Doppler ultrasound at day 5 to 7.
Treatment	Nonpharmacological:
	– Immobilization not necessary.
	– Compression leg stockings (with pressure of 30-40 mmHg at the ankle) started as soon as possible for 2 years minimum as a prophylaxis for postphlebitic syndrome in patients with symptomatic proximal DVT.
	Anticoagulation :
	Low molecular weight heparin (LMWH) or heparin IV 5000 U bolus (or 80 U/kg) then perfusion 35 000 U daily (or 18 U/kg/h) or fondaparinux s/c (or monitored s/c heparin or fixed-dose s/c heparin) + warfarin.
	LMWH treatment of choice of treatment in absence of contraindication (renal failure, morbid obesity, high risk of bleeding), as an outpatient if possible, or as inpatient if necessary.
	Continue heparin for 5 days minimum: stop heparin when INR stable and > 2 for at least 24 h.
	Continue LMWH for 3-6 months for patients with cancer.
	Warfarin for INR 2-3 for :
	– 3 months with DVT secondary to a transient risk factor or first isolated distal DVT.
	– At least 3 months with unprovoked DVT. After 3 months, evaluate the risk-benefit ratio of long term therapy. Long term therapy recommended for proximal DVT (with absent bleeding risk factors and good anticoagulant monitoring). For patients with unprovoked DVT who have a strong preference for less frequent INR testing: after the first 3 months of conventional-intensity anticoagulation, low-intensity therapy (INR 1.5-1.9) is an option.
	– Long-term treatment for a second episode of unprovoked DVT.
	– Long term treatment (or until cancer is resolved) in patients with DVT and cancer, with LMWH for the first 3 to 6 months, with subsequent therapy with warfarin or LMWH.
	Note: in patients who receive long-term anticoagulation treatment, the risk-benefit ratio of continued treatment should be periodically reassessed.
	Note: in case of isolated calf vein thrombosis and contraindication to anticoagulation, an option is to withhold therapy and follow with a venous doppler after 1 week in order to eliminate supra-popliteal extention.
	Note: A DVT should be treated before Doppler confirmation if pre-test probability of DVT is high.
	Thrombolysis in selected patients with extensive acute proximal DVT (e.g., iliofemoral DVT, symptoms for < 14 days, good functional status, life expectancy ≥ 1 year) who have low risk of bleeding, or in selected patients with upper-extremity DVT (eg, low risk of bleeding and severe symptoms of recent onset) : catheter-directed (preferred) or systemic.
	Inferior vena cava interruption: if anticoagulation contraindicated; if bleeding complications occur during anticoagulation; if recurrent thromboembolism despite adequate anticoagulation; or at the same time as a pulmonary thromboendarterectomy.
	Surgery: thrombectomy (if limb in danger) in selected patients if catheter-directed thrombolysis is not available.
	Normal D-Dimer and venous doppler at the end of anticoagulant treatment are associated with a low risk of recurrence of thromboembolic disease.

Prophylaxis	– Preoperative: See Preoperative table.
	– In patients with acute spinal cord lesion: LMWH. Alternatives: combination intermittent pneumatic compression (IPC) and heparin s/c or LMWH. Intermittent pneumatic compression and/or graded compression stockings (GCS) if anticoagulants contraindicated early post-trauma.
	– In multiple trauma patients: LMWH if not contraindicated. Intermittent pneumatic compression or graded compression stockings if LMWH delayed.
	– In burn patients with additional risk factors (advanced age, morbid obesity, extensive burns on lower extremities, concomitant trauma of lower limbs, femoral catheter and/or prolonged immobilization): heparin s/c or LMWH. If high risk of bleeding, GCS and/or IPC.
	– In patients hospitalized for an acute medical condition: if hospitalization for heart failure or severe respiratory disease, or confined to bed in presence of additional risk factors (including neoplasia, history of thromboembolic disease, sepsis, acute neurological disease, or inflammatory bowel disease) : heparin s/c or LMWH or fondaparinux. IPC or GCS if anticoagulants contraindicated.
	– For travelers who are taking flights > 8 hours :
	  - Avoidance of constrictive clothing around the lower extremities or waist, maintenance of adequate hydration, and frequent calf muscle contraction.
	  - If there are additional risk factors for thromboembolic disease, the general measures listed above are recommended: If active prophylaxis is considered, use of properly fitted below-knee GCS (providing 15-30 mmHg of pressure at the ankle) or a single prophylactic dose of LMWH injected prior to departure.

Pulmonary Embolism (PE)
Most often secondary to deep venous thrombosis.
Other causes much rarer: tumor, amniotic fluid, air, fatty, bone marrow, foreign material, septic embolism, etc.
Risk factors: see above.

Clinical findings	Pleuritic pain, dyspnea, tachypnea, cough, hemoptysis, diaphoresis, syncope, ↑ P2, signs of right heart failure, fever, tachycardia, thrombophlebitis, cyanosis, wheezing, cardiac arrhythmias.
	If massive: hypotension, right-sided heart failure.
	Differential diagnosis: pneumonia, myocardial infarction, pneumothorax, rib fracture, viral pleurodynia, exacerbated COPD, pericarditis, heart failure, etc.
	
	Wells' criteria : to evaluate the clinical probability of pulmonary embolism :
	  1. DVT symptoms or signs: 3 points
	  2. PE as likely or more likely than alternative diagnosis: 3 points
	  3. Heart rate > 100 beats/minute : 1.5 points
	  4. Immobilization or surgery in previous 4 weeks : 1.5 points
	  5. Previous DVT/PE : 1.5 points
	  6. Hemoptysis : 1 point
	  7. Cancer (treated < 6 months or palliative) : 1 point
	Low probability if ≤ 4 (12 % of EP), high if > 4 (37 %).

Workup	– See above (DVT) for routine workup and thrombophilia testing – Arterial blood gas if needed (↑ alveolo-arterial gradient, but can be normal in 20 %, hypoxemia). – ECG: tachycardia, nonspecific abnormalities, right axis deviation, right bundle branch block (RBBB), S1Q3T3, inverted T waves in anterior leads. – Chest X-ray: can be normal, or infiltrate, atelectasis, localized oligemia (Westermark's sign), prominence of pulmonary artery, wedge-shaped opacity (Hampton's hump), localised pleural effusion, cardiomegaly. – Pulmonary CT-Angio (3rd generation): If ⊕, diagnosis confirmed. If ⊖, diagnosis excluded (but consider Doppler of lower limbs if high cilinical probability). If non-diagnostic, do pulmonary scintigraphy or do lower limb Doppler to detect DVT. – Pulmonary scintigraphy as an alternative to CT-Angio, especially if allergy to contrast media or renal failure: if high probability scintigraphy and high clinical probability =

	diagnosis confirmed: if normal scintigraphy (whatever clinical probability may be) = diagnosis excluded; if scintigraphy non-diagnostic or low clinical probability and high scintigraphic probability, do an CT-Angio or a lower limb Doppler; or do a pulmonary angiography (if available) or lower limb Doppler in 7 days.
Treatment	– See above (DVT). Heparin can be continued for up to 10 days for massive pulmonary embolism. Treatment in hospital or outpatient (with LMWH). – In patients with acute nonmassive PE, LMWH is recommended (except in renal failure). In patients with massive PE, in patients in whom thrombolytic therapy is being considered or planned, or if in other situations where there is concern about s/c absorption, IV heparin is suggested. Note: PE should be treated before confirmation if pre-test probability of PE is high (Wells' score > 4). – Thrombolysis recommended for patients with hemodynamic compromise (unless major contraindications) and in selected high risk patients without hypotension (depending on the clinician's assessment of PE severity and prognosis) at low bleeding risk. – Interventional catheterization techniques (catheter extraction or fragmentation) in selected highly compromised patients unable to receive thrombolysis. – Thromboendarterectomy in selected highly compromised patients unable to receive thrombolysis if chronic pulmonary hypertension (in specialized centers).
Prognosis	Mortality of around 30 % if not treated; 2-8 % if treated. Mortality 30 % if massive PE, often occurring early. Poor prognostic factors: cancer, heart failure, prior DVT, hypotension, hypoxemia, DVT on ultrasound. Troponin ↑ and abnormal echocardiography would also confer a higher risk. Normal D-Dimer and venous doppler at the end of anticoagulant treatment seem to be associated with a low risk of recurrence of thromboembolic disease.
Thrombo-embolic Disease and Pregnancy	Overview : – First cause of maternal mortality. – Similar incidence antepartum and postpartum but postpartum considered at higher risk because over 6 weeks vs. 9 months; DVT > PE antepartum, PE > DVT postpartum. Higher risk if caesarean, especially if emergency. – Clinical diagnosis even harder because clinical manifestations similar to normal physiological changes of pregnancy; majority of patients are not hypoxemic (SaO$_2$ normal > 95 %); high clinical suspicion necessary and investigation in case of the slightest doubt. – Investigation: D-Dimer often elevated during pregnancy, therefore less useful; Doppler safe. Chest X-ray (< 0.01 mGy), ventilation-perfusion scintigraphy (not much maternal radiation, 0.9 mGy to foetus, ideal antepartum, or postpartum if not breastfeeding), CT-Angio (more maternal radiation but 0.06 mGy to foetus, no fetal complications documented with short exposition to iodine, ideal postpartum if breastfeeding or if underlying pulmonary disease) acceptable at every trimester. **Definition of the types of treatment used:** – Unfractionated heparin (UFH), prophylactic dose: 5000 U s/c every 12 hours. – UFH, intermediate-dose: s/c every 12 hours to adjust for level of anti-Xa 0.1-0.3 U/mL at mid-interval (6 h post-dose). – UFH adjusted-dose: s/c q 12 hours to adjust for therapeutic aPTT at mid-interval. – LMWH prophylactic dose: dalteparin 5000 U s/c every 24 h or tinzaparin 4500 U s/c q 24 h or enoxaparin 40 mg s/c every 24 h. – LMWH intermediate-dose: dalteparin 5000 U s/c every 12 h (anti-Xa 0.3-0.5 U/mL 4 h post-dose) or enoxaparin 40 mg s/c every 12 h. – LMWH adjusted-dose: adjusted for weight in 1 or 2 doses/day: dalteparin s/c 200 U/kg/day (anti-Xa 0.6-1.2 U/mL 4 h post-dose) or 100 U/kg every 12 h (anti-Xa 0.5-1.2 U/mL 4h post-dose) or tinzaparin 175 U/kg/day or enoxaparin 1mg/kg every 12 h

(anti-Xa 0.6-1.0 U/mL 4 h post-dose). Because the half-life of the LMWH is shorter in pregnancy, a treatment every 12 h is preferable, at least at the beginning of treatment (1-3 months) of an acute DVT/PE.
– Postpartum anticoagulation: warfarin for 4-6 weeks, INR 2-3, overlapping with UFH or LMWH until INR ≥ 2 for at least 24 h or LMWH (intensity according to indication).

Side effects: bleeding. Osteoporosis and heparin-induced thrombocytopenia (UFH >> LMWH therapeutic but ~ not with prophylactic LMWH). If heparin-induced thrombopenia, first choice of treatment = danaparoid (does not cross placenta).

Follow-up: controversial:
– CBC 2-3 x/week x 2 weeks at treatment onset then every month for platelets (probably not necessary if prophylactic LMWH only).
– aPTT or anti-Xa probably not necessary if prophylactic dose.
– aPTT or anti-Xa every trimester if intermediate dose.
– aPTT or anti-Xa every 1 month if adjusted dose.
– Some doctors adjust LMWH according to weight without monitoring except if < 40 kg or > 90 kg.

Note: Warfarin relatively contraindicated in pregnancy (teratogenicity ~ 5 % between 6-12 weeks) but safe for breastfeeding. Thrombolysis relatively contraindicated, principally peripartum.
Reserve for life-threatening situations.

Prevention of deep vein thrombosis or acute pulmonary embolism :
- For women with previous venous thromboembolism (VTE) :
– For pregnant women with a single prior episode of VTE *associated with a transient risk factor* that is no longer present and no thrombophilia (recurrence rate < 0.5 %), clinical surveillance antepartum and anticoagulant prophylaxis postpartum. If the transient risk factor associated with a previous VTE event is pregnancy or estrogen related: antepartum clinical surveillance or prophylaxis (prophylactic LMWH/UFH or intermediate-dose LMWH/UFH) plus postpartum prophylaxis, rather than routine care.
– For pregnant women with a single *idiopathic* episode of VTE but without thrombophilia and who are not receiving long-term anticoagulants (recurrence rate ~ 8 %): prophylactic LMWH/ UFH or intermediate-dose LMWH/UFH or clinical surveillance throughout pregnancy plus postpartum anticoagulants.
– For pregnant women with *thrombophilia* who have had a single prior episode of VTE and are not receiving long-term anticoagulants (recurrence rate ~ 20 %): antepartum prophylactic or intermediate-dose LMWH or prophylactic or intermediate-dose UFH or clinical surveillance throughout pregnancy; plus post-partum anticoagulants.
– For women with *"higher risk" thrombophilias* (antithrombin deficiency, antiphospholipid syndrome, homozygosity for factor V Leiden or for the prothrombin gene mutation or compound heterozygosity [factor V Leiden + prothrombin]) who have had a single prior episode of VTE and are not receiving long-term anticoagulants: antepartum prophylactic or intermediate-dose LMWH or prophylactic or intermediate-dose UFH plus postpartum anticoagulants.
– For pregnant women with *multiple* (> 2) episodes of VTE not receiving long-term anticoagulants: antepartum prophylactic, intermediate-dose, or adjusted-dose LMWH or prophylactic, intermediate or adjusted-dose UFH followed by postpartum anticoagulants.
– For pregnant women receiving long-term anticoagulants for prior VTE : LMWH or UFH throughout pregnancy (either adjusted-dose LMWH or UFH, 75% of adjusted-dose LMWH, or intermediate-dose LMWH) followed by resumption of long-term anticoagulants postpartum.

For all pregnant women with previous DVT, we suggest the use of graduated elastic compression stockings both antepartum and postpartum.

- If thrombophilia with no prior history of VTE :
– For pregnant women with no history of VTE but antithrombin deficiency: antepartum

and postpartum prophylaxis.
- For all other pregnant women with thrombophilia and no prior VTE: antepartum clinical surveillance or prophylactic LMWH or UFH according to an individualized risk assessment, plus postpartum anticoagulants.

Treatment of the deep vein thrombosis or acute pulmonary embolism :
- LMWH at adjusted-dose (1st choice) or IV heparin for a minimum of 5 days, followed by LMWH at adjusted dose (every 12 h initially) or UFH for the rest of the pregnancy.
- Stop heparin at least 24 hours prior to elective induction of labor. Many change LMWH for UFH at 36 weeks because anticoagulation monitoring is easier and protamine can be used as needed in case of spontaneous labor. IV Heparin peripartum or temporary inferior vena cava filter only in presence of extremely high risk (DVT/PE < 4 weeks).
- Resume anticoagulation postpartum with warfarin for 6 weeks minimum and until the end of treatment (for a minimum total duration of therapy of 6 months).

Long term anticoagulant treatment and pregnancy for patients with prosthetic valve :
Three possible courses of action:
1. Adjusted-dose LMWH (2 doses/day) for anti-Xa level of 1.0-1.2 U/mL 4 hours post-injection or according to weight ± anti-Xa pre-dose level of 0.65-0.7 (experts' opinion) throughout pregnancy or
2. UFH at adjusted dose (every 12 h) aiming for mid-interval aPTT ≥ 2 x control or mid-interval anti-Xa level of 0.35-0.70 U/mL throughout pregnancy or
3. UFH or LMWH (as above) until the 13th week, with warfarin substitution until close to delivery when UHF or LMWH is resumed.
For all options, resume warfarin postpartum (many days postpartum in order to avoid hemorrhage).

In women judged to be at very high risk of thromboembolism in whom concerns exist about the efficacy and safety of UFH or LMWH (e.g., older-generation prosthesis in the mitral position or history of thromboembolism), it is suggested to give warfarin throughout pregnancy with replacement by UFH or LMWH (as above) close to delivery.

For pregnant women with prosthetic valves at high risk of thromboembolism, add ASA 75-100 mg/day.

Long term anticoagulant treatment in women who are considering pregnancy:
Perform frequent pregnancy tests (every month) and replace warfarin with UFH or LMWH when pregnancy is achived (< 6 weeks safe). Alternative: change pre-conception if probable quick conception.

Regional anesthesia and anticoagulation:
According to anesthesist's evaluation, controversial:
Prophylactic doses:
- UFH: at any time (some will prefer 12 hours).
- LMWH: 12 hours after last injection (some will prefer 24 hours).
Therapeutic or moderate doses:
- UFH: 12 hours after last injection (caution: sometimes aPTT is abnormal for up to 24 hours).
- LMWH: 24 hours after last injection.

Thrombophilias and obstetrical complications (fetal loss, early severe preeclampsia, intrauterine growth restriction, abruptio placentae):
Presently, a controversial topic: association was demonstrated but treatment benefits remain uncertain.
Screening recommended:
- Antiphospholipid antibodies for recurrent early pregnancy loss (≥ 3 miscarriages) or unexplained late pregnancy loss.
Screening suggested:
- Antiphospholipid antibodies for severe or recurrent preeclampsia or intrauterine

	growth restriction.

Screening for other thrombophilias remains controversial.

Treatment:

ASA 75-100 mg/day.

Prophylactic LMWH or prophylactic or moderate-dose UFH if:
- Antiphospholipid syndrome and fetal loss (≥ 3 in 1st trimester or ≥ 1 during 2nd or 3rd trimester).
- More controversial: Other thrombophilias and ≥ 1 fetal loss at > 10 weeks of pregnancy. Obstetrical complications WITHOUT thrombophilia.
- Few/no evidence until now: other thrombophilias and early preeclampsia, intrauterine growth restriction or abruptio placentae.

Anticoagulation

Indications	**Thromboembolic Disease:** see Thromboembolic disease table. – Low molecular weight heparin (LMWH) or heparin IV 5000 U bolus (or 80 U/kg) then perfusion 35 000 U/day (or 18 U/kg/h) for heparin blood concentration between 0.3-0.7 U/mL of anti-Xa activity. Fondaparinux s/c (or monitored s/c heparin or fixed-dose s/c heparin) also available. Continue heparin for minimum 5 days: stop heparin when INR stable and > 2 for at least 24 hours. Continue LMWH for 3-6 months in patients with cancer. – Warfarin for INR 2-3 for : – 3 months for DVT secondary to a transient risk factor or first isolated distal DVT. – At least 3 months for unprovoked DVT. After 3 months, evaluate the risk-benefit ratio of long term therapy. Long term therapy recommended for proximal DVT (with absent bleeding risk factors and good anticoagulant monitoring). For patients with unprovoked DVT who have a strong preference for less frequent INR testing to monitor their therapy, after the first 3 months of conventional-intensity anticoagulation, low-intensity therapy (INR 1.5-1.9) is an option (ELATE trial). – Long-term treatment for a second episode of unprovoked DVT. – Long term treatment (or until cancer is resolved) in patients with DVT and cancer, with LMWH for the first 3 to 6 months, and subsequent therapy with warfarin or LMWH. Note: in patients who receive long-term anticoagulation treatment, the risk-benefit ratio of treatment should be reassessed at periodic intervals. Note: For isolated calf DVT and contraindication to anticoagulation, an option is to withhold therapy and do a repeat venous Doppler after one week to detect proximal extension. – Inferior vena cava interruption if contraindication or complications with anticoagulation, if recurrent thromboembolism despite adequate anticoagulation, or at the same time as a pulmonary thromboendarterectomy – Thrombolysis recommended for: patients with PE with hemodynamic compromise (unless major contraindications), in selected high risk patients without hypotension (depending on the clinician's assessment of PE severity and prognosis) at low bleeding risk: in selected patients with acute extensive proximal DVT (eg, iliofemoral DVT, symptoms for < 14 days, good functional status, life expectancy ≥ 1 year) who have low risk of bleeding: in selected patients with upper-extremity DVT (eg, low risk of bleeding and severe symptoms of recent onset) : catheter-directed (preferred) or systemic. **Atrial Fibrillation (persistent or paroxysmal) or Atrial Flutter** (recommendations ACC/AHA/ESC 2006): Stratify the cardio-embolic risk for each patient and evaluate risk-benefit ratio of anticoagulation: o High risk factors for stroke: history of TIA/stroke or prior systemic embolism, mitral

stenosis, prosthetic valve.
o   Moderate risk factors: age >75 years old, hypertension, heart failure, and/or left
     ventricular dysfunction with LVEF ≤ 35 % or diabetes.
o   Low risk factors or less well validated: age 65-74 years old, woman, CAD,
     hyperthyroidism.

- For patient with no risk factors: **ASA 81-325 mg/d.**
- For patient with one moderate risk factor: **ASA 81-325 mg/d or warfarin, INR 2-3.**
  (Warfarin rather than aspirin suggested by ACCP 2008).
- For patient with any high factor of risk or more than one moderate factor of risk: **warfarin,
  INR 2-3**, ASA only if warfarin is contraindicated.

- If non urgent cardioversion: warfarin 3 weeks before and at least 4 weeks after return to
  sinus rhythm. If no thrombus on transesophageal echocardiography, immediate
  cardioversion can be done (but anticoagulate during the pericardioversion period and at
  least 4 weeks post-cardioversion)

Note: Any precipitating factors (such as hyperthyroidism, pneumonia, heart failure) should
be treated before cardioversion.

Similar recommendations apply for cardioversion of atrial flutter.

Prosthetic Valves and Bioprosthesis :
–   Prosthetic valves :
    - Warfarin, target INR 2.5-3.5 except with bileaflet valve or with tilting disc (Medtronic)
      in aortic position who are in sinus rhythm without left atrial enlargement: target
      INR 2-3.
    - In patients with mechanical heart valves and additional risk factors (atrial fibrillation,
      anterior-apical ST-segment elevation myocardial infarction, left atrial enlargement,
      hypercoagulable state, or low ejection fraction), target INR 2.5-3.5.
    - In patients with mechanical heart valves with additional risk factors for
      thromboembolism, or with history of atherosclerotic vascular disease, add aspirin
      50-100 mg/d (except no aspirin for patients at high risk of bleeding, such as
      patients with history of GI bleed or > 80 years of age).
–   Bioprosthesis in mitral position: warfarin, target INR 2-3 for 3 months post-op, then
    ASA 50-100 mg/day.
    Bioprosthesis in aortic position in sinus rhythm: ASA 50-100 mg/day.
    Bioprosthesis and systemic embolism: warfarin, target INR 2-3 for at least 3 months
    after valve insertion, then ASA 50-100 mg/day.
    Bioprosthesis and additional risk factors for thromboembolism, including AF,
    hypercoagulable state, or low ejection fraction : warfarin, target INR 2-3 long term +
    consider aspirin (50-100 mg/d), particularly in patients with history of atherosclerotic
    vascular disease (except for patients at high risk of bleeding, such as patients with
    history of GI bleed or > 80 years of age).

Mitral Valve Disease:
    - If prior embolism, atrial fibrillation, left atrial thrombus or left atrial diameter > 55 mm:
      warfarin, INR 2-3.
    - If sinusal rhythm without dilation: no anticoagulation.
    - If recurrence of embolism despite adequate anticoagulation: add ASA 75-100 mg/day
      (or dipyridamole or clopidogrel if intolerance to ASA).
    - If mitral valvuloplasty, anticoagulation 3 weeks before and 4 weeks after.
    Mitral valve prolapse:
    - Uncomplicated: no treatment.
    - If history of unexplained TIA: ASA 50-100 mg/day.
    - If systemic embolism or atrial fibrillation or TIA despite ASA: warfarin, INR 2-3.
Infectious endocarditis:
    - Prosthetic valves: discontinue warfarin at presentation and substitute for IV heparin,
      until it is determined that no invasive procedure will be required and the patient has
      been stabilized.
    Nonbacterial thrombotic endocarditis: heparin.

| | **Post-Myocardial Infarction :** ASA 75-162 mg/day for all patients except :
– For patient at high risk of systemic embolism (previous infarction, severe left ventricular dysfunction, congestive heart failure, mural thrombus, history of thromboembolic disease): warfarin, INR 2-3 + ASA ≤ 100 mg/day for 3 months (indefinitely if permanent atrial fibrillation).
– Alternatively for post-MI patients, if optimal follow-up of INR is available: we could use: long-term (up to 4 years) warfarin (INR 3-4) **or** warfarin (INR 2-3) + ASA.
– If contraindication to ASA: clopidogrel or warfarin.
– Heparin (IV if alteplase, tenecteplase or randeplase used or with streptokinase, especially if at high risk of systemic embolism: if not, we can also give heparin s/c 12500 U s/c bid for ≥ 48 hours); low molecular weight heparin alternative acceptable if < 75 years old without renal failure or if non-ST elevation infarction (see angina table). Give heparin IV ≥ 48 hours. Heparin s/c or LMWH ad mobilisation for all patients with infarction not anticoagulated.

Stroke:
– If non-cardioembolic ischemic TIA or stroke: clopidogrel or ASA+ dipyridamole or ASA 50-100 mg/day. Anticoagulant if well documented thrombophilia.
– If cardioembolic stroke: warfarin, INR 2-3. ASA if warfarin contraindicated.
– If carotid endarterectomy: give ASA 50-100 mg/day, to start preop and to continue long term.
– If mobile aortic arch thrombus and cryptogenic CVA: warfarin or ASA 50-100 mg/day.
– If patent foramen ovale and cryptogenic CVA: antiplatelets suggested; warfarin if there is evidence of DVT or another indication for warfarin (AF), or underlying hypercoagulable state.
– If venous thrombosis: heparin IV or LMWH, followed by anticoagulation for 3-6 months, INR 2-3. |
| Side effects | **Heparin :** bleeding (reversible by protamine 1 mg for 100 U heparin : half-life heparin = 1 hour : so 50 % neutralizing dose 1 h after injection of heparin, 25 % after 2 h ...), thrombocytopenia (2 forms : **early** nonimmune, benign and **late** [4-14 days after starting treatment], immune, risk of paradoxical thrombosis : See platelet disorders table), osteoporosis, local hypersensitivity, cutaneous necrosis, anaphylaxis, alopecia, hypoaldosteronism (hyperkalemia).

Oral Anticoagulants: multiple drug interaction, cutaneous necrosis (between day 3 and 8: associated with deficiency in proteins C or S), bleeding (reversible with vitamin K or fresh frozen plasma).

Management of supra-therapeutic INR (in accordance with ACCP 2008) :
– If INR < 5 and no bleeding → ↓ or stop warfarin and no other treatment.
– If INR 5-9 and no bleeding → omit 1-2 doses of warfarin or give vitamin K 1-2.5 mg PO particularly if ↑ risk of bleeding. If rapid ↓ INR needed, give vitamin K ≤ 5 mg PO: ↓ INR in 24 hours.
– If INR > 9 and no bleeding → stop warfarin + give vitamin K 2.5-5 mg PO: ↓ INR in 24-48 hours.
– If **serious** bleeding and elevated INR → stop warfarin + vitamin K 10 mg IV (*slow* infusion) and every 12 h as needed + fresh-frozen plasma (5-8 cc/kg) or concentrate of prothrombic complex or factor VIIa recombinant, depending on the urgency of the situation.
– If **life-threatening** bleeding and elevated INR → stop warfarin + give fresh frozen plasma, prothrombic complex concentrate or recombinant factor VIIa + vitamin K 10 mg IV (*slow* infusion) and every 12 h as needed, repeated, if necessary. |

Peripheral Arterial Disease	
Overview	Peripheral arterial disease (PAD) is defined by an ankle-brachial index (ABI), i.e. the ratio of the systolic BP in lower limbs divided by systolic BP in upper limbs ≤ 0.9 (normally > 1). 20-50 % of patients with ↓ ABI are asymptomatic, 10-35 % have typical intermittent claudication, 30-40 % have atypical leg pain and 1-3 % have pain at rest or gangrene. **Intermittent claudication**: lower limb pain provoked by exercise, reproducible, relieved in a few minutes by rest. Look for pain localization, progression in time, distance before onset, position relieving the pain (sitting or standing) and resulting disability. Leriche syndrome if proximal claudication, erectile dysfunction and absent femoral pulses. **Critical ischemia**: ischemic pain at rest, presence of gangrene or painful ulcer at pressure points. Can be acute (secondary to embolism, thrombosis, trauma) or chronic. Risk factors for atherosclerosis: same as coronary risk factors. PAD is a marker of systemic disease: high prevalence of concomitant CAD, of cerebrovascular disease and of erectile dysfunction.
Differential diagnosis	Radiculopathy, spinal stenosis, osteoarthritis, chronic compartment syndrome, coarctation of the aorta, thromboangiitis obliterans, popliteal aneurysm thrombosis, compression by Baker's cyst, cystic disease of the popliteal adventitia, persistent sciatic artery, iliac dysplasia, post-radiotherapy.

Stage of severity	Fontaine's classification :
	    I: asymptomatic (ABI ≤ 0.9).
	    II: intermittent claudication.
	        a- > 200 meters.
	        b- < 200 meters.
	    III: pain at rest.
	    IV: cutaneous ischemia (ulcer, gangrene).

Workup	– Routine physical exam, cardiopulmonary, pulses, listen for bruits and palpate for pulsating abdominal masses – Basic biochemistry, lipids, glucose, ECG. – As needed : sedimentation rate, thrombophilia workup ... – Ankle-brachial Index (at bedside or via arterial lower limb Doppler): The lower the ABI, the more severe the disease, and the more reduced the survival. An ABI > 1.40 can also indicate PAD if the artery is not compressible; additional workup to do in those patients: measure of toe pressure, Doppler… – Arterial Doppler of lower limbs with or without exercise test (significant ↓ of ABI with exercise if PAD). – As needed: Lower limb plethysmography, CT-Angio, MR-Angio. – Arteriography indicated for intermittent claudication if intervention considered (depending on the disability) and if critical ischemia (except if amputation inevitable).

Treatment	For intermittent claudication :
	 – Exercise: first-line treatment for claudication. Walking program (ideally supervised), 30-60 minutes/day, ≥ 3 times a week, ≥ 3-6 months, can triple the distance to pain onset.
	 – Smoking cessation.
	 – Optimization of the diabetes and hypertension treatment.
	 – Medication : consider patient as in **secondary prevention** of atherosclerotic disease :
	     o Antiplatelets for all (aspirin 1st choice or clopidogrel if contraindication to aspirin).
	     o Angiotensin-converting enzyme inhibitors or angiotensin II receptors antagonists to consider, especially if there is hypertension.
	     o Hypolipidemic agent: as in secondary prevention.
	     o Vasodilators? few clinically significant benefits.
	 – Angioplasty: indicated if failure of exercise treatment and severe disability. Especially effective for short aorto-iliac stenosis > femoral > infra-popliteal.
	 – Surgery: rarely necessary, indicated if failure of exercise treatment and severe disability.
	
	 For critical ischemia: **vascular emergency**, quick referral to a specialist.
	 – If acute: treatment according to etiology: anticoagulation ± thrombolysis, endovascular revascularization (mechanical thrombectomy or by aspiration) or revascularization surgery or amputation.
	 – If chronic: Revascularisation if possible and other treatments same as intermittent claudication. Treatment of pain and infection as needed.

Prognosis	For intermittent claudication : good prognosis for the affected limb - after 5 years, 70-80 % remain stable or improve, 5 % need an intervention and 2 % an amputation - but bad global cardiovascular prognosis - 10-15 % die after 5 years, of which 75 % of cardiovascular cause (CAD and stroke). Prognosis equivalent to "blood vessel cancer". For critical ischemia: at 1 year, 25 % die, 30 % amputation. Prognosis equivalent to a "metastatic blood vessel cancer".

Erectile Dysfunction	
Definition: incapacity to obtain or maintain a sufficient erection for satisfactory sexual intercourse. Frequent: 50 % in 50 y.o. men, nearly 70 % in 70 y.o. men.	

Causes	Psychogenic, organic or mixed (the most frequent cause).
	
	 ▪ Psychogenic: performance anxiety, relational disorder, psychiatric disorder (depression, anxiety, schizophrenia, etc).
	 ▪ Organic:
	    - Neurogenic: Parkinson, Alzheimer, stroke, trauma, spinal cord lesion, genital sensory disorder, etc.
	    - Hormonal: hypogonadism, hyperprolactinemia, thyroid disease, etc.
	    - Vascular: penile arterial or venous insufficiency.
	    - Drug: antipsychotics, antidepressants, antihypertensive agents (beta-blockers, thiazides, spironolactone, sympatholytics, etc), benzodiazepines, narcotics, tobacco, alcohol, cimetidine, digoxin, estrogens and antiandrogens (5-α reductase inhibitors), GnRH inhibitors, ketoconazole, etc.
	    - Other systemic diseases: diabetes, chronic renal failure, prostate cancer surgery, etc.

Diagnosis	Identify associated libido, orgasm or ejaculation disorders. Psychosocial history very important. Eliminate depression, psychiatric disorder, inter-personal conflict, history of trauma or surgery… Search for sudden onset, presence of nocturnal or morning erections (suggests a psychological cause). Physical exam of breasts, body hair, penis, testes, pulses and genital and perineal sensation **Workup**: CBC, urinalysis, creatinine, glucose, lipids, TSH, testosterone (if associated with a reduction of libido). If testosterone ↓, measure free testosterone, LH and prolactin. If needed, more specialized evaluation with: penile doppler, cavernosonography, pelvic arteriography, penile nocturnal monitoring... Referral to a specialist if young or PO treatment inefficient.
Treatment	– Phosphodiesterase type 5 selective inhibitors: inactivate cyclic GMP of the cavernous body. Sildenafil (Viagra®) 25-50-100 mg or tadalafil (Cialis®) 10-20 mg or vardenafil (Levitra®) 5-10-20 mg 1x/day maximum. Side effects: headache, hot flashes, dyspepsia, abnormal vision (with sildenafil), nasal congestion, priapism (rare). Contraindicated with nitrates. Vardenafil contraindicated if use of doxazocin or terazocin. Cardiac evaluation before utilisation sometimes necessary. – Androgens: if hypogonadism present. Intramuscular or transdermic testosterone more effective than PO. Contraindicated if prostate cancer, or bladder obstruction due to benign prostate hypertrophy. Follow up with CBC, testosterone, lipids, PSA and digital rectal examination every 6 months. – Other PO treatments: trazodone, imipramine, desipramine, sertraline, clomipramine can cause delayed ejaculation (useful for early ejaculation). – Transurethral treatment: alprostadil (Muse®): prostaglandin E1. Side effects: penile or urethral pain. No systemic effect, no drug interactions. 250-1000 μg. – Intracavernosal treatments: papaverine injection, phentolamine, alprostadil or combination after education. Side effects: pain, priapism, fibrosis... Contraindicated with sickle-cell disease or psychiatric disease. – Vacuum or rings: Side effects` pain, petechia, dysesthesias... – Psychotherapy: according to cause. – Surgery: according to etiology, prosthesis or vascular surgery.

Raynaud's Phenomenon

Episodic vasospastic ischemia of the extremities.

Incidence 3- 5 %. 3-5 times more frequent in women. More frequent in cold climates, exacerbated in wintertime.

Raynaud phenomenon is characterized by a discoloration of the fingers, cyanosis and erythema following exposure to cold (or emotion). The whitening phase represents the digital vasospasm, the cyanosis, deoxygenation of the blood transporting capillaries or veinules and erythema occurs as resolution of vasoplasm takes place.

Affects mainly fingers and toes (usually, it spares thumbs), but can occur on the tongue, the tip of the nose and ears.

Causes	– Primary (or Raynaud's disease: 80 %): episodic ischemia, symmetric, for more than 2 years, absence of arterial occlusion, necrosis, gangrene, ulceration or of secondary cause. In most people, disease develops before the age of 40. Benign course. – Secondary: connective tissue diseases (scleroderma, SLE, dermatomyositis, mixed connective tissue disease, Sjögren), peripheral arterial disease (atherosclerosis, thomboangiitis obliterans, embolism, thoracic outlet syndrome, angiitis), neurologic diseases (carpal tunnel syndrome, reflex sympathetic dystrophy, spinal tumor, herniated disc, syringomyelitis), blood dyscrasias (hyperviscosity syndrome, myeloproliferative syndrome, cold agglutinine disease, cryoglobulinemia), trauma (frostbite, exposure to vibration), medication-drugs (beta-blockers, tricyclic antidepressants, ergot derivatives, chemotherapy, amphetamines), others (primary pulmonary hypertension, hypothyroidism). Differential diagnosis: – Acrocyanosis: bluish discoloration of hands and feet, exacerbated by cold, beginning at around 20-45 years old; good prognosis. – Erythromelalgia: erythematous and painful extremities after exposure to heat or post-exercise. Idiopathic or secondary (myeloproliferative syndrome, diabetes ...); treated with ASA ± non-selective beta-blockers + underlying cause. – Hypothenar hammer syndrome: arterial occlusion secondary to repeated trauma of the palm; typically, Raynaud of the 3 last fingers and distal ischemia. – Dermatological disorders: perniosis, urticaria, livedo, panniculitis, lipodermatosclerosis, neutrophilic dermatosis ...
Workup	Capillaroscopy (if available): normal in Raynaud's disease, abnormal with certain secondary causes (particularly connective tissue diseases). Patients with a normal history, normal physical examination and a normal capillaroscopy (if available) do not require further investigation. Otherwise: CBC, electrolytes, creatinine, urinalysis, sedimentation rate, ANA (look for specific auto-antibodies, according to clinical findings), rheumatoid factor, C3, C4. If needed: protein electrophoresis, TSH, cryoglobulines, cold agglutinins. Arterial Doppler of upper limbs sometimes useful if suspicion of secondary cause (e.g. asymmetry). Arteriography is sometimes useful if persistent ischemia in order to detect arterial occlusion.
Treatment	Avoid exposure to cold (gloves, warm clothes). Avoid use of vasoconstrictors: stop tobacco, avoid sympathomimetics (eg. ergotamine). Medication if not responsive to conservative treatment: calcium channel blockers, dihydropyridines, α-blockers, losartan, Fluoxetine? Response to medication: 30-40 %. Selective inhibitors of phosphodiesterase type 5 (sildenafil) if refractory. Prostaglandins IV if digital ulcers with scleroderma. Sympathectomy either proximal or peripheral if severe ischemia not responding to medical treatment: response < 20 %. In case of acute ischemic attack: nifedipine PO 10-30 mg every 8 hours, aspirin, digital-wrist block, prostaglandins IV, short-term anticoagulation, digital sympathectomy if refractory.

Edema

Pathophysiology of edema (Starling's law): can be secondary to an increase of the capillary hydrostatic pressure (e.g.: heart failure), a decrease of the plasma oncotic pressure (hypoalbuminemia), an increase of capillary permeability (e.g.: local inflammation), an increase of the interstitial oncotic pressure, or lymphatic obstruction (e.g.: lymphedema).

Determine if: the edema is localized or generalized, unilateral or bilateral, upper or lower limb, associated with weight gain, associated with features of cardiac, pulmonary, hepatic, renal disease.

Cutaneous examination of the lower limbs can demonstrate signs suggestive of venous insufficiency: lipodermatosclerosis, white atrophy, internal malleoli venous ulcers, varices, stasis dermatitis.

Causes	**Localized** edema: venous insufficiency, thrombophlebitis, cellulitis, allergic reaction, fasciitis, rupture of Baker cyst (knee), lymphedema, lipedema, post-hemiplegia, intra-muscular or intra-osseous mass, abscess, reflex sympathic dystrophy (if hyperesthesia of the whole limb ± heat ± erythema and appropriate setting). **Generalized** edema : – **Cardiac**: right ± left-sided heart failure secondary to cardiomyopathy, right ventricular infarction, valvular disease, pericardial disease (such as constrictive pericarditis). – **Pulmonary**: pulmonary hypertension; primary or secondary to embolism, COPD, sleep apnea, etc. – **Hepatic**: secondary to hypoalbuminemia + portal hypertension + secondary hyperaldosteronism: cirrhosis, etc. – **Renal**: secondary to hypoalbuminemia + water and sodium retention: nephrotic syndrome, acute or chronic renal failure, etc. – **Drugs**: vasodilators (calcium channel blockers, minoxidil, diazoxide, etc), steroids, NSAIDs, thiazolidinediones, anagrelide, etc. – Pregnancy. – Exudative enteropathy: edema secondary to hypoalbuminemia (rare). – Hypothyroidism (myxedema). – Severe malnutrition. – Idiopathic (most often affecting pre-menopausal women and involving hands, legs, face, abdomen, often cyclic).
Workup	Localized edema: according to suspected cause: biochemistry, x-ray of the site, doppler ultrasound, bone scan with flow studies (for reflex sympathic dystrophy). Generalized edema: CBC, electrolytes, creatinine, albumin, liver enzymes, TSH, urinalysis, chest X-ray, ECG. As needed according to clinical picture: protein electrophoresis, urine collection, glomerulonephritis workup, arterial blood gas, cardiac enzymes, echocardiography, ventilation-perfusion scintigraphy, pulmonary function tests, abdominal ultrasound. Follow the weight, measure input and output as needed. Note: If significative hypoalbuminemia (< 25 g/L): search for hepatic or renal disease, malnutrition or exudative enteropathy. Without significant hypoalbuminemia: search for cardiopulmonary cause.
Treatment	According to cause. In venous insufficiency, avoid diuretics. Elevation of lower limbs and compressive therapy (compression leg stockings) suggested.

Preoperative Evaluation and Perioperative Management
Cardiac Preoperative Evaluation of a Noncardiac Surgery
ACC/AHA 2007 approach:
- For urgent and necessary surgery → proceed to surgery.
- If patient presents with active cardiac disease:
  - Unstable angina or class III-IV/IV.
  - Myocardial infarction < 7 days or between 7-30 days with evidence of important residual ischemia (symptoms, non-invasive test).
  - Recent heart failure, decompensated or stage IV/IV.
  - Significant arrhythmia (eg. ventricular, uncontrolled supraventricular, high grade AV block).
  - Severe valvular disease (aortic stenosis [≈ 10 % perioperative mortality] or symptomatic mitral stenosis).
  → Treat before considering surgery.

- For low risk surgery (endoscopic intervention, superficial intervention, cataract or breast surgery or ambulatory) → proceed to surgery, except if active cardiac disease.
- If adequate functional capacity (≥ 4 METS) without cardiac symptoms → proceed to surgery.
- If poor functional capacity or unable to evaluate, or symptomatic < 4 METS: evaluate for factors increasing the risk of cardiac complications (Lee's revised cardiac risk index):
  - High risk surgery (intrathoracic, intra-abdominal).
  - Ischemic heart disease.
  - Known heart failure, even compensated.
  - Diabetes mellitus (especially insulin-dependant).
  - Renal insufficiency (creatinine > 177 μmol/L).
  - Cerebrovascular disease (TIA or stroke).
  - If no risk factor: proceed to surgery.
  - If presence of risk factors: Consider non-invasive investigation if it would change management (especially if multiple risk factors or vascular surgery).
  The treadmill test is the non invasive test of choice: if impossible, perform exercise or pharmacologic stress radionuclide myocardial perfusion imaging, or stress echocardiography.

Preoperative revascularization: There is no evidence that preoperative revascularization diminishes perioperative ischemic events (CARP study); proceed to a coronary revascularization only if indicated independently of the need for surgery (such as an acute coronary syndrome).

Management of antiplatelet therapy:
- For patients not at high risk of cardiac events, stop aspirin or clopidogrel 7-10 days before surgery. Resume aspirin or clopidogrel approximately 24 h after surgery when there is adequate hemostasis.
- For patients at high risk of cardiac events, continue aspirin. For patients receiving clopidogrel, stop clopidogrel at least 5 days (preferably 10 days) before surgery
- In patients with a bare-metal coronary stent who require surgery within 6 weeks of stent placement, continue aspirin and clopidogrel in the perioperative period.
- In patients with a drug-eluting coronary stent who require surgery within 12 months of stent placement, continue aspirin and clopidogrel in the perioperative period.

In all cases, consider uninterrupted double antiplatelet therapy in the perioperative setting for patients at high risk of thrombosis (such as previous thrombosis, revascularization of multiple vessels or of the left main stem).

Always continue beta-blockers perioperatively for patients already on therapy.
Consider addition or titration of beta-blockers to a target HR of 55-65 per minute in:
- Patients with atherosclerotic cardiac disease undergoing intermediate risk surgery (intraperitoneal, intrathoracic, carotid, head and neck, orthopedic or prostatic) or high risk surgery (vascular), especially if ⊕ non invasive test.
- Patients with at least one risk factor if high risk surgery and possibly if intermediate risk surgery
- Patients undergoing high risk surgery with no risk factors (but poor evidence; studies under way).

Contraindications: systolic BP < 100 mmHg, HR < 55/minute, high grade AV block, heart failure, bronchospasm.

Continue statins in the perioperative period; protective effect in high risk surgery.
Consider stopping ACEI and angiotensin receptor antagonists on the morning of surgery, and resuming them when patient is hemodynamically stable and euvolemic (but controversial).
Consider postponement of surgery if BP > 180/110 mmHg (but controversial).

Postoperative follow-up: patients should be investigated only if they show symptoms or signs of myocardial dysfunction, and treated accordingly.

Always consider antibiotic prophylaxis if at risk (see endocarditis table).

Pulmonary Preoperative Evaluation for Nonpulmonary Surgery

Incidence of pulmonary complications highly variable (2-19 % of surgeries): atelectasis, infections, pulmonary embolism, bronchospasm, etc.
Risk factors: COPD, age > 65 years old, active smoking, heart failure, hypoalbuminemia, sleep apnea (?)
Strategies to lower perioperative risk:
- Pulmonary expansion manoeuvres (spirometry, respiratory exercises, C-PAP)
- Thromboembolic prophylaxis (see below)
- Stop smoking before surgery (but benefit unknown).

Endocrine Preoperative Evaluation

Diabetes	Insulin usually required if: already insulin-dependant (type 1 or 2); poorly controlled diabetes; on oral antihyperglycemic agents (OH) requiring moderate-major surgery; on diet requiring major surgery; perioperative glycemia > 11 mmol/L; usually not necessary in pts with diabetes requiring minor-moderate surgery well controlled on diet or OH. → if insulin required: start before surgery D5W at 100 mL/h and subcutaneous insulin or continuous IV perfusion in Y with dextrose for better glycemic control. Measure glycemia every 2-4 hours. → if insulin not required: ...and diabetes well controlled on diet: avoid dextrose during the surgery and follow glycemia regularly every 4-6 hours perioperatively. ...and diabetes well controlled on OH: stop OH the day before surgery, start D5W at 100 mL/h on arrival at the OR, give subcutaneous insulin if glycemia > 11 mmol/L, measure glycemia every 4-6 hours (or more frequently if needed), resume OH when back on a normal diet. The perioperative glycemias should be maintained between 5 and 11 mmol/L, except for patients requiring postoperative mechanical ventilation, in which case glycemias should be maintained between 4.5-6 mmol/L.
Adrenal function	Screen for patients at risk of suppression of the hypothalamic-pituitary-adrenal axis, who should be prescribed glucocorticoids at the minimal necessary dose for the shortest possible time to avoid post-operative side effects. Perioperative supplementation usually required if patient received > 5 mg of Prednisone or its equivalent for 1 month **or** ≥ 20 mg/day for 5 days *in the past year*. If any doubt, measure cortisol or do ACTH test. 1. For superficial intervention under local anesthesia < 1 hour, give usual dose: no supplementation needed. 2. For minor surgery (e.g.: herniorraphy): the need is equivalent to 25 mg of hydrocortisone for one day. e.g.: administer 5 mg Prednisone on the day of procedure only. 3. For moderate surgery (e.g.: cholecystectomy, colon resection): 50-75 mg/day of hydrocortisone is needed for 1-2 days. e.g.: administer 10 mg Prednisone pre-op, then SoluCortef® 50mg IV per-op, then 20 mg IV every 8 hrs on day #1 then usual dose on day #2. 4. For major surgery (e.g.: cardiac, Whipple): 100-150 mg/day of hydrocortisone is needed for 2-3 days. e.g.: administer SoluCortef® 50 mg IV every 8 hours for 48-72 hrs.

Preoperative Evaluation: Antithrombotic Prophylaxis (ACCP 2008)

According to preoperative risk and type of surgery :

→ General surgery:
  - For low-risk general surgery (minor procedures and no additional thromboembolic risk factors [cancer, previous VTE, obesity, delayed mobilization, increasing age, general anesthesia, duration of surgery, postoperative infection]): early ambulation.
  - For moderate-risk general surgery (major procedure for benign disease): use LMWH, low-dose unfractionated heparin (LDUH), or fondaparinux.
  - For higher-risk general surgery (major procedure for cancer): use LMWH, LDUH tid, or fondaparinux.
  - For patients with multiple risk factors for VTE, combine a pharmacologic method (LMWH, LDUH tid, or fondaparinux) with a mechanical method (graduated compression stockings [GCS] and/or intermittent pneumatic compression [IPC]).

  - For patients with a high risk of bleeding, use mechanical thromboprophylaxis with GCS or IPC, and when the bleeding risk decreases, substitute for pharmacologic thromboprophylaxis.
  - For patients undergoing major general surgical procedures, continue thromboprophylaxis until discharge from hospital. For selected high-risk patients (including some of those with major cancer surgery or previous VTE), consider continuing thromboprophylaxis after hospital discharge with LMWH for up to 28 days.

→ Vascular surgery: for patients who do not have additional thromboembolic risk factors: early ambulation. For patients undergoing major vascular surgery with additional thromboembolic risk factors: use LMWH, LDUH, or fondaparinux.

→ Gynecologic surgery:
  - For low-risk gynecologic surgery patients (minor procedure or laparoscopic procedures with no additional risk factors): early ambulation.
  - For patients undergoing laparoscopic procedures with additional VTE risk factors: use LMWH, LDUH, IPC, or GCS.
  - For patients undergoing major gynecologic surgery for benign disease, without additional risk factors: use LMWH, LDUH, or IPC started just before surgery.
  - For patients undergoing extensive surgery for malignancy, and for patients with additional VTE risk factors: use LMWH, LDUH tid, or IPC started just before surgery. Alternative: combination of LMWH or LDUH plus mechanical thromboprophylaxis with GCS or IPC, or fondaparinux.

  - For patients undergoing major gynecologic procedures, continue thromboprophylaxis until discharge from hospital. For selected high-risk patients (including some of those with major cancer surgery or previous VTE), consider continuing thromboprophylaxis after hospital discharge with LMWH for up to 28 days.

→ Urologic surgery:
  - For patients undergoing transurethral or other low-risk urologic procedures: early ambulation.
  - For all patients undergoing major, open urologic procedures: use LDUH bid or tid, GCS, and/or IPC started just before surgery until full ambulation, LMWH, fondaparinux, or combination of pharmacologic and mechanical methods.
  - For urologic surgery patients who are actively bleeding, or who are at very high risk for bleeding: use mechanical thromboprophylaxis with GCS and/ or IPC, and when the bleeding risk decreases, substitute for or add pharmacologic thromboprophylaxis.

→ Laparoscopic surgery: for patients without additional thromboembolic risk factors: early ambulation. For patients undergoing laparoscopic surgery with additional thromboembolic risk factors: use LMWH, LDUH, fondaparinux, IPC, or GCS.

→ Bariatric surgery: for patients undergoing in-patient bariatric surgery, use LMWH, LDUH tid, fondaparinux, or the combination of one of these pharmacologic methods with optimally used IPC. Higher than usual doses for nonobese patients of LMWH or LDUH should be used.

→ Thoracic surgery: for patients undergoing major thoracic surgery, use LMWH, LDUH, or fondaparinux. For patients at high risk of bleeding, use mechanical thromboprophylaxis with GCS and/or IPC.

→ Orthopedic surgery:
- For elective hip replacement, use LMWH, fondaparinux, or warfarin, for at least 10 days, and prolongation beyond 10 days and up to 35 days is *recommended*.
- For elective knee replacement, use LMWH, fondaparinux, or warfarin, for at least 10 days, and prolongation beyond 10 days and up to 35 days is *suggested*.
- For hip fracture surgery, use fondaparinux, LMWH, warfarin, or LDUH for at least 10 days, and prolongation beyond 10 days and up to 35 days is *recommended*. If surgery is likely to be delayed, start LMWH or LDUH after hospital admission and before surgery. For patients at high risk of bleeding, use mechanical thromboprophylaxis.
- For patients undergoing knee arthroscopy without additional thromboembolic risk factors: early ambulation. For patients with additional thromboembolic risk factors: LMWH.
- For patients undergoing spine surgery without additional thromboembolic risk factors: early ambulation. For patients with additional thromboembolic risk factors, such as advanced age, malignancy, neurologic deficit, previous VTE, or anterior surgical approach: postoperative LDUH, postoperative LMWH, or perioperative IPC. Alternative: GCS. For patients with multiple risk factors for VTE, combine a pharmacological method with a mechanical method.
- For patients with isolated lower-extremity injuries distal to the knee, do not routinely use thromboprophylaxis.

→ Neurosurgery: for patients undergoing major neurosurgery: IPC. Alternative: postoperative LMWH or LDUH. For patients at particularly high thrombosis risk, combine a mechanical method with a pharmacological method.

Note: Estrogens (oral contraceptives, hormone replacement therapy), tamoxifene and raloxifene increase the risk of thromboembolic disease: stop oral contraceptive if possible 1 month preop if major surgery, stop hormone replacement therapy if possible 1 month preop and stop raloxifene 72 hours before prolonged immobilization.

Perioperative Management of Anticoagulation (ACCP 2008)

- For patients at low risk for thromboembolism (< 4%/yr: mechanical heart valve with bileaflet aortic valve prosthesis without atrial fibrillation and no other risk factors for stroke; atrial fibrillation with CHADS$_2$ score of 0 to 2 (and no prior stroke or TIA);: VTE with single VTE occurring > 12 mo ago and no other risk factors): stop warfarin 5 days before surgery and low-dose LMWH or no bridging suggested.

- For patients at moderate risk for thromboembolism (4-10%/yr: mechanical heart valve with bileaflet aortic valve prosthesis and one of the following: atrial fibrillation, prior stroke or transient ischemic attack, hypertension, diabetes, congestive heart failure, age > 75 yr; atrial fibrillation with CHADS$_2$ score of 3 or 4 ; VTE within the past 3 to 12 mo, nonsevere thrombophilic conditions [eg, heterozygous factor V Leiden mutation, heterozygous factor II mutation], recurrent VTE, active cancer [treated within 6 mo or palliative]) : stop warfarin 5 days before surgery and bridging anticoagulation *suggested* with therapeutic-dose LMWH (1st choice, in an outpatient setting), therapeutic-dose IV heparin, or low-dose LMWH.

- For patients at high risk for thromboembolism (> 10%/yr: mechanical heart valve with any mitral valve prosthesis, older [caged-ball or tilting disc] aortic valve prosthesis, recent (within 6 mo) stroke or transient ischemic attack ; atrial fibrillation with CHADS$_2$ score of 5 or 6, recent [within 3 mo] stroke or transient ischemic attack, rheumatic valvular heart disease ; VTE with recent [within 3 mo] episode, severe thrombophilia [eg, deficiency of protein C, protein S or antithrombin, antiphospholipid antibodies, or multiple abnormalities]) : stop warfarin 5 days before surgery and bridging anticoagulation *recommended* with therapeutic-dose LMWH (1st choice, in an outpatient setting) or IV heparin.

- In patients receiving bridging anticoagulation, the last dose of LMWH should be 24 h before surgery, and the last preoperative dose should be approximately half the total daily dose. If IV heparin is used, stop it 4 h before surgery. In patients undergoing a *minor* procedure, resume therapeutic-dose LMWH 24 h after the procedure when there is adequate hemostasis. In patients undergoing *major* surgery or a *high bleeding risk* surgery/procedure and for whom postoperative therapeutic-dose LMWH/IV heparin is planned, delay initiation of therapeutic-dose LMWH/IV heparin for 48-72 h after surgery when hemostasis is secured, or administer low-dose LMWH/LDUH after surgery when

hemostasis is secured, or completely avoid LMWH/heparin after surgery, depending on patient condition.
– In patients undergoing minor dermatological procedures, or cataract removal, continue warfarin.

– In patients undergoing minor dental procedures, continue warfarin and coadministrate an oral prohemostatic agent.

– In patients requiring reversal of the anticoagulation effect for an urgent surgical or other invasive procedure: vitamin K 2.5-5 mg IV or oral. For more immediate reversal: fresh-frozen plasma or another prothrombin concentrate in addition to low-dose IV or oral vitamin K.

Note: Avoid LMWH 24 hours before an epidural.

Urticaria - Angioedema

Urticaria: intensely pruritic, circumscribed, edematous wheal, erythematous and migratory, localized or disseminated (secondary to dermal involvement), each lesion persisting < 24 hours (in general 2-4 hours).
– Acute if < 6 weeks (in general 7-10 days).
– Chronic if > 6 weeks.

Angioedema: subcutaneous edema (secondary to hypodermis involvement). Affects especially face, larynx, extremities, external genital organs, GI tract.

Vasculitic urticaria: persistence of lesions > 24 hours, burning sensation, especially lower limbs. The lesions vanish leaving hyperpigmentation and/or purpura. Sometimes associated with migratory arthralgias, digestive or renal involvement. Associated with connective tissue disease or serum sickness if complement ↓. Diagnosis by skin biopsy.

40 % have urticaria and angioedema, 40 % urticaria alone, 20 % angioedema alone.

Causes	**Acute**: identifiable cause in 80 % : acute viral infection (coxsackie, EBV, hepatitis, HIV) or bacterial, foods (fish, seafood, fruits, nuts, peanuts), drugs (ACEI, aspirin, beta-lactams, opiates, NSAIDs, alteplase, local anesthetics, atropine, vancomycine, iodine contrast, pentamidine, Dextran), vaccines, inhalation, latex or other chemical products (cosmetics), insect bites. **Chronic**: idiopathic in > 80 % of cases. – Drugs (See above). – Secondary: SLE or other connective tissue diseases, internal malignancy (gastrointestinal, lymphoproliferative, breast), occult infection (bacterial, viral), thyroid disease, immunologic (hepatitis B), macroglobulinemia. – Physical urticaria: dermographism, to pressure, cold (rule-out cryoglobulinemia, cryofibrinogeninemia, cold agglutinins, cold hemolysins), solar (rule-out porphyria, SLE), cholinergic, to heat, to exercise, aquagenic. – Hereditary angioedema: autosomal dominant: rare: 10-20 years old: family history sometimes present: recurrent attack of abdominal colic, laryngeal edema: no urticaria: precipitated by trauma, infections, dental intervention, emotional stress: ↑ frequency and severity with puberty, menstruation and ovulation: Diagnosis: C4 ↓ (but sometimes normal), C1 esterase inhibitor absent (85 %) or functionally inactive (15%) where C1 esterase inhibitor is normal. – Episodic angioedema with eosinophilia (Gleich's syndrome): angioedema, urticaria, fever, leukocytosis, IgM ↑. C1 ↓. Rare. – Acquired deficiency of C1 esterase inhibitor (C1 Inh): no associated urticaria. No familial history. Rare. o Excessive activation of complement secondary to lymphoproliferative disease or neoplasia. o Antibodies against C1 Inh (SLE).

Differential diagnosis of urticaria	Insect bite. Systemic mastocytosis. Pruritus accompanied by dermographism. Maculo-papular drug eruption. Contact dermatitis. Vasculitic urticaria. Erythema multiforme Bullous pemphigoid in prodromal phase. Serum sickness. Polymorphic eruption of pregnancy (PUPPP)
Workup	– History important + + + for diagnosis (chronology, past medical history, drugs, eating habits, occupation, triggering events, accompanying signs) – CBC (eosinophilia), TSH, antithyroid antibodies, urinalysis. – If needed: sedimentation rate, C-reactive protein, C3-C4 (if suspected connective tissue disease), serum protein electrophoresis, liver enzymes, rule out *H. pylori*, hepatitis B serology, search for parasites in the stools, chest X-ray ... – C4 if suspicion of hereditary angioedema. C1 if suspicion of acquired deficiency of C1 esterase inhibitor. – Skin biopsy/direct immunofluorescence + complement assay if vasculitic urticaria suspected. – Allergy tests as needed.

Treatment	– Treatment of causal factor.
	– Acute urticaria :
	    - Anti-H1 (often at maximal doses).
	    - Corticotherapy if not controlled by anti-H1 (treat 7 days).
	
	– Chronic urticaria :
	    - Anti-H1 ± anti-H2 (often at maximal doses) 4-8 weeks.
	    - If refractory: doxepine (combined anti-H1 and anti-H2 effect but side effect = drowsiness).
	    - If refractory: steroids (but side effects - limit to 7 days of treatment).
	    - If refractory: leukotriene receptor antagonists. Cyclosporine.
	    - Change of diet? Avoid ASA-NSAIDs.
	    - Cyproheptadine for cold urticaria.
	    - NSAIDs for pressure urticaria.
	
	– Vasculitic urticaria: anti-H1 ± NSAIDs. Colchicine, dapsone, hydroxychloroquine. If resistant, steroids, azathioprine, cyclosporine, immunoglobulins IV.
	
	– Angioedema: see Anaphylaxis table.
	
	– Hereditary or acquired angioedema:
	    - Acute: concentrate of C1 Inh (500-1000 U IV: effective in 30-60 minutes). Fresh-frozen plasma (if no concentrate of C1 Inh available). Danazol.
	    - In prophylaxis: tranexamic acid or concentrate of C1 Inh for surgery or dental extraction.
	
	– Consultation in dermatology or allergy as needed.

Prognosis	40 % of urticaria persistent > 6 months is still present 10 years later. Average duration 3-5 years.

Hypothermia	
Accidental fall of the body's core temperature: under 35° C.	
Risk factors: age > 65 years old, dementia, malnutrition, homelessness, drug use, alcoholism, trauma, intellectual deficiency.	
Causes	– Environmental: exposure to cold (inside or outside: cold bath, air conditioning, perioperative period) – Dermatologic: severe psoriasis, burns, exfoliative dermatitis … – Metabolic: severe hypothyroidism, diabetic ketoacidosis, hypocorticism, hypopituitarism … – Neurological: multiple sclerosis with hypothalamic lesion, Wernicke's encephalopathy, tumor, stroke, trauma. – Sepsis. – Prolonged cardiac arrest. – Episodic hypothermia with hyperhydrosis, spontaneous periodic hypothermia syndrome (or Shapiro's syndrome). – Hodgkin's lymphoma. – Medications and drugs: beta-blockers, clonidine, meperidine, atypical antipsychotics, baclofen, organophosphates, alcohol intoxication, general anesthesia, canabinoids. – Iatrogenic: heat stroke treatment, aggressive volume repletion, multiple blood transfusions.
Severity	According to *American Heart Association:* - Mild: > 34° C. - Moderate: 30° C-34° C. - Severe: < 30° C.
Clinical findings	– Mild hypothermia: Initial phase of response to cold: hypertension, shivering, tachycardia, tachypnea, vasoconstriction. With time and fatigue: apathy, ataxia, cold diuresis, hypovolemia, ↓ judgment. – Moderate hypothermia: sinus arrhythmia, bradycardia, bradypnea, ↓ state of consciousness, mydriasis, ↓ gag reflex, hyporeflexia, hypotension, ECG - J wave (or Osborn wave: if < 32° C) Severe hypothermia: apnea, coma, non-reactive pupils, oliguria, pulmonary edema, ventricular arrhythmia, asystoly.
Workup	CBC. Electrolytes (serial), creatinine, BUN, glucose, arterial blood gas, CK. Coagulation workup. Hepatic workup. ECG. STAT capillary glycemia. If needed: TSH, infectious workup, pancreatic workup, myoglobin, toxicological screening, ethanol level, EEG.
Treatment	Usual ABC: Stabilize patient, give oxygen (humidified and heated if possible), venous access, intubation and mechanical ventilation if respiratory insufficiency. Give dextrose if capillary glycemia is not available. Adequate volume repletion (NaCl 0.9 % + D5W). Give thiamine IV + naloxone IV empirically. Urinary catheter if needed in order to evaluate urinary output ± central line. Cardiac monitoring. Move patient with care since there is risk of precipitating ventricular fibrillation. For the same reason, avoid nasogastric tube. Manage any other complications simultaneously (eg. trauma, intoxication, frostbite) If severe hypothermia: transfer to intensive care unit. For patient with preserved stable cardiac rhythm: – Mild hypothermia: passive external re-warming; take off humid clothes, put on a blanket … If no response, active external re-warming (see below). – Moderate hypothermia: active external re-warming; warming blanket, ventilated

	warming blanket (Bair Hugger®), heated IV solutions (43 °C), humidified heated oxygen (42-46 °C), and immersion in warm water – Severe hypothermia: Internal active warming; heated humidified oxygen (42-46 °C) during mechanical ventilation, gastric lavage, colonic or vesical lavage with warm saline solution. More invasive procedures:, extracorporeal circulation (↑ temperature by 7-10 °C/hour), hemodialysis / hemofiltration, pleural or peritoneal lavage with warm saline ... For patient in cardiac arrest: – Moderate hypothermia: start cardio-pulmonary reanimation, try defibrillation, establish venous access, give medication IV at longer intervals, and proceed to active internal rewarming. – Severe hypothermia: start cardio-pulmonary resuscitation, try defibrillation x 1, do not give medication until temperature > 30 ° C, proceed with active internal rewarming. Note: With treatment of hypothermia, look our for a secondary fall of core temperature (or "after-drop", when an aggravation of hypothermia can be observed as cooled blood reaches central core while peripheral vasodilatation sets in) and "re-warming shock", characterized by a decreased cardiac flow and peripheral resistance which can provoke hypotension and hypovolemic shock. The lowest temperature ever registered in an adult surviving hypothermia is 13.7 °C. So, a patient can only be considered dead if he is warm and dead (except in presence of frozen thorax, serious lesions, K^+ > 12 mEq/L, thrombosed blood or a "do not resuscitate" order).

Noninfectious Hyperthermia	
Malignant Hyperthermia	Condition encountered in a patient carrying a gene mutation for a calcium channel of the sarcoplasmic reticulum, autosomal dominant in 50 %, present in 1/15 000-1/40 000 of the general population. Clinical findings: severe hyperthermia (> 40 °C) occuring suddenly, muscular rigidity, hyporeflexia, metabolic acidosis and hemodynamic instability during or in the hours following general anaesthesia (with the use of succinylcholine, halothane). Other possible findings: tachycardia, hypotension, arrhythmia, hypoxia, lactic acidosis, DIC, ↑ CK and ↑ K^+. Treatment: stop causal agent. Rapid IV Dantrolene infusion, Cooling. Supportive cardiovascular and metabolic care.
Neuroleptic Malignant Syndrome	Clinical findings: fever, muscle rigidity ("lead pipe" type), alteration of consciousness, autonomic dysfunction (tachycardia, labile BP, diaphoresis), slow reflexes, extra-pyramidal symptoms. More progressive onset (over 1-3 days) than malignant hyperthermia or serotoninergic syndrome, occurring in general during the first 30 days of treatment. Rare (< 1 % of patients receiving neuroleptics). Cause: medication ↓ dopamine in central nervous system: haloperidol, phenothiazines, atypical antipsychotics, tricyclic antidepressants, MAOI, metocopramide, etc. Can also occur with abrupt stopping of dopaminergic agents. Workup: ↑ Na^+, acidosis, hemoconcentration, leukocytosis, ↑ CK, ↑ AST-ALT, renal failure can occur. Treatment: Stop causal agent. Cooling and supportive treatment (IV fluids, etc.). Dantrolene or bromocriptine (↓ duration of hyperthermia ?), Mechanical ventilation with muscle paralysis if needed. Mortality = 10 %. Risk of recurrence: 30 %.

Serotoninergic Syndrome	Clinical findings: hyperthermia, agitation, confusion, diaphoresis, tachycardia, diarrhea, tremor, ↑ muscular tone (especially in lower limbs), hyperreflexia, clonus, mydriasis, hypertension frequent. Shock can occur. Syndrome might be mild (even without hyperthermia), moderate or severe. Secondary to excessive stimulation of the 5-HT2A receptor, particularly by SSRI. Can also occur with tricyclics, lithium, MAOI (especially if combined with meperidine, SSRI, dextromethorphan, MDMA), L-dopa, antibiotics (linezolid), anti-emetic, LSD, natural products. The syndrome only occurs if serotoninergic agents have been taken during the last five weeks. Onset is usually rapid, most often < 6 hours after the beginning of or change of dose or after intoxication. Workup: metabolic acidosis, ↑ CK, renal failure, ↑ AST, DIC can occur. Treatment: stop causal agent. Benzodiazepine if mild syndrome or moderate hyperthermia, olanzapine 10 mg sublingual, cyproheptadine PO or via nasogastric tube (side effect = sedation). IM chlorpromazine if severe (?) (Avoid if hypotension or malignant neuroleptic syndrome). If severe hyperthermia (> 41.1 °C), immediate paralysis with non-depolarizing agents + intubation and mechanical ventilation. Hypertension/tachycardia treatment with short-acting agents (esmolol, nitroprusside). Symptoms usually resolve within 24 hours.
Drug-Induced Fever	Precise incidence unknown, 3-5 % of medication side effects. Risk factors: large number of drugs taken, HIV infection, cystic fibrosis. Clinical findings: isolated or sometimes associated with rash, urticaria, mucous membrane involvement, renal failure, hepatitis, pulmonary or hematologic involvement. Temperature-pulse dissociation. Cause: practically, any medication can cause fever, but more frequent with antibiotics (minocycline, beta-lactams, sulfonamides, nitrofurantoin), anticonvulsants, allopurinol, tricyclic antidepressants, antihistaminic drugs, amphotericin B, bleomycin, etc. Can also occur with sympathomimetics (cocaine, amphetamines, MDMA). Fever usually resolves within 72-96 hours after medication has been stopped, but may take 5-7 days.
Heat Stroke	"Classic" heat stroke or post-exercice. "Classic": occurs during summer heat waves. ↑ incidence in elderly patients, with co-morbidities or predisposing medication (anticholinergics, phenothiazines …) "Post-exercise": ↑ frequency in young athletes or with use of ephedrine or creatine. Clinical: Sudden ↑ of temperature (> 40.5 °C) with confusion, lethargy, delirium, convulsion, coma. Tachycardia, arrhythmia, myocardial ischemia, pulmonary edema, ARDS, aspiration pneumonia, oliguria, vomiting, diarrhea, hematuria, DIC: all of these can occur. Workup: hemoconcentration, leukocytosis, DIC, hematuria, myoglobinuria, proteinuria, renal failure, ↑ AST-ALT, ↑ CK, respiratory alkalosis, lactic acidosis, ↓ PO_4^{3-}, ECG abnormalities can occur. Treatment: cooling; remove clothes, immersion in ice cold water bath or use ice bags, cooling mattress. Treat complications in usual way.

Useful References: GENERAL INTERNAL MEDICINE

Alcohol-Use Disorders: Lancet 2009; 373: 492-501 (review article)
         N Engl J Med 2005; 352: 596-607 (review article)
Alcohol Withdrawal:
         JAMA 1997; 278: 144-151 & Arch Intern Med 2004 ; 164 : 1405-12 (review article)
Anaphylaxis: CMAJ 2003; 169: 307-12 (review article)
         Am J Med 2007; 120: 664-68 (review article)
Angioedema: Am J Med 2008; 121: 282-86 (review article)
Anticoagulation: Chest 2008; 133: 71S-105S (American Guidelines)
Arterial Hypertension: Can J Cardiol 2009; 25: 279-86 (Canadian Guidelines: diagnosis)
         Can J Cardiol 2009; 25: 287-98 (Canadian Guidelines: treatment)
            Annual update at www.hypertension.ca
         JAMA 2003; 289: 2560-71 (American Guidelines)
         ... Essential: Lancet 2007; 370: 591-603 (review article)
         ... Isolated Systolic: N Engl J Med 2007; 357: 789-96 (review article)
         ... Hypertensive crises: Chest 2007; 131: 1949-1962 (review article)
         ... Resistant Hypertension: Hypertension 2008; 51; 1403-1419 (AHA Guidelines)
            J Am Coll Cardiol 2008; 52: 1749-57 (review article)
Carcinoid Syndrome: Clev Clin J Med 2008 ; 75 : 849-55 (review article)
Chronic Angioedema and Urticaria: N Engl J Med 2002; 346: 175-9 (review article)
Deep Vein Thrombosis: Ann Intern Med 2007; 146: 204-10 & 454-458 (ACP Guidelines)
            CMAJ 2006; 175: 1087-92 (review article)
            Lancet 2005; 365: 1163-74 (review article)
            N Engl J Med 2004; 351: 268-77 (review article)
         ...and Pregnancy: Chest 2008; 133: 844S-886S (review article)
Drug and Alcohol Withdrawal: N Engl J Med 2003; 348: 1786-95 (review article)
Erectile Dysfunction: N Engl J Med 2007; 357: 2472-81 (review article)
         CMAJ 2004; 170: 1429-37 (review article)
Gestationnel Diabetes: Can J Diabetes 2008; 32 (suppl 1): S168-S175 (Canadian Guidelines)
         Obstet Gynecol Surv 2007; 62: 125-136 (review article)
         J Obstet Gynaecol Can 2002; 24: 904-13 (Canadian Guidelines on screening)
         Obstet Gynecol 2003; 101: 380-95 (American Guidelines on screening)
Hereditary Angioedema: N Engl J Med 2008; 359: 2025-33 (review article)
Hypertension and Pregnancy: J Obstet Gynaecol Can 2008; 30: S1-47 (Canadian Guidelines)
         Am J Obstet Gynecol 2000; 183: S1-22 (American Guidelines)
         Obstet Gynecol 2002; 100: 369-377 (review article)
Hypothermia: Am J Med 2006; 119: 297-301 (review article)
Intoxication: Chest 2003; 123: 577-92 & 897-922 (review article)
         ... Acetaminophen - Acetylcysteine: N Engl J Med 2008; 359: 285-92 (review article)
         ... Carbon Monoxide: N Engl J Med 2009; 360: 1217-25 (review article)
         ... Fomepizole: N Engl J Med 2009; 360: 2216-23 (review article)
         ... Heroin: Ann Intern Med 1999; 130: 584- (review article)
         ... Lithium: J Am Soc Nephrol 1999; 10: 666- (review article)
         ... Organophosphorus Pesticide: Lancet 2008; 371: 597-607 (review article)
Involuntary Weight Loss: Mayo Clin Proc 2001; 76: 923-9 (review article)
         ... in the elderly : CMAJ 2005 ; 172 : 773-780 (review article)
Obesity: CMAJ 2007; 176 (8 SUPPL): Online-1-117 (Canadian Guidelines)
         N Engl J Med 1997; 337: 396-407 (review article)
         ... Treatment: Mayo Clin Proc 2007; 82: 93-102 (review article)
            N Engl J Med 2002; 346: 591-602 (review article)
         ... Bariatric Surgery: N Engl J Med 2007; 356: 2176-83 (review article)
Orthostatic Hypotension: N Engl J Med 2008; 358: 615-24 (review article)
Peripheral Arterial Disease:
         J Vasc Surg 2007; 45 (Suppl S):S5A-S67A (Transatlantic Guidelines)
         Mayo Clin Proc 2008; 83: 944-950 (review article)
         Can J Cardiol 2005; 21: 997-1006 (Canadian Guidelines)
         Circulation 2006; 113: 1474-1547 (American Guidelines)
         ... Treatment: JAMA 2006; 295: 547-53 (review article)
            N Engl J Med 2001; 344: 1608-21 (review article)
         ... Intermittent Claudication: N Engl J Med 2007; 356: 1241-50 (review article)
Peripheral Edema: Am J Med 2002; 113: 580-86 (review article)
Preop: Med Clin N Am 2008; 92: 325-348 (review article)
         Cardiac Assessment: Circulation 2007; 116: 1971-1996 (ACC/AHA Guidelines)
            Mayo Clin Proc 2009; 84:79-90 (review article)
            J Am Coll Cardiol 2008; 51: 1913-24 (review article)

Pulmonary Assessment: Ann Intern Med 2006; 144: 575-580 (ACP Guidelines)
Eur Respir J 2007; 132: 1637-45 (review article)
Diabetes: Anesthesiology 2009; 110: 408-21 (review article)
Adrenal Function: Ann Surg 1994; 219: 416- (review article)
Liver Disease and Surgery: Mayo Clin Proc 1999; 74: 593- (review article)
Pulmonary Embolism: Lancet 2004; 363: 1295-305 (review article)
Circulation 2003; 108: 2726-29 & 2834-38 (review article)
Eur Heart J 2008; 29: 2276-2315 (ESC Guidelines)
… Acute: N Engl J Med 2008; 358: 1037-52 & 359: 2804-13 (review article)
Raynaud Phenomenon: N Engl J Med 2002; 347: 1001-08 (review article)
Serotoninergic Syndrome: N Engl J Med 2005; 352: 1112-20 (review article)
Thromboembolic Disease and Pregnancy: N Engl J Med 2008; 359: 2025-33 (review article)
Urticaria: Am J Med 2008; 121: 379-84 (review article)

Chapter 5

Hematology-Oncology

Disorders of Hemoglobin	
Anemia	Anemia can be subdivided according to MCV (micro-normo-macrocytic) or according to regenerative capacities (hypo or hyper-reticulocytosis).

Causes	**If reticulocytes are ↑:**
	– **MCV normal or ↑:**
	   - Acute hemorrhage.
	   - Hemolysis: see below.
	   - Spherocytosis (where mean corpuscular hemoglobin concentration is ↑ or ↓).
	– **MCV normal or ↓ :**
	   - Thalassemia (where red blood cell count is ↑).
	
	If reticulocytes are ↓:
	– **↑ MCV :**
	   - Vitamin B12 or folate deficiency, which can be secondary to pernicious anemia (see below), or secondary to malabsorption (post-gastrectomy, post-ileal resection, chronic pancreatitis, bacterial overgrowth, etc).
	   - Folate deficiency: secondary to inadequate intake, alcohol, increased requirements (pregnancy, hemolytic anemia), malabsorption or medication (see below).
	   - Medication: methotrexate, sulfamethoxazole, phenytoin, primidone, phenobarbital, sulfasalazine, oral contraceptives, triamterene, zidovudine, azathioprine, 5-FU, hydroxyurea, cytarabine, cyclophosphamide, etc.
	   - Myelodysplastic syndrome.
	   - Hypothyroidism.
	   - Hepatic disease.
	   - Other causes: HIV, multiple myeloma or other plasma cell dyscrasia, bone marrow aplasia (occasionnally), pure red cell aplasia.
	– **Normal MCV :**
	   - Anemia of chronic disease (chronic kidney disease, cirrhosis, etc).
	   - Combined micro + macrocytic anemia (where ↑ RDW).
	   - Myelodysplasic syndrome (occasionally).
	   - Marrow replacement (multiple myeloma, leukemias, solid tumors, myelofibrosis).
	   - Aplastic anemia (see Pancytopenia table).
	   - Pure red cell aplasia.
	   - Endocrine disorders: Hyper or hypothyroidism, hypopituitarism, adrenal insufficiency, hypogonadism.
	   - Other causes: HIV, medication, chemotherapy, alcohol, radiotherapy, hypersplenism, etc.
	– **↓ MCV : *with ↓ Ferritin* :**
	   - Chronic GI bleeding (ulcer, malignancy, telangiectasias, arteriovenous malformations, runner's anemia, etc).
	   - Gynecological causes (menstruations, increased need during pregnancy).
	   - Pulmonary causes (malignancy, pulmonary hemosiderosis)
	   - Malabsorption (or post-gastrectomy).
	   - Other causes: Phlebotomy (sometimes self-inflicted), chronic intravascular hemolysis, parasitic infection.
	– **↓ MCV : *with Normal or ↑ Ferritin*:**
	   - Anemia of chronic diseases (Hb rarely < 80 g/L or MCV < 75 fL): transferrin saturation > 15 % generally).
	   - Thalassemia.
	   - Secondary to chronic kidney disease.
	   - Other causes: lead poisoning, sideroblastic anemia (primary or secondary to alcohol, anticonvulsants, isoniazid, zinc deficiency, lead or copper poisoning), hemoglobin E or C, hyperthyroidism, or vitamin B6 deficiency.

Workup	CBC, blood smear (microcytosis, hypochromia, target cells, schistocytes, blasts...), reticulocytes, hemolysis workup (bilirubin, LDH, haptoglobin, Coombs test), ferritin, vitamin B12, folate, protein electrophoresis, TSH, INR, aPTT. Routine biochemistry.
	As needed: marrow aspiration + biopsy (especially if nonregenerative), Schilling test, anti-parietal cell or anti-intrinsic factor antibody levels (methylmalonic acid or homocysteinemia as needed), viral serology (parvovirus B19, others), neoplastic evaluation, fecal occult blood test, GI endoscopy, osmotic fragility test (for congenital spherocytosis), enzyme levels (glucose-6-phosphate dehydrogenase, pyruvate kinase, etc), ANA, hemoglobin electrophoresis, flow cytometry (for paroxysmal nocturnal hemoglobinuria), etc.
	Reticulocyte Production Index: reticulocytes % x (Hematocrit ÷ 0.45) x 0.5: normal = 1-2 %. Regenerative anemia if > 2.
Treatment	According to cause. Transfusions if hemodynamic instability, symptomatic or Hb < 100 g/L in cardiac patients or Hb < 70 g/L in others (controversial). Erythropoietin if chronic kidney disease, cancer on chemotherapy or chronic disease.

Hemolytic Anemia

Causes	– Intrinsic causes:
	  - Congenital:
	    • Membrane defects: congenital spherocytosis, congenital elliptocytosis, etc.
	    • Enzyme defects: pyruvate kinase or glucose-6-phosphate dehydrogenase, severe hypophosphatemia, etc.
	    • Hemoglobinopathies: sickle cell anemia, thalassemia major, unstable hemoglobins, methemoglobinemia, etc.
	  - Acquired: lead poisoning, methemoglobinemia, paroxysmal nocturnal hemoglobinuria (see Pancytopenia table).
	
	– Extrinsic causes:
	  - Immunological: autoimmune: 50 % idiopathic or secondary to SLE, chronic lymphocytic leukemia, Non-Hodgkin's lymphoma (among them: angioimmunoblastic lymphadenopathy), ovarian cancer, infections (mycoplasma, mononucleosis, severe bacteremia, medication (methyldopa, penicillin, procainamide, quinidine, ribavirin, ibuprofen, cephalosporins, tetracycline, isoniazid, rifampicine, sulfonamides, acetaminophen, hydrochlorothiazide, hydralazine, etc) sometimes with autoimmune thrombocytopenia = Evans syndrome.
	  - Cold agglutinin syndrome (primary cold hemagglutinin disease).
	  - Transfusion reactions.
	  - Microangiopathic: TTP-HUS, disseminated intravascular coagulation (see Platelet disorders table), vasculitis, valve replacement, metastatic adenocarcinoma, eclampsia, malignant hypertension, etc.
	  - Infections: malaria, *Clostridium* sp., *Borrelia* sp., parvovirus B 19.
	  - Medication: nitrofurantoin, sulfonamides (especially with glucose-6-phosphate dehydrogenase deficiency).
	  - Hypersplenism.
	  - Severe liver disease.
	  - Severe burn.

Workup	CBC, blood smear: look for schistocytes, sickle cells, Heinz bodies (suggestive of a drug-induced etiology), spherocytes. Reticulocytes, LDH, bilirubin, haptoglobin (↓ in hemolysis), direct Coombs test, INR, aPTT. As needed: enzyme levels, osmotic fragility test, hemoglobin electrophoresis, cold agglutinin, etc. Direct Coombs test: presence of **warm** antibodies with idiopathic diseases, connective tissue disease, lymphoproliferative diseases (CLL, multiple myeloma, NHL, Waldenström's macroglobulinemia), HIV, ulcerative colitis. Presence of **cold** antibodies (in 16-36 %) with cold agglutinin syndrome, mycoplasma, mononucleosis, lymphoproliferative diseases, paroxysmal cold hemoglobinuria. Hemolytic anemia with direct Coombs ⊖ is found with some drugs, toxins, trauma, some infections, microangiopathic (TTP-HUS), enzyme deficiency, hereditary spherocytosis, Wilson's disease, paroxysmal nocturnal hemoglobinuria, etc.
Treatment	Refer to specialist. Treatment according to the cause. If autoimmune: Avoid transfusion if patient is clinically stable. If necessary, transfuse the most compatible blood available. Prednisone 1-2 mg/kg/d + folic acid 1 mg/d. Effective in 1-3 weeks (⊕ in 80-90 %). If no improvement (after 6-8 weeks of treatment); splenectomy. If still no improvement; cyclophosphamide, cyclosporine, mycophenolate, danazol or IV immunoglobulins (only short term effect). Rituximab.

Pernicious Anemia

Most frequent cause of vitamin B 12 deficiency. Type A chronic atrophic gastritis.
Sometimes associated with other autoimmune diseases.
Anemia-associated symptoms, glossitis, diarrhea or malabsorption induced by megaloblastosis, subacute combined degeneration of the spinal cord (involvement of posterior and lateral columns and cerebellum), peripheral neuropathy, personality disorder, dementia. Associated with gastric adenocarcinoma and carcinoid tumor (secondary to achlorhydria).

Workup	Vitamin B 12 and folate levels. If B-12 ↓, repeat measurement once for confirmation. Anti-parietal cell and anti-intrinsic factor antibodies assays ± Schilling test to confirm diagnosis. Presence of hypersegmented neutrophiles, macro-ovalocytes and Howell-Jolly's bodies in blood smear. Homocysteine or methylmalonic acid levels may be useful if there is clinical suspicion and low to normal B12 levels. It is unclear if gastroscopy should be done for gastric tumor follow-up. Note: vitamin B 12 levels are falsely lowered in pregnancy and by oral contraceptives.
Treatment	Vitamin B 12 ≥ 100 µg IM per month or 1000 µg PO daily. If anemia is severe, treat with vitamin B12 1000 µg IM daily for 7 days, but consider risk of hypokalemia. Sub-optimal response if concomitant iron deficiency.

Sickle Cell Anemia

Autosomal codominant disorder where abnormal hemoglobin induces chronic hemolysis with its consequences.

↑ sickling with dehydration, acidosis, hypoxia (local or systemic).
8 % of the African-American population are carriers of the hemoglobin S gene (heterozygote and asymptomatic);
Sickle cell anemia (homozygote) frequency = 1/625. Prenatal genetic testing is available.

Clinical findings	Hemolysis causes jaundice, cholelithiasis, splenomegaly, leg ulcers.
	Hemolytic or aplastic crises can occur with infection (Parvovirus B 19, CMV, pneumococcus, salmonella) or folate deficiency. Hemolytic crisis can also occur with splenic sequestration or G6PD deficiency.
	Acute painful crises develop spontaneously or secondary to infection, dehydration or hypoxia, persisting for hours to days. Mainly involving long bones, back or thorax. Abdominal pain can occur. Vaso-occlusive crisis may also cause stroke (sinus thrombosis) and priapism. Appears usually between 12 months and 6 years of age.
	↑ susceptibility to osteomyelitis caused by staphylococcus and salmonella. Retinopathy can occur and cause blindness. Involvement of the heart (cardiomyopathy, murmur), lungs (restrictive disease), kidneys (papillary necrosis, nephrotic syndrome, renal failure, tubular dysfunction) can also occur.
Workup	Chronic hemolysis. Reticulocytosis (10-25 %). Sickle cells in blood smear. Howell-Jolly bodies (with hyposplenism), mild leukocytosis, thrombocytosis. Presence of erythroblasts in blood smear. Diagnosis confirmed with hemoglobin electrophoresis.
Treatment	Folic acid supplementation. Transfusion, as needed, for aplastic or hemolytic crisis. Antibiotics if infection suspected (notably in thoracic syndrome). Vaccination against pneumococcus, influenza, meningococcus, *Hemophilus influenzae* and hepatitis B. If fever: acetaminophen. Prophylactic penicillin therapy.
	For acute painful crisis: identify and treat precipitating factor. IV Hydration. Oxygen if hypoxia. Analgesia. Bed rest. Exchange transfusion indicated for stroke, recurrent acute thoracic syndrome, retinopathy, pregnancy, priapism, hematuria, chronic cutaneous ulcer: target = hemoglobin S < 30 % and hemoglobin < 100-110 g/L. Hydroxyurea to ↓ frequency of painful crises (since ↑ hemoglobin F, but long term safety?). Allogeneic stem-cell transplant? Iron chelating agent if frequent transfusions.
Prognosis	Life expectancy: 50-60 years. In adults: 78 % die from acute painful crises, chest syndrome, stroke or infections.
Polycythemia	Polycythemia vera: see Myeloproliferative Disorders table.

	Other causes of (secondary) polycythemia:
	 – With normal O_2 saturation:
	    1. Stress erythrocytosis (where lab results are normal).
	    2. Erythropoietin-secreting tumor (renal adenocarcinoma, renal adenoma, renal cyst, cerebellar hemangioblastoma, ovarian carcinoma, parathyroid carcinoma, hepatocellular carcinoma, pheochromocytoma, uterine fibroma, meningioma, etc).
	    3. Other causes: erythropoietin, androgenes, testosterone, renal artery stenosis, hydronephrosis, renal transplant, Bartter's syndrome, etc.
	 – With ↓ O_2 saturation: hypoxic polycythemia: with pulmonary disease, congenital heart disease, tobacco, sleep apnea, hemoglobinopathies … clubbing sometimes present.

Management	If hematocrit > 58 % (men) or 52 % (women) : → Measurement of O_2 saturation and leukocyte alkaline phosphatase (LAP):
	– If O_2 saturation > 92 % and LAP normal: measurement of carboxyhemoglobin (in smokers): if normal, measurement of erythropoietin and detection of the JAK2 mutation and/or perform a polysomnography. If suspicion of erythropoietin secreting tumor: abdominal ultrasound or CT.
	– If O_2 saturation < 92% and LAP normal: hypoxic polycythemia.
	– If LAP ↑: myeloproliferative disorder.
	Sometimes multiples causes present concomitantly (polycythemia vera in COPD ...). Treat according to cause.
	See Myeloproliferative Syndromes table.

Disorders of Leukocytes and Leukemia

Leukocytosis Differential diagnosis	– **Non-leukemic**: could be secondary to inflammation, infections (*C. difficile* colitis, HIV, EBV, CMV, hepatitis, influenza, tuberculosis, toxoplasmosis, cancers (leukemoid reactions), tobacco, Cushing's, medications (prednisone, lithium, G-CSF); laboratory findings: no blasts, leukocytes < 50 x 10^9/L, normal or ↑ leukocyte alkaline phosphatase, no Philadelphia chromosome, no hepatosplenomegaly (usually).
	– **Leukemic**: leukemias (see below).
	– Myeloid metaplasia (myeloid cells precursors, teardrop-shaped red blood cells): see Myeloproliferative Disorders table.
Leukopenia Differential diagnosis	Secondary to proliferation defect:
	- *bone marrow lesion*: marrow aplasia, radiotherapy, medication (chemotherapy, phenytoin, carbamazepine, sulfonamides, penicillin, cephalosporins, TMP/SMX, antiretrovirals, chloramphenicol, clozapine, cytotoxics, propylthiouracil, methimazole, indomethacin, gold compounds, tricyclic antidepressants, solvents, insecticides), paroxysmal nocturnal hemoglobinuria, hepatitis, etc.
	- *bone marrow invasion*: neoplasms, leukemias, granuloma, etc.
	Secondary to maturation defect: vitamin B12 or folate deficiency.
	Secondary to a decrease in cell survival (normal bone marrow): sepsis, HIV, autoimmune diseases (SLE, Felty), hypersplenism.
Leukemias	
Acute Lymphoid Leukemia	Most common cause of leukemia in children: 20 % of adult leukemias.
	Symptoms secondary to cytopenias (bleeding, infections, fatigue, etc), arthritis, bone pain, lymphadenopathy, visceromegaly, infiltration of gums, skin, and meninges, leukostasis if blasts > 200 x 10^9/L (with headaches, confusion, dyspnea, etc).
	Lab: pancytopenia with blasts (blasts absent in 10 % = "aleukemic leukemia").
	Bone marrow: hypercellular. Chromosomal analyses may help determine prognosis.
	Treatment: chemotherapy; bone marrow transplantation if high risk of recurrence or genetic abnormalities.
	Prognosis depends on age, chromosomal abnormalities [poor prognosis with t(9;22; t (4;11), t (8;14), t (1;19)], leukocyte count, remission with treatment : 30-40 % survival in adults.

Acute Myeloid Leukemia	Clinical features: ≈ ALL: infiltration of liver, spleen, CNS, bone, gums, lymph nodes. Leukostasis or cerebral hemorrhage if leukocytes > 100 x 10^9/L, DIC with AML M3 or M5.
	Diagnosis: Identification of leukemic myeloblasts in blood smear or marrow. 20% blasts in marrow necessary for diagnosis.
	Differentiate of primary AML from ALL, myelodysplastic syndrome, and secondary AML (secondary to hematological disease, hereditary, myelodysplastic syndrome, chemotherapy [alkylating agents, topoisomerase II inhibitors]).
	Classification (therapeutic implications): 8 AML subtypes (French-American-British classification, from M0 to M7) based of morphological, immunohistochemical, immunological and cytogenetic characteristics.
	Treatment : Induction: chemotherapy with cytarabine + anthracycline (idarubicine or daunorubicine), (complete remission 50-80 %). Post-remission: consolidation or intensification: if < 55 years: allogeneic or autologous marrow transplantation (if poor prognostic factors or recurrence) or post-remission chemotherapy with cytarabine. If > 55 years, chemotherapy if good performance status. Gemtuzumab used if AML recurrence in ≥ 60 year old, CD 33 ⊕, not eligible for cytotoxic chemotherapy. For AML M3 [t (15; 17)]: add all-trans retinoic acid (ATRA) to chemotherapy. Arsenic may be effective in case of recurrence.
	Prognosis: 5-years survival rate of 60% if favorable cytogenetic (normal chromosomes or t(8;21); t(15; 17); inv (16); 10 % if unfavorable. Poor prognosis factors: ↑ age, unfavorable karyotype (monosomy 5 or 7, trisomy 8, 11 q-, translocation 9: 22 or complex pattern), secondary AML, leukocytes > 20 x 10^9/L, ↑ LDH, poor performance status, etc.
Chronic Lymphoid Leukemia	Most common leukemia in adults (90 % > 50 years). B cell pathology in 95 % of cases.
	Clinical features: most often asymptomatic: sometimes fatigue, fever, night sweats, weight loss, lymphadenopathy, hepatosplenomegaly, recurrent infections, cytopenia-related symptoms, etc.
	Workup: mature lymphocytosis > 5 x 10^9/L and monoclonal population in flow cytometry (CD 19, 20 and 5 +): at diagnosis, anemia in 35 % (direct Coombs ⊕ in 50 %), auto-immune thrombocytopenia in 15 to 20 %: hypogammaglobulinemia in 50 %.

	Rai classification :
	      - stage 0 : lymphocytosis (> 5 x 10^9/L)
	      - stage 1 : lymphocytosis + lymphadenopathy.
	      - stage 2 : lymphocytosis + hepato and/or splenomegaly
	      - stage 3 : lymphocytosis + anemia (not autoimmune) (Hb < 100 g/L).
	      - stage 4 : lymphocytosis + thrombopenia (not autoimmune) (< 100 x 10^9/L).
	 Binet classification (in Europe).

	Differential diagnosis: reactional lymphocytosis secondary to infection (HIV, EBV, CMV, influenza, tuberculosis, toxoplasmosis, whooping cough), medication, hyperthyroidism, thymoma, autoimmune diseases, or in leukemic phase of other lymphoproliferative disorders (e.g.: mantle cell lymphoma). Treatment :
	    – No treatment if asymptomatic or mildly symptomatic.
	    – Treat when symptomatic or evidence of disease progression (weight loss, fatigue, fever, massive hepatosplenomegaly, rapidly rising lymphocytic count) or anemia or thrombopenia or if presentation at later stages (stage 3-4 or trisomy 12 or deletion 11 q and 17 p): Treatment: Fludarabine and/or rituximab

	± cyclophosphamide. Chlorambucil ± Prednisone in older patients. CVP, CHOP, 2-CDA or other possible combinations. Alemtuzumab (monoclonal antibody) under investigation. Allogeneic transplantation for young patients with poor prognosis.
	– Influenza and Pneumococcal vaccination.
	– IV immunoglobulins to ↓ recurrence of infections and if hypogammaglobulinemia.
	– Steroids or rituximab + CVP or splenectomy for autoimmune manifestations.
	– Erythropoietin for refractory anemia.
	
	Prognosis : depends on stage:
	     - 0: survival = 14.5 years.
	     - 1-2 = 7.5 years.
	     - 3-4 = 2.5 years.
	Prognosis also depends on cytogenetic analysis, leukocyte doubling-time (< or > 12 months), CD38 expression and β2 microglobulin level.
	
	Average survival = 6 years: 5 % of transformation to aggressive diffuse large B-cell lymphoma (Richter's syndrome). Can transform to prolymphocytic leukemia or myeloma. Transformation to ALL rare.
	Increased risk of secondary neoplasm (lungs, prostate, gastrointestinal) and aggressive cutaneous neoplasm.

Hairy Cell Leukemia	Rare (< 2 % leukemias). Male preponderance (4:1). Mean age 55 years. Symptoms: fatigue, bleeding, ↑ risks of infection, etc. Splenomegaly, sometimes massive. Hepatomegaly 50 %, lymphadenopathy (rare). Pancytopenia, characteristic cells (hairy cells) in blood smear. Important monocytopenia. Bone marrow: "dry tap" bone marrow aspiration. Diagnosis by bone biopsy. Treatment: 2-CDA: complete response in 85 %. Average survival > 10 years.
Chronic Myeloid Leukemia	See Myeloproliferative Disorders table.

Eosinophilia	
\multicolumn{2}{l}{Absolute eosinophil count > 0.5 x 10^9/L (or > 500/µL).}
\multicolumn{2}{l}{Note any history of allergies, travel, medication, and systemic disease symptoms.}

Causes	**Low to moderate (0.5-5 x 10^9/L):** *Frequent*: – Atopy: asthma, allergic rhinitis and other atopic diseases. – Medications: leukotriene receptor antagonists, GM-CSF, sulfonamides, nitrofurantoin, gold compounds, sulfasalazine, NSAIDs, aspirin, penicillin, cephalosporin, tetracycline, ranitidine, allopurinol, phenytoin, venlafaxine, L-tryptophan. – Parasites: helminthes (worms, schistosomiasis, trichinosis, Strongyloides, filariasis, toxocariasis ...), *Isospora belli, Dientamoaba fragilis*, etc. *Rare*: – Infections: scarlet fever, tuberculosis, aspergillosis, coccidioidomycosis, etc. – Neoplasms: leukemia, lymphoma, Sézary syndrome, lung tumor, stomach, colon, bladder, cervix, vagina, penis tumor, etc. – Hematological diseases: polycythemia vera, myelodysplasia, hyper-IgE syndrome, Omenn's syndrome, etc. – Inflammatory diseases: inflammatory bowel disease, Churg-Strauss syndrome, polyarteritis nodosa, rheumatoid arthritis, sarcoidosis, etc. – Dermatological diseases: dermatitis herpetiformis, psoriasis, pemphigus, fasciitis, panniculitis, cellulitis, folliculitis, eosinophilic ulcer, etc. – Hypereosinophilic syndrome: see below. – Other: chronic eosinophilic pneumonia, eosinophilic gastroenteritis, adrenal insufficiency, cholesterol embolism, mastocytosis, primary immunodeficiency, chronic active hepatitis, thymoma, etc. **Severe (> 5 x 10^9/L):** – Hypereosinophilic syndrome: myeloproliferative syndrome with eosinophils > 1.5 x 10^9/L for 6 months without other cause, with organic involvement (heart, lung, skin, nervous system, spleen, liver, etc). Affects males > females, 20-50 years of age. – Eosinophilic leukemia (> 10 % of blasts in marrow).
Workup	CBC and blood smear. As needed: stool ova and parasites exam ± serology for parasites, duodenal aspiration for strongyloides, cutaneous biopsy for toxocariasis, muscular biopsy for trichinosis, etc. For hypereosinophilic syndrome: bone marrow aspiration + biopsy, leukocyte alkaline phosphatase, vitamin B12 level, karyotype, ECG, echocardiography, etc. Note: If mild eosinophilia (≤ 1.5 x 10^9/L), repeat CBC in 6 months. If > 1.5 x 10^9/L, repeat CBC in 1-2 months; if remains ↑, refer to a hematologist for further investigation.
Treatment	Treatment according to cause. Treatment for hypereosinophilic syndrome: steroids, imatinib, cyclosporine, chemotherapy. Treatment specific to affected organs.

Platelet Disorders

Thrombocytopenia

Rule out pseudothrombocytopenia (decrease in platelet number in automated cell counter but not in a blood smear) by collecting specimen with citrate (anticoagulant) or by using a fingerstick source.

Causes	1. **↓ production :** Bone marrow failure: − Suppression: aplastic or megaloblastic anemia, myelodysplasia, alcohol, radiotherapy, vitamin B12 or folate deficiency, viral infection (HIV, EBV, HCV, Parvovirus, rubella), etc. − Invasion: leukemias, lymphomas, myelofibrosis, solid tumors, sarcoidosis, etc. − Hereditary disorders (rare): Wiskott-Aldrich, May-Hegglin, etc. 2. **↑ destruction:** *Immunological:* − Idiopathic thrombocytopenic purpura (ITP): see below. − Medication: heparin (heparin-induced thrombopenia - see below), quinine, quinidine, acetaminophen, gold compounds, sulfonamides, valproic acid, carbamazepine, amphotericin B, thiazides, vancomycin, glycoprotein IIb/IIIa inhibitor, procainamide, rifampicin, natural products, etc. − Posttransfusion purpura: 5-8 days post-transfusion: platelet antigen HPA-1a ⊕ transfused to a HPA-1a ⊖ patient: treatment: IV immunoglobulins, plasmapheresis + steroids. − Extracorporeal circulation. − Systemic autoimmune diseases: systemic lupus erythematosus, polyarteritis nodosa, antiphospholipid syndrome, etc. − Malignancies: chronic lymphocytic leukemia, lymphomas, etc. − Viral infections: HIV, EBV, CMV, etc. − Allo-immunity: HPA-1a incompatibility between mother and fetus. *Non-immunological:* − Thrombotic thrombocytopenic purpura and hemolytic-uremic syndrome (TTP-HUS): see below. − Infections: sepsis, malaria, ehrlichiosis, etc. − Disseminated intravascular coagulation (DIC): see below. − HELLP syndrome. − Microangiopathic hemolytic anemia: (heart valve prosthesis). − Paroxysmal nocturnal hemoglobinuria. 3. **Sequestration**: hypersplenism, hemangioma, etc. 4. **Dilutional**: pregnancy, etc.
Workup	CBC, INR, aPTT, blood smear. As needed: vitamin B12 + folate levels, DIC workup (fibrinogen, D-Dimers, etc), hemolysis workup (bilirubin, LDH, direct Coombs test, haptoglobin, etc), renal function tests, abdominal ultrasound (to rule out hypersplenism), ANA, HIV, anticardiolipin antibodies, lupus anticoagulant, heparin-induced thrombocytopenia testing. If not diagnostic: bone marrow biopsy and myelogram: hypocellular myelogram (aplasia), myelophthisic (neoplasm, leukemia, myelofibrosis) or hypercellular (myelodysplasia or megaloblastic): biopsy with normal or ↑ megakaryocytes (with destruction/sequestration).

Treatment	Treatment according to cause. Platelet transfusion if bleeding, platelets < 10 or < 20 x 10^9/L in association with fever. Do not transfuse platelets in TTP-HUS, ITP or heparin-induced thrombopenia. Administer folates as needed. Note: In general, thrombocytopenias secondary to medications improves within in 4-14 days (gold salts may take longer), and those induced by a viral infection within 2-12 weeks.
Idiopathic Thrombocyto-penic Purpura (ITP)	Asymptomatic or presenting with mucosal, cutaneous, or less frequently cerebral/meningeal bleeding. Splenomegaly in 10 %. 40-60 % of adults develop chronic ITP. Diagnosis of exclusion ("isolated thrombocytopenia without apparent associated pathology"). Anti-platelet glycoprotein IIb-IIIa antibodies. MPV ↑ and giant platelets in blood smear. 10 % have concomitant hemolytic anemia (Evans syndrome). Normal marrow with normal or ↑ megakaryocytes (bone marrow examination suggested in patients > 60 years old or requiring splenectomy). Rule out presence of *H. pylori* and HIV. Treatment: indicated if mucosal or cutaneous bleeding, if there is a bleeding risk factor, or if platelets < 30 X 10^9/L. Steroids (Prednisone 1 mg/kg/day or dexamethasone 40 mg PO daily for 4 days: 50 % response in 2-4 weeks) ± immunoglobulins if platelets < 10 x 10^9/L : splenectomy if refractory (effective in 60-70 %: 10 % have accessory spleen): if hemorrhage, IV immunoglobulins 1 g/kg x 2 days + IV SoluMedrol® 1 g daily x 3. Other treatments: danazol, vincristin, vinblastin, azathioprin, cyclophosphamide, rituximab, anti-D, plasmapheresis, etc. Eradication of *H. pylori*: 50 % response to treatment (mechanism unknown). No platelet transfusions except in life-threatening hemorrhage (5 units every 4-6 hours).

Thrombotic Thrombocyto-penic Purpura and Hemolytic-Uremic Syndrome (TTP-HUS)	TTP pathophysiology: deficiency of a vWF-cleaving protease ADAMTS 13 that reduces the size of large vWF multimers, in some cases due to an antibody directed against the protease.
	
	Causes: idiopathic (> 90 %) or secondary to infection by *E. coli* O157H7, Shigella, pneumococci, HIV, malignancy, pregnancy, autoimmune diseases, bone marrow transplantation, quinine, estrogens, clopidogrel, cyclosporine, tacrolimus, mitomycin C, cisplatin, etc.
	
	Pentad: (only 40 % have a complete pentad):
	    1- Microangiopathic hemolytic anemia.
	    2- Thrombopenia.
	    3- Fever.
	    4- Acute renal failure.
	    5- Neurological involvement (headaches, confusion, aphasia, lethargy, seizures, paresis, syncope, coma, etc): frequently dominate clinical presentation.
	
	Occasionally present with abdominal pain, pancreatitis, etc. Patients usually present a poor clinical state. Prodrome often present in preceding 1-2 weeks.
	
	Treatment: plasmapheresis or fresh frozen plasma ± steroids. If no response after 3 days: cryosupernatant or ↑ plasma exchange volume: if failure, chemotherapy or splenectomy.
	Do not give heparin or platelet (except in life-threatening hemorrhage).
	Full response in 80-90 %. 20 % chronic or recurrent. 25 % mortality and 50 % chronic kidney disease development in patients with HUS.

Disseminated Intravascular Coagulation (DIC)	Causes: infectious, obstetrical (amniotic fluid embolism, abruptio placentae), traumatic (muscular, fat embolism, cerebral), malignancy (myeloproliferative-lymphoproliferative syndromes, solid tumors – pancreas, prostate), medications and toxins (venom, quinine, amphetamines, etc), pancreatic or severe hepatic failure, vascular (shock, giant hemangioma, aortic aneurism), immunological (severe allergy, transfusion reactions, graft rejection). Acute or chronic. Bleeding and/or systemic thrombosis. ↓ platelets, ↑ INR, ↑ aPTT, ↑ D-Dimers, ↓ fibrinogen, schistocytes ⊕. Treatment according to cause (sepsis, malignancy, etc). Heparin if thrombosis (antithrombin level > 50 %). Fresh frozen plasma, cryoprecipitates or platelets as needed. Activated protein C with sepsis (if platelets > 30 x 10^9/L). Antifibrinolytics as needed if bleeding is associated with with malignancy.
Heparin-Induced Thrombocytopenia	2 types: Type 1: **early**, nonimmune < 4 days after the start of heparin therapy, benign; Type 2: **late** 4-14 days after beginning heparin, autoimmune, severe and associated with systemic thrombosis (heparin-induced thrombocytopenia – HIT). Develops in 0.1-3 % of patients exposed to heparin. If past exposure to heparin (especially < 120 days), autoimmune type (type 2) can develop earlier. Low molecular weight heparins cause less HIT. Clinically: arterial or venous thrombosis (in 25-50 % of HIT patients). Can occur up to 19 days after the cessation of heparin. Venous gangrene can occur if concomitant treatment with warfarin. Acute platelet activation syndrome (fever, chills, transitory amnesia 5-30 minutes after starting heparin), cutaneous lesions at heparin injection site. Workup: ↓ platelet > 50 %. Functional or antigenic heparin-induced thrombocytopenia test (false negative in 10-15%). Treatment: stop heparin immediately if suspected. Danaparoid (< 5 % cross-reactivity: follow factor Xa level for adequacy of anticoagulation), lepirudin, argatroban, etc. Start warfarin when platelet count > 100-150 x 10 ^{9}/L. Avoid administering low molecular weight heparin. Stop warfarin if already administered and reverse with vitamin K. Anticoagulation for at least 2-4 weeks for HIT without associated thrombosis.
Thrombocytosis	

Causes	• Primary thrombocytosis: see Myeloproliferative Disorders table.
	• Secondary thrombocytosis :
	  - Infectious diseases or chronic inflammation (connective tissue disease, vasculitis, allergy, etc).
	  - Surgery - tissue damage.
	  - Malignancy: lymphomas, solid tumors.
	  - Iron deficiency anemia, hemolytic anemia, acute bleeding.
	  - Post-splenectomy.
	  - Recovery phase of chemotherapy-induced thrombocytopenia or immune thrombocytopenia.
	  - Renal diseases: renal failure, nephrotic syndrome.
	  - Medication : vincristine, tretinoin, cytokines, etc.
	• Hereditary thrombocytosis (rare)

Management	See Myeloproliferative Disorders table. Differentiation between primary and secondary thrombocytosis: chronicity, history of thrombosis or hemorrhage, splenomegaly, blood smear, platelet function test, myelogram compatible with primary thrombocytosis, cause of secondary thrombocytosis identified and increased acute phase reactants associated with reactive thrombocytosis.

Pancytopenia	
Definition: simultaneous ↓ in erythrocytes, leukocytes and platelets. Symptoms related to cytopenias (hemorrhage, infection, etc).	

Causes	**Bone marrow cell count ↓ :**
	- *Aplastic anemia*: idiopathic (40-70 %: autoimmune), congenital (Fanconi syndrome) or secondary: toxins (benzene, toluene, insecticides, radiotherapy), medications (chemotherapy, methotrexate, azathioprin, chloramphenicol, sulfonamides, gold compounds, arsenic, trimethadione, linezolid, anti-TNF antibodies, indomethacin, diclofenac, etc) post viral infection (hepatitis, CMV, EBV, Parvovirus B19, mycoplasma, influenza, HIV, etc), malignancies (leukemia), SLE, pregnancy, graft-versus-host disease, paroxysmal nocturnal hemoglobinuria, copper deficiency in total parenteral nutrition, etc.
	- Some myelodysplastic syndromes (10-15 %).
	- Aleukemic leukemia, rarely (AML).
	- Some bone marrow lymphomas.
	- Infections : Q fever, legionnaires' disease, mycobacteria.
	- Anorexia nervosa, fasting.
	
	Bone marrow cell count ↑ or cellular replacement :
	– Primary medullary disorders:
	 - *Myelodysplastic syndromes* : primary or secondary (to chemotherapy or radiotherapy): primary syndrome subtypes :
	  - Refractory anemia.
	  - Refractory anemia with ringed sideroblasts.
	  - Refractory anemia with excess blasts (5-19 % blasts in bone marrow).
	  - Refractory cytopenia with multilineage dysplasia and ringed sideroblasts.
	  - 5q- syndrome.
	  - Myelodysplastic syndrome, unclassified.
	  - Chronic myelomonocytic leukemia (myelodysplastic/myeloproliferative disease).
	 - Myeloid metaplasia.
	 - Some aleukemic leukemias.
	 - Myelophthisis (with malignancy of breast, prostate, lung, etc.).
	 - Bone marrow lymphoma.
	 - Hairy cell leukemia.
	 - Large granular lymphocyte leukemia.
	 - Hemophagocytic lymphohistiocytosis (primary hemophagocytic syndrome).
	 - Paroxysmal nocturnal hemoglobinuria: intravascular hemolysis (hemoglobinuria, hemoglobinemia, hemosiderinuria), thrombophilia: bone marrow aplasia and leukemia are also possible etiologies.
	– Secondary to systemic diseases:
	 - Systemic lupus erythematosus.
	 - Hypersplenism.
	 - Vitamin B12 or folate deficiency.
	 - Severe infection, AIDS, brucellosis, histoplasmosis, tuberculosis, leishmaniasis, *Bartonella* sp.
	 - Hemophagocytic syndrome secondary to infection, cancer, autoimmune disease: ↑ ferritin and ↑ triglycerides.
	 - Alcohol.
	 - Sarcoidosis.
	
	Note: several other medications are associated with pancytopenia without aplasia: carbamazepine, zidovudine, etc.

Workup	CBC with differential, blood smear, reticulocyte count, myelogram (unless cause is obvious). As needed: hepatic enzymes, viral serology (HBV, HCV, EBV, CMV, HIV, Parvovirus B19), vitamin B12 + folate levels, hemolysis workup, erythropoietin levels, karyotype, abdominal ultrasound. Flow cytometry for paroxysmal nocturnal hemoglobinuria (absence of GPI-linked antigen).

Treatment	Treatment according to cause. Avoid antiplatelet drugs. For aplastic anemia: if mild, transfusions as needed (careful evaluation required since transfusions negatively affect the prognosis of an eventual allogeneic bone marrow transplant). If severe (if 3 or 4 of following criteria are present: neutrophils < 0.5 x 10^9/L, platelets < 20 x 10^9/L, reticulocytes < 1 % and bone marrow cell count < 20 %) and < 40 years with compatible donor: allogeneic bone marrow transplant. If > 40 years or no compatible donor: antithymocyte globulins + steroids + cyclosporine. High dose of cyclophosphamide? Androgens sometimes useful. IV immunoglobulins if secondary to Parvovirus. 15 % will suffer another hematological disease several years after antithymocyte globulin treatment (acute leukemia, myelodysplasia, paroxysmal nocturnal hemoglobinuria, etc). For myelodysplastic syndrome: supportive treatment (marrow transplant if < 55 years). Androgens or steroids sometimes useful. Cell lineage growth factors (erythropoietin and G-CSF) as needed. If no response to growth factors, azacytidine or decitabine. Cyclosporine for hypocellular bone marrow. Pyridoxine for sideroblastic anemia. Lenalidomide for 5q- syndrome.
Prognosis	For aplastic anemia: long term survival 75 % with intensive immunosuppressive therapy, 65 % with bone marrow transplant and < 25 % with androgenes only. For myelodysplastic syndrome: subtype-dependant: average survival is 12-36 months.

Myeloproliferative Diseases

Clonal hematopoetic stem cell diseases.
One type of myeloproliferative syndrome may transform to another.

Polycythemia Vera Clinical features	Weakness, aquagenic pruritus, headaches, dizziness, weight loss, joint pain, erythromelalgia, dyspnea, epigastric pain, thromboembolism (presenting symptom in 20-30 %), bleeding, hyperviscosity syndrome, hypertension, claudication, angina, peptic ulcers, peripheral neuropathy, tinnitus, etc. Median age at presentation is 60 years.
Diagnosis	Diagnostic criteria : JAK2 mutation ⊕ in 95 %. Serum erythropoietin ↓, sedimentation rate ↓↓. Spontaneous erythroid stem cell growth (BFU-E). Also, thrombocytosis, leukocytosis, leukocyte alkaline phosphatase > 100, vitamin B12 > 900 ng/L, splenomegaly. Myelogram: hypercellularity and hyperplasia, atypical megakaryocytic hyperplasia (normal in 10 %). Absence of iron stores in 95 % of patients. 11 % of cytogenetic anomaly. Absent Philadelphia chromosome. Diagnosis approach: measurement of erythropoietin level and JAK2 mutation testing if hematocrit > 58 % in men and 52 % in women, with normal saturation and normal carboxyhemoglobin levels: – If JAK2 ⊕ and EPO ↓: probable polycythemia vera (PV) (bone marrow examination not essential). – If JAK2 ⊕ and EPO normal or ↑: probable PV (but repeat both tests and bone marrow examination is necessary if results remain unchanged). – If JAK2 ⊖ and EPO ↓: possible PV: consider bone marrow examination + JAK2 exon 12 mutation analysis. – If JAK2 ⊖ and EPO normal or ↑: PV unlikely. Look for other cause.

Treatment	Treatment according to patient's individual risk :
	– If < 60 years of age without cardiovascular risk factors, without thrombocytosis > 1 500 x 10^9/L and with no history of thrombosis: phlebotomy for hematocrit < 42 % (women) or < 45 % (men) ± aspirin.
	– In presence of cardiovascular risk factor or thrombocytosis > 1 500 x 10^9/L: phlebotomy ± interferon α or anagrelide ± aspirin.
	– If > 60 years or history of thrombosis: phlebotomy ± aspirin ± hydroxyurea or interferon α.
	Other possible treatments: anagrelide (especially if thrombocytosis), ^{32}P (if > 60 ans). Avoid hydroxyurea in pregnant women.
	If thrombosis or bleeding: heparin, warfarin, hydroxyurea or platelet apheresis (if platelets > 800 x 10^9/L), phlebotomy and allopurinol.
Prognosis	Risk of transformation to myeloid metaplasia in 10-30 % over a period of 10-25 years, or less frequently to leukemia (although ↑ frequency with chemotherapy or ^{32}P). 2 % thrombosis risk annually if < 40 years of age and 5 % if > 70 years. Median survival in phlebotomized patients > 12 years.
Essential Thrombocytosis	Presentation: asymptomatic, hemorrhage (especially if platelets > 2 000 x 10^9/L), arterial or venous thrombosis or vasomotor symptoms (erythromelalgia). Median age 60 years. Risk of thrombosis 20 %: hemorrhage 3 %.
Diagnosis	Platelets > 600 x 10^9/L: splenomegaly: normal erythrocytic mass: myelogram with megakaryocytic hyperplasia + absence of Philadelphia chromosome or BCR/ABL fusion gene. Absence of fibrosis in bone marrow. Normal bone marrow iron stores. Spontaneous stem cell growth. JAK2 mutation in 30 %.
	Absence of other causes of thrombocytosis (acute or chronic inflammatory disease, acute or chronic bleeding, iron deficiency, hemolysis, disseminated cancer, splenectomy or hyposplenism/asplenia, post-operative, pregnancy, adrenaline, other myeloproliferative disorder, etc): C-reactive protein should be ↓ in essential thrombocytosis.
Treatment	Platelet apheresis in case of emergency (hemorrhage or thrombosis), if urgent surgery or delivery. Chronic treatment indicated if active or previous thrombosis, cardiovascular risk factors or if > 60 years old with platelets > 600 x 10^9/L: anagrelide (if < 65 years old or intolerance to hydroxyurea), hydroxyurea, radioactive phosphorus, interferon α (aim for platelets < 400 x 10^9/L). Note: Anagrelide raises arterial thrombosis risks. Hydroxyurea is the 1st choice in high risk patients.
	Aspirin if > 60 years of age or cardiovascular risk factors or history of thrombosis. Anticoagulants as needed.
	Watchful waiting for asymptomatic patient (without prior thrombosis or hemorrhage) < 60 years of age, without cardiovascular risk factors and with platelets < 1 500 x 10^9/L.
Prognosis	Risk of thrombosis is 30 %/year in patients with prior thrombosis and 3 %/year in patients without prior thrombosis. Risk of thrombosis is 15 %/year if > 60 years of age and < 2 %/year if < 40 years. Leukemia or myeloid metaplasia transformation in < 5 %.

Myeloid Metaplasia	Splenomegaly in 100 %: hepatomegaly in 70 %. Lymphadenopathy. Abdominal symptoms in 23 % (abdominal discomfort, early satiety, diarrhea, etc). Portal hypertension 7 %. Constitutional symptoms. Splenic infarct. Bone pain. Differential diagnosis: fibrosis secondary to metastatic cancer, lymphomas, chronic myeloid leukemia, myelodysplastic syndrome, hairy cell leukemia, infectious diseases, hyperparathyroidism, SLE, Paget's disease, radiotherapy, benzene, etc.
Diagnosis	Leukoerythroblastosis, teardrop-shaped red cells. "Dry tap" bone marrow aspiration. Myelogram: hypocellular, fibroblastic proliferation. JAK2 mutation in 50 %. Possible disseminated intravascular coagulation.
Treatment	Watchful waiting if asymptomatic. Treat if symptomatic (palliative): transfusion as needed, androgens + Prednisone if insufficient erythropoiesis: erythropoietin. Steroids if hemolysis or thrombocytopenia. Hydroxyurea if hepatosplenomegaly, ↑ leukocyte or platelet count. Vitamin B12 + folic acid as needed. Splenectomy if symptoms of hepatosplenomegaly are resistant to hydroxyurea, portal hypertension, severe hemolysis, severe or refractory thrombocytopenia (Vaccination before surgery). If surgery not possible: radiotherapy. For young patient with poor prognosis: allogeneic marrow transplant, potentially curative. Mean survival is 3.5-5.5 years (↓ with age or anemia).
Chronic Granulocytic Leukemia (Chronic Myeloid Leukemia)	20 % of leukemias. Mean age 50 years. Philadelphia chromosome ⊕ in > 95 %. Clinical features: *Chronic phase* (median 4 years) asymptomatic or associated with malaise, dyspnea, anorexia, fever, nocturnal diaphoresis, weight loss, abdominal discomfort and early satiety, bleeding, gout, splenomegaly in 85 %. *Accelerated or blastic phase:* headaches, fever, bone pain, hemorrhage, splenomegaly, lymphadenopathy.
Diagnosis	In chronic phase: ↑ leukocytes > 50 x 10^9/L (all stages of maturation), < 10 % blasts. Basophilia, eosinophilia, ↓ leukocyte alkaline phosphatase. ↑ Vitamin B12. Thrombocytosis. Hyperplastic bone marrow, with myelofibrosis in 10-40 %, cytogenetics, molecular biology (Q-PCR). In blastic phase: myelofibrosis, blasts > 20 %, anemia, thrombocytopenia, ↑ basophilia, ↑ leukocyte alkaline phosphatase, new cytogenetic anomalies, ↓ response to treatment.
Treatment	Imatinib mesylate (standard for chronic phase in the absence of bone marrow donor), interferon α, hydroxyurea. Only curative treatment: allogeneic bone marrow transplant, for patients < 60 years old (success rate 40-60 %). If failure or intolerance to imatinib: dasatinib or nilotinib. Blastic crisis treatment: increased dosage of imatinib, dasatinib, IV hydration, allopurinol, aggressive chemotherapy (7-3), hydroxurea, leukocyte apheresis, cerebral radiotherapy. Survival without treatment = 3.5 years, with treatment 5-7 years or more.

Disorders of Coagulation

Hypocoagulability

Overview	– Bleeding time ↑ with qualitative or quantitative platelet disorders or vascular defects. – PT-INR evaluates extrinsic coagulation pathway (factor VII) + common pathway. – aPTT evaluates intrinsic coagulation pathway (factors VIII, IX, XI, XII) + common pathway. – Thrombin time evaluates fibrinogen levels. – Factor XII deficiency does not provoke bleeding. – Factor XIII deficiency: provokes post-operative bleeding: does not alter any paraclinical coagulation parameter. – Factor II, V, or VII deficiencies are extremely rare. – α2-antiplasmin and plasminogen activator inhibitor deficiencies are rare.

von Willebrand's disease (vWD)	– Most common inherited bleeding disorder.
	– Autosomal dominant disease with variable penetrance or recessive disease.
	– Factor VIII + von Willebrand factor (vWF) complex cause platelet aggregation and adhesion.
	– Classification: type 1 (75 %) quantitative ↓ of vWF; type 2 (10-30 %) qualitative defect of vWF (subtypes 2A, 2B, 2M, 2N); type 3 (1-5 %) vWF nearly absent.
	– Sometimes secondary to lymphoproliferative or myeloproliferative diseases, medications (valproic acid, ciprofloxacin, etc), autoimmune diseases (SLE), malignancy, severe aortic stenosis, etc.
	– Clinical features: mucosal bleeding (epistaxis, ecchymosis, hematoma), gastrointestinal bleeding, post-operative bleeding, menorrhagia. Rarely as severe as hemophilia.
	– Workup : bleeding time (or PFA-100) usually ↑, normal platelets, aPTT normal or slightly ↑, ↓ vWF antigen, ↓ factor VIII, ↓ ristocetin cofactor activity, ↓ platelet aggregation with ristocetin, multimer analysis.
	– Treatment: DDAVP releases stores of vWF: useful for non-severe type 1 vWD.
	    o Factor VIII concentrates rich in vWF for types 2b and 3 or 1 resistant to DDAVP – Anti-fibrinolytic agents as needed - Cryoprecipitates as needed.
	    o Oral contraceptives for menorrhagia.
	– Avoid antiplatelet therapy and NSAIDs.

Hemophilia A (factor VIII deficiency)	– X-linked recessive disease. Spontaneous mutation in 3 %. Factor VIII:C deficiency. – Severe if factor VIII < 1 %, moderate if factor 1-5 %, mild if > 5 %. – Clinical features: joint, muscular, gastro-intestinal bleeding if severe; bleeding associated with trauma or surgery if mild or moderate deficiency. – Workup: aPTT ↑. Factor VIII: C ↓. Normal INR + bleeding time. Normal vWF. – aPTT will normalize if combined with normal plasma unless anti-factor VIII antibodies are present. HIV, HBV, HCV often ⊕. – Differential diagnosis: acquired anti-factor VIII antibodies (with ↑ age, post-partum, connective tissue disease, malignancy, medication, idiopathic, etc). – Treatment: factor VIII concentrates as needed: ↑ factor VIII to 25 % if minor bleeding, to 50 % if moderate bleeding, to 100 % if surgery or cranial trauma; – 1 U/kg increases circulating VIII of 2 % VIII (½ life = 12 h). – Recombinant factor VIII available. – If mild hemophilia: DDAVP useful before surgery or for minor bleeding. – If bleeding is persistent despite treatment, antifibrinolytic agents may be used. – Always measure anti-factor VIII antibodies before surgery (⊕ in 5-20 % of patients). – Avoid trauma, antiplatelets, NSAIDs.

Hemophilia B (Factor IX deficiency)	– X-linked recessive disease. Quantitative (but 1/3 qualitative) factor IX deficiency. – 15 % of hemophiliacs. – aPTT ↑, factor IX levels ↓. – Treatment: factor IX concentrates as needed (1 U/kg increases circulating factor IX of 1 %: ½ life 18 h), recombinant factor IX or fresh frozen plasma. Avoid antiplatelets, NSAIDs.
Hemophilia C (factor XI deficiency)	– Autosomal recessive disease, particularly common in Ashkenazi Jews. – Clinical features: mild bleeding, especially post-operative. – aPTT ↑, factor XI levels ↓. – Treatment: fresh frozen plasma as needed. Avoid antiplatelets, NSAIDs.

Hypercoagulability	
Causes	Acquired causes of hypercoagulable state: malignancy, immobilization, surgery, estrogens, pregnancy, nephrotic syndrome, chemotherapy, antiphospholipid syndrome*, DIC, heparin-induced thrombocytopenia, myeloproliferative syndromes, inflammatory bowel diseases, foreign bodies (catheter, etc), obesity, Behçet's disease, paroxysmal nocturnal hemoglobinuria, etc. Inherited causes: protein C, protein S and antithrombin III deficiencies, activated protein C resistance, factor II 20210A mutation, ↑ factors VIII, IX and XI (> 150 % normal), factor XII deficiency, fibrinogen ↑*, dysfibrinogeninemia, deficiencies in t-PA and heparin cofactor II, histidine-rich glycoprotein, etc. Combined causes: hyperhomocysteinemia*. * causes of arterial or venous thrombosis.
Workup for thrombophilia	Workup for thrombophilias is indicated for idiopathic thromboembolic event and: positive family history or patient < 50 years of age or thrombophlebitis at an unusual site or recurrent thromboembolism (but controversial). Proteins C, S, antithrombin III levels. Resistance to activated protein C: biochemical and genetic testing (factor V Leiden). Genetic testing for mutation of factor II 20210A. Plasma homocysteine (rule out vitamin B12 + folate deficiency). Screening for mutation MTHFR C677T? Lupus anticoagulant, anticardiolipin antibodies, anti-β2-glycoprotein-1. Factor VIII levels. Quantification of factors IX and XI still controversial. Thrombin time (to rule out dysfibrinogenemia). Fibrinogen levels. Avoid testing during acute thrombotic event (false ↓ in protein levels acutely). Repeat abnormal tests to confirm deficiency. Proteins C and S levels must be assayed without warfarin use (2-4 weeks after cessation of warfarin), but possible under LMWH if anticoagulation cannot be stopped. Antithrombin and activated protein C resistance (biochemical test) must be assayed without heparin use. Family screening if inherited thrombophilia. Screen for thrombophilia and anticardiolipin antibodies in women with repeated spontaneous abortions (3 or more), or if severe or recurrent preeclampsia, placenta abruptio, or if unexplained intrauterine death.
Treatment	For 1st thrombotic event, treat as you would any other patient. Long term anticoagulation for recurrent event. – If heterozygous for factor V Leiden or for factor II 20210A: avoid oral contraceptives: treatment same as above. – If malignancy or antithrombin deficit: treatment for ≥ 12 months (long term ?) at 1st episode.

	– If factor V Leiden homozygous, protein C or S deficiency, multiple thrombophilias, or recurrent thrombotic episodes in the presence of risk factors: optimal treatment and duration unclear. – If hyperhomocysteinemia: optimal treatment and duration unclear. Folic acid ± vitamin B12 or B6 aiming for normal homocysteine level (but no evidence that ↓ homocysteine level leads to ↓ thrombotic events). – If antiphospholipid syndrome: see below.
Thrombophilia and pregnancy	– Proven association between hereditary thrombophilia and following obstetrical complications: fetal loss (≥ 3 during 1st trimester or ≥ 1 during 2nd or 3rd trimester), severe/early preeclampsia (< 34 weeks), placenta abruptio >> intrauterine growth restriction. – Screen for hereditary thrombophilia in women with spontaneous abortions. Screening is more controversial for women with preeclampsia, placenta abruptio, and especially in cases of intrauterine growth restriction. Treatment : – For women with hereditary thrombophilia and spontaneous abortions: low-dose aspirin + low-dose prophylactic unfractionated heparin or prophylactic LMWH during pregnancy + post-partum anticoagulation. – For women with hereditary thrombophilia and preeclampsia, placenta abruptio ± intrauterine growth restriction: *consider* prophylactic LMWH during pregnancy ± low-dose aspirin + post-partum anticoagulation (very controversial, no controlled study). – For women with anticardiolipin antibodies: see below.

Antiphospholipid Syndrome (APS)

Includes antiphospholipid antibodies, lupus anticoagulant and others.
Lupus anticoagulants are immunoglobulins, which interfere (in vitro) with coagulation phospholipids, causing ↑ aPTT. Associated with procainamide, quinidine, chlorpromazine, HIV, connective tissue diseases, lymphoproliferative syndromes, etc.

Clinical findings	Arterial or venous thrombosis, repeated spontaneous abortions, thrombocytopenia, hemolytic anemia, livedo reticularis, chorea, repeated TIA or CVA, transverse myelitis, etc.
Workup	↑ aPTT secondary to lupus anticoagulant is not normalized when combined (1:1) with normal plasma. Anticardiolipin antibodies, lupus anticoagulant, and anti-ß2-glycoprotein-1 levels. These tests must be positive (moderate to high titer) on a minimum of two occasions ≥ 12 weeks apart.
Diagnostic criteria	At least one clinical criteria *and* one laboratory criteria from the following: – Arterial thrombosis, venous thrombosis, or obstetrical complication. – Anticardiolipin IgG and/or IgM antibodies, lupus anticoagulant and/or anti-ß2-glycoprotein-1: ≥ 2 occasions at ≥ 12 weeks interval < 5 years after initial clinical manifestations. "Catastrophic" antiphospholipid syndrome if multiple vascular occlusions in ≥ 3 organs or affected systems (kidney, lungs, central nervous system, heart, DIC), developing simultaneously or within a week.
Treatment	Controversial. No treatment if asymptomatic. If thrombotic event, warfarin for at least 12 months (lifelong?). Target INR: 2-3. In patients with a recurrent thrombotic event with therapeutic INR or with additional risk factors for thrombotic events, target INR: 2.5-3.5. Follow-up of INR and aPTT sometimes difficult with lupus anticoagulants. If aPTT ↑ initially and treatment is needed, favour low molecular weight heparin (no need to follow aPTT).

APS and pregnancy	– For pregnant women with antiphospholipid syndrome: presence of antibodies AND...
	- A history of multiple spontaneous abortions (≥ 3 in 1ʳˢᵗ trimester or ≥ 1 in 2ⁿᵈ or 3ʳᵈ trimester): antepartum unfractionated heparin at prophylactic or intermediate-dose or prophylactic LMWH + ASA (see Thromboembolic Diseases table for definition).
	- Prior thromboembolic manifestations and anticoagulated: replace warfarin with heparin during pregnancy (see Thromboembolic Diseases table) and give low-dose ASA.

Splenomegaly

Overview	Normal spleen usually: 12 x 7 cm (normal limit up to 13 cm): 250 g.
	Pathophysiology: **C**ongestive, **R**eactive or **I**nfiltrative.
Causes	– Secondary to portal hypertension: cirrhosis, portal vein thrombosis, right-sided cardiac failure, etc.
	– Secondary to hematological disorders: myeloproliferative syndromes, leukemias, lymphomas, hemolytic anemia, metastases (rare).
	– Secondary to infiltrative diseases: sarcoidosis, amyloidosis, Gaucher's disease, glycogen storage disease, etc.
	– Secondary to infection: infectious mononucleosis, CMV, toxoplasmosis, tuberculosis, endocarditis, mycotic infections, malaria, etc.
	– Secondary to inflammatory diseases: Felty's syndrome (rheumatoid arthritis, SLE).
	– Secondary to hemorrhage (hematoma).
	If massive (if ≥ 8 cm below costal margin): myelofibrosis (myeloid metaplasia or bone marrow infiltration), chronic lymphocytic leukemia, chronic myeloid leukemia, hairy cell leukemia, congestive, visceral leishmaniasis, malaria.
Management	Workup: CBC, blood smear (rule out hemolysis, leukemia, etc), reticulocyte count, liver function tests, abdominal ultrasound ± doppler, liver-spleen scan, endoscopy, myelogram, etc.
	Possible resection (with pneumococcal, *Hemophilus influenzae* and meningococcus vaccines before surgery) for diagnosis (rarely: Hodgkin, lymphoma, sarcoidosis, etc) or for treatment (spherocytosis, immune thrombocytopenic purpura or congestive symptoms).

Lymphadenopathy

History taking: age, localization, duration, localized vs generalized, pain, associated signs and symptoms (decreased performance status, splenomegaly, fever and other B symptoms, malabsorption, joint pain, etc).
Pathophysiology: **R**eactive or **I**nfiltrative.

Differential diagnosis in 3 general categories: infections, malignancies and immune diseases (as for fever of unknown origin).

Causes of *localized* lymphadenopathy	– Occipital: scalp pathology.
	– Pre-auricular: conjunctivitis, cat-scratch disease (Parinaud's syndrome).
	– Cervical : bacterial or gonococcal pharyngitis, dental abscess, otitis, infectious mononucleosis, CMV, toxoplasmosis, hepatitis, adenovirus, rubella, Kikuchi's disease (young women with indolent unilateral posterior cervical lymphadenopathy regressing within 3 months), head and neck malignancies, metastasis, lymphomas.
	– Axillary: breast or lung cancer, melanoma, arm infection, tularemia, cat-scratch disease, sporotrichosis.
	– Supra-clavicular and pre-laryngeal: pulmonary neoplasm (left lung = right lymphadenopathy), genital infections, tuberculosis, fungi, sarcoidosis, toxoplasmosis. Virchow's node: left supra-clavicular node: classically associated with gastrointestinal or thoracic malignancy. Delphian node (prelaryngeal) classically associated with thyroid or laryngeal malignancy, possible association with lymphomas.
	– Epitrochlear: lymphoma, chronic lymphocytic leukemia, infectious mononucleosis, sarcoidosis, HIV, dermatological disease, connective tissue diseases.
	– Hilar and mediastinal: vascular distension sometimes taken for a lymphadenopathy.
	   ○ Unilateral hilar lymphadenopathy: pneumonia, granulomatous disease, mycobacteria, fungi, tularemia, psittacosis, whooping cough, lymphomas, carcinoma, metastasis, etc.
	   ○ Bilateral hilar lymphadenopathy: sarcoidosis, lymphomas, metastases, granulomatous diseases, berylliosis, silicosis, tuberculosis, fungi.
	   ○ Mediastinal lymphadenopathy: verify that increased size of mediastinum not secondary to another cause (mediastinitis, hemorrhage, lipoma, etc). Differential diagnosis similar to hilar lymphadenopathy.
	– Abdominal: malignancy (lymphomas, metastasis, urinary, chronic lymphocytic leukemia, hairy cell leukemia), tuberculosis. Sister Mary Joseph's nodule (umbilical) classically associated with gastric cancer (possible association with other cancers).
	– Inguinal: benign inflammatory reaction (walking barefoot), lymphomas, melanoma, malignancy of rectum, penis or vulva (not testicular which metastasize via retroperitoneum), cellulitis, sexually transmitted diseases. Cloquet's node (near femoral canal) sometimes mistaken for inguinal hernia.

Causes of *generalized* lymphadenopathy	– Inflammatory: connective tissue diseases, sarcoidosis, histiocytosis, serum sickness, graft-vs-host disease, celiac disease, Crohn's disease, mastocytosis, etc. – Drug-induced: phenytoin, carbamazepine, primidone, gold compounds, allopurinol, indomethacin, sulfonamides, post-vaccination, etc. – Endocrine-metabolic: hyperthyroidism (secondary to reactional hyperplasia). – Malignancies: hematological neoplasms (lymphomas, leukemias, multiple myeloma, Waldenström's macroglobulinemia, systemic mastocytosis), metastasis. – Infectious: bacterial (cutaneous, syphilis, cat-scratch disease, brucellosis, Whipple, etc), viral (mononucleosis, CMV, hepatitis, HIV, adenovirus, post-vaccination, etc), toxoplasmosis, chlamydia, mycobacteria, fungal diseases (histoplasmosis, cryptococcus, coccidioidomycosis), malaria, filariasis, etc. – Other causes: Wegener's granulomatosis, amyloidosis, angioimmunoblastic lymphadenopathy, lymphomatoid granulomatosis, angiocentric immunoproliferative lesions, Castleman's disease, inflammatory pseudotumor of the lymph node, etc. Note: lymphadenopathy associated with splenomegaly typically in lymphomas, infectious mononucleosis, acute leukemias or chronic lymphocytic leukemia.
Workup	In accordance with suspected cause. Precise measurement of lymphadenopathy. Biopsy (needle or excisional), especially if lymphadenopathy > 1 cm (other than inguinal) for > 1 month.

Monoclonal Gammopathies	
MGUS	– *Monoclonal Gammopathy of Unknown Significance.* – Most frequent gammopathy (prevalence 3 % at > 50 years of age: 5 % at > 70 years). – Diagnosis: M protein (monoclonal) < 30 g/L, < 10 % plasma cells in bone marrow, no myeloma-related organ or tissue impairment (normal creatinine, no anemia, no bone lesion). – 69 % IgG, 17 % IgM, 11 % IgA, 7 % light chain only. – Differential diagnosis of monoclonal gammopathies: hematological malignancies, solid tumors, cirrhosis, sarcoidosis, parasites, Gaucher's disease, pyoderma gangrenosum, autoimmune diseases, etc. – 25 % progress to malignant gammopathy within 25 years (myeloma, amyloidosis, Waldenström, other lymphoproliferative diseases). – Bone marrow aspirate and biopsy indicated if M protein > 15 g/L, or if there is typical laboratory or radiological abnormalities. Consider bone marrow biopsy and aspirate for non-IgG MGUS, or when there is doubt about the diagnosis. Skeletal survey (for all or only if M-protein > 15 g/L) is controversial. – Follow-up protein and urine electrophoresis, CBC, creatinine and Ca^{++} every 6-12 months. – No treatment necessary.
Multiple Myeloma	Approximately 1 % of the malignancies. Mean age at presentation is 65 years. More frequent in men and in the African-American population. Diagnostic criteria according to *International Myeloma Working Group* (2003) : – Presence of an M protein in blood and/or urine. – Medullary plasmocytosis (generally > 10 %) or presence of plasmacytoma. – Presence of related organ or tissue impairment ("**CRAB**": hyper**C**alcemia, **A**nemia, **R**enal failure, lytic **B**one lesions, hyperviscosity syndrome, amyloidosis, recurrent infections). Monoclonal peak: IgG (55 %), IgA (20 %), IgD (1 %), IgM (0.5 %), IgE (rare) or light-chain only (in urine - 20 %). 3 % is nonsecretory (no detectable monoclonal peak). Clinical features: bone pain, acute renal failure, hypercalcemia, fatigue, weight loss, spinal cord compression, ↑ susceptibility to infections (pneumococci, staphylococci, shingles, Gram negative rods), secondary amyloidosis, bleeding, hyperviscosity syndrome. May be asymptomatic (*smoldering*) in 15 %: M protein > 30 g/L, > 10 % of medullary plasmocytosis, but no myeloma-related organ or tissue impairment. May be nonsecretory in 3 % with no detectable M-protein, but with medullar plasmocytosis and myeloma-related organ or tissue impairment. Can be localized = plasmacytoma. Rarely with POEMS syndrome: *p*olyneuropathy, *o*rganomegaly, *e*ndocrinopathy, *m*onoclonal gammopathy, *s*kin.
Staging	International Staging System: – Stage 1: β2-microglobulin < 296 µmol/L and albumin > 35 g/L. – Stage 2: β2-microglobulin 296-465 µmol/L and/or albumin < 35 g/L. – Stage 3: β2-microglobulin > 465 µmol/L.	Durie-Salmon Staging : – I: if Hb > 100 g/L and normal Ca^{++} and normal bone and low M protein production (IgG < 50 g/L, IgA < 30 g/L, urinary κ or λ < 4 g/day). – II: if does not correspond to stages I or III. – III: 1 or more of following criteria: Hb < 85 g/L or Ca^{++} > 3 mmol/L or > 3 lytic lesions or high M protein production (IgG > 70 g/L, IgA > 50 g/L, urinary κ or λ > 12 g/day). Sub classification: A if creatinine < 177 or B if creatinine > 177 µmol/L.

Workup	CBC (anemia? rouleaux formation?), electrolytes, calcium, creatinine, BUN, LDH, C-reactive protein, uric acid, serum and urinary protein electrophoresis. Protein immunoelectrophoresis or immunofixation. β2-microglobulins. Serum viscosity if needed. Skeletal survey. Bone scan not reliable. Bone marrow biopsy of an involved site.
Treatment	Chemotherapy: dexamethasone + thalidomide or lenalidomide. Melphalan + prednisone ± thalidomide. Several other protocols (VAD, cyclophosphamide + prednisone, etc). Thalidomide if refractory (post-melphalan + prednisone, VAD or graft). Proteasome inhibitors (Bortezomib) if refractory or recurrent. If renal failure: VAD or dexamethasone only.
	Bisphosphonates for all patients with myeloma (evidence of ↓ mortality). Bone marrow autograft (for patients < 60-65 years with good performance status, not curative but ↑ survival). Bone marrow autograft followed by mini-allogeneic graft under investigation. Allogeneic bone marrow transplant for patients < 60 years (experimental). Plasmapheresis for hyperviscosity or nephropathy.
	Supportive treatment: erythropoietin for anemia, anti-influenza and anti-pneumococcal vaccinations. Antibioprophylaxis with chemotherapy. Immunoglobulins as needed. Radiotherapy for pain or spinal compression.
	Asymptomatic multiple myeloma: wait for progression before treating. Good prognosis (10 %/year progression towards symptomatic myeloma for 5 years then 3 %/year for the next 5 years, and 1 %/year for the following 10 years). Plasmocytoma: radiotherapy.
Prognosis	Overall prognosis = 2-3 years. Prognosis according to the International Staging System: median survival for Stage 1 = 62 months; stage 2 = 45 months; stage 3 = 29 months.
Waldenström's Macroglobulinemia	– IgM monoclonal gammopathy. – Clinical-paraclinical features: hyperviscosity syndrome (visual disturbance, papilledema, mucous membrane bleeding, fatigue, dizziness), cryoglobulinemia, neuropathy, cold agglutinin hemolytic anemia, chronic kidney disease (nephrotic syndrome), lymphadenopathy, splenomegaly, etc. No bone lesions (generally). – IgM peak > 30 g/L. Rouleaux formation + + +. – Treatment: R-COP or fludarabine, chlorambucil, rituximab + 2-CDA + cyclophosphamide or R-CHOP. – Several other protocols possible. – Plasmapheresis for hyperviscosity. – Better prognosis than most other myelomas.
Amyloidosis	Primary in 90 % (AL amyloid fibrils) vs secondary (AA amyloid fibrils: with chronic infection, autoimmune disease, age, medullary thyroid carcinoma and *multiple endocrine neoplasia* II) vs familial (transthyretin amyloid fibrils - ATTR) vs secondary to dialysis vs "localized". Clinical manifestations: weakness, weight loss, hepatosplenomegaly, macroglossia, "shoulders pads", nail dystrophy, alopecia, chronic kidney disease, proteinuria, nephrotic syndrome, heart failure, carpal tunnel syndrome, peripheral polyneuropathy (progressive, painful, symmetric,demyelinating), dysautonomia (orthostatic hypotension, diarrhea), bleeding (secondary to ↓ transformation from fibrinogen → fibrin or secondary to ↓ in factor X), post-proctoscopy periorbital purpura. Involvement in order of frequency: renal, cardiac, carpal tunnel, peripheral neuropathy ± orthostatic hypotension. Workup: Monoclonal peak on serum or urinary protein electrophoresis present in 90 %.

	Abdominal fat biopsy (⊕ 70-80 %), salivary glands biopsy (⊕ 80 %), rectal biopsy (⊕ 75 %), bone marrow biopsy (⊕ 56 %) with Congo red **staining**. Fibril analysis by electron microscopy. ECG: low voltage (despite LVH). Echocardiography: LVH, diastolic dysfunction ± "granular" myocardial appearance. Treatment: melphalan + prednisone (18 % response). β-blockers, calcium channel blockers, and digoxin contraindicated. For secondary causes: treat the underlying inflammatory cause. Hepatic transplant for ATTR amyloidosis (familial: transthyretin mutation). Consider bone marrow autograft. Prognosis: if only neuropathy = 42 months: if renal involvement = 27 months: if heart failure = 6 months.

Lymphoma

Hodgkin's Lymphoma

Characterized by the presence of Reed-Sternberg cells.
Pathology of lymphocytes. Association with Epstein-Barr virus.
Bimodal peak in incidence: around 25 years of age and after 50.

WHO/REAL Classification:
–   "Classic" Hodgkin's lymphoma, with 4 pathological subtypes: nodular sclerosis (more frequent), mixed-cellularity, lymphocyte-depleted, lymphocyte-rich.
–   "Nodular lymphocyte predominant" Hodgkin's lymphoma (distinguishable from "classic" Hodgkin's lymphoma by flow cytometry).

Clinical	Lymphadenopathy, constitutional symptoms (B symptoms: fever, weight loss ≥ 10 % within 6 months, night sweats), fatigue, pruritus, painful lymphadenopathy following alcohol consumption, jaundice. ↑ risk of infection with CMV and VZV.
Staging	Cotswolds staging : – Stage I: 1 lymph node region or lymphoid structure involved, or involvement of a single extralymphatic site. – Stage II: 2 or more lymph node regions involved on the same side of the diaphragm. – Stage III: Involvement of lymph node regions on both sides of the diaphragm. – Stage IV: Diffuse or disseminated involvement of one or more extralymphatic organs or tissues (bone, liver, etc), with or without associated lymph node involvement. "X" for large mass (bulky disease). "E" for extra-nodal sites. Subdivided into stage A (no B symptoms) or B (B symptoms present).
Workup	– CBC, ESR, calcium, LDH, uric acid, protein levels, protein electrophoresis, hepatorenal workup, alkaline phosphatase, etc. – Bone marrow biopsy/aspirate. – Thoracic, abdominal and pelvic CT scan. – Gallium scan or PET scan if available. – Exploratory laparoscopy as needed (not necessary for already documented stages IIIb and IV). – Tissue biopsies as needed.

Treatment	In early disease (stages I-II):
	- "Favorable prognosis": in the absence of the following risk factors: B symptoms, extranodal disease, bulky disease (≥ 10 cm or > 33 % of the chest diameter on chest X-ray), ≥ 3 sites of nodal involvement, sedimentation rate ≥ 50: ABVD chemotherapy (2 cycles) + involved-field radiotherapy. For nodular lymphocyte-predominant Hodgkin's, radiotherapy only for early disease.
	- "Unfavorable prognosis" in presence of risk factors: 4-6 cycles of ABVD ± radiotherapy.
	In advanced disease (stages III-IV):
	- "Favorable prognosis" if ≤ 3 IPI adverse risk factors (see below, Prognosis): ABVD for 6-8 cycles ± radiotherapy if extensive.
	- "Unfavorable prognosis" if ≥ 4 adverse risk factors: ABVD for 6-8 cycles or BEACOPP.
	If progression: autologous bone marrow transplant.
	If emergencies (superior vena cava syndrome, airway obstruction, tamponade, spinal cord compression), proceed with radiotherapy or chemotherapy.
	Treatment complications: infertility, amenorrhea, secondary neoplasms (leukemias, non-Hodgkin's lymphomas, solid tumors of lung, breast, head and neck, colon, stomach, thyroid, melanoma), cardiomyopathy, radiation pneumonitis, radiation-induced constrictive pericarditis, myelodysplastic syndrome, hypothyroidism, pulmonary fibrosis, avascular necrosis, post-splenectomy pneumococcus sepsis, etc.
Prognosis	Depends on age, stage, B symptoms presence, histology, PET scan findings. Treatment is curative in 75 % of patients (generally). Stages I-IIA: 80 % 10-year survival rate. Stages IIB-IV: 50-60 % 5-year survival rate.
	International Prognostic Index (IPI) for patients with advanced-stage Hodgkin's based on the presence or absence of 7 factors: Albumin level < 40 g/L, hemoglobin level < 105 g/L, male sex , age ≥ 45 years, stage IV disease, white blood cell (WBC) count ≥ 15 x 10^9/L, absolute lymphocytic count < 0.6 x 10^9/L and/or < 8% of the total WBC count: 60-84 % freedom from progression at 5 years for advanced favorable disease, 42-51 % freedom from progression at 5 years for advanced unfavorable disease.
Non-Hodgkin's Lymphoma (NHL)	Malignancy of lymphocytes. ↑ frequency with HIV. Generally: indolent lymphomas are slowly growing but incurable, intermediate grade lymphomas are curable but more aggressive and grow rapidly.
Clinical features	Diffuse low-grade lymphadenopathy. B symptoms. Compressive symptoms (spinal cord, ureter, etc). Isolated lymphoma possible (bone, testicles, thyroid, intestines, orbits, lungs, central nervous system, gastric, cutaneous, etc).
Classification	Evolving: WHO/REAL Classification: B-cell, T-cell or putative NK-cell malignancies, Hodgkin's lymphoma (multiple subtypes).
	The most common lymphomas are the follicular lymphomas (45 %) and the diffuse large B-cell lymphomas (40 %) Lymphomas can be clinically divided into indolent, aggressive, or very aggressive (rare).

Workup	– CBC, ESR, calcium, LDH, proteins level, protein electrophoresis, hepatorenal workup, alkaline phosphatase, uric acid, HIV, etc. – Bone marrow biopsy/aspirate. – Thoracic, abdominal and pelvic CT scan. – Gallium scan or PET scan if available. – Karyotype analysis. – Tissue biopsies as needed. – Lumbar puncture in some cases (with involvement of spinal cord or suspicion of central nervous system involvement). – Spinal or head MRI in the presence of neurological symptoms. – Isotopic ventriculography as needed, prior to chemotherapy.
Treatment	According to type of lymphoma. – For follicular lymphoma: Watchful waiting if asymptomatic and low tumor burden. If symptomatic, disease progression or important tumor burden: Rituximab + CVP, chlorambucil, or rituximab + CHOP (R-CHOP). For recurrence: fludarabine, rituximab or ibritumomab or tositumomab. – Maintenance treatment with rituximab every 3 months for 2 years: increases disease-free survival. – For diffuse large B-cell lymphoma: R-CHOP. Bone marrow transplant for recurrence. – For MALT lymphoma (associated with *H. pylori*): antibiotics ± radiotherapy or chlorambucil.
Prognosis	International Prognostic Index (IPI) useful for aggressive lymphoma, based on the presence or absence of 5 factors: age > 60 years, Ann-Arbor stages III-IV, ≥ 2 extranodal sites, LDH ↑, performance status (ECOG 2-4/4): 5-year survival rate of 73 % with 0-1 factors, 51 % with 2, 43 % with 3, 26 % with 4-5 (but these numbers were obtained prior to the use of rituximab). Average survival of 6-8 years with follicular lymphoma; for more aggressive lymphomas, it depends on the response to chemotherapy. FLIPI Index for follicular lymphoma (*Follicular Lymphoma International Prognostic Index*) based on 5 factors: age > 60 years, stage III-IV, hemoglobin < 120 g/L, LDH ↑, > 4 lymph node regions involved: Survival at 5 years of 91 % with 0-1 factor, 78 % with 2 factors and 53 % with at least 3 factors.

Breast Cancer

Most common cancer in women: 1 in 8 women will develop this cancer during her lifetime.
2nd cause of cancer mortality in women.

Risk factors: personal or familial breast cancer history, ↑ age, nulliparity, precocious menarche, ↑ age at first full-term pregnancy, late menopause, diet, exogenous estrogens, alcohol, benign breast disease, obesity, radiotherapy, past history of endometrial or ovarian cancer.
These risk factors are present in 21 % of 30-54 years old women affected by breast cancer and 29 % of those between 55-84 years of age.
BRCA 1 and BRCA 2 genes also ↑ risk: ⊕ in 5-10 % of women but those ⊕ have 50-80 % risk of breast cancer in their lifetime.

Staging	See table
Workup	– Mammography, tumor biopsy, estrogen and progesterone receptor expression, HER-2 status (⊕ in 25 %). – Breast ultrasound as needed. PET scan as needed if available. – Basic biochemistry, liver function testing, calcium, alkaline phosphatase. Chest X-ray, abdominal ultrasound. – Bone scan if symptoms, ↑ alkaline phosphatase or stages II-III. Head or liver CT scan if metastasis suspected. – Screen for BRCA1 and BRCA2 genes in high-risk families.

Treatment	According to stage: stages I -II -III potentially curable.
	■ Surgery: tumorectomy + axillary dissection + radiotherapy for stages I-II-III. Mastectomy for more advanced stage or in patients for whom radiotherapy is contraindicated.
	
	■ Adjuvant therapy:
	- If lymph node ⊖: assess risk according to: tumor size, histologic or nuclear grade (I to III), estrogen receptor status (ER), lymphatic and vascular invasion, level of HER-2/neu expression.
	    – low risk if tumor ≤ 1 cm and all good prognostic factors present (i.e. : ER ⊕, grade I and no lymphatic or vascular invasion).
	    – high risk if tumor > 3 cm or > 1 cm and 1 poor prognostic factor (i.e. : ER ⊖, grade III or lymphatic or vascular invasion).
	    – intermediate risk if neither low nor high risk.
	    → If low risk: no adjuvant treatment.
	    → If intermediate risk: if ER ⊕: hormonotherapy ± chemotherapy.
	        If ER ⊖: chemotherapy.
	    → If high risk: premenopausal, ER ⊕ or ⊖: chemotherapy (+ tamoxifen if ER ⊕).
	        If postmenopausal, ER ⊕: chemotherapy + tamoxifen (or anastrozole or letrozole).
	        If postmenopausal, ER ⊖: chemotherapy.
	
	- If lymph node ⊕ and T1,T2 or T3 :
	    – If premenopausal: chemotherapy; tamoxifen ± LHRH analogue or ovarian ablation for patients who decline chemotherapy and are ER ⊕.
	    – If postmenopausal and 50-69 years old and ER ⊖: chemotherapy.
	    – If postmenopausal and 50-69 years old and ER ⊕: chemotherapy, letrozole or anastrozole (consider tamoxifen if severe osteoporosis).
	    – If > 70 years old (physiological) ER ⊕ : letrozole, anastrozole or tamoxifen if severe osteoporosis.
	
	- If stage IV: with minimal visceral involvement and ER ⊕ : letrozole or anastrozole (1st line) or tamoxifen; otherwise chemotherapy (depending on patient's condition). Anti-Her-2 monoclonal antibodies tratuzumab if expression ⊕ . Bisphosphonates if bone metastasis visible through standard radiography.

	Note: Anastroxole or letrozole adjuvant treatment last 5 years. If tamoxifen is administered, after 2 years change for exemestane or anastrozole for 3 more years (disease-free survival advantage). If tamoxifen is administered for 5 years, consider 5 years of letrozole afterwards (disease-free survival advantage and potentially on overall survival).

	- Chemotherapy :
	   - If lymph node ⊖: 4 cycles of AC (cyclophosphamide, doxorubicin), 4 cycles of TC (taxotere,cyclophosphamide) or 6 cycles of FEC 100 (cyclophosphamide, epirubicine, 5-FU).
	   - If lymph node ⊕: FEC 100/D (FEC 100 x 3 cycles and docetaxel x 3 cycles) or AC x 4 and paclitaxel x 4 administered every 2 weeks.
	   - If HER-2 ⊕ and lymph node ⊕ or tumor ≥ T 1c: add trastuzumab every 3 weeks for 1 year.
	   - If metastasis ⊕ (depending on metastasis site, severity of involvement, and adjuvant therapy previously received): hormonotherapy (if ER ⊕), CMF, AC, epirubicine, docetaxel, paclitaxel, abraxane, capecitabine, vinorelbine, gemcitabine, etc. Anti-HER-2/neu monoclonal trastuzumab antibodies if expression ⊕.
	
	 - Radiotherapy: adjuvant to tumorectomy or for localized symptomatic disease (with > 3 axillary lymphadenopathies) or advanced (with tumor ≥ 5 cm or skin invasion, pectoral muscle or thoracic wall invasion). Useful for palliation (control of a painful site, etc).

Prognosis	Depends on the number of lymph nodes involved, tumor size, hormone receptor expression, tumor grade, HER-2/neu expression, etc. Survival rate for stage 0 : 98 % at 5 years, 95 % at 10 years ; stage I 85 % at 5 years, 70 % at 10 years ; stage IIA 70 % at 5 years, 50 % at 10 years ; stage IIB 60 % at 5 years, 40 % at 10 years ; stage IIIA 55 % at 5 years, 30 % at 10 years ; stage IIIB 30 % at 5 years, 20 % at 10 years ; stage IV 5-10 % at 5 years, 2 % at 10 years. For low-risk neoplasm without lymph nodes invasion: recurrence at 10 years < 10 %. For high-risk neoplasm without lymph nodes invasion: recurrence at 10 years > 20 %.
Screening and prevention	Mammography every 2 years for women of age 50-69. Controversial for 40-49 years old (except if elevated risk) and > 70 years old. With ⊕ family history, start mammography 5-10 years before age of first breast cancer diagnosis in family. Note: Mammography may miss 10 % of palpable mass at physical examination; always evaluate palpable mass through breast ultrasound. Screen for BRCA1 and BRCA2 genes in women at risk (should probably test if one 1st degree relative < 40 years or two 1st degree relatives < 50 years are affected). Chemoprophylaxis (with tamoxifen) could be considered as primary prevention in high-risk patients (Gail index ≥ 1.66 % at 5 years) but controversial (no evidence of ↓ in mortality).

Breast Cancer: TNM Classification

Primary tumor (T)

TX: Primary tumor cannot be assessed

T0: No evidence of primary tumor

Tis: Carcinoma in situ; intraductal carcinoma, lobular carcinoma in situ, or Paget's disease of the nipple with no associated tumor. Note: Paget's disease associated with a tumor is classified according to the size of the tumor.

T1: Tumor 2.0 cm or less in greatest dimension

   T1mic: Microinvasion 0.1 cm or less in greatest dimension

   T1a: Tumor more than 0.1 but not more than 0.5 cm in greatest dimension

   T1b: Tumor more than 0.5 cm but not more than 1.0 cm in greatest dimension

   T1c: Tumor more than 1.0 cm but not more than 2.0 cm in greatest dimension

T2: Tumor more than 2.0 cm but not more than 5.0 cm in greatest dimension

T3: Tumor more than 5.0 cm in greatest dimension

T4: Tumor of any size with direct extension to (a) chest wall or (b) skin, only as described below.

   Note: Chest wall includes ribs, intercostal muscles, and serratus anterior muscle but not pectoral muscle.

   T4a: Extension to chest wall

   T4b: Edema (including peau d'orange) or ulceration of the skin of the breast or satellite skin nodules confined to

the same breast
T4c: Both of the above (T4a and T4b)
T4d: Inflammatory carcinoma

Regional lymph nodes (N)
NX: Regional lymph nodes cannot be assessed (e.g., previously removed)
N0: No regional lymph node metastasis
N1: Metastasis to movable ipsilateral axillary lymph node(s)
N2: Metastasis to ipsilateral axillary lymph node(s) fixed or matted, or in clinically apparent ipsilateral internal mammary nodes in the *absence* of clinically evident lymph node metastasis
    N2a: Metastasis in ipsilateral axillary lymph nodes fixed to one another (matted) or to other structures
    N2b: Metastasis only in clinically apparent* ipsilateral internal mammary nodes and in the absence of clinically evident axillary lymph node metastasis
N3: Metastasis in ipsilateral infraclavicular lymph node(s) with or without axillary lymph node involvement, or in clinically apparent* ipsilateral internal mammary lymph node(s) and in the *presence* of clinically evident axillary lymph node metastasis; or metastasis in ipsilateral supraclavicular lymph node(s) with or without axillary or internal mammary lymph node involvement
    N3a: Metastasis in ipsilateral infraclavicular lymph node(s)
    N3b: Metastasis in ipsilateral internal mammary lymph node(s) and axillary lymph node(s)
    N3c: Metastasis in ipsilateral supraclavicular lymph node(s)

Pathologic classification (pN)
pNX: Regional lymph nodes cannot be assessed (e.g., not removed for pathologic study or previously removed)
pN0: No regional lymph node metastasis histologically, no additional examination for isolated tumor cells (ITC)
    pN0(I-): No regional lymph node metastasis histologically, negative IHC
    pN0(I+): No regional lymph node metastasis histologically, positive IHC, no IHC cluster >0.2 mm
    pN0(mol-): No regional lymph node metastasis histologically, negative molecular findings (RT-PCR)
    pN0(mol+): No regionally lymph node metastasis histologically, positive molecular findings (RT-PCR)
pN1: Metastasis in 1 to 3 axillary lymph nodes, and/or in internal mammary nodes with microscopic disease detected by sentinel lymph node dissection but not clinically apparent
    pN1mi: Micrometastasis (>0.2 mm but =2.0 mm)
    pN1a: Metastasis in 1 to 3 axillary lymph nodes
    pN1b: Metastasis in internal mammary nodes with microscopic disease detected by sentinel lymph node dissection but not clinically apparent
    pN1c: Metastasis in 1 to 3 axillary lymph nodes and in internal mammary lymph nodes with microscopic disease detected by sentinel lymph node dissection but not clinically apparent. (If associated with >3 positive axillary lymph nodes, the internal mammary are classified as pN3b to reflect increased tumor burden)
pN2: Metastasis in 4 to 9 axillary lymph nodes, or in clinically apparent internal mammary lymph nodes in the absence of axillary lymph node metastasis to ipsilateral axillary lymph node(s) fixed to each other or to other structures
    pN2a: Metastasis in 4 to 9 axillary lymph nodes (at least 1 tumor deposit >2.0 mm)
    pN2b: Metastasis in clinically apparent internal mammary lymph nodes in the absence of axillary lymph node metastasis
pN3: Metastasis in 10 or more axillary lymph nodes, or in infraclavicular lymph nodes, or in clinically apparent* ipsilateral internal mammary lymph node(s) in the presence of 1 or more positive axillary lymph nodes; or in more than 3 axillary lymph nodes with clinically negative microscopic metastasis in internal mammary lymph nodes; or in ipsilateral supraclavicular lymph nodes
    pN3a: Metastasis in 10 or more axillary lymph nodes (at least one tumor deposit >2.0 mm), or metastasis to the infraclavicular lymph nodes
    pN3b: Metastasis in clinically apparent ipsilateral internal mammary lymph nodes in the presence of 1 or more positive axillary lymph node(s); or in more than 3 axillary lymph nodes and in internal mammary lymph nodes with microscopic disease detected by sentinel lymph node dissection but not clinically apparent
    pN3c: Metastasis in ipsilateral supraclavicular lymph nodes

Distant metastasis (M)
MX: Presence of distant metastasis cannot be assessed
M0: No distant metastasis
M1: Distant metastasis present

Stage AJCC	Stage IIA	Stage IIIA	Stage IIIB
	T0, N1, M0	T0, N2, M0	T4, Any N, M0
Stage 0	T1,* N1, M0	T1,* N2, M0	
Tis, N0, M0	T2, N0, M0	T2, N2, M0	**Stage IIIC**
		T3, N1, M0	Any T, N3, M0
Stage I	**Stage IIB**	T3, N2, M0	
T1,* N0, M0	T2, N1, M0		**Stage IV**
	T3, N0, M0		Any T, Any N, M1

*T1 includes T1mic
Breast. In: American Joint Committee on Cancer.: AJCC Cancer Staging Manual. 6th ed. New York, NY: Springer, 2002, pp 171-180.

Central Nervous System Cancer

1.5 % of all neoplasms. 48 % are metastasis.
Origin of primary CNS tumors: 35 % glial cells, 40 % meninges, 25 % neurons, Schwann cells, lymphocytes and pituitary, ependyma, choroid plexus, neuroectoderm, vessels, or germ cells. Tumors often heterogeneous, with high and low-grade regions.

WHO histologic grade of CNS tumors:
Grade I tumors have a low replication potential with good response to surgery alone.
Grade II tumors usually infiltrating but with a low mitotic activity, however may recur.
Grade III tumors are lesions with evident histologic malignancy (mitotic activity, infiltration, anaplasia).
Grade IV tumors are lesions with active mitotic activity, associated with rapid growth.

Classification	**I. Neuroepithelial tissue tumors:**

I. Neuroepithelial tissue tumors:
- Astrocytic Tumors: pilocytic astrocytoma* (grade I), diffuse astrocytoma (grade II), anaplastic astrocytoma (grade III), glioblastoma (grade IV), subependymal giant cell astrocytoma (grade I).
- Oligodendroglial Tumors: oligodendroglioma (grade II), anaplastic oligodendroglioma (grade III).
- Oligoastrocytic Tumors: oligoastrocytoma (grade II), anaplastic oligoastrocytoma (grade III).
- Ependymal Tumors: subependymoma (grade I), myxopapillary ependymoma (grade I), ependymoma (grade II), anaplastic ependymoma (grade III).
- Choroid Plexus Tumors: papilloma (grade I) or carcinoma (grade III).
- Other Neuroepithelial Tumors: astroblastoma (grade I), chordoid glioma of the 3rd ventricle (grade II), angiocentric glioma (grade I).
- Neuronal and Mixed Neuronal-Glial Tumors: gangliocytoma (grade I), ganglioglioma (grade I-III), dysembryoplastic neuroepithelial tumors (grade I), central neurocytoma (grade II), cerebellar liponeurocytoma (grade II), paraganglioma (grade I).
- Tumors of the Pineal Region: pineocytoma (grade II), pineoblastoma* (grade IV), of intermediary differentiation.
- Embryonal Tumors: medulloblastoma* (grade IV), primitive neuroectodermal tumor (including ependymoblastoma*) (grade IV), atypical teratoid/rhabdoid tumor.

II. Tumors of cranial and paraspinal nerves: schwannoma (grade I), neurofibroma, perineurioma, malignant peripheral nerve sheath tumor.

III. Tumors of the meninges: meningioma (grades I-III, with breast cancer history, neurofibromatosis, cerebral irradiation, etc), mesenchymal tumors, primary melanocytic lesions, other (capillary hemangioblastoma - grade I).

IV. Lymphoma and hemopoietic neoplasms: lymphoma (including primary CNS lymphoma, especially in immunosuppressed, HIV: 40 % multifocal, plasmacytoma, granulocytic sarcoma.

V. Germ cell tumors*: germinomas, embryonal carcinoma, yolk sac tumor, choriocarcinoma, teratoma, etc.

VI. Tumors of the sellar region: craniopharyngioma (grade I), granular cell tumor (grade I), pituicytoma (grade I), etc.

VII. Metastases: lung, breast, melanoma, renal, gastrointestinal, gynecological.

* Especially in children.

Clinical findings	Headaches 40 %, typically when waking up, ↓ in one hour. Localized headaches possible. Convulsions, hemiparesia, decreased level of consciousness, elevated intracranial pressure with nausea - vomiting - cranial nerve VI paralysis ± diplopia, papilledema, aphasia, altered visual field, impaired cognition, etc. Focal neurologic deficits according to tumor localization. Transient symptoms like visual loss, paresis, headaches, or altered level of consciousness can occur. Meningeal carcinomatosis sometimes associated.
Workup	MRI. PET scan as needed. HIV serology in presence of lymphoma. Lumbar puncture if meningeal carcinomatosis or lymphoma suspected (but risk of herniation). Vitrectomy sometimes useful if ocular involvement of suspected lymphoma (if lumbar pucture negative). Chest X-ray, abdominal ultrasound, bone scan if suspect cerebral metastasis. Mammography in women. In men < 50 years, exclude germinal tumor. Stereotactic biopsy of mass as needed. Arteriography sometimes useful (pituitary tumor vs aneurysm).
Treatment	According to histologic type, expansion, and patient's condition. – Steroids (but avoid if possible when there is no pathologic diagnosis because it could make lymphoma diagnosis more difficult): dexamethasone 10 mg IV then 4 mg qid. – Surgery if possible. Controversial for asymptomatic meningioma. For solitary metastasis, surgery or radiosurgery as needed. Stereotaxic radiosurgery as needed for metastasis < 3 cm, schwannoma, meningioma, some hypophyseal tumors and as adjuvant treatment for glioma. – Radiotherapy for high-grade glioma or for metastasis. – Chemotherapy according to type of tumor. Useful for oligodendroglioma, germinal cell tumor and medulloblastoma and lymphomas. ↑ survival when combined with radiotherapy in high-grade gliomas (nitrosourea, temozolomide). – Mannitol for elevated intracranial pressure. Anticonvulsants as needed.
Prognosis	Pilocytic astrocytoma: good prognosis with surgery. Low-grade astrocytoma: mean survival of 5-8 years. Low-grade oligodendroglioma: mean survival of 12-16 years. Anaplastic astrocytoma: median survival of 2-3 years. Glioblastoma: mean survival of 1 year, survival < 10 % at 5 years. Anaplastic oligodendroglioma: mean survival of 3 years. Lymphoma: median survival of 40 months in immunocompetent, and 2-6 months in immunocompromised.

Colorectal Cancer

2nd cause of cancer mortality: incidence men ≈ women, increases with age. Rare < 50 years.
Risk factors: age, family history, personal history, inflammatory bowel disease, environmental (calcium-deficient diet, high-fat diet, alcohol, tobacco) and genetic factors.
Hereditary syndromes :
- Familial adenomatous polyposis: > 100 polyps, malignant transformation before age 40, autosomal dominant. Includes Gardner and Turcot syndromes.
- HNPCC (*hereditary nonpolyposis colon cancer*) or Lynch syndrome: ≥ 3 relatives with colorectal cancer within 2 generations with one < 50 years (Amsterdam criteria): autosomal dominant : Lynch I and Lynch II (latter associated with cancer of uterus, breast, ovary) : predominantly right-sided cancer.
- Peutz-Jeghers and Ruvalcaba-Myhre-Smith syndromes, Cowden disease, familial juvenile polyposis, etc.

Clinical findings	Proximal lesion: weight loss, microcytic anemia, abdominal mass, melena. Distal lesion: hematochezia, obstruction, tenesmus, change in intestinal bowel habits.
Staging	See table.
Workup	– CBC, INR, aPTT, CEA, alkaline phosphatase, AST, ALT. – ECG, chest X-ray. – Colonoscopy ± biopsy: barium enema if endoscopy not available. – Thoracic and abdominal CT scan. – For rectal neoplasia: pelvic CT scan, transrectal ultrasound or pelvic MRI.
Treatment	According to staging. – Stage I: Curative surgery. – Stage II: Curative surgery ± adjuvant chemotherapy if high risk of recurrence (T4, poorly differentiated histology, intestinal perforation or occlusion, etc). Neoadjuvant radiochemotherapy for advanced rectal neoplasia (T3, T4, N +). – Stage III: Curative surgery + adjuvant chemotherapy (5-FU + leucovorin + oxaliplatin [FOLFOX] or capecitabine), because mortality ↓ by 33 %. Neoadjuvant chemotherapy for rectal neoplasia ± adjuvant chemotherapy. – Stage IV: 5-FU + leucovorin + irinotecan ("FOLFIRI" 1st line) ± bevacizumab or 5-FU + leucovorin + oxaliplatin ("FOLFOX") ± bevacizumab. Capecitabine PO ± oxaliplatin ("CapeOX") ± bevacizumab. Cetuximab or panitumumab if available and K-ras wild type. Consider palliative surgery to ↓ risk of obstruction. Metastasectomy as needed for relatively isolated hepatic or pulmonary lesions in patients in overall good condition (with primary tumor resection).

Follow-up	For stages I-III :
	   - Complete colonoscopy after surgery if not done before.
	   - Complete colonoscopy 1, 3 years and every 5 years afterwards.
	 For stages II and III:
	   - History + physical examination + CEA every 3 to 6 months for 3 years, then every 6 months for a total of 5 years.
	   - Thoracic and abdominal CT scan annually x 3 for high-risk patients.
	
	 If CEA increases twofold:
	 - Control levels and colonoscopy ± thorax and abdominal CT scan ± PET scan (if available) ± laparotomy for investigation of recurrence.

Prognosis	Overall survival 35 %: 55 % cured by surgery. 5-year survival rate: stage 0 > 95 %: stage I 93 %: stage II 72-85 %: stage III 44-83 %: stage IV 8 %.

Screening	**Individuals □ 50 years of age without risk factors:**
	2004 Canadian recommendations:
	– Hematest every 2 years ± sigmoidoscopy every 5 years;
	– Double contrast barium enema every 5 years or complete colonoscopy every 10 years.
	Individuals with 1st degree relative affected after age 60:
	– Total colonoscopy every 10 years from age 40.
	Individuals with 1st degree relative before age 60 or □ 2 1st degree relatives affected:
	– Total colonoscopy every 5 years from age 40 or 10 years before age at which youngest relative was diagnosed.
	Familial adenomatous polyposis:
	– Genetic testing. Sigmoidoscopy every year from age 10-12.
	HNPCC or ⊕ Amsterdam criteria:
	– Genetic testing. Total colonoscopy every 1-2 years from age 20-25.
	Inflammatory bowel disease with colitis:
	– Total colonoscopy + random biopsies throughout colon every 2 years after 8 years if pancolitis or after 15 years if left colitis.

Colorectal Cancer: TNM Classification

Primary tumor (T)	Regional lymph nodes (N)	Distant metastasis (M)	Stage AJCC
TX: Primary tumor cannot be assessed	**NX**: Regional nodes cannot be assessed	**MX**: Distant metastasis cannot be assessed	**Stage 0** Tis, N0, M0
T0: No evidence of primary tumor	**N0**: No regional lymph node metastasis	**M0**: No distant metastasis	**Stage I** T1, N0, M0 T2, N0, M0
Tis: Carcinoma in situ: intraepithelial or invasion of the lamina propria*	**N1**: Metastasis in 1to 3 regional lymph nodes	**M1**: Distant metastasis	**Stage IIA** T3, N0, M0
T1: Tumor invades submucosa	**N2**: Metastasis in 4 or more regional lymph nodes		**Stage IIB** T4, N0, M0
T2: Tumor invades muscularis propria	A tumor nodule in the pericolorectal adipose tissue of a primary carcinoma without histologic evidence of residual lymph node in the nodule is classified in the pN category as a regional lymph node metastasis if the nodule has the form and smooth contour of a lymph node. If the nodule has an irregular contour, it should be classified in the T category and also coded as V1 (microscopic venous invasion) or as V2 (if it was grossly evident), because there is a strong likelihood that is represents venous invasion		**Stage IIIA** T1, N1,M0 T2,N1,M0
T3: Tumor invades through the muscularis propria into the subserosa, or into nonperitonealized pericolic or perirectal tissues			**Stage IIIB** T3,N1,M0 T4,N1,M0
T4: Tumor directly invades other organs or structures, and/or perforates visceral peritoneum **,***			**Stage IIIC** Any T, N2, M0 **Stage IV** Any T, Any N, M1

* Note: Tis includes cancer cells confined within the glandular basement membrane (intraepithelial) or lamina propria (intramucosal) with no extension through the muscularis mucosae into the submucosa.
** Note: Direct invasion in T4 includes invasion of other segments of the colorectum by way of the serosa; for example, invasion of the sigmoid colon by a carcinoma of the cecum.
*** Note: Tumor that is adherent macroscopically to other organs or structures is classified T4. If no tumor is present in the adhesion microscopically, however, the classification should be pT3. The V and L substaging should be used to identify the presence or absence of vascular or lymphatic invasion.

Colon and rectum. In: American Joint Committee on Cancer.: AJCC Cancer Staging Manual. 6th ed. New York, NY: Springer, 2002, pp 113-124.

Esophageal Cancer	
Overview	Progressive dysphagia (solids → liquids) with weight loss. Dyspnea, cough, hoarseness or chest pain can occur. **Adenocarcinoma** causes > 50 % of esophageal neoplasms in Canada: associated with Barrett's esophagus, tobacco, GERD, obesity, develops mainly in lower third of esophagus. **Squamous cell carcinoma** causes < 50 % of esophageal neoplasms: associated with alcohol, tobacco, achalasia, caustic oesophagitis, palmoplantar tylosis. Rarely other causes: other carcinomas, melanomas, leiomyosarcomas, carcinoid, lymphomas, etc.
Workup	Diagnostic: esophagogastroduodenoscopy with biopsy. Workup for extension: routine biochemistry, thoracic and abdominal CT scan, positron emission tomography scan (if available), endoscopic ultrasound if localized tumor with fine needle aspiration if indicated and surgical candidate ± bronchoscopy for advanced mid-esophageal tumor.
Staging	See table.
Treatment	According to stage: stages 0, I, IIA curable: stages IIB, III and IVA rarely curable: stage IV: palliative. – Stage I: surgery only. – Stage IIA, IIB and III good surgical candidates: neoadjuvant radiochemotherapy (5-FU and cisplatin-based) then surgery vs definitive radiochemotherapy only, especially for stages IIB and III; consider per-op chemotherapy if adenocarcinoma of distal esophagus. – Stages IVA: potentially resecable if isolated celiac lymphadenopathy < 1.5 cm (controversial). – If non-resectable tumor or stage IVB: chemotherapy ± palliative radiotherapy for patient in good condition. Otherwise: endoprosthesis, radiotherapy or laser therapy or absolute alcohol for severe dysphagia. Enteral nutrition as needed.

Prognosis	10-13 % 5-year overall survival rate. If tumor is resected: 5-year survival rate of 20-30 %.
	5-year survival rate according to stage: Stage 0: 95 %.
	        Stage I: 50-80 %.
	        Stage IIA: 30-40 %.
	        Stage IIB: 10-30 %
	        Stage III: 10-15 %.
	        Stage IV: 4 %

Esophageal Cancer: TNM Classification

Primary tumor (T)	Regional lymph nodes (N)	Distant metastasis (M)	Stage AJCC
TX: Primary tumor cannot be assessed	**NX**: Regional lymph nodes cannot be assessed	**MX**: Distant metastasis cannot be assessed	**Stage 0** Tis, N0, M0
T0: No evidence of primary tumor	**N0**: No regional lymph node metastasis	**M0**: No distant metastasis	**Stage I** T1, N0, M0
Tis: Carcinoma in situ		**M1**: Distant metastasis	**Stage IIA** T2, N0, M0 T3, N0, M0

T1: Tumor invades lamina propria or submucosa	**N1**: Regional lymph node metastasis	Tumors of the lower thoracic esophagus:
		  M1a: Metastasis in celiac lymph nodes
		  M1b: Other distant metastasis
			Stage IIB
			T1, N1, M0
			T2, N1, M0

T2: Tumor invades muscularis propria		Tumors of the midthoracic esophagus:
		  M1a: Not applicable
		  M1b: Nonregional lymph nodes and/or other distant metastasis
			Stage III
			T3, N1, M0
			T4, Any N, M0

T3: Tumor invades adventitia			**Stage IV** Any T, Any N, M1

T4: Tumor invades adjacent structures		Tumors of the upper thoracic esophagus:
		  M1a: Metastasis in cervical nodes
		  M1b: Other distant metastasis
			-- Stage IVA --
			Any T, Any N, M1a

		For tumors of midthoracic esophagus use only M1b, since these tumors with metastasis in nonregional lymph nodes have an equally poor prognosis as those with metastasis in other distant sites	-- Stage IVB -- Any T, Any N, M1b
Esophagus. In: American Joint Committee on Cancer.: AJCC Cancer Staging Manual. 6th ed. New York, NY: Springer, 2002, pp 91-98.			

Gastric Cancer

Pathology: adenocarcinoma 90 %, lymphoma 5 %, sarcoma 2 %, mesenchymal tumor (gastro-intestinal stroma tumor, leimyoma, neurinoma, schwannoma) 1-3 %, or carcinoid < 1 %.
Incidence varies throughout the world: 1st cause of mortality in Japan. Risk ↑ in Native Americans, Hispanics, African-Americans, etc. World global incidence ↓ but noticeable increase of proximal cancer.

Gastric Adenocarcinoma

Overview	Symptoms include malaise, dyspepsia, dysphagia (proximal tumor), early satiety, pain, weight loss, obstruction or metastases in patients > 40 years. Acute or chronic bleeding can occur. Known risk factors: *H. pylori* infection (for distal neoplasm), intestinal metaplasia, atrophic gastritis, pernicious anemia, adenomatous polyp, diet, tobacco, and hereditary (1-3 % of cases). Probable risk factors: history of partial gastrectomy > 20 years ago. 75% have unresectable disease at the time of diagnosis. 3 % of gastric ulcers are cancer.
Workup	Routine biochemistry, hepatic enzymes, endoscopy with biopsy, thoraco-abdominal CT scan and CT or ultrasound of pelvis (females) ± endoscopic ultrasound if available ± positron emission tomography scan if available ± diagnostic laparoscopy.
Stage	See table
Treatment	According to stage: stages I-II-III are potentially curable. - Stage Tis or T1a limited to mucosa: consider endoscopic mucosal resection. - Stages I-II-III: for surgical candidate, resection with extended lymphadenectomy. For stage ≥ T2 or N +, consider pre-op and post-op chemotherapy or pre-op chemoradiotherapy or post-op chemoradiotherapy: total parenteral nutrition or feeding jejunostomy post-op as needed. Follow vitamin B12 levels after gastrectomy. Treat *H. pylori* if positive. - Stage IV or non-surgical candidate: palliative endoscopic treatment (laser, absolute alcohol, etc) vs dilation and endoprosthesis vs gastrostomy. Chemotherapy (cisplatin-based or 5-FU) or palliative radiotherapy.

Prognosis	5-year survival: average = 20 % in North America: worse for proximal than distal lesion (because asymptomatic).
	         Stage 0: > 90 %.
	         Stage I: 52-85 %.
	         Stage II: > 20 % if distal: < 20 % if proximal.
	         Stage IIIA: 17 % : stage IIIB : 15 %
	         Stage IV: < 5 %.

Gastric Lymphoma	− Most frequent extranodal site. 5 % of gastric neoplasms. − 90 %: high-grade B cell non-Hodgkin's lymphoma. − 10 % MALT lymphoma (MALToma) caused by *H. pylori* infection. − Treatment according to stage: stage IE = surgery or chemotherapy: stages IIE to IV = chemotherapy. − Antibiotic treatment for *H. pylori* with low-grade MALToma. − Prognosis: 5-year survival rate of 50 %: > 80 % for stage IE.
Gastric Carcinoid Tumor	Rare: type I associated with pernicious anemia or atrophic gastritis: type II associated with Zollinger-Ellison syndrome: type III sporadic. Development of classical symptoms in the presence of hepatic metastasis. Surgical or endoscopic treatment depending on type.

Gastrointestinal Stromal Tumor	Rare tumor. Average age: 58 years. Rare before 40 years old. 50-70 % of stromal tumors occur in the stomach. Tumors may grow quite large before becoming symptomatic, mainly severe hemorrhage or chronic bleeding. Risk of metastases ↑ if tumor > 3 cm. Liver or peritoneal metastases. **Diagnosis**: with gastroscopy, CT scan (characteristic image) or endoscopic ultrasound. Positron emission tomography sometimes useful if available. Biopsy only necessary for atypical lesion. **Treatment**: Surgery. If metastasis, imatinib. Sunitinib if refractory to imatinib. **Prognosis:** Depends on tumor diameter and mitotic index. Excellent chance of survival if a localized tumor is completely resected and poor 5-year survival rate if metastatic.

Gastric Cancer: TNM Classification

Primary tumor (T)	Regional lymph nodes (N)	Distant metastasis (M)	Stage AJCC
TX: Primary tumor cannot be assessed	The regional lymph nodes are the perigastric nodes, found along the lesser and	**MX**: Distant metastasis cannot be assessed	**Stage 0** Tis, N0, M0
T0: No evidence of primary tumor	greater curvatures, and the nodes located along the left gastric, common hepatic, splenic, and celiac arteries. For	**M0**: No distant metastasis	**Stage IA** T1, N0, M0
Tis: Carcinoma in situ: intraepithelial tumor without invasion of the lamina propria	pN, a regional lymphadenectomy specimen will ordinarily contain at least 15 lymph nodes. Involvement of other intra-abdominal lymph nodes, such as	**M1**: Distant metastasis	**Stage IB** T1, N1, M0 T2, N0, M0
T1: Tumor invades lamina propria or submucosa	the hepatoduodenal, retropancreatic, mesenteric, and para-aortic, is classified as distant metastasis.		**Stage II** T1, N2, M0 T2, N1, M0 T3, N0, M0
T2: Tumor invades the muscularis propria or the subserosa* T2a: Tumor invades muscularis propria T2b: Tumor invades subserosa	**NX**: Regional lymph node(s) cannot be assessed **N0**: No regional lymph node metastasis ****		**Stage IIIA** T2, N2, M0 T3, N1, M0 T4, N0, M0
T3: Tumor penetrates the serosa (visceral peritoneum) without invading adjacent structures**,***	**N1**: Metastasis in 1 to 6 regional lymph nodes **N2**: Metastasis in 7 to 15 regional lymph nodes		**Stage IIIB** T3, N2, M0
T4:Tumor invades adjacent structures***	**N3**: Metastasis in more than 15 regional lymph nodes		**Stage IV** T4, N1, M0 T4, N2, M0 T1, N3, M0 T2, N3, M0 T3, N3, M0 T4, N3, M0 Any T, Any N, M1

* Note: A tumor may penetrate the muscularis propria with extension into the gastrocolic or gastrohepatic ligaments or into the greater or lesser omentum without perforation of the visceral peritoneum covering these structures. In this case, the tumor is classified T2. If there is perforation of the visceral peritoneum covering the gastric ligaments or omentum, the tumor should be classified T3.
** Note: The adjacent structures of the stomach include the spleen, transverse colon, liver, diaphragm, pancreas, abdominal wall, adrenal gland, kidney, small intestine, and retroperitoneum.
*** Note: Intramural extension to the duodenum or esophagus is classified by the depth of greatest invasion in any of these sites, including stomach.
**** Note: A designation of pN0 should be used if all examined lymph nodes are negative, regardless of the total number removed and examined.

Stomach. In: American Joint Committee on Cancer.: AJCC Cancer Staging Manual. 6th ed. New York, NY: Springer, 2002, pp 99-106.

Lung Cancer	
Clinical findings	1st cause of cancer mortality in men and women. Cough, dyspnea, wheezing, hemoptysis. obstructive pneumonitis. Systemic symptoms. Regional symptoms: parietal pain, superior vena cava syndrome, brachial plexopathy, dysphonia secondary to recurrent laryngeal nerve lesion, diaphragmatic paralysis secondary to phrenic nerve lesion, dysphagia secondary to esophageal obstruction, cardiac tamponade. Symptoms due to metastases. Paraneoplastic syndrome: ectopic secretion of ACTH, SIADH, myasthenic syndrome (Eaton-Lambert): independent of tumor stage. Hypercoagulability, dermatomyositis, and membranous glomerulonephritis are sometimes associated.
Non-Small Cell Lung Carcinoma	Adenocarcinoma 40 %: squamous cell carcinoma 30-35 %: large cell carcinoma 10 %. – Adenocarcinoma: peripheral tumor (in 65 %), clubbing and hypertrophic osteoarthropathy. Most frequent type in non-smokers. – Bronchioalveolar carcinoma is a distinct subtype of adenocarcinomas with better prognosis than other types of pulmonary neoplasm: secondary bronchorrhea in 20 %. Sometimes multifocal tumor. Less association with tobacco. – Large cell carcinoma: clubbing and possible hypertrophic osteoarthropathy (but less frequent than with adenocarcinoma). – Squamous cell carcinoma: proximal tumor (in 2/3 cases), cavitary (in 5-35 % cases), associated paraneoplasic hypercalcemia. Metastases: brain, liver, bone, adrenals, etc.
Stages	See table Diagnosis: 10 % will be in stage I; 20 % in stage II; 15 % in stage IIIA; 15 % in stage IIIB; and 40 % in stage IV.
Workup	– Basic biochemistry (CBC, Na^+, K^+, creatinine, Ca^{++}, alkaline phosphatase, liver enzymes, etc). – Sputum cytology: ⊕ in < 50 %. More frequently ⊕ in central tumor. – Look for nodules on previous chest X-rays: look for nodule development or progression. – Chest CT scan including adrenals. – Bronchoscopy: diagnostic in 10 % if nodule < 15 mm; 40-60 % if > 2 cm. – Cytologic analysis of pleural effusion if present. – Transthoracic biopsy (⊕ > 85 %; risk of pneumothorax 25-30 %) or endoscopic (esophageal or endobronchial) if no diagnosis with above workup. If biopsy not possible, consider thoracoscopy. Biopsy of lymphadenopathy or metastasis if available and easier access. – Positron emission tomography (PET) scan if available. Possible false ⊖ with carcinoid or bronchioloalveolar. – If PET scan not available and according to stage/workup: abdominal ultrasound, bone scan, head CT scan or MRI. – If mediastinal involvement suspected (mediastinal lymphadenopathy > 1 cm or ⊕ PET scan): mediastinoscopy or endoscopic ultrasound depending on anatomy; non-operability has to be proven in general since possible false ⊕. – Pre-op evaluation with full pulmonary function testing (predicted post-op FEV1 and DLCO must be > 40 %). Arterial blood gas as needed (surgery relatively contraindicated if $PaCO_2$ > 45 mmHg). Quantitative pulmonary scan (if FEV1 < 60-80 % or DLCO pre-op < 60-80 %). Exercise test: if FEV1 borderline, ensure VO_2max in general > 15 mL/kg/min (pre-op) according to extent of surgery.

Treatment	According to stage: – Stages I-II: surgery (if operable). Radiotherapy if contraindication or as adjuvant treatment if incomplete macroscopic resection. Consider adjuvant chemotherapy for stage II (cisplatin-based). – Stage IIIA: surgery (if operable) + chemotherapy ± radiotherapy. If not operable, treat as a Stage IIIB lung cancer. – Stage IIIB: radiotherapy + chemotherapy (concomitant > sequential). If stage IIIB with neoplastic effusion, treat as Stage IV with chemotherapy. – Stage IV: palliative chemotherapy (according to patient's general condition) ± radiotherapy (palliative) ± surgery (palliative). If solitary cerebral metastasis: metastasis excision on a case-by-case basis (or via stereotaxic surgery, according to case); afterwards, consider cerebral radiotherapy. Palliative endobronchial treatment (electrocauterization, cryosurgery, brachytherapy).
Prognosis	Disease potentially curable if stages I-II-IIIa. 5-year survival depends on stage: mean of 15 %. For Stage IA 67 %; stage IB 57 %; stage IIA 55 %; stage IIB 38-39 %; stage IIIA 23-25 %; stage IIIB 3-7 %, and stage IV 1 %.
Small Cell Lung Carcinoma	15 % of pulmonary neoplasms, typically proximal (in > 80 % of cases). Highly associated with tobacco. Paraneoplastic syndromes (see above). Metastasis ⊕ in 70 %: bone 35 %, liver 25 %, central nervous system 10-15 %, bone marrow 20 %, lymph nodes, subcutaneous, pleura, etc.
Staging	– Limited stage disease (33 % of patients): confined to one hemithorax; includes involvement of mediastinal, contralateral hilar, and/or supraclavicular and scalene lymph nodes. Malignant pleural effusion is excluded – Extensive stage: disease has spread beyond the definition of limited stage, or malignant pleural effusion is present.
Workup	See non-small cell lung carcinoma workup.
Treatment	According to staging: Surgery + chemotherapy for very localized lesion, nonmetastatic T1-2N0M0 (rare). Chemotherapy for other cases if no contraindications (usually etoposide and cisplatin). Thoracic radiotherapy for limited stage. Prophylactic cerebral radiotherapy indicated for extensive stage if response to chemotherapy or for limited stage if complete response to chemotherapy. If symptomatic metastasis: radiotherapy as needed.
Prognosis	Survival without therapy: 2-4 months. If extensive, mean survival of 9 months, with 1-year survival rate of 10 %, and 5-year of 1 %. If limited, mean survival of 18 months, with 5-year survival rate of 20 %.
Other Histologic Types	Malignant epithelial tumors 5 % of pulmonary neoplasms (carcinoid tumor, sarcomatoid, salivary glands, etc). With typical or atypical carcinoid tumor: possible ectopic ACTH secretion.
Malignant Mesothelioma	Insidious onset of dyspnea, thoracic pain, weight loss. History of asbestos exposure in 70-80 % (but could be minimal). Not tobacco related. 20-40 year latency between exposure and disease. Chest X-rays + CT scan may suggest diagnosis. Exudative or hemorrhagic pleural effusion. Pleural biopsy for histologic diagnosis: cytology often non-diagnostic. Treatment not very effective: consider pleurodesis and palliative chemotherapy. Median survival of 8-12 months.

Lung Cancer: TNM Classification

Primary tumor (T)	Regional lymph nodes (N)	Distant metastasis (M)	Stage AJCC
TX: Primary tumor cannot be assessed, or tumor proven by the presence of malignant cells in sputum or bronchial washings but not visualized by imaging or bronchoscopy	**NX**: Regional lymph nodes cannot be assessed	**MX**: Distant metastasis cannot be assessed	**Occult carcinoma** TX, N0, M0
T0: No evidence of primary tumor	**N0**: No regional lymph node metastasis	**M0**: No distant metastasis	**Stage 0** Tis, N0, M0
Tis: Carcinoma in situ	**N1**: Metastasis to ipsilateral peribronchial and/or ipsilateral hilar lymph nodes, and intrapulmonary nodes including involvement by direct extension of the primary tumor	**M1**: Distant metastasis present	**Stage IA** T1, N0, M0
T1: A tumor that is 3 cm or less in greatest dimension, surrounded by lung or visceral pleura, and without bronchoscopic evidence of invasion more proximal than the lobar bronchus (i.e., not in the main bronchus)*		Note: M1 includes separate tumor nodule(s) in a different lobe (ipsilateral or contralateral).	**Stage IB** T2, N0, M0
			Stage IIA T1, N1, M0
T2: A tumor with any of the following features of size or extent: - More than 3 cm in greatest dimension - Involves the main bronchus, 2 cm or more distal to the carina - Invades the visceral pleura - Associated with atelectasis or obstructive pneumonitis that extends to the hilar region but does not involve the entire lung	**N2**: Metastasis to ipsilateral mediastinal and/or subcarinal lymph node(s)		**Stage IIB** T2, N1, M0 T3, N0, M0
	N3: Metastasis to contralateral mediastinal, contralateral hilar, ipsilateral or contralateral scalene, or supraclavicular lymph node(s)		**Stage IIIA** T1, N2, M0 T2, N2, M0 T3, N1, M0 T3, N2, M0
T3: A tumor of any size that directly invades any of the following: chest wall (including superior sulcus tumors), diaphragm, mediastinal pleura, parietal pericardium; or tumor in the main bronchus less than 2 cm distal to the carina but without involvement of the carina; or associated atelectasis or obstructive pneumonitis of the entire lung			**Stage IIIB** Any T, N3, M0 T4, Any N, M0
T4: A tumor of any size that invades any of the following: mediastinum, heart, great vessels, trachea, esophagus, vertebral body, carina; or separate tumor nodules in the same lobe; or tumor with a malignant pleural effusion **			**Stage IV** Any T, Any N, M1

* Note: The uncommon superficial tumor of any size with its invasive component limited to the bronchial wall, which may extend proximal to the main bronchus, is also classified as T1.

** Note: Most pleural effusions associated with lung cancer are due to tumor. However, there are a few patients in whom multiple cytopathologic examinations of pleural fluid are negative for tumor. In these cases, fluid is non-bloody and is not an exudate. When these elements and clinical judgment dictate that the effusion is not related to the tumor, the effusion should be excluded as a staging element and the patient should be staged as T1, T2, or T3.

Lung. In: American Joint Committee on Cancer.: AJCC Cancer Staging Manual. 6th ed. New York, NY: Springer, 2002, pp 167-181.

Melanoma (Cutaneous)

Overview	Melanoma incidence is increasing.
	Risk factors include:
	    - fair skin.
	    - high number of nevi (> 50).
	    - clinically atypical nevi.
	    - solar lentigo.
	    - sun exposure during childhood.
	    - presence of actinic keratosis.
	    - family history of melanoma.
	    - others: blistering sunburn.
	                regular sunbed use.
	                higher social class.

Clinical features	ABCD rules can suggest development of a melanoma.
	A melanoma is usually characterized by asymmetry (A), border irregularity (B), color variegation (C), a diameter (D) > 6 mm and an evolving (E) lesion (a new lesion or history of change in size, shape or color).
	
	Dermatoscopy is becoming increasingly popular among dermatologists, as it adds complementary information to the clinical examination and can be performed with relative ease in the outpatient setting with a hand-held device.
	
	There are 4 major clinical melanoma subtypes :
	  - Superficial spreading melanoma (60-70 %).
	  - Nodular melanoma (15-30 %).
	  - Lentigo maligna melanoma (5-15%).
	  - Acral lentiginous melanoma (5-10 %).

Staging	See table.
Workup	A lesion suspected of being melanoma must be excised completely for histopathological analysis. Melanoma diagnosis must include measurement of the Breslow thickness. This is the distance from the granular layer of the epidermis to the lower most invasive cell. This measurement predicts the risk of metastasis, and therefore survival. Complete patient history and physical exam. Laboratory exams and imaging (CT scan and/or positron emission tomography scan) are indicated for a tumor whose Breslow thickness is > 4 mm and when sentinel lymph node is ⊕. In symptomatic patients, the evaluation is oriented toward symptoms and signs.

Treatment	Definitive treatment of melanoma involves excision of a safety margin of normal surrounding skin to deep muscle fascia. The size of the wider margin is determined by the Breslow thickness.			

	Tumor thickness			
	In situ	≤ 1 mm	> 1-4 mm	> 4 mm
Suggested surgical margins	5 mm	1 cm	2 cm	2-3 cm
Lymph node dissection	No	No #	Sentinel lymph node biopsy, dissection if ⊕	If clinically ⊕
Adjuvant therapy (Interferon)	No	Only if increased risk	To be considered	To be considered

Sentinel lymph node biopsy if melanoma is ulcerated or if Clark level ≥ IV.

Prognosis	Breslow thickness is the best indicator of prognosis. 10-year survival rate for an early stage melanoma (≤ 1 mm) is 88 % vs 54 % for an advanced melanoma (> 4 mm).

Melanoma: TNM Classification

Primary tumor (T)	Regional lymph nodes (N)	Distant metastasis (M)	AJCC clinical staging
TX: Primary tumor cannot be assessed	**NX**: Regional lymph nodes cannot be assessed	**MX**: Distant metastasis cannot be assessed	**Stage 0** Tis, N0, M0
T0: No evidence of primary tumor	**N0**: No regional lymph node metastasis	**M0**: No distant metastasis	**Stage I** T1a, N0, M0
Tis: Melanoma in situ			
T1: Tumor 1,0 mm or less in thickness with or without ulceration	**N1**: Metastasis to 1 lymph node	**M1**: Distant metastasis	**Stage IB** T1b, N0, M0 T2a, N0, M0
T1a: Tumor 1,0 mm or less in thickness and Clark's level II or III, no ulceration	**N1a**: Clinically occult (microscopic) metastasis *	**M1a**: Metastasis to skin, subcutaneous tissues, or distant lymph nodes	**Stage IIA** T2b,N0,M0 T3a, N0, M0
T1b: Tumor 1,0 mm or less in thickness and Clark's level IV or V or with ulceration	**N1b**: Clinically apparent (macroscopic) metastasis	**M1b**: Metastasis to lung	
T2: Tumor more than 1,0 mm but not more than 2,0 mm in thickness with or without ulceration	**N2**: Metastasis to 2 or 3 regional nodes or intralymphatic regional metastasis without nodal metastasis	**M1c**: Metastasis to all other visceral sites or distant metastasis at any site associated with an elevated serum lactic dehydrogenase (LDH)	**Stage IIC** T4b, N0, M0
T2a: Tumor more than 1,0 mm but not more than 2,0 mm in thickness, no ulceration	**N2a**: Clinically occult (microscopic) metastasis		**Stage III** **Any T, N1, M0** Any T, N2, M0 Any T, N3, M0
T2b: Tumor more than 1,0 mm but not more than 2,0 mm in thickness, with ulceration	**N2b**: Clinically apparent (macroscopic) metastasis		
T3: Tumor more than 2,0 mm but not more than 4 mm in thickness with or without ulceration	**N2c**: Satellite or in-transit metastasis *without* nodal metastasis		**Stage IV** Any T, Any N, M1
T3a: Tumor more than 2,0 mm but not more than 4 mm in thickness, no ulceration	**N3**: Metastasis in 4 or more regional nodes, or matted lymph nodes, or in-transit metastasis or satellite(s) *with* metastatic regional node(s)		
T3b: Tumor more than 2,0 mm but not more than 4 mm in thickness, with ulceration			
T4: Tumor more than 4,0 mm in thickness with or without ulceration			
T4a: Tumor more than 4,0 mm in thickness, no ulceration			
T4b: Tumor more than 4,0 mm in thickness, with ulceration			

* Note: Micrometastasis are diagnosed after elective or sentinel lymphadenectomy; macrometastasis are defined as clinically detectable lymph nodes metastasis confirmed by therapeutic lymphadenectomy, or when any lymph node metastasis exhibits gross extracapsular extension.

Melanoma of the skin. In: American Joint Committee on Cancer.: AJCC Cancer Staging Manual. 6th ed. New York, NY: Springer, 2002, pp 209-220.

Ovarian Cancer

6th cause of cancer in women but 5th cause of mortality since it is the most lethal gynecologic cancer.
Peak incidence at approx. 60 years of age.
Many types of ovarian tumors exist, most often benign.
Predictive factors of malignancy: age, tumor size, echographic characteristics, symptoms, ↑ CA-125, bilaterality, ascites.
Exact cause unknown: theory of continual ovulation with LH stimulation, trauma and epithelial repair, associated with exposition to environmental agents (industrialized countries, higher socio-economic status).
Risk factors: ovarian or breast cancer in the family (5-15 %) ("hereditary breast ovarian cancer syndrome", Lynch syndrome II, others), advanced age, nulliparity, infertility and ovulation inducers, early menarche, late menopause, hormone replacement therapy.
Risk ↓ with oral contraceptives, pregnancy, lactation, hysterectomy and tubal ligation.
Women with BRCA1 (constitute 5-10 % of ovarian cancer) have a 20-40 % risk of developing an ovarian cancer during their lifetime (versus < 10 % for women with BRCA2).

Clinical features	– Asymptomatic or nonspecific gastrointestinal or pelvic symptoms (abdominal or pelvic girdle discomfort, such as sensation of perpetual pressure, swelling or bloating). Change in urination habits (urinary symptoms) or defecation (intestinal symptoms such as constipation, early satiety, unexplained weight change, flatulence, nausea or indigestions). Abnormal vaginal bleeding, dyspareunia or lumbago. – Fatigue or fever – On occasion discovery of abdominal or pelvic mass with ascites (peritoneal carcinomatosis). Inguinal, supraclavicular or axillary lymphadenopathy possible findings. – Dyspnea secondary to pleural effusion (neoplastic or not). – Subacute cerebellar degeneration, Leser-Trelat sign (sudden seborrheic keratosis), Trousseau's syndrome (superficial migratory thrombophlebitis and hypercoagulability), plantar fasciitis, dermatomyositis and polyarthritis can occur.
Histology	– Epithelial tumors from ovarian surface cells in 80-90 % (including papillary serous, endometrioid, mucinous, Brenner or clear cell). Sometimes borderline (or epithelial ovarian tumor low malignant potential). – Germinal tumors in young patients, usually benign (dermoid cyst or mature teratoma), sometimes malignant and aggressive (dysgerminoma with LDH ↑, endodermic sinus tumor with α-fetoproteins ↑, choriocarcinoma with HCG ↑ and immature teratoma). – Mullerian mixed tumor (or carcinosarcoma). – Stromal tumors: hormonal secretions with precocious puberty, virilization, or endometrial hyperplasia. Thecoma usually benign. Sertoli-Leydig may secrete androgens leading to virilization. – Ovarian metastasis from endometrial, gastrointestinal (Krukenberg), or breast cancer can occur (usually bilateral).
Staging	See table
Workup	Basic biochemistry. AST, ALT, alkaline phosphatase. Calcium. Chest X-ray. Tumor marker CA-125 ↑ in 85 % of ovarian neoplasms but only 50 % in earlier stages. Transvaginal ultrasound, abdominal ultrasound, abdominal CT scan or PET scan. Evaluation of metastases based on clinical suspicion (gastroscopy, colonoscopy, mammography, etc). Bone scan, head MRI as needed if symptoms, signs or workup suggestive. If possible avoid paracentesis to prevent tumor dissemination. Diagnostic exploratory laparoscopy (surgical exploration to be performed usually if post-menopause). Note: Premenopausal women with tumor of cystic appearance, unilateral, mobile, asymptomatic, and < 6-10 cm can remain under observation for 4-6 weeks before intervention (frequent spontaneous regression, around 70 %).

Treatment	– For early stage: total abdominal hysterectomy with bilateral salpingo-oophorectomy and omental resection and selective lymphadenectomy + chemotherapy (except for stage IA-IB). If the patient desires to remain fertile and in certain other circumstances, we can preserve the uterus and the other ovary if not involved.
	– For advanced stage: same type of surgery and a cytoreduction (reduce remaining tumoral volume up to < 1 cm in diameter) + platinum-based chemotherapy (paclitaxel + carboplatin or cisplatin + paclitaxel or docetaxel). If optimal cytoreduction (residual disease < 1 cm), best response to chemotherapy. Intraperitoneal chemotherapy can be used with optimal cytoreduction for stage II-III (but side effects are much more frequent). If a primary cytoreduction was suboptimal, repeat surgery could be considered after 3-4 cycles of chemotherapy, particularly in patients responding to chemotherapy. Possible intraperitoneal chemotherapy for stage II-III with optimal cytoreduction (but side effects are much more frequent).
	– If disease recurrence ($\uparrow$ CA-125), but asymptomatic and absence of tumor on CT scan: patient follow-up or hormonal therapy (tamoxifen or aromatase inhibitor). If symptomatic or CT scan $\oplus$ or progression on hormonal therapy: platinum-based retreatment or taxane if treatment was > 6 months ago. Consider a secondary cytoreduction. If no response to treatment and/or platinum or taxane-based therapy within the past 6 months, 2nd-line chemotherapy: doxorubicine, navelbine, thalidomide, bezacizumab. May be a candidate for a clinical trial.
	– For women carrying BRCA mutation, prophylactic bilateral salpingo-oophorectomy, with or without total or subtotal hysterectomy, is a valuable option as a preventive measure.
Prognosis	At diagnosis, 70 % have advanced stage disease (stage III or IV). 5-year survival rates: 82 % for stage I, 65 % for stage II, 38 % for stage III, and 14 % for stage IV.
	Most important general prognostic factors are the following: histologic type (other than mucinous or clear cell tumors), grade (1 > 3), absence of ascites, and early stage. Among other prognostic factors: young age, treatment response, good health and physical condition, good functional status (WHO or ECOG). Most important specific prognostic factors are the following: tumor volume before surgery and tumor residual volume after surgery.
Screening	Early detection measures with annual clinic examination, CA-125, and endovaginal ultrasound are not effective in the general population.
	Screening of patients with family history is probably more useful in presence of familial ovarian cancer syndrome.

Ovarian Cancer

Stage I

Stage I ovarian cancer is limited to the ovaries.

- Stage IA: Tumor limited to 1 ovary; capsule intact, no tumor on ovarian surface. No malignant cells in ascites or peritoneal washings.*
- Stage IB: Tumor limited to both ovaries; capsules intact, no tumor on ovarian surface. No malignant cells in ascites or peritoneal washings.*
- Stage IC: Tumor limited to 1 or both ovaries with any of the following: capsule ruptured, tumor on ovarian surface, malignant cells in ascites or peritoneal washings.

Stage II

Stage II ovarian cancer is tumor involving 1 or both ovaries with pelvic extension and/or implants.

- Stage IIA: Extension and/or implants on the uterus and/or fallopian tubes. No malignant cells in ascites or peritoneal washings.
- Stage IIB: Extension to and/or implants on other pelvic tissues. No malignant cells in ascites or peritoneal washings.
- Stage IIC: Pelvic extension and/or implants (stage IIA or IIB) with malignant cells in ascites or peritoneal washings.

Different criteria for allotting cases to stages IC and IIC have an impact on diagnosis. In order to evaluate this impact, it would be of value to know if rupture of the capsule was (1) spontaneous or (2) caused by the surgeon, and if the source of malignant cells detected was (1) peritoneal washings or (2) ascites.

Stage III

Stage III ovarian cancer is tumor involving 1 or both ovaries with microscopically confirmed peritoneal implants outside the pelvis. Superficial liver metastasis equals stage III. Tumor is limited the true pelvis but with histologically verified malignant extension to small bowel or omentum.

- Stage IIIA: Microscopic peritoneal metastasis beyond pelvis (no macroscopic tumor).
- Stage IIIB: Macroscopic peritoneal metastasis beyond pelvis 2 cm or less in greatest dimension.
- Stage IIIC: Peritoneal metastasis beyond pelvis more than 2 cm in greatest dimension and/or positive retroperitoneal or inguinal nodes.

Stage IV

Stage IV ovarian cancer is tumor involving 1 or both ovaries with distant metastasis. If pleural effusion is present, there must be positive cytologic test results to designate a case to stage IV. Parenchymal liver metastasis equals stage IV.

* Note: malignant ascites is not classified. The presence of ascites does not affect staging unless malignant cells are present.

Ovary. In: American Joint Committee on Cancer: AJCC Cancer Staging Manual. 6th ed. New York, NY: Springer, 2002, pp 275-284.

Pancreatic Cancer

90 % adenocarcinoma. 75 % head, 20 % body, and 5 % tail.
5th cause of cancer mortality.
Risk factors: chronic pancreatitis, hereditary pancreatitis, tobacco, high-fat diet, diabetes?

Jaundice (90 % if head, 10 % if tail), Courvoisier's gallbladder, weight loss (malabsorption and ↓ intake), pain (epigastric or left upper quadrant, vague, sometimes irradiating to the back), discomfort, anorexia, new-onset diabetes, nausea and vomiting secondary to obstruction or gastroparesis following neural invasion; less frequently acute pancreatitis, superficial thrombophlebitis, marantic endocarditis, psychiatric disorders, gastrointestinal bleeding, ascites, perirectal metastasis, etc.

Exocrine cancer in > 95 % of cases, rarely endocrine.

Staging	See table
Workup	– Basic biochemistry, liver enzymes, chest X-ray. – Abdominal ultrasound + CT scan (except if ultrasound indicates metastases) + thoracic CT scan. – Percutaneous biopsy only for non-surgical candidates. – Endoscopic ultrasound and fine needle aspiration (if available) and/or ERCP ± positron emission tomography scan ± laparoscopy as needed for surgical candidates. – Tumor markers: CA 19-9, CEA.
Treatment	15-20 % of patients are candidates for pancreatectomy. Surgical candidates if absence of metastasis, absence of extensive lymph node involvement, patency of the portal vein and superior mesenteric vein, absence of celiac axis and superior mesenteric artery involvement. Discuss neoadjuvant radiochemotherapy (5-FU-based) vs adjuvant chemotherapy (gemcitabine-based). Non-surgical candidates with locally advanced cancer without distance metastases: radiochemotherapy vs chemotherapy alone gemcitabine-based. Stage IV: palliative treatment or gemcitabine-based chemotherapy. – Jaundice: surgical biliary and duodenal bypass if patient in good condition. Otherwise, ERCP with endoprosthesis vs percutaneous transhepatic prosthesis when ERCP impossible. – Pain: narcotics. If ineffective, celiac block. – Exocrine insufficiency: pancreatic enzymes.
Prognosis	5-year survival rates of 20-30 % if surgery with negative margins and absence of lymph node involvement, and 10 % if nodes positive. 3-5 % 5-year overall survival.

Pancreatic Cancer: TNM Classification

Primary tumor (T)	Regional lymph nodes (N)	Distant metastasis (M)	Stage
TX: Primary tumor cannot be assessed	**NX**: Regional lymph nodes cannot be assessed	**MX**: Distant metastasis cannot be assessed	**Stage 0** Tis, N0, M0
T0: No evidence of primary tumor	**N0**: No regional lymph node metastasis	**M0**: No distant metastasis	**Stage IA** T1, N0, M0
Tis: In situ carcinoma	**N1**: Regional lymph node metastasis	**M1**: Distant metastasis	
T1: Tumor limited to the pancreas 2 cm or less in greatest dimension			**Stage IB** T2, N0, M0
T2: Tumor limited to the pancreas more than 2 cm in greatest dimension			**Stage IIA** T3, N0, M0
T3: Tumor extends beyond the pancreas but without involvement of the celiac axis or the superior mesenteric artery			**Stage IIB** T1, N1, M0 T2, N1, M0 T3, N1, M0
T4: Tumor involves the celiac axis or the superior mesenteric artery (unresectable primary tumor)			**Stage III** T4, Any N, M0 **Stage IVB** Any T, Any N, M1

Exocrine pancreas. In: American Joint Committee on Cancer.: AJCC Cancer Staging Manual. 6th ed. New York, NY: Springer, 2002, pp 157-164.

Prostate Cancer	
	Most frequent cancer in men: 3rd cause of cancer mortality in men. Risk factors: age, family history, race (African-American), hormones, testosterone, high-fat diet.

Clinical features	– Asymptomatic indurated nodule discovered by digital rectal examination. – Prostatism (with large tumor: rare), erectile dysfunction, hematospermia, painful ejaculation, metastatic symptoms (bone pain, back pain, pelvic pain, lymphadenopathy, weight loss, acute urinary retention, spinal cord compression, etc).
Workup	– Prostate specific antigen (PSA): cancer incidence = 20-25 % if 4-10 μg/L ; 50 % if > 10 μg/L. 15 % of cancers have normal PSA (therefore, rectal exam is necessary). – Basic biochemistry, calcium, alkaline phosphatase. Disseminated intravascular coagulation can occur if metastatic. – Urology consultation if PSA > 4 μg/L or if PSA < 4 μg/L and ↑ of > 0.75 μg/L-year on 3 separate measures at least 18 months apart or if abnormal digital rectal examination when patient is a candidate for treatment. – Prostate ultrasound with biopsy. – Bone scan if symptoms, advanced disease (T3, T4), PSA > 15-20 μg/L or Gleason score ≥ 8. – Pelvic CT or MRI if T3, T4 or if the estimated risk of lymph node involvement > 20 %.
Staging	See table.

Treatment	If life expectancy ≤ 5 years and asymptomatic, no other workup or treatment until symptoms develop, except for patients with high risk of complications (high risk of hydronephrosis or metastasis within 5 years, like bulky T3-T4 tumors or Gleason score of 8-10, for whom radiotherapy or hormonotherapy could be considered.)
	
	If life expectancy > 5 years or symptomatic, management according to risk of recurrence:
	– If low risk (T1-T2a and Gleason 2-6 and PSA < 10 μg/L):
	  - If survival estimated < 10 years: Watchful waiting or radiotherapy (external or brachytherapy).
	  - If survival estimated >10 years: Watchful waiting or radiotherapy (external or brachytherapy) or radical prostatectomy* ± lymph node dissection.
	– If intermediate risk: (T2b-T2c or Gleason 7 or PSA 10-20 μg/L):
	  - If estimated survival < 10 years: Watchful waiting or radiotherapy (external ± brachytherapy) ± short-term hormonotherapy or radical prostatectomy* ± lymph node dissection.
	– If high risk (T3a or Gleason 8-10 or PSA > 20 μg/L): hormonotherapy# (long-term drug vs orchiectomy) + radiotherapy or radiotherapy alone or radical prostatectomy* + lymph node dissection.
	– If very high risk (T3b-T4): radiotherapy + hormonotherapy or hormonotherapy only.
	– If metastatic N1: hormonotherapy or radiotherapy + hormonotherapy.
	– If metastatic M1: hormonotherapy. If refractory to hormonal treatment: Chemotherapy (docetaxel + prednisone slight ↑ in survival) or radiotherapy to site of metastases to control pain. Ketoconazole ± steroids or estrogens if antiandrogen not used before. Bisphosphonates (zoledronic acid) for bone involvement refractory to hormonotherapy (reduced risk of fracture).
	
	*If radical prostatectomy with ⊕ resection margins, give radiotherapy as needed.
	If radical prostatectomy and lymph node involved (N1), hormonotherapy as needed.
	
	# Always administer antiandrogen before or concomitant to LHRH analogue (since there is a risk of increased testosterone and pain). Do bone density testing at regular intervals and give calcium supplement and vitamin D ± bisphosphonates if osteopenia/osteoporosis.

	Post-op follow-up with PSA levels twice within 3 months then every 6 months. Post-op PSA must remain < 0.1 and post-radiotherapy ≤ 0.5-1 µg/l. If post-radiotherapy biochemical failure (= nadir + 2), look for recurrence. Note: post-op complications: > 50 % erectile dysfunction and < 5 % urinary incontinence.
Prognosis	Depends on PSA level pretreatment (better prognosis if < 10 µg/L). Survival ↓ if Gleason score ≥ 5, with ↓ proportional to score. 15-year survival rate for stages I-II 85-90 %. Stage IV mean survival: 2-3 years.
Screening	Controversial. PSA level measurement after doctor-patient discussion regarding advantages and disadvantages, according to risk factors.

Prostate Cancer: TNM Classification

Primary tumor (T)	Regional lymph nodes (N)	Distant metastasis # (M)	Stage AJCC
TX: Primary tumor cannot be assessed **T0**: No evidence of primary tumor **T1**: Clinically unapparent tumor not palpable nor visible by imaging **T1a**: Tumor incidental histologic finding in 5% or less of tissue resected **T1b**: Tumor incidental histologic finding in more than 5% of tissue resected **T1c**: Tumor identified by needle biopsy (e.g., because of elevated PSA) **T2**: Tumor confined within prostate* **T2a**: Tumor involves one half of 1 lobe or less **T2b** : Tumor involves more than one half of 1 lobe but not both lobes **T2c**: Tumor involves both lobes **T3**: Tumor extends through the prostatic capsule** **T3a**: Extracapsular extension (unilateral or bilateral) **T3b**: Tumor invades seminal vesicle(s) **T4**: Tumor is fixed or invades adjacent structures other than seminal vesicles: bladder neck, external sphincter, rectum, levator muscles, and/or pelvic wall	Regional lymph nodes are the nodes of the true pelvis, which essentially are the pelvic nodes below the bifurcation of the common iliac arteries. They include the following groups (laterality does not affect the N classification): pelvic (not otherwise specified [NOS]), hypogastric, obturator, iliac (internal, external, NOS), and sacral (lateral, presacral, promontory (Gerota's), or NOS). Distant lymph nodes are outside the confines of the true pelvis. They can be imaged using ultrasound, computed tomography, magnetic resonance imaging, or lymphangiography, and include: aortic (para-aortic, periaortic, lumbar), common iliac, inguinal (deep), superficial inguinal (femoral), supraclavicular, cervical, scalene, and retroperitoneal (NOS) nodes. Although enlarged lymph nodes can occasionally be visualized, because of a stage migration associated with PSA screening, very few patients will be found to have nodal disease, so false-positive and false-negative results are common when imaging tests are employed. In lieu of imaging, risk tables are generally used to determine individual patient risk of nodal involvement. Involvement of distant lymph nodes is classified as M1a. **NX**: Regional lymph nodes cannot be assessed **N0**: No regional lymph node metastasis **N1**: Metastasis in regional lymph node or nodes	**MX**: Distant metastasis cannot be assessed **M0**: No distant metastasis **M1**: Distant metastasis **M1a**: Nonregional lymph node(s) **M1b**: Bone(s) **M1c**: Other site(s) **Histopathologic grade (G)** **GX**: Grade cannot be assessed **G1**: Well differentiated (slight anaplasia) (Gleason 2-4) **G2**: Moderately differentiated (moderate anaplasia) (Gleason 5-6) **G3-4**: Poorly differentiated or undifferentiated (marked anaplasia) (Gleason 7-10)	**Stage I** T1a, N0, M0, G1 **Stage II** T1a, N0, M0, G2, 3-4 T1b, N0, M0, Any G T1c, N0, M0, Any G T1, N0, M0, Any G T2, N0, M0, Any G **Stage III** T3, N0, M0, Any G **Stage IV** T4, N0, M0, Any G Any T, N1, M0, Any G Any T, Any N, M1, Any G

*Note: Tumor found in 1 or both lobes by needle biopsy, but not palpable or reliably visible by imaging, is classified as T1c.
**Note: Invasion into the prostatic apex or into (but not beyond) the prostatic capsule is not classified as T3, but as T2.
*** NOS, not otherwise specified.
# Note: When more than 1 site of metastasis is present, the most advanced category (pM1c) is used.
Prostate. In: American Joint Committee on Cancer.: AJCC Cancer Staging Manual. 6th ed. New York, NY: Springer, 2002, pp 309-316.

Renal Cancer	
	Male preponderance (2:1). Median age: 60 years old.

Renal Cancer

Male preponderance (2:1). Median age: 60 years old.
Risk factors: tobacco, obesity, hypertension, dialysis, renal transplant, genetics (von Hippel-Lindau syndrome).

Pathology: adenocarcinoma (most frequent, 80-85 %), transitional cell cancer of the renal pelvis (= 5 %), lymphoma, sarcoma, germinal tumor, metastasis (lung, breast, stomach, lymphomas), oncocytoma or angiomyolipoma (benign tumor), Wilms' tumor (rare in adults).

Differential diagnosis for solid renal mass: angiomyolipoma, adrenal tumor, inflammatory mass, (renal abscess, tuberculosis, xanthogranuloma pyelonephritis), complex renal cyst, Wilms' tumor (children).

Clinical features	Classic triad: flank pain, hematuria, and palpable mass in 10 %. Metastatic symptoms at presentation in 20-30 %. Other nonspecific symptoms (fever, night sweats, malaise, weight loss). Hypertension also can occur with vascular compression. Left varicocele. Paraneoplastic syndromes: hypercalcemia (secondary to ectopic PTH secretion), polycythemia (secondary to ectopic erythropoietin production) anemia, hyponatremia (secondary to SIADH), Cushing's syndrome (secondary to ectopic ACTH secretion), hypercoagulable state. Rarely: amylosis, Stauffer's syndrome (i.e.: reversible hepatic dysfunction in absence of hepatic metastasis), limbal encephalitis, myopathy, polymyalgia rheumatica. 20-30 % incidentally discovered during radiologic imaging.
Workup	– Basic biochemistry, CBC, calcium, liver enzymes, alkaline phosphatase, LDH, chest X-ray. Urinalysis. – Bone scan as needed (if bone pain or ↑ alkaline phosphatase). – Abdominal CT scan. – CT-angio, MRI or angiography if vascular involvement suspected. – Cerebral CT scan/MRI if neurologic symptoms or large tumor. – Chest CT scan as needed.
Staging	See table Only 40 % have tumor confined to the kidney at diagnosis.
Treatment	For Stages I- III: Radical nephrectomy. Nephron-sparing surgery (partial nephrectomy) can be done if technically feasible. Radiofrequency ablation or cryoablation possible for patient with small tumor (< 3 cm) not candidate for nephrectomy (being investigated). For Stage IV: Nephrectomy if candidate for surgery. Resection of solitary metastasis as needed (increases survival up to 15-30 % at 5 year). If histology shows predominance of clear cells (in 75 %): give sunitinib (1st line) or immunotherapy (interleukin-2). Temsirolimus 2nd line treatment or 1st line in patients with poor prognosis. For other histology: chemotherapy (gemcitabine, 5-FU, etc: less effective)? Sunitinib? Temsirolimus, bevacizumab and sorafenib being studied. Radiotherapy for pain, bleeding, bone or cerebral metastasis. Stereotactic radiosurgery for cerebral metastasis as needed. Consider bisphosphonates if bone metastasis.
Prognosis	5-year survival rates: Stage I: 95 %; stage II: 88 %; stage III: 59 %; stage IV: 20 %.

Renal Cancer: TNM Classification

Primary tumor (T)	Regional lymph nodes (N)	Distant metastasis (M)	Stage

TX Primary tumor cannot be assessed
T0 No evidence of primary tumor
T1 Tumor 7 cm or less in greatest dimension, limited to the kidney
  T1a Tumor 4 cm or less in greatest dimension, limited to the kidney
  T1b Tumor more than 4 cm but not more than 7 cm in greatest dimension, limited to the kidney
T2 Tumor more than 7 cm in greatest dimension, limited to the kidney
T3 Tumor extends into major veins or invades adrenal gland or perinephric tissues but not beyond Gerota's fascia
  T3a Tumor directly invades the adrenal gland or perirenal and/or renal sinus fat but not beyond Gerota's fascia
  T3b Tumor grossly extends into the renal vein or its segmental (muscle-containing) branches, or vena cava below the diaphragm
  T3c Tumor grossly extends into vena cava above diaphragm or invades the wall of the vena cava above diaphragm
T4 Tumor invades beyond Gerota's fascia
	NX: Regional lymph nodes cannot be assessed
	
	N0: No regional lymph node metastasis
	
	N1: Metastasis in a single regional lymph node
	
	N2: Metastasis in more than 1 regional lymph node
	
	Note: Laterality does not affect the N classification.
	
	If a lymph node dissection is performed, then pathologic evaluation would ordinarily include at least eight nodes.
		MX: Distant metastasis cannot be assessed
		
		M0: No distant metastasis
		
		M1: Distant metastasis
			Stage I
			T1, N0, M0
			
			Stage II
			T2, N0, M0
			
			Stage III
			T1, N1, M0
			T2, N1, M0
			T3a, N0, M0
			T3a, N1, M0
			T3b, N0, M0
			T3b, N1, M0
			T3c, N0, M0
			T3c, N1, M0
			
			Stage IV
			T4, N0, M0
			T4, N1, M0
			Any T, N2, M0
			Any T, Any N, M1

Kidney. In: American Joint Committee on Cancer.: AJCC Cancer Staging Manual. 6th ed. New York, NY: Springer, 2002, pp 323-28.

Testicular Cancer

Frequent cancer in men 15-35 years of age.

5-10 % occurs in extragonadal sites (retroperitoneal, mediastinal, pineal gland).

Risk factor: cryptorchidism, Klinefelter's syndrome, HIV.

Clinical: Asymptomatic testicular mass (most frequent presentation), non-specific symptoms (asthenia, fever, diaphoresis, etc), local pain, gynecomastia, symptomatic metastasis (lower back pain, abdominal pain, pulmonary and cerebral symptoms).

Pathology: seminoma 40-50 % vs nonseminoma (choriocarcinoma, teratoma, embryonal carcinoma) vs nongerminal tumor (rare: gonadoblastoma, Leydig cells, Sertoli cells). If mixed tumor (seminoma and nonseminoma), consider and treat like nonseminoma.

Tumor markers: α- fetoprotein (AFP) and hCG for nonseminoma (5-7 % of seminomas have ↑ beta-hCG, but they never have ↑ α- fetoprotein).

Staging	See Table.
Workup	Tumor markers (α-fetoprotein and beta-hCG). Basic biochemistry (and LDH). Abdominal + pelvic CT scan. Chest X-ray ± thoracic CT scan (if abnormal chest X-ray or abdominal CT scan). Cerebral CT scan or MRI if beta-hCG > 10 000 UI/L or if multiple pulmonary metastasis. Bone scan if symptoms. If available, Positron emission tomography useful for seminomas if residual tumor post-chemotherapy.

Management Stage	Seminoma	Nonseminoma
I	Orchiectomy ± radiotherapy (or chemotherapy).	Orchiectomy ± watchful waiting or chemotherapy and/or retroperitoneal lymph node dissection.
II	Orchiectomy + radiotherapy (or chemotherapy) ± surgery if residual tumor if PET scan ⊕.	Orchiectomy + chemotherapy and/or retroperitoneal lymph node dissection for residual tumor.
III	Orchiectomy + chemotherapy ± radiotherapy on residual tumor.	Chemotherapy ± radiotherapy ± surgery.
	Chemotherapy: etoposide, cisplatin ± bleomycin or other protocols. Side effects: infertility (usually reversible), nausea, myelosuppression, neuropathy, pneumopathy, anemia, ototoxicity, etc. Post-radiotherapy, ↑ risk of secondary neoplasms (stomach, bladder, pancreas?).	

Prognosis	For seminoma: stage I: 95-97 % 5-year survival rate; stage II: 85-90 %; stage III: 80-85 %. For nonseminoma: stage III: 95 % 5-year survival rate if minimal metastatic disease, but 50 % if significant metastatic disease.

5-year prognosis according to *International Germ Cell Collaboration Group Prognostic Clasification* (1997):

	Seminoma	Non-seminoma
Good prognosis (91 %)	No visceral metastasis other than pulmonary.	Primary testicular/retroperitoneal; no visceral metastases other than pulmonary; and AFP < 1000 IU/L, hCG < 5000 IU/L and LDH < 1.5 times normal.
Intermediate prognosis (79 %)	Visceral metastasis other than pulmonary	Primary testicular/retroperitoneal; no visceral metastases other than pulmonary; and AFP 1000-10 000 IU/L, hCG 5000-50 000 IU/L or LDH 1.5-10 times normal.
Poor prognosis (48 %)	Patient not classified as above.	Primary mediastinal; or visceral metastases other than pulmonary; or AFP > 10 000 IU/L, hCG > 50 000 IU/L or LDH > 10 times normal.

Testicular Cancer: TNM Classification

Primary tumor (T)

The extent of primary tumor is classified after radical orchiectomy, and for this reason a pathologic stage is assigned.

pTX: Primary tumor cannot be assessed*

pT0: No evidence of primary tumor (e.g., histologic scar in testis)

pTis: Intratubular germ cell neoplasia (carcinoma)

pT1: Tumor limited to the testis and epididymis without lymphatic/vascular invasion; tumor may invade into the tunica albuginea but not the tunica vaginalis

pT2: Tumor limited to the testis and epididymis with vascular/lymphatic invasion, or tumor extending through the tunica albuginea with involvement of the tunica vaginalis.

pT3: Tumor invades the spermatic cord with or without vascular/lymphatic invasion.

pT4: Tumor invades the scrotum with or without vascular/lymphatic invasion.

* Note: Except for pTis and pT4, the extent of primary tumor is classified by radical orchiectomy. TX may be used for other categories in the absence of radical orchiectomy.

Regional lymph nodes (N)

NX: Regional lymph nodes cannot be assessed.

N0: No regional lymph node metastasis.

N1: Metastasis with a single lymph node mass 2 cm or less in greatest dimension; or multiple lymph nodes, 2 cm or less in greatest dimension.

N2: Metastasis with a single lymph node mass larger than 2 cm but no more than 5 cm in greatest dimension; or multiple lymph nodes, no more than 5 cm in greatest dimension.

N3: Metastasis with a lymph node mass 5 cm or more in greatest dimension.

Distant metastasis (M)

MX: Presence of distant metastasis cannot be assessed.

M0: No distant metastasis.

M1: Distant metastasis present.

    M1a : Nonregional nodal or pulmonary metastasis.

    M1b : Distant metastasis other than to nonregional lymph nodes and lungs.

Serum tumor markers (S)

SX: Marker studies not available or not performed.

S0: Marker study levels within normal limits.

S1: Lactate dehydrogenase (LDH) less than $1.5 \times N^*$ and Human chorionic gonadotropin (hCG) less than 5,000 (mIU/mL), and α-fetoprotein (AFP) less than 1,000 (ng/mL).

S2: LDH $1.5–10 \times N^*$ or hCG 5,000-50,000 (mIU/mL), or AFP 1,000-10,000 (ng/mL).

S3: LDH more than $10 \times N^*$ or hCG > more than 50,000 (mIU/mL), or AFP more than 10,000 (ng/mL).

* Note: N indicates the upper limit of normal for the LDH assay.

Stage AJCC	Stage I pT1-4, N0, M0, SX	Stage II : Any pT/TX, N1-3, M0, SX	Stage III : Any pT/TX, Any N, M1, SX
	Stage IA pT1, N1, M0, S0	**Stage IIA** Any pT/TX, N1, M0, S0-1	**Stage IIIA :** Any pT/TX, Any N, M1a, S0-1
Stage 0 pTis, N0, M0, S0	**Stage IB :** pT2, N1, M0, S0 pT3, N1, M0, S0 pT4, N1, M0, S0	**Stage IIB** Any pT/TX, N2, M0, S0-1 **Stade IIC** Any pT/TX, N3, M0, S0-1	**Stage IIIB** Any pT/TX, N1-3, M0, S2 Any pT/TX, Any N, M1a, S2
	Stage IS Any pT/TX, N0, M0, S1-3		**Stade IIIC** Any pT/TX, N1-3, M0, S3 Any pT/TX, Any N, M1a, S3 Any pT/TX, Any N, M1b, Any S

Testis. In: American Joint Committee on Cancer.: AJCC Cancer Staging Manual. 6th ed. New York, NY: Springer, 2002, pp 317-322.

Thyroid Cancer	
Causes	Papillary 70-85 %, follicular 10-20 %, medullary 2-3 %, anaplastic 0.5-1 %, lymphoma < 1 %, metastasis (kidney, lung, breast, esophagus). Risk factors for malignancy of a nodule: age < 20 years or > 60 years, male (but women have thyroid cancer overall), rapid growth, hoarseness, progressive dysphagia, dyspnea, history of head or neck irradiation, positive family history (thyroid cancer - higher likelihood with a family history of medullary cancer, MEN II), firmness, diameter > 4 cm, hard and/or fixed lymphadenopathy, cold nodule on thyroid scan, solid or mixed composition by ultrasound, hypoechoic, irregular borders, microcalcifications, central vascularization by doppler, round rather than oval shape, absence of eggshell calcification, absence of a thin echolucent halo.
Management	**Papillary**: surgery (total thyroidectomy): radioiodine treatment for all (controversial when low-risk papillary neoplasm: < 1 cm without capsular or vascular invasion and no lymph node). Stop L-T4 3 weeks before treatment. Confirm TSH > 25-50 mU/L before radioiodine treatment. L-T4 suppressive therapy for life (decrease in local recurrence but no evidence of ↓ in mortality). When low-risk tumor, aim for lower limit of normal TSH level 0.1-0.5 mU/L. When high-risk tumor, aim for TSH < 0.1 mU/L. **Follicular**: surgery (total thyroidectomy) + thyroid ablation by radioiodine treatment + L-T4 suppressive therapy for life. For papillary and follicular: post-ablation follow-up of TSH-suppressed thyroglobulin levels (and under TSH stimulation [Thyrogen®] if low level), at 6 and 12 months, then according to risk (high risk: every 1-2 years; others every 3-5 years). Rule out interfering antithyroglobulin antibodies. Neck ultrasound every year, chest X-ray every year for high-risk tumor. Less frequently for low-risk papillary tumor. Note: Thyroglobulin is TSH-dependent and can be suppressed with the suppressive therapy. Follow-up whole-body thyroid scanning using I^{131} (stopping L-T4 or using rh-TSH to avoid stopping L-T4) every 6-12 months the first year then according to severity of tumor. If ↑ thyroglobulin but normal whole-body scan, proceed to PET scan plus conventional imagery of neck, thorax, and bone. **Medullary**: Rule out pheochromocytoma and hyperparathyroidism pre-op. Surgical treatment with cervical lymph node dissection. Follow-up with calcitonin and CEA post-op. Radiotherapy ± useful if nonresectable. 25 % of medullary are hereditary with MEN II or non-MEN: evaluate family members at risk (RET proto-oncogene mutations in 1st degree relatives). **Anaplastic**: most lethal solid tumor: surgery to prevent obstruction. Radiotherapy if symptomatic. Chemotherapy rarely useful. **Lymphomas**: non-Hodgkin, especially with rapidly ↑ goiter in women with Hashimoto's thyroiditis. Treat according to stage. Excellent prognosis with papillary and follicular (80-100 % 5-year survival rate depending on stage) but local recurrence (approximately 20 %) can occur up to 20 years after diagnosis. Average for medullary (82 % 5-year survival rate), anaplastic rapidly fatal (10 % 1-year survival rate). Risk factors for thyroid cancer mortality: age ≥ 45 years, diameter ≥ 4 cm, local, capsular, or vascular invasion, lymph node metastasis, distant metastasis (bone, lungs, liver, brain).

Cancer of Unknown Origin

3 % of neoplasms have no identifiable primary site regardless of history, physical exam (including head and neck, rectal, testicular, gynecological, breast) and workup (CBC, urinalysis, fecal occult blood test, chest X-ray, abdominopelvic CT scan, mammography).
Average age of 60 years.

Histology: adenocarcinoma 60 %, poorly differentiated carcinoma 30 %, squamous cell carcinoma 5 %, neuroendocrine carcinoma 5 %.
Sites involved: lymph nodes 40 %, liver 30 %, bone 30 %, lung 30 %, pleura 10 %, peritoneum 10 %, brain 5 %, adrenal 5 %, skin 5 %, bone marrow 5 %. Only one site in 40 %, 2 sites in 30 %, 3 or more sites in 30 % of cases.

In 85 % of cases, the primary site will be identified either after diagnostic investigation (20 %), during follow-up, or at autopsy (65 %).

Most frequent sites of primary lesions: pancreas 25 %, lung 20 %, stomach 10 %, colon 10 %, kidney 5 %, breast and ovaries 2-3 % ...

Workup: biopsy with pathological analysis, immunohistochemistry, electron microscopy and chromosomal analysis as needed. Tumor markers (PSA, hCG, α-fetoprotein, etc) as needed.

Adeno-carcinoma of unknown primary site	4 groups of patients to identify: women with axillary lymphadenopathy, women with peritoneal carcinomatosis, women with bone metastasis from adenocarcinoma, and men with bone metastasis from adenocarcinoma.
	Immunohistochemical analysis for prostate-specific antigen in men and estrogen receptors in women.
	  – Women with axillary lymphadenopathy: considered as breast cancer: measure CA 15-3, mammography ± breast MRI. Mastectomy ⊕ in 2/3. Treated as stage II breast cancer. Five-year survival of 50 %.
	  – Women with peritoneal carcinomatosis: considered as ovarian cancer: measure CA-125. Refer to gynecologist for surgical debridement and chemotherapy. Survival similar to stage III ovarian cancer.
	  – Women with bone metastasis from adenocarcinoma: evaluate as for women with axillary lymphadenopathy. Biopsy analyzed for estrogen and progesterone receptors and CA 15-3. If ⊕, treat as breast cancer.
	  – Men with bone metastasis from adenocarcinoma: evaluation of prostate and PSA levels. If ⊕, treat as prostate cancer.

Poorly differentiated carcinoma of unknown primary site	Detailed immunohistochemical analysis to exclude melanoma, sarcoma, lymphoma, and others. In young man, exclude germinal tumor: measure hCG and α-fetoprotein levels. Chest X-ray and lung/abdominal CT scan, testicular ultrasound. Treat with chemotherapy even with unidentfied primary tumor, 5-year survival 30 %.

Squamous cell carcinoma of unknown primary site	– If squamous cell involvement of cervical nodes, consider and treat as head and neck cancer. 5-year survival of 40 %.
	  Perform physical exam, chest X-ray, CT scan of neck and lungs, positron emission tomography (PET scan), ENT panendoscopy (and multiple blind biopsies if primary lesion not identified).
	  30 % of primary lesions discovered on ENT evaluation, and 25% of patients will eventually reveal tumor on follow-up (2/3 ENT, 1/3 pulmonary).
	  Treatment is surgery (if primary lesion identified) + radiotherapy.
	– If squamous cell at lower cervical or supraclavicular node levels, lung cancer probable. Conventional evaluation and treatment (see lung cancer table).
	– If squamous cell and inguinal lymphadenopathy, exclude vulva, vagina, cervix, and anus cancer in women and anus and penis cancer in men. Refer women to gynecologist for abdominopelvic CT scan + anuscopy. For men, penile exam and anuscopy. Radiotherapy with a 5 % 5-year survival rate.

Neuro-endocrine carcinoma of unknown primary site	Metastatic carcinoid, endocrine tumor or small-cell cancer. Treatment with cisplatin-based chemotherapy with > 1 year survival.
If primary tumor unidentifiable, platinum-based ± paclitaxel empiric chemotherapy. Mean survival 4-6 months.	

Useful References: HEMATOLOGY-ONCOLOGY

Amyloidosis: Mayo Clin Proc 1999; 74: 490-94 (review article)
    N Engl J Med 1997; 337: 898-909 (review article)
Anemia: Aplastic: Lancet 2009 ; 363 : 324-39 (review article)
    … Iron Deficiency: Cleve Clin J Med 2008; 75: 793-801 (review article)
    … of Chronic Disease: N Engl J Med 2005; 352: 1011-23 (review article)
    … Pernicious: N Engl J Med 1997; 337: 1441-48 (review article)
        Arch Intern Med 1999; 159: 1289-98 (review article)
    … Sickle cell: N Engl J Med 1999; 340: 1021-30 (review article)
Antiphospholipid Syndrome: JAMA 2006; 295: 1050-1057 (review article)
    N Engl J Med 2002; 346: 752-63 (review article)
Blood Smear: N Engl J Med 2005; 353: 498-507 (review article)
Cancer, Breast: Lancet 2005; 365: 1727-41 (review article)
    Mayo Clin Proc 2007; 82: 999-1012 & 1131-1140 (review article)
    … Early: Lancet 2009; 373: 1463-79 (review article)
    … Inherited Predisposition: N Engl J Med 2007; 357: 154-62 (review article)
Cancer, Central Nervous System: Mayo Clin Proc 2007; 82: 1271-86 (review article)
    Lancet 2003; 361: 323-31 (review article)
Cancer, Colorectal: Mayo Clin Proc 2007; 82: 114-129 (review article)
    Lancet 2005; 365: 153-65 (review article)
    … Follow-up: N Engl J Med 2004; 350: 2375-82 (review article)
    … Hereditary: N Engl J Med 2003; 348: 919-32 (review article)
    … Screening: Gastroenterology 2005; 128: 1685-95 (review article)
        Can J Gastroenterol 2001; 18: 93- (Canadian Guidelines)
        Can J Gastroenterol 2001; 18: 509- (Québec Guidelines)
   …Systemic Therapy: Gastroenterology 2008; 134: 1296-1310 (review article)
    … Therapy: Mayo Clin Proc 2007; 82: 114-129 (review article)
Cancer, Esophageal: N Engl J Med 2003; 349: 2241-52 (review article)
    Am J Gastroenterol 1999; 94: 20- (American Guidelines)
Cancer, Esophagus and Stomach: Mayo Clin Proc 2008; 83: 712-22 (review article)
Cancer, Gastric: Lancet 2009; 374: 477-90 (review article)
Cancer, Lung: Chest 2007; 132: 1S-19S (ACCP American Guidelines)
    Treatment: N Engl J Med 2004; 350: 379-92 (review article)
    … Non-Small Cell: Mayo Clin Proc 2008; 83: 584-94 (review article)
    … Small Cell: Mayo Clin Proc 2008; 83: 355-367 (review article)
        Lancet 2005; 366: 1385-96 (review article)
Cancer of Unknown Origin: Med Clin North Am 1996; 80: 153-71 (review article)
Cancer, Ovarian: Mayo Clin Proc 2007; 82:751-770 (review article)
    N Engl J Med 2004; 351: 2519-29 (review article)
Cancer, Pancreatic: Lancet 2004; 363: 1049-57 (review article)
    Gastroenterology 1999; 117: 1464-84 (American Guidelines)
    … Treatment: Mayo Clin Proc 2007; 82: 628-637 (review article)
Cancer, Prostate: Lancet 2008; 371: 1710-21 (review article)
    … Localized: N Engl J Med 2007; 357: 2696-705 (review article)
    … Treatment: Mayo Clin Proc 2007; 82: 243-249 (review article)
Cancer, Renal: Lancet 2009; 373: 1119-32 (review article)
    N Engl J Med 2005; 353: 2477-90 (review article)
Cancer, Testicular: Lancet 2006; 367: 754-65 (review article)
    JAMA 2008; 299: 672-684 (review article)
Cancer, Thyroid: Lancet 2003; 361: 501-11 (review article)
    Europ J Endocr 2004; 150: 105-112 (review article)
Disseminated Intravascular Coagulation: N Engl J Med 1999; 341: 586-92 (review article)
Eosinophilia: Mayo Clin Proc 2005; 80: 75-83 (review article)
G6PD Deficiency: Lancet 2008; 371: 64-74 (review article)
Gastrointestinal Stromal Tumor: Lancet 2007; 369: 1731-41 (review article)
Hemophilia: N Engl J Med 2001; 344: 1773-80 (review article)

Heparin-Induced Thrombocytopenia (HIT): Chest 2009; 135:1651-64 (review article)
    N Engl J Med 2006; 355: 809-17 (review article)
    … Treatment: Arch Intern Med 2004; 164: 361-9 (review article)
Hereditary Spherocytosis: Lancet 2008; 372: 1411-26 (review article)
Immune Thrombocytopenic Purpura: Mayo Clin Proc 2004; 79: 504-22 (review article)
    N Engl J Med 2002; 346: 995-1008 (review article)
    Blood 1996; 88: 3-40 (American Guidelines)
Leukemia, Acute Lymphoblastic: Lancet 2008; 371: 1030-43 (review article)
    Treatment: N Engl J Med 2006; 354:166-178 (review article)
Leukemia, Chronic Lymphocytic: Lancet 2008; 371: 1017-29 (review article)
    Mayo Clin Proc 2006; 81: 1105-1129 (review article)
Leukemia, Acute Myeloid: Mayo Clin Proc 2006; 81: 247-260 (review article)
    Lancet 2006; 368: 1894–907 (review article)
Leukemia, Chronic Myeloid: Lancet 2007; 370: 342-50 (review article)
    Mayo Clin Proc 2006; 81: 973-988 (review article)
Lymphadenopathy: Mayo Clin Proc 2000; 75: 723-32 (review article)
Lymphoma: Hodgkin's: Mayo Clin Proc 2006; 81: 419-26 (review article)
    Non-Hodgkin : Lancet 2003; 362: 139-46 (review article)
    … Monoclonal Antibody Therapy: N Engl J Med 2008; 359: 613-26 (review article)
Malignant Glioma: N Engl J Med 2008; 359: 492-507 (review article)
Malignant Mesothelioma: N Engl J Med 2005; 353: 1591-1603 (review article)
    Chest 2004; 126: 1318-29 (review article)
Melanoma: Mayo Clin Proc 2007; 82: 364-380 & 490-513 (review article)
Monoclonal Gammopathy of Unknown Significance (MGUS):
    Mayo Clin Proc 2006; 81: 693-703 (review article)
    N Engl J Med 2006; 355: 2765-70 (review article)
Multiple Myeloma: Mayo Clin Proc 2005; 80: 1371-82 (review article)
    Lancet 2009; 363: 324-39 (review article)
    … Treatment: N Engl J Med 2004; 351: 1860-73 (review article)
    Mayo Clin Proc 2007; 82: 323-341 (review article)
Myelodysplasia: Mayo Clin Proc 2006; 81: 104-130 (review article)
Myelofibrosis with Myeloid Metaplasia: N Engl J Med 2000; 342: 1255-65 (review article)
Oncologic Emergencies: Mayo Clin Proc 2006; 81: 835-848 (review article)
Polycythemia Vera: Mayo Clin Proc 2003; 78: 174-94 (review article)
    … and JAK2 Mutation : Mayo Clin Proc 2007; 82: 599-604 (review article)
Stem-Cell Transplantation: N Engl J Med 2006; 354: 1813-26 (review article)
Superior Vena Cava Syndrome: N Engl J Med 2007; 356: 1862-9 (review article)
Thrombocytosis: N Engl J Med 2004; 350: 1211-1219 (review article)
Thrombotic Microangiopathies: N Engl J Med 2002; 347: 589-600 (review article)
Thrombotic Thrombocytopenic Purpura: N Engl J Med 2006; 354: 1927-35 (review article)
    Clev Clin J Med 2008; 75: 369-375 (review article)
Trastuzumab: N Engl J Med 2007; 357: 39-51 (review article)
Transfusions: Lancet 2007; 370: 415-26 (review article)
    N Engl J Med 1999; 340: 438-47 & 525-33 (review article)
    …of Coagulation Factor Concentrates: Lancet 2007; 370: 439-48 (review article)
    … Platelet: Lancet 2007; 370: 427-38 (review article)
    … Reactions: CMAJ 2007; 170: 141-47 (review article)
von Willebrand's disease: NHLBI Health Information Center, publication n° 08-5832, Dec 2008, 126 p (NHLBI
    Guidelines)
    Thromb Haemost 2000; 84: 160-74 (review article)
    … Treatment: N Engl J Med 2004; 351: 683-694 (review article)
Waldenström's Macroglobulinemia: J Clin Oncol 2000; 18: 214-26 (review article)

Useful Web Sites in Oncology: www.nccn.org (*National Comprehensive Cancer Network*)
    www.cancer.gov/cancerinfo/pdq/treatment (*National Cancer Institute*)

Chapter 6

Infectious Diseases

Sepsis

Severe sepsis is associated with multi-organ dysfunction and ranks first among causes of mortality in the intensive care unit.

Sepsis generates an inflammatory and hormonal response, as well as activates the coagulation cascade and suppresses fibrinolysis.

Risk factors for multi-organ dysfunction include: advanced age, metabolic disorders, cancer, immunosuppression, diabetes, cirrhosis, and the need for pressors despite adequate volume repletion.

Definitions	– **Systemic inflammatory response syndrome** ("*SIRS*") : if ≥ 2 following clinical criteria are present in the context of a major physiological insult: temperature > 38°C or < 36°C, heart rate > 90/minute, tachypnea > 20/minute or hyperventilation with $PaCO_2$ < 32 mmHg, WBC count > 12 x 10^9/L or < 4 x 10^9/L or > 10% immature (band) cells. – **Sepsis**: "SIRS" + suspected or confirmed infection. **Severe** sepsis: sepsis associated with organ dysfunction, hypotension or hypoperfusion (lactic acidosis, oliguria, altered mental status). – **Septic shock** : sepsis-induced hypotension (systolic BP < 90 mmHg or ↓ in mean BP > 40 mmHg if pre-existing hypertension) unresponsive to 500 mL of fluid challenge + peripheral hypoperfusion. – **Multi-organ dysfunction** ("MOD"): progressive but reversible dysfunction of ≥ 2 organs.
Causes	Lower respiratory tract infections (50 %). Primary bacteremia (25 %). Intra-abdominal infections (20 %). Complicated genito-urinary infections (15 %) Central nervous system infections. Skin and soft tissue infections (wounds, necrotizing fasciitis, cellulitis). Ear, nose, throat infections (sinusitis, otitis, etc). Osteo-articular infections. Endovascular infections (catheter-related, infectious endocarditis, septic thrombophlebitis, etc). Fungemia.
Clinical findings	Cardiovascular effects: persistent hypotension, decreased O_2 delivery, myocardial depression. Pulmonary effects: ↑ pulmonary capillary leak and adult respiratory distress syndrome. Oliguria, anuria, acute renal failure. Hepatic dysfunction: ischemic hepatitis, cholestasis, hyperbilirubinemia… Coagulopathy: disseminated intravascular coagulation. Hyperglycemia and adrenal insufficiency. Delirium, encephalopathy or central nervous system depression.

Workup	Two sets of blood cultures from peripheral sites (prior to antibiotics). If endocarditis suspected, draw a third set. Blood cultures may be taken via central as well as peripheral catheter if catheter infection is suspected (see table on Catheter-related sepsis). Other cultures (as indicated): respiratory secretions, urine, wound, cerebro-spinal fluid, cutaneous lesions, catheter if present > 48 hours, etc. CBC, electrolytes, glucose, creatinine, BUN, aPTT, INR, fibrinogen, D-dimers, AST, ALT, alkaline phosphatase, bilirubin, amylase, lipase, lactate, C-reactive protein, urinalysis, blood gas, ECG, Chest X-ray. As required: Abdominal/thoracic CT, cortisol, ACTH stimulation test, CK, troponin, pregnancy test, *C. difficile* assay (endoscopy in patients with ileus), echocardiography, lumbar puncture, etc. Note: 5-30 % of ⊕ blood cultures are contaminants (suspect if bacterium is part of normal skin flora and in only one bottle: Coagulase neg. Staphylococcus, *Micrococcus* sp., *Propionibacterium* sp., *Bacillus* sp., *Corynebacterium* sp). Monitoring: Urinary catheter. Arterial line in pts on pressors. Heart monitor. Central venous catheter ± pulmonary arterial catheter (Swan-Ganz) in order to optimize filling pressures with colloids and/or cristalloids as needed.

Management	Treatment: secure the ABC's (*Airway, Breathing, Circulation*) as usual :
	– 100 % oxygen. Mechanical ventilation as needed.
	– Immediate and agressive volume replacement if hypotension or ↑ lactate: Aim for:
	     Central venous pressure (CVP) : 8-12 mmHg.
	     Mean arterial pressure ≥ 65 mmHg.
	     Urine output ≥ 0.5 mL/kg/h.
	     Central venous or mixed venous O_2 saturation ≥ 70 %.
	– Generous fluid repletion: 500-1000 mL of cristalloids or 300-500 mL of colloid in 30 minutes then repeat as needed to maintain BP or urine output in the absence of fluid overload.
	– Use pressors when hydration alone fails to restore BP and/or organ perfusion, or temporarily until volume re-establishes adequate perfusion: Norepinephrine and dopamine through a central line are the drugs of choice. In cases of shock refractory to volume and high dose pressors, consider vasopressin (0.01-0.04 U/minute).
	– Dobutamine should be considered if cardiac output is insufficient despite adequate volume.
	– If cental venous or mixed venous O_2 saturation is < 70 % despite a CVP 8-12 mmHg, consider transfusions to attain a hematocrit ≥ 30 %.
	
	Removal of the source of sepsis: urinary catheter, I.V. catheters if suspected of being the source of infection, debridement of wounds or drainage of abscesses, etc.
	
	Antibiotics STAT: given in accordance with the suspected etiology, the immune status, the source, the past medical or surgical history, medication, recent trips, etc.
	If the etiology is unknown and presence of a life-threatening infection: piperacillin-tazobactam or carbapenem (meropenem or imipenem) ± tobramycin or cipro IV (if *P. aeruginosa* suspected). Add vancomycin or linezolid if MRSA suspected. Add linezolid if vancomycin resistant enterococcus (VRE) suspected.
	If pt asplenic: cefotaxime, ceftriaxone or moxifloxacin.
	If biliary tract suspected: piperacillin/tazobactam or ticarcillin/clavulanate.
	If IV drug use: cloxacillin or vancomycin.
	If intra-abdominal origin suspected:
	     Community acquired: piperacillin/tazobactam or ticarcillin/clavulanate.
	     Hospitalized: piperacillin/tazobactam or carbapenem (meropenem or imipenem) ± tobramycin or cipro IV (sepsis of abdominal origin if multiple abdominal operations and exposure to antibiotics)
	     If urinary tract suspected: ampicillin + gentamicin or piperacillin/tazobactam or ticarcillin/clavulanate or carbapenem (meropenem or imipenem), or fluoroquinolone IV.

	Early enteral nutritional support if possible (otherwise parenteral).
	Activated C protein given to patients at high risk of mortality (APACHE II ≥ 25, multi-organ dysfunction secondary to sepsis, septic shock or ARDS secondary to sepsis) in the absence of contra-indications related to the risk of bleeding or risk not outweighing estimated benefits. Drip of 24 µg/kg/h IV for 96 hours. Proven ↓ mortality (PROWESS study).
	Steroids: Consider in patients requiring vasopressors despite adequate volume replacement (hydrocortisone 200-300 mg/day in 3-4 doses or IV for 7 days) but controversial.
	Supportive treatment: analgesia, sedation, paralysis, transfusions (aim Hb 70-90 g/L in the absence of CAD or active bleeding), DVT prophylaxis, stress ulcer prophylaxis, continuous veno-venous hemofiltration or intermittent hemodialysis as needed, stop all BP-lowering medication, etc.
Prognosis	Mortality of septic shock 30-70 %. Mortality is correlated with the number of failing organs in MOD: 54 % if 2 organs involved, 100 % if 5.

Catheter-Related Sepsis

Causes up to 50 % of nosocomial bacteremia.
80-90 % source is a central line.
In order of frequency: femoral line > jugular > sub-clavian.
More frequent with hemodialysis or TPN line.

Etiology	Coagulase neg. *Staphylococcus*, *S. aureus*, *Enterococcus* sp., *Corynebacterium jeikeium*, *Bacillus* sp., Gram neg. rods (*Klebsiella sp., Enterobacter sp., E. coli, Pseudomonas sp., Acinetobacter sp., Serratia sp.*), *Candida albicans* or others, atypical mycobacteria.
Clinical findings	Fever, chills, malaise … non-specific symptoms. Erythema around site of catheter in 10 % of cases, neither sensitive nor specific.
Diagnosis	Many diagnostic methods: - Catheter culture by Maki semi-quantitative method (⊕ if growth of ≥ 15 CFU/segment of catheter in presence of same pathogen in blood cultures): validated for peripheral IV lines only. - Differential time for positivity: growth of the same pathogen from blood cultures taken through the catheter two hours earlier than peripheral blood cultures suggests catheter-related sepsis. If negative blood culture via catheter, catheter-related sepsis not likely. Useful when removal of the central line is not desirable. - Culture of catheter site with peripheral blood cultures ⊕ for same pathogen.
Treatment	Immediate removal of catheter if easy to insert a new one or if patient is very ill, if ⊕ repeat blood cultures at 48 hours, in the presence of *S. aureus*, Gram neg. rods, *Corynebacterium* sp. or *Bacillus* sp. or fungi, if pt is neutropenic, for local complications (catheter tunnel infection, septic thrombophlebitis), for metastatic infections (endocarditis …) or in the presence of abnormal heart valves. A potentially infected catheter may also be changed over a guidewire (esp. in patients in whom instrumentation is likely to be difficult), while waiting for catheter culture results; if ⊖ culture, leave new catheter in place; if ⊕ culture, remove new catheter and replace it in a new site. Empiric antibiotic therapy with vancomycin (± Gram neg. rods coverage in patients who appear very ill or in immunosuppressed pts) while waiting for culture results: - For *S. aureus*: treat for 2 weeks if there is no complicated infection, without underlying valvular disease, and who respond adequately to antibiotics in < 3 days following

	removal of catheter.
	- If complicated by septic phlebitis, endocarditis or other, treat for 4 weeks.
	- For coagulase neg. *Staphylococcus*: treat for 5-7 days (14 if catheter not removed).
	- For *Candida albicans*: if not complicated, fluconazole for ≥ 14 days.
	- For *Candida glabrata/krusei*: amphotericin B or caspofungin.
	In *S. aureus* infections, always rule out an associated endocarditis (⊕ in 25 %).
	Repeat blood cultures after stopping treatment if catheter is not removed.
	Antibiotic lock therapy for catheter tunnel infection to be considered in an attempt to preserve the catheter (combined with systemic antibiotics).
Prevention	Use sterile technique (cap, gown, gloves, mask, sterile drapes, 2 % chlorhexidin desinfectant) when inserting catheter. Antibiotic-impregnated catheter as needed for catheters remaining in place > 5 days if incidence of catheter infection is ↑. There is no advantage to routinely changing central lines. Change peripheral catheters every 48-72 hours. Keep duration of use of catheters at a minimum.

Fever of Unknown Origin	
Definition	1. Fever > 3 weeks.
	2. Over to 38.3 °C on several measurements.
	3. Diagnosis remains unknown after a full week of in-hospital investigation.
Causes	Infectious 30-40 %.
	Neoplastic 20-30 %.
	Rheumatologic 10-20 %.
	Miscellaneous 15-20 %.
	No diagnosis 5-15 %.
	Most frequent etiologies: 50 % caused by the 7 following diseases: tuberculosis, endocarditis, lymphoma, solid tumors, adult Still's disease, vasculitis, common rheumatologic diseases (SLE, Sjögren's).
	Other frequent causes: intra-abdominal abscess, urinary tract infection, drug-related fever, inflammatory bowel disease, pulmonary embolism.
	Infectious:
	– Infectious endocarditis.
	– Intra-abdominal abscess (hepatic, splenic, sub-phrenic, pancreatic, biliary, psoas, pelvic).
	– Urinary tract infection (acute pyelonephritis, renal abscess, obstructive, prostatic abscess, etc).
	– Osteomyelitis.
	– Upper respiratory tract infection (oral, sinusitis).
	– Vascular infection (septic phlebitis).
	– Systemic infections :
	- Bacterial : salmonellosis, brucellosis, chronic meningococcemia, Whipple's disease, yersiniosis, tularemia, syphilis, disseminated gonococcal infection, Q fever, psittacosis, borreliosis, leptospirosis, cat-scratch disease, melioidosis (South-East Asia).
	- Mycobacterial: tuberculosis.
	- Fungal : histoplasmosis, coccidioidomycosis (South-West American), *Pneumocystis jiroveci* pneumonia (in immunosuppressed patient), etc.
	- Viral: CMV, EBV, HIV, etc.
	- Parasitic: malaria, toxoplasmosis, babesiosis.

Neoplastic :
- Lymphoproliferative disorders: lymphoma, Langherhans cell histiocytosis, angioimmunoblastic lymphadenopathy, Kikuchi's histiocytic necrotizing lymphadenitis, Castleman's disease, etc.
- Leukemia.
- Myelodysplastic syndromes.
- Solid tumors: renal, lung, breast, ovarian, stomach, esophagus, colon, biliary, pancreas, sarcoma, primary hepatic, atrial myxoma.

Rheumatologic :
- Adult Still's disease.
- Giant cell arteritis.
- Polymyalgia rheumatica.
- Vasculitis: Wegener's, Takayasu's, polyarteritis nodosa, cryoglobulinemia.
- Connective tissue disease: SLE, rheumatoid arthritis, Sjögren's.

Miscellaneors:
- Granulomatous diseases: Crohn's, sarcoidosis, granulomatous hepatitis.
- Alcoholic hepatitis.
- Hematoma.
- Pulmonary embolism or deep vein thrombosis.
- Drug fever.
- Familial Mediterranean fever.
- Hyperthyroidism, subacute thyroiditis.
- Adrenal insufficiency.
- Schnitzler syndrome.
- Factitious fever.

Diagnosis	Medical history:
	   - describe the fever (duration, pattern).
	   - complete medical, surgical and family history.
	   - travel history, animal contact, food, work.
	   - HIV risk factors.
	   - exposure to tuberculosis.
	   - age (in a young patient suspect Still's disease, factitious, CMV, EBV : In older patients, polymyalgia rheumatica, temporal arteritis).
	   - symptoms of connective tissue disease.
	
	Complete physical examination including:
	   - skin.
	   - eyes (fundoscopic).
	   - lymphadenopathy.
	
	Workup :according to clinical context:
	   - CBC.
	   - Urinalysis and urine culture.
	   - Hepatic and renal workup.
	   - Blood cultures.
	   - Chest X-ray.
	   - Abdominal CT.
	   - Laparoscopy.
	   - Bone marrow biopsy, liver biopsy and, in patients > 50 y.o., temporal artery biopsy.
	   - Positron emission tomography (PET scan).
	   - Gallium scan or radio-labelled WBC scan.
	   - Doppler ultrasound of lower extremities, V/Q scan.
	
	Stop all non-essential medication.

FUO and special groups	With cancer: 50 % of FUO's are infectious, the rest are paraneoplastic. With HIV: 75 % infectious: mycobacteria, CMV, toxoplasmosis, *Pneumocystis jiroveci*, cryptococcus, salmonellosis, Leishmaniasis, aspergillosis, varicella zoster, HIV alone rare. Most frequent non infectious is lymphoma and drug fever: 15 % remain undetermined.

Cellulitis	
Cellulitis	Infection reaching dermis (contrary to erysipelas: see below). **Causes**: β-hemolytic streptococci (groups A, B, C, and G), *Staphylococcus aureus*, Gram neg. rods ... Some bacteria are associated with specific exposures (*Aeromonas hydrophila* with water, *Pseudomonas aeruginosa* with pools/hot tubs, *Pasteurella multocida* with cat/dog bites, *S. aureus* with IV drug users, MRSA with hospital-acquired wound infections, community-acquired MRSA (CA-MRSA) in intravenous drug users, jail, sports teams, etc). Polymicrobial infections (Gram neg. rods, anaerobic bacteria, Gram positive cocci): diabetic foot, human bites, abdominal wound infections, IV drug use, chronic vascular insufficiency, etc. **Risk factors**: dermatitis, burns, wounds, trauma, venous or lymphatic stasis, tinea pedis, history of cellulitis, IV drug use, surgery for breast cancer, etc. Differential diagnosis: acute dermatitis, crystal arthropathy, drug reaction, shingles, Sweet's syndrome, sting, thrombophlebitis, gangrenous dermatitis, Kawasaki's syndrome. **Clinical features**: either sudden or progressive onset, toxicity, pain, erythema with either distinct or imprecise margins, predisposing lesion may be present (must be looked for). Streptococcal infection (erysipelas) tends to begin suddenly, with rapid progression of the cutaneous lesions (< 6 hours), well defined borders, associated lymphangitis, cutaneous breach often absent (sometimes associated with saphenous vein dissection). **Workup**: CBC, blood cultures, wound culture (if purulent discharge). Needle aspiration or cutaneous biopsy for cultures if deemed necessary (30 % positivity), to be considered in immunosuppressed or neutropenic patients; in the presence of severe systemic symptoms; in the setting of a bite; for a recurrent infection; or when there is no response to antibiotic therapy. **Treatment**: for erysipelas: penicillin for 10 days. Alternatives: first generation cephalosporins (cefazolin, cephalexin, cefadroxil, etc), clindamycin or vancomycin. Other presentations: cloxacillin or first generation cephalosporins. Alternatives: clindamycin, vancomycin, macrolides. If human or animal bite, amoxicillin-clavulanate + rabies prophylaxis (if indicated) and tetanus immunization as needed. Alternative: moxifloxacin or ertapenem. Surgery if intra-articular penetration suspected. Bedrest and elevation of the extremity. Streptococcal infections respond rapidly, however with lymphatic obstruction a slower response is expected, the extremity should be elevated, and a longer treatment course given as needed.
Necrotizing fasciitis due to group A streptococcal infection	**Definition**: invasive streptococcal infection reaching subcutaneous tissues and fasciae. **Cause**: group A streptococci (recently a few cases reported with groups B and G). **Differential diagnosis**: Meleney's progressive bacterial synergistic gangrene, Fournier's gangrene (perineum), anaerobic cellulitis, gas gangrene (*Clostridium perfringens*), post-operative necrotizing fasciitis (mixed flora), myonecrosis (muscle tissue infection and necrosis). **Clinical features**: Abrupt onset, severe toxicity, intense pain (essential to diagnosis), erythema, edema, hypotension or shock, vesicular or necrotizing lesions. Frequently associated with toxic shock (hypotension and dysfunction of at least 2 target organs). **Workup**: CBC, blood cultures, CK (advanced stages), AST, ALT, bilirubin, DIC workup, culture of lesions with Gram stain STAT, throat swab. CT or MRI sometimes useful. **Treatment**: Depends on the rapidity of intervention. Admission to the ICU STAT. **Urgent consultation of surgery team and Infectious Diseases specialist.**

	Antibiotics: penicillin G 4 MU IV every 4 h + clindamycin 900 mg IV every 8 h. Potentially effective adjuvant treatments: IV gammaglobulins 1 g/kg every 24 hours x 2 doses. Debridement of necrotic tissues. Contact prophylaxis: immediate family members, health care workers with significant exposure (ressuscitation, contact with respiratory secretions, etc) → penicillin, cephalexin or erythromycin for 10 days. **Prognosis**: mortality > 30 %, amputation in 20 %.
Erysipelas	Superficial skin infection (epidermis and dermis), usually affecting face or extremities with a sharply demarcated and raised border, associated with serious infection of cutaneous lymphatics. Risk factors: venous or lymphatic stasis, previous erysipelas. **Clinical features**: fever, chills, acute onset of pain. Lymphatic involvement often present. **Cause**: group A streptococci (rarely, group C or G streptococci). **Workup**: CBC, throat swab (optional). **Treatment**: Penicillin for 10 days. Alternatives: first generation cephalosporins (cefazolin, cephalexin, cefadroxil, etc.), clindamycin (risk factor for *C. difficile*), vancomycin. Some recurrent cases require antibiotic prophylaxis.

Endocarditis

- Can occur with mechanical valves, mitral valve prolapse, degenerative valvular disease, congenital heart disease (bicuspid valves), in IV drug users (tricuspid), with invasive monitoring, in hemodialysis patients, in patients with diabetes, or with patients with poor oral hygiene.
- Source of the bacteremia: manipulations of oropharyngeal, gastro-intestinal or genito-urinary sites and active infections.

Clinical features	Infective endocarditis (IE) can be acute (e.g.: *S. aureus*) or subacute (e.g.: *Streptococcus viridans*).
	Fever, a heart murmur, heart failure, cutaneous lesions (petechiae, Osler's nodes [subacute], Janeway lesions, splinter hemorrhages, conjunctival hemorrhages), Roth spots (subacute), anorexia, weight loss, malaise, night sweats, musculoskeletal manifestations (arthralgia, arthritis, myalgia, lower back pain), splenomegaly.
	Endocarditis in IV drug users: on native valve. Mainly tricuspid. Pulmonary manifestations frequent (septic emboly, pleuritic pain, etc): good prognosis (mortality < 10 %).
	Complications : valvular (perforation, vegetations), valve ring abscess, myocardial infarction (secondary to emboli), conduction disturbances, pericarditis, prosthetic valve dysfunction, heart failure, peripheral vascular disease, mycotic aneurysms (in central nervous system, aorta, coronary, mesentary ... : in subacute cases), neurological complications (embolism, mycotic aneurysms, seizures, abscesses), renal complications (glomerulonephritis, renal emboli with infarction).
Causes	– Native valve: streptococci (viridians group, *S. bovis*), staphylococci (*S. aureus*, coagulase neg.), enterococci, Gram neg. rods, others. – Prosthetic early post-operative (≤ 60 days): staphylococci (coagulase neg., *S. aureus*), Gram neg. rods, diphtheroids, fungi, others. – Prosthetic late post-operative (> 60 days): staphylococci (coagulase neg., *S. aureus*), streptococci (viridians group, *S. bovis*), Gram neg. rods, enterococci, diphtheroids, fungi, others. – IV drug users: *S. aureus*, streptococci, *Pseudomonas aeruginosa*, polymicrobial, *Corynebacterium* sp, fungi. – 5 % are culture negative: secondary to recent antibiotic use, rare pathogens (*Coxiella burnetti*, *Chlamydophilia* sp., *Bartonella* sp., *Legionella* sp., *Brucella* sp., *Tropheryma whippelii*, fungi …).

Workup	– CBC, electrolytes, creatinine, urinalysis, rheumatoid factor, sedimentation rate, C-reactive protein.
	– Blood cultures ⊕ in 95 %: incubation for 3-4 weeks needed to grow fastidious pathogens. Repeat blood cultures after 5-7 days of antimicrobial therapy.
	– The MIC for the pathogen with respect to the administered antibiotics must be determined.
	– Chest X-ray.
	– Serial ECGs.
	– Echocardiography (transthoracic or transesophageal): to be performed as soon as possible after the diagnosis is suspected, to be repeated after 7-10 days if patient at high risk of complications or if first echocardiogram was not diagnostic (and clinical suspicion persists), and to be performed again at the end of treatment.
Diagnosis	Modified Duke Criteria :
	Major criteria :
	1. Positive blood culture (≥ 2) for infective endocarditis :
	a. Typical microorganisms from two separate blood cultures (viridians group streptococci, *Streptococcus bovis*, HACEK* group, *S. aureus* or community-acquired enterococci without a primary focus);
	b. Microorganisms consistent with IE from persistently positive blood cultures defined as: 2 positive cultures of blood samples drawn >12 hours apart, or all of 3 or a majority of 4 separate cultures of blood (with first and last sample drawn 1 hour apart);
	c. Single positive blood culture for *Coxiella burnetti* **or** phase 1 IgG antibody titer for *C. burnetti* > 1:800.
	2. Evidence of endocardial involvement:
	a. New valvular regurgitation;
	b. Positive echocardiogram for endocarditis: oscillating intracardial mass on valve **or** periannular abscess **or** a new partial dehiscence of a prosthetic valve.
	Minor criteria :
	1. Predisposing factors: predisposing cardiac conditions **or** IV drug use.
	2. Fever ≥ 38 °C.
	3. Vascular phenomena: major arterial emboli, mycotic aneurysms, septic pulmonary infarct, intracranial hemorrhage, conjunctival hemorrhage, Janeway lesions.
	4. Immunologic phenomena: presence of rheumatoid factor, glomerulonephritis, Osler's nodes, Roth spots.
	5. Microbiological findings: positive blood culture, but not meeting the major criteria or serological evidence of active infection with plausible organism.
	Infective endocarditis is **definite** → if 2 major criteria fulfilled **or** 1 major and 3 minor **or** 5 minor criteria or with the demonstration of a microorganism by either culture or with characteristic histopathological changes on a vegetation, a vegetation that has embolized, or an intracardiac abscess.
	Infective endocarditis is **possible** if 1 major criterion and 1 minor criterion **or** 3 minor criteria are fulfilled.
	Diagnosis rejected if: An alternative diagnosis explains the signs of infective endocarditis **or** resolution of the endocarditis syndrome within four days or less of antibiotic therapy **or** absence of pathological evidence for infective endocarditis at surgery or autopsy, after 4 days or less of antibiotic treatment.
	* Fastidious pathogens classically associated with culture negative infective endocarditis: *Haemophilus* sp., *Actinobacillus actinomycetemcomitans*, *Cardiobacterium hominis*, *Eikenella corrodens* and *Kingella kingae*.

| Treatment of frequent pathogens | If microorganism not yet identified :
     For acute endocarditis: cloxacillin + gentamicin ± vancomycin (if risk of MRSA).
     For subacute endocarditis on native valve: ampicillin + gentamicin.
     For prosthetic valve endocarditis: vancomycin + gentamicin + rifampicin.

For native valve endocarditis caused by highly penicillin-sensitive viridans group streptococci or *S. bovis* (MIC ≤ 0.12 μg/mL):
     Penicillin G 12-18 million IU/d for 4 wk **OR** ceftriaxone 2 g/d for 4 wk **OR**
     Penicillin G 12-18 million IU/d + gentamicin 3 mg/kg/d (single daily dose) for 2 wk
     OR ceftriaxone 2 g/d + gentamicin 3 mg/kg/d (single daily dose) for 2 wk **OR**
     vancomycin 15 mg/kg q 12 h (max 2 g/24 h) for 4 weeks.

For native valve endocarditis caused by strains of viridans group streptococci and *S. bovis* relatively resistant to penicillin (MIC > 0.12-≤ 0.5 μg/mL)* :
     Penicillin G 24 million IU/d for 4 wk + gentamicin 3 mg/kg/d (single daily dose) for
     2 weeks **OR** ceftriaxone 2 g/d for 4 wk + gentamicin 3 mg/kg/d (single daily dose)
     for 2 weeks **OR** vancomycin 15 mg/kg q 12 h (max 2 g/24 h) for 4 weeks.
* Patients with endocarditis caused by penicillin-resistant (MIC > 0.5 μg/mL) strains should be treated with regimen recommended for enterococcal endocarditis.

For endocarditis on prosthetic valves or other prosthetic material caused by viridans group streptococci and *S. bovis* :
– If penicillin-susceptible strain (MIC ≤ 0.12 μg/mL) :
     Penicillin G 24 million IU/d for 6 wk ± gentamicin 3 mg/kg/d (single daily dose) for
     2 wk **OR** ceftriaxone 2 g/d for 6 wk ± gentamicin 3 mg/kg/d (single daily dose) for
     2 wk **OR** vancomycin 15 mg/kg q 12 h for 6 weeks.
– Penicillin relatively or fully resistant strain (MIC > 0.12 μg/mL) :
     Penicillin G 24 million IU/d + gentamicin 3 mg/kg/d (single daily dose) for 6 wk **OR**
     ceftriaxone 2 g/d + gentamicin 3 mg/kg/d (single daily dose) for 6 wk **OR**
     vancomycin 15 mg/kg q 12 h for 6 weeks.

For endocarditis caused by staphylococci in the absence of prosthetic materials :
– Methicillin-susceptible strains: cloxacillin 2 g IV q 4 h for 6 wk (or 2 wk for
     uncomplicated right-sided IE) ± gentamicin 3 mg/kg/d (in 2 or 3 divided doses) for 3-5
     days. Penicillin G 24 million IU/d IV may be used in place of cloxacillin if strain is
     penicillin susceptible (MIC ≤ 0.1 μg/mL) and does not produce β-lactamase.
– For penicillin-allergic patients (nonanaphylactoid type): cefazolin 2 g IV q 8 h for 6 wk
     ± gentamicin 3 mg/kg/d (in 2 or 3 divided doses) for 3-5 days: for patients with
     anaphylactoid-type hypersensitivity to β-lactams, vancomycin should be used.
– Methicillin-resistant strains: vancomycin 15 mg/kg q 12 h for 6 weeks.

For prosthetic valve endocarditis caused by staphylococci :
– Methicillin-susceptible strains: cloxacillin 2 g IV q 4 h + rifampin 300 mg IV/PO q 8 h
     for ≥ 6 wk + gentamicin 3 mg/kg/d (in 2 or 3 divided doses) for 2 wk. Penicillin G 24
     million U/d IV may be used instead of cloxacillin if strain is penicillin-sensitive (MIC ≤
     0.1 μg/mL); vancomycin should be used in patients with immediate-type
     hypersensitivity reactions to β-lactams; cefazolin may be substituted for cloxacillin in
     patients with non-immediate-type hypersensitivity reactions to penicillins.
– Methicillin-resistant strains : vancomycin 15 mg/kg q 12 h + rifampin 300 mg IV/PO q
     8 h for ≥ 6 wk + gentamicin 3 mg/kg/d (in 2 or 3 divided doses) for 2 weeks.

For native valve or prosthetic valve enterococcal endocarditis caused by strains **susceptible** to penicillin, gentamicin, and vancomycin :
     Ampicillin 2 g IV q 4 h + gentamicin 1 mg/kg q 8 h for 4-6 wk (4-wk therapy
     recommended for patients with symptoms of illness ≤ 3 mo and 6-wk therapy
     recommended for patients with symptoms > 3 mo) **OR** penicillin G 18-30 million
     IU IV/d + gentamicin 1 mg/kg q 8 h for 4-6 wk **OR** vancomycin 15 mg/kg q 12 h +
     gentamicin 1 mg/kg q 8 h for 6 weeks. For prosthetic valve or other prosthetic
     cardiac material: minimum of 6 wk of therapy recommended. |

For native or prosthetic valve enterococcal endocarditis caused by strains **susceptible** to penicillin, streptomycin, and vancomycin and **resistant** to gentamicin :

> Ampicillin 2 g IV q 4 h + streptomycin 7.5 mg/kg q 12 h for 4-6 wk (4-wk therapy recommended for patients with symptoms of illness ≤ 3 mo and 6-wk therapy recommended for patients with symptoms > 3 mo) **OR** penicillin G 24 million IU IV/d + streptomycin 7.5 mg/kg q 12 h for 4-6 wk **OR** vancomycin 15 mg/kg q 12 h + streptomycin 7.5 mg/kg q 12 h for 6 weeks.

For native or prosthetic valve enterococcal endocarditis caused by strains **resistant** to penicillin and **susceptible** to aminoglycoside and vancomycin :

- β-Lactamase-producing strain: Ampicillin 2 g IV q 4 h + gentamicin 1 mg/kg q 8 h for 6 wk **OR** vancomycin 15 mg/kg q 12 h + gentamicin 1 mg/kg q 8 h for 6 weeks.
- Intrinsic penicillin resistance: vancomycin 15 mg/kg q 12 h + gentamicin 1 mg/kg q 8 h for 6 weeks. Consultation with an Infectious Diseases specialist is recommended.

For native or prosthetic valve enterococcal endocarditis caused by strains **resistant** to penicillin, aminoglycoside, and vancomycin : Patients with endocarditis caused by these strains should be treated in consultation with an Infectious Diseases specialist :

E. faecium: Linezolid, daptomycin **OR** quinupristin-dalfopristin for ≥ 8 weeks.
E. faecalis: Imipenem + ampicillin **OR** ceftriaxone + ampicillin for ≥ 8 weeks.

For native and prosthetic valve endocarditis caused by HACEK organisms :

> Ceftriaxone 2 g/d for 4 wk **OR** ciprofloxacin 500 mg PO bid or 400 mg IV q 12 h for 4 weeks (fluoroquinolones recommended only for patients unable to tolerate cephalosporins).

For culture-negative endocarditis including *Bartonella* endocarditis: Patients with endocarditis caused by these strains should be treated in consultation with an Infectious Diseases specialist :

- Native valve: ampicillin-sulbactam + gentamicin **OR** vancomycin + gentamicin + ciprofloxacin for 4-6 wk.
- Prosthetic valve (early, ≤ 1 y): vancomycin + gentamicin + cefepime + rifampin.
- Prosthetic valve (late, > 1 y) :
  o Suspected *Bartonella*, culture negative : ceftriaxone + gentamicin ± doxycycline.
  o Documented *Bartonella*, culture positive : doxycycline + gentamicin.

Surgery: refractory congestive heart failure, recurrent serious systemic embolic episodes, uncontrolled infection, evidence of intracardiac progression of infection, prosthetic valve dehiscence.

Prophylaxis	In accordance with the 2007 *American Heart Association* Guidelines: **Cardiac conditions at high risk of endocarditis:** - Prosthetic cardiac valve (including bioprosthetic and homograft) or prosthetic material used for cardiac valve repair. - Previous infective endocarditis. - Congenital heart disease (unrepaired cyanotic CHD, including palliative shunts and conduits; completely repaired congenital heart defect with prosthetic material or device, whether placed by surgery or by catheter intervention, during the first 6 months after the procedure; repaired CHD with residual defects at the site or adjacent to the site of a prosthetic patch or prosthetic device - which inhibit endothelialization). - Cardiac transplantation recipients who develop cardiac valvulopathy. Procedures for which antibiotic prophylaxis is reasonable: - **Dental:** For all dental procedures that involve manipulation of gingival tissue or the periapical region of teeth or perforation of the oral mucosa. - **Respiratory:** For any invasive procedure of the respiratory tract that involves incision or biopsy of the respiratory mucosa, such as tonsillectomy and adenoidectomy. - **Others:** Antibiotic prophylaxis could be recommended for patients who undergo a surgical procedure that involves infected skin, skin structure, or musculoskeletal tissue. Note: Antibiotic prophylaxis is not recommended for gastrointestinal or genitourinary tract procedures, except for patients who have an established GI or GU tract infection. **Prophylactic regimen** for dental (or respiratory tract) procedures (adults): - Standard: amoxicillin 2 g 30-60 minutes pre-op. - If pt unable to take oral medication: ampicillin 2 g IM/IV 30 minutes before operation or cefazolin or ceftriaxone 1 g IM/IV 30-60 minutes pre-op. - Allergic to penicillin or ampicillin: cephalexin* 2 g 30-60 min before operation or clindamycin 600 mg 30-60 min before operation or azithromycin or clarithromycin 500 mg 30-60 min pre-op. - Allergic to penicillins and unable to take oral medication: cefazolin* or ceftriaxone* 1 g IM/IV 30-60 min before operation or clindamycin 600 mg IM/IV - 60 min pre-op. * Cephalosporins should not be used in a patient with a history of anaphylaxis, angioedema, or urticaria with penicillins.

Central Nervous System Infections	
Meningitis	
Clinical findings	Presentation of bacterial meningitis: 25 % fulminant, 50 % evolving over 1-7 days: 25 % over 1-3 weeks. More subtle in elderly or immunosuppressed patients. Acute meningitis caused by bacteria or viruses; subacute with tuberculosis; chronic with fungi, tumor, etc. May be primary or secondary to ENT infection, pneumonia, infectious endocarditis … Fever, headache, malaise, ↓ level of consciousness, seizure, vomiting, nausea, photophobia. Signs of menigeal irritation (stiff neck, Kernig's and Brudzinski's), cranial nerve palsies, papilledema, Cushing reflex. Rash in 50 % with meningococcemia. Seizures, focal deficits, nystagmus, ataxia, cranial nerve palsies with *Listeria monocytogenes*
Causes	Bacterial : age 18-50: *S. pneumoniae* and *N. meningitidis*: 　　Age > 50: as above + Gram neg. rods and *Listeria monocytogenes*. 　　With cellular immune deficiency: Gram neg. rods and *Listeria monocytogenes*. 　　With neurosurgery, head trauma, CSF shunt: *S. aureus*, Gram neg. rods, *S. pneumoniae* (with CSF leak). 　　***Streptococcus pneumoniae:*** Gram ⊕ diplococcus. Causes 50 % of meningitis in adults. Risk factors: splenectomy, sickle-cell anemia, myeloma, alcoholism, hypogammaglobulinemia: if recurrence, rule out CSF leak or immunoglobulin deficiency. 　　***Neisseria meningitidis:*** Gram neg. diplococcus. Causes 35 % of adult meningitis: with deficits in C5-C9 complement. Associated with rash and Waterhouse-Friderichsen syndrome (necrotic hemorrhage of adrenal glands). 　　***Listeria monocytogenes:*** Gram ⊕ bacillus. Causes 4 % of meningitis. Risk factors: extremes of age, immunosuppression, pregnancy, milk or ice-cream consumption, cheese, contaminated water or salads. 　　**Gram negative rods** (*E. coli, K. pneumoniae, P. aeruginosa*, etc): secondary to bacteremia, complications of head trauma or neurosurgery or chronic disease (diabetes, alcoholism, chronic urinary infection). 　　**Others:** *S.aureus, H. influenzae* (3 %), *S. agalactiae* (aged patients), *Nocardia* sp., *Enterococcus* sp., anaerobic flora, diphtheroids. Viral: enterovirus, coxsackie, echovirus, mumps, arbovirus, lymphocytic choriomeningitis, HSV, VZV, CMV, HIV, EBV, etc. Mainly seen in summer-autumn. Others: fungi (*Cryptococcus* sp., *Candida* sp., *Coccidioides immitis*, histoplasmosis), tuberculosis, syphilis, Lyme disease, cysticercosis (secondary to *Tænia solium*), sarcoidosis, amebiasis, other unicellular parasites (*Naegleria fowleri* with swimming: severe + + +), tumor, drug, vasculitis, etc.
Workup	CBC, blood cultures STAT. Head CT if focal neurologic deficit, papilledema or other signs of intra-cranial hypertension, new onset seizure, various space-occupying lesions, recent neurosurgery, immunosuppression, CSF shunts, trauma or moderate to severe altered consciousness (Glasgow < 10). Note: If cerebral CT scan is indicated, give antibiotics + dexamethasone before!!! Lumbar puncture with CSF fluid analysis : －　Opening pressure: elevated (> 18 cm H_2O) with bacteria, tuberculosis, *Cryptococcus* sp., syphilis... normal or slightly elevated with viruses, sarcoidosis, carcinomatous meningitis. －　WBC differential: **Neutrophilic** predominance with bacteria (from 100 x 10^6/L to > 60 000 x 10^6/L) or with the initial presentation of tuberculosis or viral infections.

	Lymphocytic predominance with viruses, *Cryptococcus* sp., syphilis or tuberculosis (maximum 500-1000 cells x 10^6/L). **Monocytic** predominance with sarcoidosis or carcinomatous meningitis (occasionally *L. monocytogenes*).
	– Protein: increased < 1 g/L with viruses, ≈ 1 g/L with tuberculosis, *Cryptococcus* sp., syphilis, > 1-5 g/L with bacteria or carcinomatous meningitis.
	– Glucose: ↓ with bacteria, tuberculosis, cryptococcus, sarcoidosis (50 %), carcinomatous meningitis. Normal with viruses, carcinomatous meningitis, syphilis.
	– Gram and culture: Gram is positive in 60-90 % of bacterial infections (specificity ≥ 97 %) except with *L. monocytogenes* (25 % ⊕). Culture ⊕ in 80 %.
	– Antigens: *S. pneumoniae, N. meningitidis, H. influenzae* type B, *Cryptococcus* sp. (controversial, sensitivity ↓).
	– Others: neoplastic cells with carcinomatous meningitis, viral serologies ...
	Repeat lumbar puncture in any patient who has not responded clinically after 48 hours of appropriate antimicrobial therapy.
Treatment of bacterial meningitis	– Before CSF analysis, patient 18-50 years old: vancomycin + ceftriaxone or cefotaxime (± ampicillin if *L. monocytogenes* suspected).
	– Before CSF analysis, patient > 50 years old or alcoholic or immunosuppressed: vancomycin + ampicillin + cephalosporin (ceftriaxone or cefotaxime).
	– If nosocomial meningitis, post neurosurgery, or post-trauma: vancomycin + meropenem OR vancomycin + ceftazidime. If immunosuppressed or neutropenic : same + ampicillin (for listeriosis).
	– For Gram ⊕ cocci in chains (*S. pneumoniae*): vancomycin + ceftriaxone (until susceptibility determined) + dexamethasone (see Note below). If allergic to penicillin: vancomycin + moxifloxacin IV or desensitization.
	– For Gram neg. cocci (*N. meningitidis*): penicillin. If allergic: cefotaxime, ceftriaxone moxifloxacin IV or chloramphenicol (not vancomycin): treat close contacts with rifampicin, ceftriaxone, ciprofloxacin or azithromycin. Vaccine available against following serotypes A-C-Y-W135. Respiratory isolation for 24 hours.
	– For Gram ⊕ rods (*L. monocytogenes*): penicillin or ampicillin + gentamicin (or TMP/SMX).
	– For Gram neg. rods: meropenem or cephalosporin (ceftriaxone or cefotaxime) + aminoglycoside.
	– For neurosurgery, recent head trauma or presence of CSF shunts: vancomycin + either meropenem or ceftazidime.
	Note: Dexamethasone (10 mg IV before first dose of antibiotic and every 6 hours for 4 days) has been proven effective as adjuvant therapy in meningitis caused by *S. pneumoniae*. Its use in meningitis caused by other agents should be discussed *a priori* with a specialist.
	Specific organisms :
	S. pneumoniae: antibiotics as above. Duration 10-14 days.
	N. meningitidis: antibiotics as above. Duration 7 days.
	L. monocytogenes: antibiotics as above. Duration ≥ 21 days.
	H. influenzae: ceftriaxone. Duration 7 days.
	Enterobacteriaceae: cephalosporin (cefotaxime or ceftriaxone) + gentamicin (IV or intrathecal). Duration 21 days.
	Pseudomonas sp., *Acinetobacter* sp.: meropenem or ceftazidime + aminoglycoside. Duration 21 days.
	P.S.: These are initial treatments which should be modified depending on susceptibility tests.
	Admission in intensive care unit if: Glasgow coma scale < 10, shock, neurological deterioration, pulmonary infiltrates or seizures.

Prognosis	*S. pneumoniae* meningitis: Mortality 19-37 %, neurological deficit up to 30 %. *N. meningitidis* meningitis: mortality 3-13 %, neurological deficit: 3-7 %. *L. monocytogenes* meningitis: mortality 20 %. Bad prognostic factors: sepsis, altered conciousness, ↓ leukocytes in CSF.
Encephalitis	– Clinical features similar to meningitis however earlier and greater reduction level of consciousness: seizures occur more frequently. – Causes: HSV-1 > HSV-2, VZV. Enteroviruses, arboviruses, rubella, mumps, Japanese encephalitis (Asia), West Nile virus … – Diagnosis: Suggestive CSF: hypercellularity with lymphocytosis < 500 cells x 10^6/L in 90 % (red blood cells seen with HSV in 20 %) and pleocytosis. – PCR *(polymerase chain reaction)* on CSF diagnostic for HSV (also available for CMV, VZV, EBV, HIV, enterovirus, JC virus, rubella). – EEG with PLEDS *(periodic lateralizing epileptiform discharges)* with HSV: CT or MRI reveals temporal lesions in HSV in close to 90 % of cases. – IgM of West Nile virus in CSF for diagnosis. – Cerebral biopsy for herpes encephalitis is rarely necessary since the development of PCR.
Treatment	– HSV: acyclovir 10 mg/kg every 8 h for 14-21 days. – VZV: acyclovir if risk of progression (even if no trials have shown benefit). – Discuss treatment of other types of encephalitis with a specialist.
Prognosis	Mortality from herpetic encephalitis 19 %, important neurological sequelae 42 %.
Brain abscess	Often associated with underlying infection or risk factor (sinusitis, otitis, mastoiditis, periodontal abscess, trauma, neurosurgery, chronic pulmonary infection, esophageal dilation, immunosuppression). 20-30 % are cryptogenic. If in frontal lobes: sinusitis probable or periodontal abscess. In cerebellum or temporal lobes: otitis media or mastoiditis probable. Pathogenesis: cerebritis → capsule formation → definitive capsule (abscess). Mixed aerobic and anaerobic (frequently with *Streptococcus* sp.): *S. aureus* wih trauma or neurosurgery. In HIV ⊕ patients and imaging suggests abscess: rule out toxoplasmosis. For patients from endemic areas (e.g.: Mexico): rule out neurocysticercosis. Clinical findings: headache, altered level of consciousness, meningismus. Fever in 50 %. Papilledema 25 %, convulsion 25 %.
Treatment	– If related to sinusitis or otitis: 3rd gen. cephalosporin + metronidazole. – If penetrating trauma or post-operative: vancomycin + ceftazidime or meropenem + vancomycin. – Surgery indicated for abscess with air-fluid levels, loculated abscess, mycotic abscess or encapsulated abscess > 2.5 cm. Needle-guided aspiration for other abscesses is controversial. – Dexamethasone if mass effect or ↓ level of consciousness.

Bone and Joint Infections	
Septic Arthritis	Most often due to hematogenous spread. Risk factors: immunosuppression, diabetes, cancer, joint abnormalities (rheumatoid arthritis), extra-articular infections (endocarditis, urinary ...: present in 75 %). Post-infectious arthritis encountered with hepatitis B, meningococcemia, sexually transmitted infections, and enteric infections. Differential diagnosis: suppurative tenosynovitis, cellulitis, bursitis, osteomyelitis, crystal-induced arthropathy.
Clinical findings	Pain and decreased range of motion. Usually low grade fever. Involvement of knee > hip - shoulder > wrist, ankle, elbow, interphalangial. Involvement of sacro-iliac and sternoclavicular joints with IV drug users. Polyarticular involvement in 10 % (especially in men with rheumatoid arthritis: also associated with diabetes, steroids and SLE): viral arthritis is typically polyarticular.
Causes	**Acute bacterial arthritis :** - *Staphylococcus aureus* most frequent. - Group A streptococcus (or group B in diabetics). - Gram neg. rods with elderly or immunosuppressed patients: *Pseudomonas aeruginosa* in IV drug users, brucellosis in immigrants (sacro-iliac, knee, hip). - Gonococcus with adults < 40 y.o. sexually active with multiple partners, gonococcal infections disseminated with migratory arthritis and knees, hands, wrists, feet predominant tenosynovitis, maculo-papular cutaneous lesions with a necrotic center (extremities); gonococcal septic arthritis follows disseminated infection most of the time; cultures of articular fluid ⊕ < 40 % of cases; blood cultures often negative. Genital and pharyngeal cultures are specimens of choice. - *Pasteurella multocida* after cat or dog bites. *Eikenella corrodens* after human bites. - Lyme disease: caused by *Borrelia burgdorferi*. History of travel to the North-Eastern United Sates and bite from May to August, erythema migrans in 80% 3-30 days post-tick fever and arthritis in weeks to many months after onset of initial symptoms. Fluctuating arthritis. Involvement of heart as well as the nervous system (neuropathy, meningitis ...) also occurs. **Chronic monoarticular arthritis :** *Mycobacterium tuberculosis, M. kansasii, M. marinarum.* Fungi: sporotrichosis, coccidioidomycosis, blastomycosis, *Candida* sp.. **Viral arthritis :** Parvovirus B19, hepatitis B and C, rubella, mumps, LCM, HIV, chikungunya ...
Workup	– ↑ ESR and C-reactive protein. – Synovial fluid: purulent, turbid or serosanguinous: WBC > 2 x 10 ^{9}/L up to > 50 x 10 ^{9}/L: Gram stain ⊕ in 50 %. – Serology for Lyme disease: ⊕ 4-6 weeks after infection. – Draw blood cultures (⊕ in 1/3). LP if neurological symptoms. If gonococcus, perform pharyngeal, rectal, urethral and cervical swabs. – If mycobacteria/fungi suspected, culture synovial tissue. – Joint X-ray, CT or MRI as needed. – Consultation in orthopedics surgery.
Treatment	Depending on Gram stain : - For Gram ⊕ cocci in clusters: cloxacillin (vancomycin if allergic, with prosthesis or resistance to methicillin). - For Gram ⊕ cocci in chains: penicillin or cephalosporin (if allergic to penicillin, clindamycin or vancomycin). For Gram neg. organisms: 3rd generation cephalosporin, imipenem or ticarcillin/clavulanate or piperacillin/tazobactam. If Gram non-contributory: - Cloxacillin (or vancomycin) + 3rd gen cephalosporin until culture results.

	- If risk factor for gonococcal arthritis: ceftriaxone 1 g IV daily for 7-10 days + doxycycline or azithromycin. If bites: ticarcillin/clavulanate, piperacillin/tazobactam or ertapenem (if allergic to penicillin: clindamycin + ciprofloxacin or moxifloxacin). According to culture: - If *B.burgdorferi*: doxycyclin 100 mg bid for 1 month. If no response, 2nd cycle PO antibiotic or ceftriaxone 2 g daily for 14-28 days. If refractory, athroscopic synovectomy as needed. - If mycobacteria or fungi: treatment according to pathogen and Infectious Diseases consultation. Duration of antibiotic therapy: - 2 weeks for *Haemophilus influenzae*, Gram neg. cocci, streptococci. - 3 weeks for staphylococci or Gram neg. rods. Serial synovial fluid aspirations for the first 5-7 days: if fluid reaccumulates persistently after seven days proceed to surgical drainage. Arthritis of the hip or shoulder requires surgical drainage.
Osteomyelitis	Disease of the two extremes of age. Can occur as a complication of septic arthritis or mechanical prosthesis. Caused by hematogenous seeding (especially in the pediatric population), contiguous extension, traumatic or surgical inoculation of bacteria. Classified as chronic or acute osteomyelitis.
Clinical findings	Fever, chills, malaise, local pain, edema.
Causes	– *Staphylococcus aureus* most frequent. – *Pseudomonas aeruginosa* (with permanent urinary catheter, IV drug use, "mal perforans" foot ulcer, penetrating trauma), *Pasteurella multocida* (cat/dog bites), anaerobic flora (vascular insufficiency, diabetes or decubitus ulcers), fungi (IV drug use, prolonged neutropenia). – With immunosuppression or sickle-cell anemia: S*almonella* sp.. – With foreign body: coagulase neg. *Staphylococcus*, *Propionibacterium acnes*. – With soil contamination = *Clostridium* sp., *Bacillus* sp., *Nocardia* sp. – With water contamination = *Aeromonas hydrophila* or *P. aeruginosa*.
Diagnosis	– ESR/C-reactive protein (if normal: osteomyelitis unlikely). – Bone radiography: cortical destruction after > 2 weeks. – Technetium scan: sensitive but not specific. Radio-labelled WBC scan: higher specificity but lower sensitivity (difficult to distinguish from cellulitis). Gallium scan: small number of studies. – CT or MRI: good diagnostic modalities, especially for vertebral infection. – Pre-treatment biopsy for precise diagnosis (except with diabetic foot).
Treatment	General principles: vertebral osteomyelitis usually does not require surgery; chronic osteomyelitis requires surgical treatment; prosthetic infections usually require surgical removal of foreign material. For *S. aureus*: penicillin if sensitive (rare); cloxacillin or cefazolin if sensitive to methicillin; vancomycin if methicillin resistant; adding rifampin is optional (encouraged if foreign body removal impossible). For *Streptococcus* sp.: penicillin, ceftriaxone or cefotaxime. For *Pseudomonas aeruginosa*: ciprofloxacin or ceftazidime ± tobramycin for 2 weeks. Adjustment according to sensitivities. For mixed flora: piperacillin/tazobactam or ticarcillin/clavulanate, imipenem or clindamycin + ciprofloxacin. Optimal length of treatment not defined: 6 weeks suggested. For vertebral osteomyelitis: surgery reserved for complications (spinal cord compression, spinal instability, and abscess) or treatment failure.

Urinary Tract Infection

Most frequent bacterial infection.

Clinical manifestations:
- **Cystitis:** Dysuria, urgency, supra-pubic pain with cloudy urine, foul-smelling urine or hematuria. In women, when dysuria and frequency are present in the absence of vaginal symptoms → the probability of cystitis = 90%.
- **Uncomplicated pyelonephritis:** fever, chills, nausea, vomiting, diarrhea ± cystitis symptoms. Altered level of consciousness in elderly. Costovertebral angle tenderness sometimes ⊕.
- **Complicated pyelonephritis:** When acute pyelonephritis is associated with structural or functional abnormalities (obstruction, stone, reflux, neurological disease), to urological manipulation (catheter, renal transplant) or to underlying disease (diabetes, immunosuppression, polycystic kidney disease).

Differential diagnosis :
- *Prostatitis*: rule out if symptoms of cystitis in male patient: digital rectal examination painful.
- *Urethritis*: chlamydial, gonorrheal, HSV. Pyuria without hematuria. Gradual onset of symptoms, vaginal or urethral discharge (worse before first morning micturition).
- *Vaginitis*: *Candida* sp. or *Trichomonas vaginalis*. Urine culture ⊖. Vaginal discharge. No urgency or frequency

Causes	*E. coli, K. pneumoniae, P. mirabilis, E. faecalis/faecium, S. saprophyticus, S. aureus, S. epidermidis, P. aeruginosa, Candida* sp., etc. Note: *S.aureus* infection should raise possibility of bacteremia of non-renal origin. Risk of urinary infection with urinary catheter of 3-10 %/day

Management	– Asymptomatic bacteriuria: treat pregnant women, patients requiring an invasive genitourinary procedure or renal transplant patients in the early post-operative period. *Do not treat* young women (without vesico-ureretal reflux), diabetics or the institutionalized elderly.
	
	 – Acute uncomplicated cystitis in women : treat three days with TMP-SMX, or ciprofloxacin (or nitrofurantoin for 7 days)
	   - For diabetic, symptomatic > 7 days, age > 65 years, use of diaphragm or recent cystitis : consider treatment for 7 days
	   - For pregnant women: treat 7 days with amoxicillin, nitrofurantoin or TMP/SMX.
	   - If relapse after 3 days: sub-clinical pyelonephritis probable: treat for 14 days.
	
	 – Acute uncomplicated cystitis in men: treat for 7-14 days (6 weeks if persistent or recurrent).
	
	 – Pyelonephritis, complicated or not: treat in outpatient setting if not severe (no nausea or vomiting): hospitalize if severe or urosepsis possible (recommended during pregnancy). Perform blood cultures if inpatient. Urine culture in all cases.
	
	 – Acute uncomplicated pyelonephritis:
	   Ciprofloxacin or TMP/SMX (according to local resistance level).
	   Evaluate clinical response after 3 days:
	   - If OK, continue treatment.
	   - If no response: consider resistance and abscess formation (imaging studies to be done)
	
	 – Acute complicated pyelonephritis: ampicillin + gentamicin or fluoroquinolone (ciprofloxacin or levofloxacin, no moxifloxacin since not excreted in urine) with early adjustment of antibiotherapy according to culture results:
	   - For *Enterococcus* sp.: ampicillin or amoxicillin (for penicillin-allergic patients, vancomycin).
	   - For Gram neg. rods: stop ampicillin and continue ciprofloxacin or gentamicin.
	   → Immediate imaging studies if severe (hypotension) or if stone suspected:
	      → If ⊕ = consultation with urologist as needed (nephrostomy tube).
	      → If ⊖: assess response to treatment: consider resistance ± perform CT

	if no response (to rule out abscess).
	– Pyelonephritis during pregnancy: treatment as above with ceftriaxone, gentamicin ± ampicillin, aztreonam or TMP/SMX IV then amoxicillin, cephalosporin or TMP/SMX PO (to be avoided during the third trimester). Length of treatment for pyelonephritis = 14 days (or 7 days if "mild" pyelonephritis treated with fluoroquinolone). Treatment for 21 days is an option for severe pyelonephritis. Treatment for 6 weeks if prostatitis or underlying polycystic kidney disease. Perform urine culture 2 weeks after the end of treatment of pyelonephritis if patient is pregnant, has history of recurrent pyelonephritis, is immunosuppressed or after complicated acute pyelonephritis. Pregnancy test in all women of childbearing age. Take into consideration interactions between antibiotics and oral contraceptives!
Recurrence	If cystitis relapses early (i.e.: same pathogen): rule out occult source of infection or urological lesion: prolonged treatment (2-6 weeks). For reinfection cystitis (i.e.: different pathogen) : ...and diaphragm or spermicide use: change method of contraception. If ≥ 3 infections/year and no relation with sexual intercourse: prophylaxis daily or 3x/week with TMP/SMX, nitrofurantoin or ciprofloxacin. If ≥ 3 infections/year and relation to intercourse: postcoital prophylaxis with TMP/SMX, nitrofurantoin or ciprofloxacin. If < 3 infections/year: treat only symptomatic episodes.

Upper Respiratory Tract Infection, Influenza and ENT Infections

Viral Infection of Upper Respiratory Tract	The common cold may be caused by more than 200 viruses: rhinovirus (more frequent), respiratory syncytial virus, parainfluenza, adenovirus, metapneumovirus, coronavirus, etc. Clinical findings: acute rhinitis, fever (< 10 % of cases in adults), cough, malaise, mild headache. Average duration: 7 days. No work-up necessary. Symptomatic treatment (analgesia, nasal vaporization, antitussives). No antibiotics!
Influenza	Infection caused by RNA viruses, appearing generally between December and end of March. Responsible for ± 5000 deaths annually in Canada. 90 % in people ≥ 65 years old. 3 types of influenza: Type A (responsible for pandemics), Type B and Type C (which is rarely pathogenic in humans). Droplets are the most frequent mode of transmission. Incubation period 1-4 days. Could be contagious 2 days before and up to 5 days after symptoms. **Clinical findings:** Sudden-onset fever, myalgia, cough, headache, sore throat, nasal congestion, chills, malaise, and ocular symptoms. Possible viral complications: viral complications (viral pneumonia) or secondary bacterial (*S. pneumoniae* superinfection, *H. influenzae*, *S. aureus,* typically after transient improvement). Other complications: rhabdomyolysis, Guillain-Barré syndrome. ↑ risk of complication in older patients, in patients with heart disease or chronic pulmonary diseases, asthma, cystic fibrosis, diabetes, cancer, CKD, etc. Respiratory syncytial virus (RSV), parainfluenza or adenovirus may present like influenza.

Diagnosis: Quick antigen influenza test (Influenza A and B) and PCR. Viral culture of nasopharynx secretions for epidemiological purposes. Leukocytosis (up to 15×10^9/L) frequent or leucopenia. CK ↑ can occur.

Treatment: Neuraminidase inhibitors (oseltamivir *per os*, inhaled zanamivir) for 5 days. It is essential to start treatment < 48 hours after onset of symptoms. Oseltamivir to be adjusted in case of renal insufficiency, zanamivir contraindicated in asthmatic patients. Prophylaxis for contacts at high risk of complication.
To be kept in respiratory isolation up to 5 days after onset of symptoms.
Oseltamivir resistance is now a concern.

Prevention: Vaccine indicated for patients over 60 or patients at high risk of complications (cardiac disease or chronic pulmonary disease, diabetes, cancer, immunosuppression, nephropathy) or patients who may transmit influenza to patients at risk (health center workers, day-care workers).
Effective in 80-85 % of healthy adults (after 2 weeks), in about 50 % in elderly.
↓ 85 % of hospitalizations and 50 % of deaths linked to influenza with vaccine.
Contraindicated if known egg allergy or vaccine-triggered anaphylaxis.
WHO guidelines suggest both droplets and contact precautions (still controversial).

Pharyngitis	Etiology: Viral (90 % of cases: adenovirus, coronavirus, adenovirus, influenza, enterovirus, EBV, HSV, HIV, measles, etc), bacterial (group A, other ß-hemolytic streptococci, diphtheria, meningococcus, secondary syphilis, *Arcanobacterium haemolyticum, Fusobacterium necrophorum*). *Mycoplasma, Chlamydophilia* or fungi. Exudative pharyngitis is in general due to group A streptococcus (or EBV, HSV, diphtheria, *Candida, Fusobacterium*).

Clinical: Sore throat. Presence of rhinitis, conjunctivitis, cough, and diarrhea suggest viral etiology. Winter or springtime infection with a history of contact, sudden fever, headaches, abdominal pain, exudates, anterior cervical lymphadenopathy and a scarlatiniform rash is compatible with group A streptococcus, though not diagnostic.

Differential diagnosis of throat pain: peritonsilar abscess (with trismus), epiglottitis (see below), infectious mononucleosis, parapharyngeal infections.

Workup: Quick antigenic test or throat culture if high probability of group A streptococcus.
Throat culture for gonococcus if suspected.
As needed: Monotest ± specific serology for EBV, HIV or others.

Complications: With untreated group A streptococcus pharyngitis, possible risk of acute rheumatic fever (approx. 3 %), occurring mostly 19 days after pharyngitis. Acute glomerulonephritis can occur, depending on strain (up to 10-15 % if nephritogenic strain). Post-streptococcus reactive arthritis can occur. *Erythema nodosum* (2-4 weeks post infection). Scarlet fever, toxic shock, otitis media, lymphadenitis, sinusitis, or peritonsillar abscess can occur.

Treatment:
– For group A streptococcus: emergency treatment for very ill patient or patient with rheumatic heart disease. Otherwise, await culture results. Penicillin V for 10 days. For penicillin-allergic patients: macrolides, 1st generation cephalosporin (cefadroxil or cephalexin). Clinical response to antibiotics within 24 hours in general.
– For non group A streptococcus: no treatment in general.

No indication to culture or treat asymptomatic contacts except in rare cases.

Acute Rhinosinusitis	Etiology: viral (80 % of cases: rhinovirus, influenza, parainfluenza) or bacterial (*S. pneumoniae*, *H. influenzae*, *S. aureus*, *M. catarrhalis*, goup A streptococcus, anaerobes). Nosocomial sinusitis with nasal obstruction by nasogastric tube or nasotracheal tube. Mucormycosis to be considered in a patient with diabetic keto-acidosis, neutropenia, renal failure or on desferroxamine.
	Clinical findings: facial pain, fever, purulent nasal discharge. Headache, nasal obstruction, anosmia.
	Diagnosis: clinical: sinus X-ray as needed (may show an air-fluid level, sinus opacification, mucosal thickening > 5 mm). Sinus CT sometimes useful, especially with chronic sinusitis refractory to treatment, in immunosuppressed patients or if intracranial complications or orbital mucormycosis suspicion. Nasal endoscopy if symptoms remain despite treatment or recurrent sinusitis. Direct aspiration of sinuses in patients not responding to initial treatment, in immunosuppressed patients, or in nosocomial sinusitis, etc.
	Treatment: Symptomatic if low probability of bacterial cause (if ≤ 1 of 3 following criteria: upper respiratory tract infection > 7 days, facial pain, purulent discharge) with nasal mucolytic agent, decongestant, antihistamine and intra-nasal steroid. Antibiotic therapy indicated if high likelihood of bacterial etiology (if ≥ 2/3 of above mentioned criteria) or if failure of symptomatic treatment after 7-10 days. Treat with amoxicillin, TMP/SMX, clavulanic acid/amoxicillin, 2nd generation cephalosporin, macrolides, fluoroquinolones ... combined with a decongestant (oxymetazoline intra-nasal for 2-3 days, pseudoephedrin PO). Nasal topical steroids sometimes useful. Duration of antibiotic therapy: 10-14 days (depending on antibiotic). ENT consultation if no response.
Otitis	Otitis **media**: bacterial infection of middle ear usually brought on by an upper respiratory tract viral infection causing auditory canal edema, resulting in liquid and mucus accumulation, superinfected with bacteria. Rare in adults, more frequent in patients with diabetes or cystic fibrosis. Causes earache, pressure in the ear, frequent fever ± hearing loss. In examination: erythema and ↓ mobility of tympanic membrane. Diagnostic tympanocentesis to be performed in immunosuppressed host or if infection persistent or recurrent.
	Otitis **externa**: superficial infection of the external auditory canal, causing pain, pruritus, exudate, erythema, edema of the canal, discharge. Tympanic membrane moves well (as opposed to otitis media). Frequent in swimmers.
	Malignant external otitis: *Pseudomonas aeruginosa* severe infection associated with high mortality (20 %). Seen in diabetic older patient. May extend to deep tissues and to bony structures. Frequent facial nerve paralysis. To be suspected in patients with diabetes and who do not respond to topical treatment. Diagnosis is difficult to establish. CT sometimes useful.
	Treatment: – Otitis media: antibiotic therapy (amoxicillin, 2nd generation cephalosporin) often combined with nasal decongestant. Myringotomy if severe earache or complicated otitis (mastoiditis, meningitis). – Otitis externa: Topical treatment. Canal cleansing ± antibiotic drops. If there is significant canal edema, insert cotton wickdipped in Burrow's solution. If concomitant cellulitis, systemic antibiotic. – Malignant otitis externa: hospitalization and antipseudomonal antibiotics (e.g.: ticarcillin + tobramycin). Consultation with ENT ± Infectious Diseases suggested. Treat for 4-6 weeks, according to antibiotic sensitivities. For early malignant external otitis that is not too severe, treatment with ciprofloxacin can be considered.

Epiglottitis	Severe and acute cellulitis of the epiglottis and adjacent tissues usually caused by *H. influenzae* type b (rarely by *H. parainfluenzae* or β-hemolytic streptococci). Very rare since *H. influenzae* type b universal vaccination. Occurs most frequently in children between 3-7 years old, sometimes in adults. **Clinical:** Sudden fever, sore throat and systemic toxicity. Odynophagia. Hoarseness. Obstruction of respiratory tract is rare in adults. The patient assumes the sitting position, remains bent forward, with mouth open, and drools. Edema of pharynx with secretions. Oropharyngeal examination sometimes normal in adults. **Diagnosis:** Through visualization of epiglottis by qualified personnel. Lateral X-ray of soft tissues sometimes useful in less severe cases. Leukocytosis. Blood culture to be done. **Treatment**: Potential medical emergency. Immediate transfer to a hospital. Antibiotics IV STAT with cephalosporin 2nd and 3rd generations (if allergy: respiratory fluoroquinolone). Antibiotic total duration: 10-14 days. Surveillance of airway during hospitalization (bedside tracheostomy equipment). Adjuvant steroid useful? Intubation if dyspnea or quick progression of sore throat.

Community-Acquired Pneumonia

Clinical findings: fever and respiratory symptoms: more often atypical in elderly.

Risk factors for community-acquired pneumonia (CAP): Advanced age, tobacco, alcoholism, malnutrition, chronic disease (COPD, cystic fibrosis, heart failure, cirrhosis, diabetes), intravenous drug users, anatomic or functional asplenia, immunosuppression: HIV, congenital (hypogammaglobulinemia), chronic kidney disease, nephrotic syndrome, leukemia, lymphoma, multiple myeloma, chemotherapy, transplantation.

Differential diagnosis: heart failure, pulmonary embolism, cancer, sarcoidosis, drug reaction, pulmonary hemorrhage, cryptogenic organizing pneumonia (COP), eosinophilic pneumonia, aspiration pneumonitis, etc.

Causes	> 100 causes of pneumonia. 50 % of pneumonias requiring hospitalisation are of unknown etiology (no pathogen isolated).
	S. pneumoniae: Gram ⊕ diplococcus. Specific risk factors: military barracks, diabetic ketoacidosis, alcoholism, COPD, organ transplant, sickle-cell anemia, myeloma, HIV. Brownish sputum. 10-20 % penicillin resistant. Vaccine available. *H. influenzae*: Gram neg. coccobacillus. In transplant patients, HIV. *Legionella pneumophila*: exposure to air-conditioning, outbreaks. In transplant patients, diabetics, COPD, elderly. Consider in severe cases of pneumonia. May have neurologic and gastrointestinal manifestations, bradycardia, hyponatremia, rhabdomyolysis… *Mycoplasma pneumoniae*: Frequent pathogen in young or ambulatory patients. Presents with predominant cough, low grade fever, pharyngitis, bullous myringitis, encephalitis, hepatitis, hemolytic anemia and erythema multiforme. History can reveal index case. Spontaneous resolution in 2-6 weeks. *Chlamydophila pneumoniae*: In military barracks. Associated with pharyngitis and erythema nodosum: atypical pneumonia, splenomegaly, neutropenia. *C. psittaci*: exposure to birds, ducks and turkeys. *S. aureus*: Gram ⊕ cocci in clusters. With diabetic ketoacidosis, alcoholism, post-influenza. Severe pneumonia complicated with abscesses. *K. pneumoniae*: Large Gram neg. rod: in alcoholics. *Moraxella catarrhalis*: Gram neg. intracellular diplococcus: with COPD. *Pseudomonas aeruginosa*: Severe pneumonia. With cystic fibrosis, bronchiectasis and immunosuppression. *Coxiella burnetti* (Q fever): Exposure to infected parturient cat, sheep, goat. Atypical pneumonia of variable severity, endocarditis, hepatitis, ↑ aPTT. *Anaerobes*: Periodontal disease and poor buccal hygiene. Infection of right lung > left. Empyema ⊕. *Virus*: Influenza (autumn - winter), respiratory syncytial virus, adenovirus, varicella, hantavirus (very rare and severe). **Chronic** pneumonia if symptoms > 1 month: fungi or tuberculosis. *Nocardia sp.*: Cutaneous nodules and central nervous system involvement may occur. *M. tuberculosis*: In prisoners or homeless, immigrants, HIV exposure, sometimes erythema nodosum ⊕. *Fungal pneumonia*: coccidioidomycosis (Arizona desert), histoplasmosis (diffuse disease), blastomycosis (cutaneous involvement): opportunistic fungi (*Cryptococcus* sp., *Aspergillus* sp., *Candida* sp.). *P. jiroveci* pneumonia (formely *P.carinii*) with HIV or chronic steroid therapy. **Recurrent** pneumonia: with bronchiectasis, bronchial obstruction, aspiration (underlying conditions: esophageal diverticulum, achalasia, esophageal or gastric motility disorder, tracheo-esophageal fistula), immune disorder (↓ immunoglobulins), bronchopulmonary sequestration.
Workup	– Standard workup: CBC, electrolytes, creatinine, hepatic enzymes, INR, aPTT, arterial blood gas or oxymetry, Chest X-ray. – Two blood cultures drawn for all hospitalized patients. – Sputum Gram stain and culture. – Pleural tap as needed (pH, proteins, LDH, pleural and plasma glucose, cell count, Gram stain ± auramine or Ziehl-Neelsen, bacterial culture ± fungi ± mycobacteria). – Serology as needed: *M. pneumoniae*, *L. pneumophila*, *C. pneumoniae/psittaci*, adenovirus, RSV, influenza, fungi … Cold agglutinins as needed (50 % ⊕ with mycoplasma however non specific and not recommended). – Urinary antigen detection for *L. pneumophila* serogroup 1 if severe pneumonia or severe immunosuppression. – Urinary antigen detection for pneumococcus if available. – Consider HIV serology. – Invasives procedures as needed, especially with fulminant pneumonia, immunosuppressed patient (e.g.: severe neutropenia) or lack of response to treatment: bronchoscopy with bronchoalveolar lavage ± protected brushing, transthoracic needle aspiration, open lung biopsy.

Management	Evaluation of disease seriousness with following score "**CURB-65**" **C:** **C**onfusion. **U:** ↑ **U**rea (BUN) > 7 mmol/L. **R:** **R**espiratory rate ≥ 30/minute. **B:** **B**lood Pressure: systolic BP < 90 mmHg or diastolic BP ≤ 60 mmHg. **65:** age **65** or older. If 0-1: out-patient treatment. If 2 : in-patient treatment If ≥ 3, intensive care unit. Note: Score is to be used along with clinical judgment, taking into account patient's compliance, home support, etc.

Empiric treatment of community acquired pneumonia	In accordance with the 2007 IDSA/ATS Guidelines.
	
	– Outpatient treatment:
	  1. Previously healthy and no use of antibiotics within the previous 3 months: use as 1st choice: **macrolide**, 2nd choice: **doxycycline (but see point 3).**
	  2. In patients with underlying conditions such as chronic heart, lung, liver or renal disease, diabetes, alcoholism, cancer, asplenia, immunosuppression, or use of antimicrobials within the previous 3 months (in which case an alternative from a different class should be selected), use a **respiratory fluoroquinolone** (moxifloxacin or levofloxacin 750 mg) or a **ß-lactam** (amoxicillin/clavunalic acid or cefuroxime axetil) + **macrolide**.
	  3. In areas where > 25 % of strains of pneumococcus have high-level (MIC ≥ 16 µg/mL) macrolide resistance, consider use of alternative agents listed above in point 2 for patients without underlying conditions. **In Québec, this rate is often over 25 %.** Prior exposure to macrolides increases significantly the risk of resistance.
	
	– Inpatients, non-ICU treatment:
	  Respiratory fluoroquinolone or ß-lactam (cefuroxime, ceftriaxone, cefotaxime) **+ macrolide**.
	
	– Inpatients, ICU treatment:
	  ß-lactam (cefotaxime or ceftriaxone) + either azithromycin IV or "respiratory" fluoroquinolone IV (for penicillin-allergic patients, respiratory fluoroquinolone + aztreonam).
	
	– If *Pseudomonas* is a consideration:
	  Antipneumococcal antipseudomonal ß-lactam (piperacillin/tazobactam, cefepime, imipenem, meropenem) **+ either ciprofloxacin or levofloxacin** (750 mg) *or* **antipseudomonal ß-lactam + aminoglycoside + azithromycin** *or* **antipseudomonal ß-lactam + aminoglycoside + antipneumococcal fluoroquinolone** (for penicillin-allergic patients, substitute aztreonam for above ß-lactam).
	
	– If community-acquired MRSA is a consideration: add vancomycin or linezolid.
	
	– If macro-aspiration suspected: 1st choice: amoxicillin/clavunalic acid, timentin/tazocin if IV or moxifloxacin. 2nd choice: cefuroxime axetil + either clindamycin or metronidazole.
	
	– For pneumonia acquired in a nursing home: *S. pneumoniae,* coliforms, *H. influenzae*: 1st choice: **respiratory fluoroquinolone alone or amoxicillin/clavunalate + macrolide.** 2nd choice: **2nd generation cephalosporin + macrolide.**
	  → If hospitalized: similar to any other hospitalized patient.
	
	Note: Despite published guidelines, the best approach remains to rely on local profiles of

	reisistance and then try to identify the pathogen (Gram stain and sputum culture) and rapidly tailor the treatment accordingly. The emergence of resistance, the side effects of antibiotics and the risk for *C. difficile* colitis are some of the considerations behind this approach. – If no response to treatment within 3-5 days: consider bronchoscopy. – Parapneumonic effusion: thoracentesis if significant (> 10 mm on lateral decubitus) or no response to treatment: chest tube if pH < 7.2 (complicated pleural effusion). – Resolution: afebrile in 3-4 days. Radiological resolution normally occurs in 4 weeks in an otherwise healthy patient: 12 weeks or more if > 50 y.o. ± COPD or alcoholism. – Repeat chest X-ray in 7-12 weeks if cancer suspected, > 60 y.o., smoker or with constitutional symptoms. – Anti-pneumococcal vaccine for patients > 65 years and those with chronic diseases, whatever their age.

Treatment of community acquired pneumonia (CAP) according to pathogen	– *S. pneumoniae*:
	    Penicillin sensitive (CMI < 0.1 mg/L): penicillin, amoxicillin, cephalosporin.
	    Intermediate resistance (CMI ≤ 0.1-1 mg/L): amoxicillin (500-1000 mg tid) or cefuroxime axetil (500 mg PO bid).
	    High-level resistance (CMI ≥ 2 mg/L): high-dose penicillin G (3 MU every 4 h IV), cefotaxime (1-2 g IV every 8 h) or ceftriaxone (1-2 g IV every 24 h) or respiratory fluoroquinolone.
	    High-level resistance (with concurrent meningitis): vancomycin or respiratory fluoroquinolone.
	    Length of treatment for CAP with *S.pneumoniae* can be reduced to 3 days once fever is resolved (IDSA).
	– *H. influenzae*: ß-lactamase ⊖: ampicillin IV, amoxicillin, TMP/SMX, macrolides.
	– *H. influenzae* ß-lactamase ⊕: cephalosporin 2nd-3rd or ß-lactam/ß-lactamase inhibitor, respiratory fluoroquinolone, azithromycin or clarithromycin.
	– *M. catarrhalis*: cephalosporin 2nd-3rd-or ß-lactam/ß-lactamase inhibitor or macrolide.
	– Respiratory anaerobes: ß-lactam/ß-lactamase inhibitor or moxifloxacin, 3rd-gen fluoroquinolone (i.e.: levofloxacin) + metronidazole or 3rd-gen cephalosporin + metronidazole.
	– *S. aureus*:
	    Methicillin sensitive: cloxacillin, cefazolin.
	    Methicillin resistant : vancomycin, linezolid.
	– Coliforms: ß-lactam/ß-lactamase inhibitor, carbapenem, 3rd-4th-gen. cephalosporin. If wide-spectrum ß-lactamase: carbapenem, cefepime or ciprofloxacin.
	– *P. aeruginosa*: antipseudomonal β-lactam + ciprofloxacin or antipseudomonal aminoglycoside.
	– Legionella: fluoroquinolone or macrolide ± rifampin.
	– *C. pneumoniae*: macrolide, doxycycline or fluoroquinolone.
	– *M. pneumoniae*: macrolide, doxycycline or fluoroquinolone.
	– *C. Burnetii* (Q fever): doxycycline or erythromycin.
	
	In general, length of treatment is at least 5 days for a patient who has been afebrile for 48-72 hours and is clinically stable, depending on pathogen and type of antibiotic used.

Prognosis	See chart on next page.

Prognosis Model for Patients with Community-Acquired Pneumonia

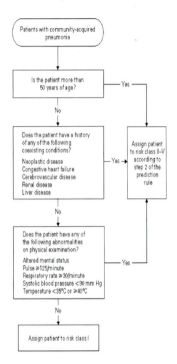

This model can help the clinician choose an initial intervention decision but may not be applicable to all patients. The clinician must rely on his/her judgment. From Fine MJ, Auble TE, Yearly DM et al. A prediction rule to identify low-risk patient with community-acquired pneumonia. *N Engl J Med* 1997;336:243-50.

Scoring system

Patient characteristics	Points assigned[1]
Demographic factors	
Age : men	age (in years)
women	age (in years) -10
Nursing home resident	+ 10
Coexisting illnesses	
Neoplastic disease	+ 30
Liver disease	+ 20
Congestive heart failure	+ 10
Cerebrovascular disease	+ 10
Renal disease	+ 10
Physical examination findings	
Altered mental status	+ 20
Respiratory rate ≥ 30/minute	+ 20
Systolic BP < 90 mmHg	+ 20
Temperature < 35 °C or ≥ 40 °C	+ 15
Pulse ≥ 125/minute	+ 10
Laboratory and radiographic findings	
pH < 7.35	+ 30
Uree > 10.7 mmol/L	+ 20
Sodium <130 mEq/L	+ 20
Glucose > 13.9 mmol/L	+ 10
Hematocrit < 30 %	+ 10
PO_2 < 60 mmHg[2]	+ 10
Pleural effusion	+ 10

[1] The patient's risk score is obtained by summing the patient's age in years (age minus 10 for women) and the points for each applicable characteristic.
[2] An oxygen saturation < 90 % is also considered abnormal.

Mortality rate from pneumonia according to risk class

Validation cohort

Risk class	Score	Number of patients	Mortality (%)
I	No risk factors	3 034	0.1
II	≤ 70	5 778	0.6
III	71-90	6 790	2.8
IV	91-130	13 104	8.2
V	> 130	9 333	29.2

Hospital-Acquired Pneumonia

Definition: pneumonia occuring ≥ 48 hours after admission.
Nosocomial infection associated with greatest morbidity and mortality. 33 to 50 % mortality attributed to infection.

Sub-categories:
- Hospital-acquired pneumonia: developing ≥ 48 hours after hospital admission.
- Early hospital-acquired pneumonia: < 5 days, late onset: ≥ 5 days.
- Ventilator-associated pneumonia: developing ≥ 48 hours after intubation.
- Healthcare-associated pneumonia: ≥ 2 days hospital stay within the past 90 days; living in a long-term care facility; outpatient intravenous therapy (like chemotherapy or antibiotics); home wound care within the past 30 days; or attending a hospital clinic or dialysis center in the past 30 days.

Risk factors: endotracheal intubation, mechanical ventilation (risk of pneumonia 3%/day during first 5 days of mechanical ventilation, 2%/day between day 5 and day 10 and 1 %/day afterwards), microaspiration.

Risk factors	Risk factors for multidrug-resistant hospital-acquired pneumonia : antimicrobial therapy in preceding 90 days, current hospitalization of 5 days or more, high frequency of antibiotic resistance in the community or in the specific hospital unit, presence of risk factors for healthcare-associated pneumonia (hospitalization for 2 days or more in the preceding 90 days, residence in a nursing home or extended care facility, home IV therapy-including antibiotics, chronic dialysis within 30 days, home wound care, family member with multidrug-resistant pathogen), immunosuppressive disease and/or therapy. **Risk factors** for specific pathogens: **Anaerobes** = aspiration or recent abdominal surgery: ***S. aureus*** = coma, head trauma, diabetes, renal failure: ***Legionella pneumophila*** = high dose steroids: ***P. aeruginosa*** = prolonged intensive care stay, steroids, antibiotics, structural lung disease. With pneumonia occuring early (< 5 days) without risk factors for multi-drug resistant pathogens: caused by the following pathogens: *Enterobacter* sp., *E. coli, Klebsiella* sp., *Proteus* sp., *Serratia* sp., *H. influenzae, S. aureus, S. pneumoniae.* If pneumonia with risk factors for multi-drug resistant pathogens or late-onset severe pneumonia (≥ 5 days): suspect pathogens listed above + *P. aeruginosa, Acinetobacter* sp., methicillin resistant *S. aureus* (MRSA) and *L. pneumophila.*
Workup	– CBC, electrolytes, creatinine, liver enzymes, sputum, chest X-ray, two blood cultures, arterial blood gas or oxymetry. – Thoracentesis if effusion > 10 mm or patient appears toxic. – Bronchoscopy as needed with bronchoalveolar lavage (⊕ if > 10^4 *colony-forming unit*/mL) or bronchial brushings (⊕ if > 10^3 *colony-forming units*/mL).
Treatment	Definition of acuteness: admission to ICU, respiratory failure (PaO_2 < 60 mmHg with FIO_2 > 35 %, except COPD), severe sepsis with hypotension or evidence of organ dysfunction (shock, inotropes required > 4 h, oliguria, dialysis), progression, cavitation or multilobar infection. Admit to the ICU if: O_2 saturation < 90 % with FIO_2 ≥ 50 %, mechanical ventilation, inotropic support, frequent supervision by nursing staff required. Begin an antibiotic empirically in the presence of a new or progressive radiographic infiltrate plus at least two of three clinical features (fever > 38°C, leukocytosis or leukopenia, and purulent secretions): – If pneumonia occuring < 5 days after admission without risk factors for multi-drug resistant pathogens: empirical treatment suggested: **ceftriaxone or respiratory fluoroquinolone or ertapenem.** – If pneumonia ≥ 5 days after admission **or** risk factors for multi-drug resistant

	pathogens: empirical treatment suggested: **antipseudomonal cephalosporin or imipenem/meropenem or ß-lactam/ß-lactamase inhibitor + either antipseudomonal fluoroquinolones (ciprofloxacin or levofloxacin) or an aminoglycoside.** ⇒ If MRSA suspected or locally prevalent, add vancomycin (alternative = linezolid). ⇒ If *L. pneumophila* suspected: include a macrolide or a fluoroquinolone rather than an aminoglycoside. Length of treatment: 8 days, except for *Pseudomonas aeruginosa* or *Acinetobacter* sp. (because ↑ risk of recurrence) where a 14-day treatment is recommended.
Prevention	Strategies to lower risk of nosocomial pneumonia in intubated patients: raise head of bed 30-45°, check position of feeding tube, reduce duration of intubation (noninvasive positive-pressure ventilation if needed) and blood transfusions, control hyperglycemia, prevent ongoing aspiration of sub-glottic secretions.

Tuberculosis

- Infection caused by *Mycobacterium tuberculosis*.
- Population at risk: immunosuppressed (AIDS, HIV, CKD/hemodialysis, organ transplant, other), silicosis, head and neck tumor, diabetic, immigrant, First Nations, homeless, IV drug users, prisoners, contact with tuberculosis, elderly, living in an area with high prevalence, healthcare workers, HIV, alcoholism, steroids (> 15 mg, > 2 weeks), gastrectomy, malnutrition, radiotherapy, recent tuberculin skin test conversion.
- Recrudescence with HIV.
- Tuberculosis (TB) is multidrug-resistant if resistant to > 1 anti-TB agent.
- Classified as either active tuberculosis if the patient has symptoms or latent tuberculosis if tuberculin skin test ⊕ without evidence of active disease.
- Active disease can be *primary* if no evidence of active TB in the past or *reactivation* if there is a history of active TB in the past followed by a period of inactivity.

Clinical findings	- Primary infection is usually asymptomatic. - Systemic hematogenous dissemination. - 90 % of TB patients have reactivation disease of latent infection. - Fatigue, ↓ weight, anorexia, night sweats, fever. Pulmonary symptoms are usually insidious and chronic (cough, hemoptysis, dyspnea, chest pain). Atypical presentation more frequent in HIV/older patient. - Occasionally extra-pulmonary manifestations: lymph nodes, genitourinary, skeletal, miliary, central nervous system, abdominal, pericardial ...
Screening	Tuberculin skin test (PPD 5TU) 0.1 mL intradermal, read within 48-72 hours. Positive if: - ≥ 5 mm in the following: HIV* patient or at risk for HIV; close contact with an active case of tuberculosis; Chest X-ray compatible with old TB; immunosuppression (prednisone > 15 mg/d). - ≥ 10 mm otherwise. * In patients with HIV living in populations with very high prevalence of tuberculosis, any reaction between 0 and 4 mm can be considered positive. Repeat tuberculin skin test during pre-employment screening to avoid the "booster" effect. - False negatives with anergy secondary to HIV, viral infection, recent vaccination, malnutrition, chronic kidney disease, sarcoidosis, steroids. - False positives with non-tuberculous mycobacteria or previous BCG vaccination (rarely > 10 mm after 2 years).

	Note: conversion requires 3-7 weeks: repeat as needed if recent contact.
Diagnosis	– Sputum: culture morning sputum daily x 3 + acid-fast (AFB, Ziehl-Neelsen) smear or auramine-rhodamine (to evaluate contagiousness). Sputum induction as needed.
	– Bronchoscopy with broncho-alveolar lavage ± transbronchial biopsy.
	– Gastric aspiration for culture. Blood cultures for tuberculosis. Bone marrrow cultures, urine culture, pleural fluid culture (25 % ⊕)...as needed. Pleural biopsy and culture, bone marrow biopsy and liver biopsy.
	– Needle aspiration of nodule or mass lesion.
	– Culture (with sensitivities) in 3-4 weeks. Use of PCR allows rapid identification of AFB ⊕ samples but with AFB ⊖ samples, it is less sensitive than culture.
	– Chest X-ray: With reactivation, apical fibrosis and cavitation are seen. Atypical involvement pattern with HIV.
	– If tuberculin skin test ⊕: rule out active infection with culture and chest X-ray.
	– Always identify contacts of patients with active disease.
	– Reportable infectious disease and compulsory treatment.
	– Ask for HIV test within 2 months of a diagnosis of TB.
Treatment	Treatment of **"latent"** infection: treatment with isoniazid 300 mg daily for 9 months or rifampin 600 mg daily for 4 months or rifampicin + pyrazinamide for 2 months (for HIV patients only, because fatal hepatitis reported in immunocompetent patients). Isoniazid treated patients must be advised of symptoms/signs of hepatitis and transaminases must be measured every 1-2 months.
	Treatment of **active** disease: **isolation if AFB smear on sputum positive**, confirmed TB or suspected TB: follow sputum until three consecutive ⊖ samples on 3 separate days: stop isolation if clinical improvement and three ⊖ AFB smears. Patients with multi-drug resistant tuberculosis must remain in isolation during the whole admission due to risk of non-response or recurrence on treatment.
	Agents:
	– Isoniazid (INH): 5 mg/kg (max 300 mg) daily or 15mg/kg (max 900 mg) 2x/week. Side effects: neuropathy, hepatitis, hypersensitivity, lupus. Give pyridoxine if pregnant, epileptic or patient at risk for neuropathy (diabetic, alcoholic, CKD). Interaction with phenytoin, warfarin ...
	– Rifampicin (RIF): 10 mg/kg (max 600 mg) daily or 2x/week. Side effects: fever, hepatitis, hypersensitivity, renal insufficiency, thrombocytopenia, orange coloration of secretions. Interaction with oral contraceptives, warfarin, steroids, digoxin, phenytoin, protease inhibitors, oral antihyperglycemic agents...
	– Rifapentin (RPT): 10 mg/kg (max 600 mg) every week. Use only in non HIV patients without cavitary TB, in the continuation phase (after 2 months of RIF-INH-PZA). Side effects: same as RIF.
	– Pyrazinamide (PZA): 15-30 mg/kg (max 2 g) daily or 50-70 mg/kg (max 4 g) 2x/ week. Side effects: hepatitis, ↑ uric acid, joint pain. Teratogen.
	– Ethambutol (ETB): 15-25 mg/kg (max 2.5 g) daily or 50 mg/kg (max 2.5 g) 2x/ week. Side effects: optic neuritis (blurred vision; reversible with rapid withdrawal of medication), rash. Essential to have follow-up with ophthalmologist every month. Adjust dosage for renal failure.
	– Streptomycin (SM): 15 mg/kg (max 1 g) daily or 25-30 mg/kg (max 1.5 g) 2x/ week. Side effects: nephrotoxicity, dammage to cranial nerve VIII. Teratogen.
	– Other agents : capreomycin, kanamycin, ethionamide, para-aminosalicylic acid, cycloserine, fluoroquinolones, etc.
	Note: Combinations exist (Rifater® = INH + RIF + PZA) but are more costly.
	Treatment options :
	– INH, RIF, PZA for 8 weeks, then INH + RIF for 16 weeks. If patient from group at risk for INH resistance: add ETB or SM until sensitivity to INH + RIF is demonstrated.
	– INH + RIF + PZA daily for 2 weeks then DOT (directly observed therapy) 2x / week for 6 weeks: then INH + RIF 2x/week for 16 weeks: first line treatment with four drugs suggested if resistance is a possibility. Consult an expert if cultures remain ⊕ after 2 months.

– INH + RIF + PZA + SM or ETB via DOT 3x/ week for 6 months: consult an expert if cultures remain ⊕ after 2 months.

Chest X-ray must be done after completion of treatment.
AFB smear + sputum culture taken after 2 months of treatment. If culture ⊖, complete 6 months: if culture ⊕/without cavitation, complete 6 months, but if culture ⊕/with cavitation extend treatment to 9 months.
"Directly observed therapy (DOT)" should be standard, especially if compliance is in doubt.

For treatment failure after 2 months: consult an expert.
For tuberculosis with HIV: refer to above options but treat 6-9 months total.
For resistant or multi-drug resistant tuberculosis: ≥ 3 agents to which the strain is sensitive for 18-24 months.
For extrapulmonary tuberculosis: treatment with same agents except, 12 months for miliary, meningeal or skeletal. Steroids for pericarditis or tuberculous meningitis ± miliary.
For tuberculosis during pregnancy: avoid pyrazinamide and streptomycin (if possible), and consult an expert.

During treatment of active disease, see the patient once a month in order to assess adequate response, compliance and side effects of medication.

Infectious Mononucleosis and Mononucleosis-Like Syndrome

Infectious Mononucleosis	Epstein-Barr Virus infection (EBV), a herpesvirus. **Clinical findings:** Fever, sore throat, malaise, fatigue, headache, myalgias, diaphoresis, anorexia, chest pain, cough … Frequent prodrome 1-2 weeks. More specifically with infectious mononucleosis: pharyngitis/tonsillitis (⊕ in 80 %: quite specific for EBV), lymphadenopathy (mostly posterior cervical), hepatitis-splenomegaly, maculopapular eruption. It could also be asymptomatic (especially in children). More atypical presentation is seen in older individuals. Resolution in 1-3 weeks, but fatigue and malaise may be persistent for weeks and months. **Differential diagnosis:** CMV infection, toxoplasmosis, HIV primary infection, viral hepatitis, leptospirosis, rubella, HHV-6 infection, cat scratch disease, drug hypersensitivity reaction (carbamazepine), lymphoma … Differential diagnosis of pharyngitis: group A streptococcal infection, adenovirus, herpes simplex, diphtheria, gonococcus, infections of the soft tissues of the neck. **Diagnosis:** leukocytosis, lymphocytosis, with atypical lymphocytes (non specific). Heterophil antibodies ⊕ (e.g.: Mono test) but false ⊖ in 10-15 %, especially at the beginning of disease (become ⊕ in 60 % after 2 weeks) and young children. Anti-EBV antibodies: mostly useful if heterophil antibodies ⊖: look for EBV specific antigen: VCA (*viral capsid antigen*) and EBNA (*Epstein-Barr nuclear antigen*). VCA-IgM ⊕ in acute, and disappears within 1-2 months. VCA-IgG ⊕ acute, it remains ⊕ lifelong. EBNA ⊕ at 3-4 weeks and it remains lifelong (so EBNA ⊕ rules out the diagnosis of acute mononucleosis). Throat culture to be done in order to rule out group A streptococcal pharyngitis. **Complications:** Coombs ⊕ hemolytic anemia (1-3 %), thrombocytopenia, neutropenia, hemophagocytic syndrome, hepatitis (with ↑ alkaline phosphatase > ALT), splenic rupture, neurologic complications (Guillain-Barré syndrome, encephalitis, meningitis, mononeuritis, cerebellar attacks, transverse myelitis), airway obstruction, rash with ampicillin or amoxicillin (in 90-100 % of patients), other (myositis, myopericarditis, pneumonitis, pancreatitis …).

	Treatment: usual analgesia ± steroids if severe tonsillitis/pharyngeal edema with imminent or beginning airway obstruction, acute hemolytic anemia or severe thrombocytopenia, neurological complications, myocarditis or pericarditis. Avoid contact sports for many months in order to lower risk of spleen rupture. **Prognosis:** Symptoms persist for 2-4 weeks, but 3 % > 1 month. No re-infection. Chronic EBV infection is rare but severe.
Cytomegalo-virus	Causes 5-10 % of mononucleosis-like syndromes, and is the most frequent cause of a mononucleosis-like syndrome with negative heterophil antibodies. Orally transmitted, sexually transmitted, by transfusion, or post-transplant. **Clinical findings:** Often asymptomatic, or symptoms of fever, malaise, hepatitis, splenomegaly … but pharyngitis and cervical lymphadenopathy are less frequent than in infectious mononucleosis. Resolution: in 2-4 weeks. **Diagnosis:** Anti-CMV antibodies IgM with acute infection. **Complications:** hepatitis, hemolytic anemia, thrombocytopenia, neurological complications, interstitial pneumonia, chorioretinitis. **Treatment:** treatment not usually necessary. Indications for steroids: similar to infectious mononucleosis.
Toxoplasmosis	Protozoal infection frequently found in warm blooded animals, especially felines. **Clinical:** 3 clinical syndromes in immuno-competent patient: 1 - mononucleosis-like syndrome identical to infectious mononucleosis, but pharyngitis and splenomegaly are less significant, 2 - ocular toxoplasmosis, 3 - congenital toxoplasmosis. **Diagnosis:** IgG which rises with time (but may require 3 weeks to become positive, so must be repeated as needed. IgM detects acute disease (but false ⊕). **Treatment:** Usually no treatment. Treatment indicated if constitutional symptoms are severe or persistent, involvement of a vital organ (pneumonia, myocarditis, encephalitis), immunosuppressed state, congenital toxoplasmosis: sulfadiazine or pyrimethamine: Consultation with Infectious Diseases recommended.
HIV Primary Infection	See HIV table.

HIV-AIDS

Immunodeficiency syndrome caused by HIV-1 virus (rarely HIV-2).

Sexually transmitted (1/250 to 1/1000 according to type of relation), acquired by contaminated needle (0.3 % if HIV ⊕), through blood transfusion (risk is: < 1/500 000 at present) or through neonatal transmission (30 % if not treated, < 1 % with antiretroviral therapy and viral load < 50 copies/mL).

Clinical features	Primary infection: mononucleosis-like syndrome occuring 1-3 weeks, post exposure (symptomatic in 50-70 %). Spontaneous clinical resolution until later progression of disease. Clinical presentation of the asymptomatic phase or AIDS: diffuse lymphadenopathy, cytopenias, *Pneumocystis* pneumonia, localised candidiasis, constitutional symptoms, bacterial infections by encapsulated pathogens, tuberculosis, sexually transmitted diseases, neurological syndromes, Kaposi's sarcoma → see complications: below. AIDS defining diseases: *Pneumocystis jiroveci* pneumonia, esophageal candidiasis, cytomegalovirus infection, cerebral toxoplasmosis, *Herpes simplex* (chronic ulcers, lasting > 1 month), invasive cervical cancer, recurrent pneumonia (> 2 episodes in 12 months), Kaposi's sarcoma, disseminated infection by atypical mycobacteria (*M. avium complex*, etc), chronic cryptosporidiosis (> 1 month), extrapulmonary cryptococcosis, disseminated histoplasmosis, lymphoma, progressive multifocal leukoencephalopathy, tuberculosis, HIV related encephalopathy, recurrent *Salmonella* sp. septicemia.
Workup	HIV serology: screen with ELISA and confirm with Western Blot. Seroconversion within 2-12 weeks in 95 % of patients. CD4: indirect indicator of the degree of immunodeficiency: useful in guiding antiretroviral therapy as well as prophylaxis. There can be diurnal variation in counts and among different laboratories, can also be ↓ in any acute infections, steroids… Measure every 3-6 months. Viral load: measure HIV RNA. Used for initial evaluation of untreated patient and follow-up of infection in treated and untreated individuals : 2 baseline values must be obtained, 4-8 weeks after initiation of treatment or modification of treatment, then measured every 3-4 months : always use the same laboratory method. Also useful if suspicion of primary infection; but be careful with false positives. p24 antigen: indicates active viral replication. ⊕ before seroconversion. Useful if acute infection suspected. Genotyping of HIV (virtual phenotype): measures resistance to antiretrovirals. Indicated for untreated patients (including pregnant women), in primary infection and in cases of virologic failure. Drug level measurements: plasma concentrations of non-nucleosidic inhibitors of reverse transcriptase and of protease inhibitors. Indicated in cases of virologic failure, drug toxicity, drug interactions, liver failure and in children. Tropism test: determines whether circulating viruses are using CCR5, CXCR4 or both to enter cells. Indicated when the use of entry inhibitors such as maroviroc is considered.

Management	– Initial evaluation: history, assess infectious exposures (drug addiction, homosexuality, tuberculosis, HSV, histoplasmosis, previous vaccination ...), mental and physical examination, education and prevention of transmission, psychosocial support.
	– Basic workup: CBC, biochemistry, urinalysis, triglycerides + cholesterol, chest X-ray, CD4 count, viral load, tuberculin skin test, serology for syphilis, toxoplasmosis (IgG), HBV, HCV, CMV, PAP test every 6 months, genotype if viral load > 1000 copies/mL.
	– Immunization with vaccines for pneumococcus, hepatitis A and B, influenza.
	If opportunistic disease, if CD4 ≤ 350/mm³, HIV nephropathy, pregnant woman, co-infected with HBV and treatment is indicated for HBV: start antiretroviral treatment: see below.
	If CD4 < 200: prophylaxis for *Pneumocystis*.
	If CD4 < 100: prophylaxis for toxoplasmosis if seropositive ± fungal infection.
	If CD4 < 50: prophylaxis for *M. avium complex* ± CMV if seropositive.
	Note: Co-infection with hepatitis C is frequent and can complicate treatment.
Treatment	– Treatment should be initiated and followed by an expert in this disease.
	– Network of HIV experts in Quebec (Consultation AIDS) : 1-800-363-4814
	– Treatment indications: AIDS or HIV symptomatic disease or CD4 ≤ 350 or post-exposure (bi- or tri-therapy for 4 weeks), or in HIV ⊕ pregnant woman, or if HIV nephropathy, or if co-infected with HBV and treatment for HBV is clinically indicated.
	– Indications for modifying treatment: treatment failure (viral load reduction < 1 log after 4-8 weeks or ↓ CD4 or clinical progression) or toxicity or non-compliance to treatment.
	Drugs :
	– Nucleoside reverse transcriptase inhibitors: zidovudine, stavudine, didanosine, abacavir, lamivudine, tenofovir, emtricitabine. Fixed dose pills: Trizivir ® (AZT+ABC+3TC), Combivir® (AZT+3TC), Kivexa® (ABC+3TC), Truvada® (TDF + FTC).
	– Nonnucleoside reverse transcriptase inhibitors: nevirapine, delavirdine, efavirenz, etravirin.
	– Protease inhibitors: saquinavir, indinavir, ritonavir, Kaletra® (lopinavir + ritonavir), nelfinavir, fosamprenavir, atazanavir, tipranavir, darunavir.
	– Integrase inhibitor: raltegravir, elvitegravir.
	– Fusion inhibitor: enfuvertide (T-20).
	– CCR5 Entry inhibitors: maraviroc.
	– Combination: Atripla® (efavirenz + FTC + TDF).
	Side effects are specific to each drug.
	First line combination therapy : 2 nucleoside reverse transcriptase inhibitors + 1 protease inhibitor combined with low dose ritonavir (100 or 200 mg) **or** 2 nucleoside reverse transcriptase inhibitors + 1 nonnucleoside reverse transcriptase inhibitor (efavirenz) **or** other options possible but less effective or more toxic (avoid certain combinations: see relevant text).
	Treatment interruptions should be discouraged. Risk of clinical events increased with treatment interruption.

HIV-AIDS Complications

Pulmonary	– Infectious: bronchitis, sinusitis, bacterial pneumonia, *Pneumocystis jiroveci* pneumonia, tuberculosis, *Mycobacterium avium intracellulare*, fungal pneumonia (dimorphic). – Non infectious: Kaposi's sarcoma, non-specific interstitial pneumonitis, pulmonary hypertension, etc.
Neurological	– Meningitis due to HIV (in primary infection), cryptococcal, tuberculous or aseptic, histoplasmosis. – Intracerebral mass lesion : toxoplasmosis, primary lymphoma, progressive multifocal leukoencephalopathy. – Encephalitis, CMV, HSV, syphilis, toxoplasmosis. – HIV related dementia. – Vacuolar myelopathy. – Polyneuropathy, mononeuritis multiplex, myopathy, etc.
Gastro-intestinal	– Esophageal: candidiasis, CMV, HSV, HIV, drug-induced esophagitis. – Diarrhea: bacterial: *Mycobacterium avium intracellulare*, *C. difficile* ... Viral: CMV, HSV, HIV ... Parasitic: cryptosporidiosis, *Isospora belli*, microsporidiosis ... Drug-induced (didanosine, clindamycin, nelfinavir, ritonavir, Kaletra®, tripanavir, etc). – Hepatic: *Mycobacterium avium intracellulare*, CMV, hepatic peliosis (*B. henselae*), tuberculosis, cryptococcus, Kaposi, *Pneumocystis*, hepatitis ... Multiple drugs. – Biliary tract : CMV, *Cryptosporidium*. – Pancreatitis : drugs (didanosine, pentamidine, stavudine, cotrimazole, etc). – Proctitis: *N. gonorrheae*, *C. trachomatis* type LGV, HSV, CMV, syphilis. – Anorexia: antiretroviral agents.
Others	– Lipodystrophy: symdrome that include lipoaccumulation, lipoatrophy, dyslipidemia, insulin resistance and/or diabetes. Protease inhibitors have been associated mostly with lipoaccumation, dyslipidemia, and insulin resistance. Nucleoside and non-nucleoside reverse transcriptase inhibitors are associated with lipoatrophy (except for tenofovir, abacavir and 3TC/FTC). – Malignancies: Kaposi's sarcoma, lymphoma, cervical cancer in women, anal cancer in men. – The following systems can also be involved: dermatologic, ophtalmologic, cardiac, renal, rheumatologic (osteopenia, osteoporosis), endocrine, hematologic, etc. – Kaletra, fosamprenavir and indinavir have been associated with an increased risk of cardiovascular diseases. – Recent data also suggest a possible association with cardiovascular diseases and Abacavir.

Useful References: INFECTIOUS DISEASES

Acute Bronchitis: Ann Intern Med 2001; 134: 518-521
    Ann Intern Med 2000; 133: 981-91 (review article)
Acute and Chronic Prostatitis: Med Clin North Am 2004; 88: 483-94 (review article)
Acute Pharyngitis: N Engl J Med 2001; 344: 205-211 (review article)
    Group A streptococcus: Clin Infect Dis 2002; 35: 113-25 (American Guidelines)
Acute rheumatic fever: Lancet 2005; 366: 155–68 (review article)
Acute Sinusitis: N Engl J Med 2004; 351: 902-10 (review article)
    Am J Med 2007; 120: 289-94 (review article)
Aspiration Pneumonia: N Engl J Med 2001; 344: 665-72 (review article)
Blastomycosis: Clin Infect Dis 2008; 46: 1801-12 (IDSA Guidelines)
Brain Abscess: Clin Infect Dis 1997; 25: 763-81 (review article)
Catheter-Related Infection: Clin Infect Dis 2009; 49: 1-45 (IDSA Guidelines)
Candidiasis: Clin Infect Dis 2009; 48: 503-35 (IDSA Guidelines)
C. difficile Colitis:
    Cleve Clin J Med 2006; 73: 187-197 (review article)
    … Recurrent: Gastroenterology 2006; 130: 1311-16 (review article)
    … Fulminant Infection: Am J Gastroenterol 2008; 103: 3195-3203 (review article)
Cellulitis: Clin Infect Dis 2005; 41: 1373-1406 (IDSA Guidelines)
    N Engl J Med 2004; 350: 904-912 (review article)
Chronic Prostatitis: N Engl J Med 2006; 355: 1690-8 (review article)
    Coccidioidomycosis: Mayo Clin Proc 2008; 83: 343-349 (review article)
Community-Acquired MRSA infection - Treatment:
    N Engl J Med 2007; 357: 380-90 (review article)
Community-Acquired Pneumonia: Clin Infect Dis 2007; 44: S27-72 (consensus IDSA-ATS)
    N Engl J Med 2002; 347: 2039-45 (review article)
Complicated Intra-Abdominal Infections:
    Clin Infect Dis 2003; 37: 997-1005 (American Guidelines)
Diabetic Foot Infections: Clin Infect Dis 2004; 39: 885-910 (review article)
Encephalitis: Clin Infect Dis 2008; 47: 303-27 (IDSA Guidelines)
    … West Nile Virus: Mayo Clin Proc 2003; 78: 1137-44 (review article)
Endocarditis: N Engl J Med 2001; 345: 1318-30 (review article)
    Lancet 2004; 363: 139-49 (review article)
    Eur Heart J 2004; 25: 267-76 (European Guidelines)
    Prophylaxis: Circulation 2007; 116: 1736-54 (American Guidelines)
    Treatment: Circulation 2005; 111: 3167-84 (American Guidelines)
Fever in the ICU: Clin Infect Dis 1998; 26: 1042-59 (review article)
    Chest 2000; 117: 855-69 (review article)
Fever in the Immunocompromised Patients: N Engl J Med 1999; 341: 893-900 (review article)
Fever of Unknown Origin: Clin Infect Dis 1997; 24: 291- (review article)
    Arch Intern Med 2003; 163: 545-51 (review article)
Fungal Infections: Clin Infect Dis 2000; 30: 652-718 (IDSA Guidelines)
Histoplasmosis: Clin Infect Dis 2007; 45: 807-25 (IDSA Guidelines)
HIV Infection: Lancet 2006; 368: 489-504 (review article)
    … Newly Diagnosed: N Engl J Med 2005; 353: 1702-10 (review article)
    … Opportunistic infections - prevention and treatment:
        MMWR Recomm Rep 2009; 58: 1-207 (CDC-IDSA Guidelines)
    … Treatment: JAMA 2008; 300: 555-570 (AIDS Society Guidelines)
        JAMA 2006; 296: 827-843 (review article)
    See following web site: www.hivatis.org
Hospital-Acquired Pneumonia:
    Am J Respir Crit Care Med 2005; 171: 388-416 (American Guidelines)
HSV Infections - Treatment: Arch Intern Med 2008; 168: 1137-44 (review article)
Infection in Solid-Organ Transplant Recipients:
    N Engl J Med 2007; 357: 2601-14 (review article)
Influenza: Clin Infect Dis 2009; 48: 1003-32 (IDSA Guidelines)

    N Engl J Med 2008; 359: 2579-85 (review article)
Lyme Disease: Mayo Clin Proc 2008; 83: 566-571 (review article)
    N Engl J Med 2006; 354: 2794-801 (review article)
    Clin Infect Dis 2006; 43: 1089-134 (IDSA Guidelines)
Malaria: JAMA 2007; 297: 2264-2277 (review article)
    Lancet 2005; 365: 1487-98 (review article)
    CMAJ 2004; 170: 1693-702 (review article)
    … Prevention: N Engl J Med 2008; 359: 603-12 (review article)
    See following web site: www.cdc.gov/malaria/
Meningitis: N Engl J Med 2006; 354: 44-53 (review article)
    Clin Infect Dis 2004; 39: 1267-84 (IDSA Guidelines)

Mononucleosis-Like Syndrome - Diagnostic Evaluation:
    Am J Med 2007; 120: 911.e1-911.e8 (review article)
Neutropenia in the Oncology Patient: Clin Infect Dis 2002; 34: 730-51 (IDSA Guidelines)
Necrotizing Infections of Soft Tissues: Clin Infect Dis 2007; 44: 705-10 (review article)
Osteomyelitis: Lancet 2004; 364: 369-79 (review article)
Pneumocystis Pneumonia: N Engl J Med 2004; 350: 2487-98 (review article)
Prosthetic-Joint Infections: N Engl J Med 2004; 351: 1645-54 (review article)
Q Fever: Mayo Clin Proc 2008; 83: 574-579 (review article)
    Lancet 2006; 367: 679-88 (review article)
Sepsis: Am J Med 2007; 120: 1012-1022 (review article)
    … Severe - management: Intensive Care Med 2008; 34: 17-60 (Guidelines)
    … Treatment: N Engl J Med 2006; 355: 1699-713 (review article)
Septic Arthritis: Clin Infect Dis 1995; 20: 225-30 (review article)
Septic Shock: Lancet 2005; 365: 63-78 (review article)
    CMAJ 2005; 173: 1054-65 (review article)

Tuberculosis: Lancet 2007; 370: 2030-43 (review article)
    CMAJ 1999; 160: 837-9 & 1025-8 & 1185-90 &1344-8 & 1597-603 & 1725-9.
    CMAJ 1999; 161: 47-51 & 405-11 & 717-24 & 1271-7.
    CMAJ 2000; 162: 57-61 & 351-5 (review article)
    Treatment: JAMA 2005; 293: 2776-84 (review article)
        Am J Respir Crit Care Med 2003; 167: 603-62 (American Guidelines)
    Tuberculosis with HIV: N Engl J Med 1999; 340: 367-73 (review article)
        CMAJ 1999; 161: 47-51 (review article)
    "Latent" Tuberculosis: N Engl J Med 2002; 347: 1860-66 (review article)
Typhoid Fever: Clin Infect Dis 2005; 41: 1467-72 (review article)
    N Engl J Med 2002; 347: 1770-82 (review article)
    … and Paratyphoid Fever: Lancet 2005; 366: 749-62 (review article)
Urinary Tract Infections:
    Uncomplicated Urinary Tract Infections in Women:
        N Engl J Med 2003; 349: 259-66 (review article)
    Asymptomatic Bacteriuria in Adults: Clin Infect Dis 2005; 40: 643-54 (IDSA Guidelines)
Ventilator-Acquired Pneumonia: Am J Respir Crit Care Med 2002; 165: 867-903 (review article)

Chapter 7

Nephrology

Disorders of Serum Sodium	

Hypernatremia - Na^+ > 145 mEq/L

Clinical findings: Mainly neurological manifestations: severe thirst, lethargy, hyperreflexia, spasticity, irritability, ataxia, coma, seizures, respiratory arrest.

Causes
 	
See algorithm
	1. Hypovolemic hypernatremia: water losses > loss of Na^+:
	  – If UNa^+ > 20 mEq/L: *renal losses*: diuretic or osmotic diuresis, nephropathy.
	  – If UNa^+ < 20 mEq/L: *extrarenal losses*: GI, skin, lung, etc.
	
	2. Isovolemic hypernatremia : water losses:
	  – If urinary osmolality ↑ (> 400 mosm/kg H_2O): insensible loss, osmotic diuresis.
	  – If urinary osmolality ↓ (< 250 mosm/kg H_2O): diabetes insipidus:
	    o Central: idiopathic 50 %, tumor, trauma, cyst, granuloma, aneurysm, meningitis, encephalitis, congenital, sarcoidosis, Langerhans' cell histiocytosis, etc.
	    o Nephrogenic: ↓ K^+, ↑ Ca^{++}, obstructive uropathy, renal failure, tubulointerstitial renal disease (e.g.: sickle cell disease, amyloidosis, Sjögren's syndrome), gestational, drug-related (lithium, demeclocycline, amphotericin B), hereditary.
	
	3. Hypervolemic hypernatremia: gain of Na^+ > gain of water (rare):
	Hypertonic solution, $NaHCO_3$, NaCl tablets, hypertonic dialysis, primary hyperaldosteronism, Cushing's syndrome, etc.

Management	Workup: serum and urinary osmolality, urinary Na^+.
	Water restriction test to differentiate between central diabetes insipidus, nephrogenic diabetes insipidus and psychogenic polydipsia (when facing a polyuria of unknown cause).
	
	Treatment : depending on cause:
	Calculate water deficit (L) = 0.5 (0.4 for women) x ideal weight x [(Na^+/140) - 1].
	  – If symptomatic: correct to a normal serum sodium at a rate of 0.5-1 mEq/L/h until symptom resolution (not more than 12 mEq/L during the first 24h).
	  – If asymptomatic: correct to a normal serum sodium at a rate of 0.5 mEq/L/h (because of risk of cerebral edema).
	Give free water (orally, nasogastric tube) or D5W and/or NaCl 0.45 % if isovolemic or hypervolemic. Give NaCl 0.9% if hypovolemic until hemodynamically stable: then give NaCl 0.45 % and/or D5W.
	Monitor Na^+ every 2-4 hours (at first). Monitor blood glucose.
	
	Other treatments: depending on cause:
	    If central diabetes insipidus: complete = DDAVP: partial = DDAVP, chlorpropamide, carbamazepine, etc.
	    If nephrogenic diabetes insipidus: amiloride (for lithium toxicity), thiazides, NSAIDs, etc.

Hypernatremia

Fluid volume status assessed by physical examination

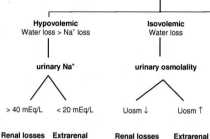

Hypovolemic Water loss > Na$^+$ loss	**Isovolemic** Water loss	**Hypervolemic** Water and Na$^+$ gain
urinary Na$^+$	**urinary osmolality**	**urinary Na$^+$**

> 40 mEq/L	< 20 mEq/L	Uosm ↓	Uosm ↑	> 20 mEq/L

Renal losses
- Diuretic
- Osmotic diuresis (glucose, urea, mannitol)
- Post-obstructive diuresis

Extrarenal losses
- GI losses (diarrhea, vomiting)
- Insensible losses: skin, lung

Renal losses
Central, nephrogenic diabetes insipidus

Extrarenal losses
Insensible losses: skin, lung

Iatrogenic :
- Hypertonic solutions
- NaCl tablets, NaHCO$_3$

Mineralocorticoid:
- Primary hyperaldosteronism
- Cushing's syndrome

Hypertonic dialysis

Treatment
Treatment depending on origin of sodium loss. Isotonic, then hypotonic solutions.

Treatment
Oral water replacement. D5W and/or NaCl 0.45 % at a rate of 0.5-1 mEq/L/h ± vasopressin (5 U every 6 h) for central diabetes insipidus.

Treatment
Diuretics ± dialysis.

Hyponatremia - Na^+ < 135 mmol/L

Clinical findings: According to cause, rate of development of hyponatremia and age: GI manifestations if Na^+ 125-130 mEq/L: nausea, vomiting.

Neurological manifestations if < 125 mEq/L: headaches, muscle weakness or cramps, lethargy, cerebral edema, seizures, coma, respiratory depression.

Note: Young women with symptomatic hyponatremia may be at greater risk of complications.

Causes
 	
See algorithm
	1. Pseudohyponatremia, isosmotic or hyperosmotic hyponatremia (or translocational): related with ↑ blood glucose, ↑ triglycerides, ↑ protein, maltose, irrigation solution without Na^+ (transurethral prostate resection, hysterectomy) with glycine or sorbitol.
	2. **Hypovolemic** hyposmotic hyponatremia :
	   - If UNa^+ > 20 mEq/L: renal losses: salt-losing nephropathy (with advanced CKD, polycystic kidney, analgesic nephropathy, chronic pyelonephritis, obstructive uropathy), Na^+ loss of central origin (*Cerebral salt-wasting* - after subarachnoid hemorrhage), type II renal tubular acidosis, diuretics (thiazides), osmotic diuresis, mineralocorticoid deficiency, etc.
	   - If UNa^+ < 20 mEq/L: extrarenal losses: vomiting, diarrhea, bleeding, 3rd space, excessive sweating, extensive skin lesions, etc.
	3. **Isovolemic** hyposmotic hyponatremia: psychogenic polydipsia, low dietary solute intake (tea and toast diet), beer potomania, hypotonic saline, thiazides, hypothyroidism, glucocorticoid deficiency; SIADH: with CNS or lung lesion, tumors, post-operative state, pain, nausea or drugs: DDAVP, psychoactive agents (SSRIs), phenothiazines, tricyclics, clozapine, *ecstasy*), chemotherapy (vincristine, cyclophosphamide), carbamazepine, oxacarbazepine, bromocriptine, chlorpropamide, ACEI, omeprazole, etc.
	4. **Hypervolemic** hyposmotic hyponatremia: acute or chronic renal failure, nephrotic syndrome, pregnancy, cirrhosis, heart failure.

Management	Workup: urinary Na^+, serum and urinary osmolality, BUN, creatinine, uric acid (↓ in SIADH and psychogenic polydipsia), monitor Na^+ every 2-3 h (at first).
	Always rule out adrenal insufficiency (especially if hyperkalemia is present), hypothyroidism and kidney failure if SIADH is suspected.
	
	Note: Each ↑ 5.6 mmol/L of serum glucose = ↓ Na^+ 1.7 mmol/L.
	
	Treatment : depending on cause :
	* If urine is **concentrated** (i.e. : urinary osmolality > 200 mOsm/kg H_2O) and no hypervolemia :
	   - if symptomatic: correct to a normal serum sodium at a rate of 1-2 mEq/L/h until symptom resolution (not more than 12 mEq/L during the first 24h because of the risk of central pontine myelinolysis).
	   - if asymptomatic: correct to a normal serum sodium at a rate of 0.5 mEq/L/h (because of the risk of central pontine myelinolysis).
	Example: Female 60 kg - Na^+ 115 mEq/L and asymptomatic.
	Note: Total body water = weight (kg) multiplied by 0.6 for male, 0.5 for female.
	Na^+ correction at a rate of 0.5 mEq/L/h x total body water (L), (i.e.: 60 x 0.5) = 15 mEq/h. NaCl 3 % = 1 mEq/2 mL (513 mEq/L), so give NaCl 3 % at a rate of 30 mL/h.
	
	* If urine is **diluted** (i.e.: urinary osmolality < 200 mOsm/kg H_2O): water restriction except only if presence of severe symptoms (coma or seizures) for which hypertonic solution is needed.
	
	* Other treatments: depending on cause.
	   If SIADH: water restriction (< 1.2 L/day), demeclocycline, NaCl + furosemide.
	   If hypovolemic hyponatremia: give iso or hypertonic solution.
	   If hypervolemic hyponatremia: water restriction and furosemide.

Hyponatremia

Serum osmolality

Normal

Isosmotic hyponatremia
Pseudohyponatremia
- Severe hyperlipidemia
- Severe hyperproteinemia

Low

High

Hyperosmotic hyponatremia
1. Hyperglycemia
2. Hypertonic infusions
   - Mannitol
   - Glycine
   - Glycerol
   - Sorbitol
   - Ethanol, methanol
   - Contrast dye

**Assess extracellular fluid
volume state**

Hypovolemic hyposmotic
hyponatremia

Urinary Na$^+$

Isovolemic hyposmotic
hyponatremia

Urinary Na$^+$

Hypervolemic hyposmotic
hyponatremia

Urinary Na$^+$

**< 20 mEq/L
Extrarenal
losses**
- GI (diarrhea, vomiting, bleeding).
- 3rd space (pancreatitis)
- Insensible losses: skin, lung

**> 40 mEq/L
Renal losses**
- Diuretics
- Osmotic diuresis
- Renal damage
- Renal tubular acidosis
- Adrenal insufficiency

< 20 mEq/L
- Water intoxication (psychogenic polydipsia)
- Low dietary solute intake

> 40 mEq/L
- SIADH
- Hypothyroidism
- Stress
- Adrenal insufficiency

< 20 mEq/L
- Cirrhosis
- Heart failure
- Nephrotic syndrome
- Pregnancy

> 40 mEq/L
- Acute/chronic renal failure

Treatment
Isotonic or hypertonic
saline

Treatment
According to cause

Treatment
Water restriction
Diuretic

Disorders of Serum Potassium	
Hyperkalemia - K⁺ > 5.0 mmol/L	
Clinical findings: muscle weakness, paralysis, irritability, confusion, ventricular arrhythmia, atrioventricular block, cardiac arrest.	
Causes See algorithm	Rule out pseudohyperkalemia: hemolysis (tourniquet effect), WBC > 100 x 10⁹/L, ↑ platelet > 1 000 x 10⁹/L. 1. ↓ excretion: acute or severe chronic renal failure, interstitial nephritis, hypoaldosteronism (Addison's disease, type IV renal tubular acidosis due to diabetes mellitus, HIV, obstructive uropathy, hyperkalemic type I renal tubular acidosis), drugs (potassium supplements, NSAIDs, ACEI, ARB, antibiotics [trimethoprim, pentamidine], heparin, potassium-sparing diuretics, cyclosporine, tacrolimus, natural products), Gordon's syndrome (with hypertension). 2. Redistribution: acute acidosis, familial periodic paralysis, drugs (succinylcholine, α-adrenergic agonist, severe digoxin intoxication, beta-blockers, IV amino acids), intense exercise. 3. ↑ intake (rare and associated with renal excretion problems) or tissue release with cell lysis (tumor, rhabdomyolysis) or stored blood.
Management	Workup: ECG (peaking T waves, sometimes complete intraventricular block), creatinine, arterial blood gas, TTKG (UK⁺ / PK⁺ x Posm/Uosm): value ≤ 5 is suggestive of hypoaldosteronism: not useful if Uosm < 300 mosm/kg H₂O. Treatment : If moderate (6-7 mmol/L): cardiac monitoring, correct related factors, stop intake, treat the cause. If severe (> 7 mmol/L or ECG abnormalities): cardiac monitoring, stop intake. - Calcium gluconate: 10 mL 10 % IV in 2 minutes if abnormal ECG (contraindicated if taking digoxin). - Dextrose 50 % 50 mL followed by insulin R 5-10 U IV over 60 minutes. - Salbutamol (Ventolin®) 10-20 mg/2-4 mL saline (5 mg/mL) over 10 minutes by nebulizer. - Bicarbonate 1-2 vials of 50 mmol IV over ≤ 10 minutes for metabolic acidosis. - Combination glucose-insulin-salbutamol or glucose-insulin-HCO₃ to be considered. - Kayexalate 15-30 g PO every 4-6 h as needed (not to be given if ileus present): enema 30-50 g /100-200 mL of water every 4 h as needed. - Hemodialysis. Monitor K⁺ every 2 hours until K⁺ ≤ 5.5 mmol/L.

Hyperkalemia

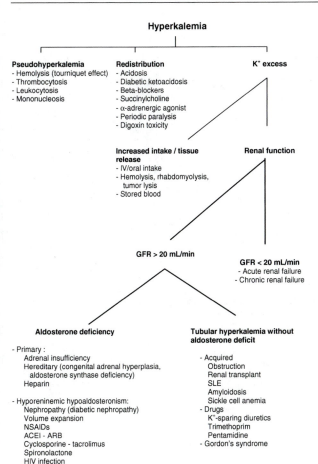

Pseudohyperkalemia
- Hemolysis (tourniquet effect)
- Thrombocytosis
- Leukocytosis
- Mononucleosis

Redistribution
- Acidosis
- Diabetic ketoacidosis
- Beta-blockers
- Succinylcholine
- α-adrenergic agonist
- Periodic paralysis
- Digoxin toxicity

K⁺ excess

Increased intake / tissue release
- IV/oral intake
- Hemolysis, rhabdomyolysis, tumor lysis
- Stored blood

Renal function

GFR > 20 mL/min

GFR < 20 mL/min
- Acute renal failure
- Chronic renal failure

Aldosterone deficiency

- Primary :
    Adrenal insufficiency
    Hereditary (congenital adrenal hyperplasia, aldosterone synthase deficiency)
    Heparin

- Hyporeninemic hypoaldosteronism:
    Nephropathy (diabetic nephropathy)
    Volume expansion
    NSAIDs
    ACEI - ARB
    Cyclosporine - tacrolimus
    Spironolactone
    HIV infection
    Obstructive uropathy (sometimes)

Tubular hyperkalemia without aldosterone deficit

- Acquired
    Obstruction
    Renal transplant
    SLE
    Amyloidosis
    Sickle cell anemia
- Drugs
    K⁺-sparing diuretics
    Trimethoprim
    Pentamidine
- Gordon's syndrome

Hypokalemia - K$^+$ < 3.5 mmol/L

Non-specific symptoms: anorexia, nausea, vomiting, ileus, muscle weakness, arrhythmia.
Digoxin toxicity ↑.
Rarely: Secondary diabetes insipidus, rhabdomyolysis, hyperglycemia, worsening of hepatic encephalopathy.

Causes
 	
See algorithm
	1. ↑ extrarenal loss: gastrointestinal, biliary, skin losses, etc.
	2. ↑ renal loss: measure arterial blood pressure:
	    - BP ↑ in hypermineralocorticoid state:
	        o With renin ↓: primary hyperaldosteronism (where aldosterone is ↑): black licorice, Cushing's syndrome, Liddle's syndrome (in which aldosterone is ↓).
	        o With renin ↑: secondary hyperaldosteronism: with malignant hypertension, renal artery stenosis, renin-producing tumor ...
	    - Normal BP if diuretic (# 1 cause), vomiting (# 2 cause), drugs (amphotericin, penicillin, aminoglycosides, cisplatin, levodopa), nasogastric suction, Bartter's syndrome, Gitelman's syndrome, osmotic diuresis, hypomagnesemia, type I and II renal tubular acidosis, lysozymuria (with leukemia).
	3. Redistribution: acute alkalosis, familial periodic paralysis, medication (insulin, β-adrenergic agonist [bronchodilator, epinephrine], bicarbonate ...), catecholamines (stress), hypokalemic periodic paralysis, cell proliferation secondary to the treatment of megaloblastic anemia, hypothermia, barium or theophylline intoxication.
	4. ↓ intake (rare).
	
	Rule out related hypomagnesemia.

Management	Workup: ECG (decreased or inverted T waves, increased U waves: ST segment depression can occur), creatinine, arterial blood gas, CK (secondary rhabdomyolysis), Mg^{++}. TTKG (UK$^+$ / PK$^+$ x Posm/Uosm): value > 3 suggests renal potassium loss: not useful if Uosm < 300 mosm/kg H$_2$O. Note: total estimated K$^+$ deficit; for K$^+$ = 3 mmol/L ≈ 200-400 mEq, for K$^+$ = 2 mmol/L ≈ 400-800 mEq (non applicable to a redistribution problem). Treatment depending on cause: PO if K$^+$ ≥ 3 mmol/L, IV if < 3 mmol/L or symptomatic : KCl 10-20 mEq/100 mL NaCl 0.9 % IV in 1 hour. KCl 20 mEq/50 mL NaCl 0.9 % IV in 2-4 hours by central venous catheter, repeat as needed. KCl 20-40 mEq PO tid. Very important to correct hypovolemia (in order to counter secondary hyperaldosteronism) and hypomagnesemia if present.

Hypokalemia

Exclude redistribution:
- Alkalosis
- Insulin
- Periodic paralysis
- Barium or theophylline toxicity
- Vitamin B12 therapy
- Catecholamine excess (stress, ß-agonists ...)
- Hypothermia
- ↑ production of blood cells.

Extrarenal K⁺ losses
$UK^+ < 20$ mEq/L, TTKG < 2

- GI losses, biliary, skin, fistula ...
- Plasmapheresis

Renal K⁺ losses
$UK^+ > 20$ mEq/L, TTKG > 3-4

High blood pressure

Plasma renin

↑
- Malignant hypertension
- Renovascular disease
- Renin-secreting tumor

↓

Normal blood pressure

Plasma HCO₃⁻

↓
- RTA (type I or II)
- DKA

↑

Plasma Aldosterone

↑
- Primary hyperaldosteronism

↓
- Mineralocorticoid ingestion
- Congenital adrenal hyperplasia
- Cushing's syndrome
- Liddle's syndrome

Urinary chloride

< 10 mEq/L
- Vomiting
- Gastric drainage

> 10 mEq/L
- Bartter's syndrome
- Gitelman's syndrome
- Diuretics
- Mg⁺⁺ deficiency

Disorders of Serum Calcium	
Hypercalcemia – ionized Ca^{++} > 1.32 mmol/L.	

Symptoms: Nocturia, polydipsia, polyuria, fatigue, constipation, anorexia, headaches, muscle weakness …
History of nephrolithiasis, peptic ulcer, pancreatitis, delirium.
Signs: ↑ blood pressure, band keratopathy, hyporeflexia.
ECG: ↓ QT interval.

| Causes | **1. Endocrine:**
– Primary hyperparathyroidism: most frequent cause of asymtomatic hypercalcemia: Pathology = 80% adenoma, 10-15 % hyperplasia, < 5 % cancer: 20 % have PTH at upper limit of normal. Rule out MEN (present in 1-2 %) and familial hypocalciuric hypercalcemia (FHH) since presentation is sometimes identical (20 % of FHH have ↑ PTH).
– Tertiary hyperparathyroidism: with chronic kidney disease and autonomous parathyroid function (when ↑ PTH).
– Familial hypocalciuric hypercalcemia: autosomal dominant, ↑ Cl$^-$, 50 % have ↑ Mg^{++}.
– Hyper or hypothyroidism.
– Adrenal insufficiency.
– Pheochromocytoma.
– Acromegaly.
– Vipoma.

2. Cancer:
– Bone metastases.
– Multiple myeloma.
– Secretion of PTH related peptide (PTHrP): lung cancer (squamous cell), renal cancer, ovarian cancer, etc.
– Secretion of 1.25 (OH)$_2$ D$_3$ with lymphoma.
– Ectopic PTH (with cancer: very rare).

3. Granulomatous diseases:
Sarcoidosis, tuberculosis, berylliosis, fungal infection (histoplasmosis), leprosy, etc.

4. Drugs:
Thiazides, lithium, theophylline, estrogens and antiestrogens, vitamin A or D toxicity, milk-alkali syndrome, aluminum toxicity, etc.

5. Immobilization: especially among teenagers or Paget's disease.

6. Other causes: after acute renal failure secondary to rhabdomyolysis, severe chronic liver disease, AIDS with disseminated CMV, severe dehydration, TPN, iatrogenic. |
| Management

See algorithm | Corrected Ca^{++} = (Ca^{++} measured) + 0.025 (40 - albumin [g/L]).

Basic workup: Ca^{++} (to be rechecked), albumin, PO$_4^{3-}$, Cl$^-$, Mg^{++}, creatinine, alkaline phosphatase, ECG (↓ QT), TSH, PTH, urinary calcium.

→ Workup according to suspicion of primary hyperparathyroidism versus cancer based on clinical findings.

For primary hyperparathyroidism: PTH, bone densitometry (rule out associated osteoporosis), 24 h urinary calcium (measure fractional excretion of Ca^{++} in order to rule out hypocalciuric hypercalcemia, in which it is < 0.01), 24 h urine phosphate (in order to measure rate of phosphate reabsorption which is < 60 % in primary hyperparathyroidism), protein electrophoresis (rule out associated myeloma), rule out associated MEN. |

	De visu localisation of adenoma by surgery or by ^{99m}Tc Sestamibi, MRI, CT or abdominal U/S. **For cancer:** Chest X-ray, bone series (search for metastasis), mammography, abdominal U/S, bone scan, serum + urine protein electrophoresis, etc. **If diagnosis remains unclear:** 25-OHD, PTHrP, 1.25(OH)$_2$ D$_3$, vitamin A, etc.

Treatment	***Treatment of severe and/or symptomatic hypercalcemia (serum calcium > 3 mmol/L):***
	 - Hydration 3-6 L/24 h. NaCl 0.9 % ± furosemide 20-80 mg IV after correction of hypovolemia.
	 - Calcitonin 4-8 UI/kg IM or s/c every 6-12 hours: unsustained effect.
	 - Bisphosphonates: pamidronate (Aredia®) 60 to 90 mg/1L over 2 hours every 5-7 days or zoledronic acid (Zometa®) 4 mg IV over 15 minutes or clodronate (Bonefos®) 300 mg IV over ≥ 2 hours or PO, especially for paraneoplastic hypercalcemia: slow but sustained effect.
	 - PO steroids as needed 0.5 to 1 mg/kg/day (if ↑ 1.25(OH)$_2$D$_3$, myeloma, lymphoma, some metastases, Addison's, non-infectious granulomatous diseases like sarcoidosis).
	 - Hemodialysis to be considered if serum calcium > 4.5-5 mmol/L and patient has neurologic symptoms.
	
	 Treatment of mild, chronic hypercalcemia (serum calcium 2.8-3 mmol/L):
	 - Treat if hypercalciuria present because of risk of nephrolithiasis and nephrocalcinosis.
	 - Treatment depends on etiology: Oral hydration and NaCl rich diet.
	                         Avoid thiazide diuretics.
	                         Steroids if lymphoma, granulomatous diseases…
	                         Cinacalcet.
	
	 Treatment of primary hyperparathyroidism:
	 - Medical follow-up for Ca < 0.25 mmol/L above upper limit of normal, no history of acute hypercalcemia, normal creatinine and normal bones: serum calcium and creatinine every year and bone density every 1-2 years.
	 - If surgery indicated but patient refuses surgery = treat with bisphosphonates. Cinacalcet to be considered. PO phosphorus (for nonoperable pregnant women).
	 - Surgical treatment indicated if Ca^{++} > 0.25 mmol/L above upper limit of normal, history of life-threatening hypercalcemia, if creatinine clearance < 60 mL/min, nephrolithiasis, osteoporosis (bone densitometry with T-score < -2.5 and/or previous fracture fragility), age < 50, patient accepting surgery, patient unreliable for an adequate medical follow-up. Surgical risk = morbidity 17 % (hypoparathyroidism, recurrent hypercalcemia, true vocal cord paralysis), mortality = 0 %.
	 - Consequences of hypercalcemia: nephrolithiasis, pancreatitis, peptic ulcer, osteitis fibrosa cystica (alkaline phosphatase > 2 x normal).

Hypercalcemia

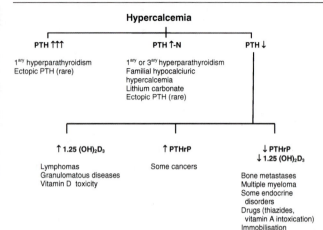

PTH ↑↑↑

1^{ary} hyperparathyroidism
Ectopic PTH (rare)

PTH ↑-N

1^{ary} or 3^{ary} hyperparathyroidism
Familial hypocalciuric
hypercalcemia
Lithium carbonate
Ectopic PTH (rare)

PTH ↓

↑ 1.25 (OH)$_2$D$_3$

Lymphomas
Granulomatous diseases
Vitamin D toxicity

↑ PTHrP

Some cancers

↓ PTHrP
↓ 1.25 (OH)$_2$D$_3$

Bone metastases
Multiple myeloma
Some endocrine
   disorders
Drugs (thiazides,
   vitamin A intoxication)
Immobilisation
Paget's disease
Milk-alkali syndrome

Hypocalcemia

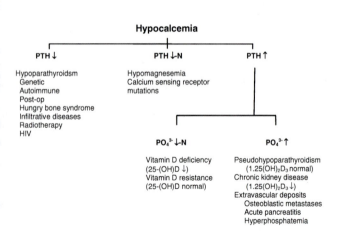

PTH ↓

Hypoparathyroidsm
   Genetic
   Autoimmune
   Post-op
   Hungry bone syndrome
   Infiltrative diseases
   Radiotherapy
   HIV

PTH ↓-N

Hypomagnesemia
Calcium sensing receptor
mutations

PTH ↑

PO$_4$$^{3-}$ ↓-N

Vitamin D deficiency
   (25-(OH)D ↓)
Vitamin D resistance
   (25-(OH)D normal)

PO$_4$$^{3-}$ ↑

Pseudohypoparathyroidism
   (1.25(OH)$_2$D$_3$ normal)
Chronic kidney disease
   (1.25(OH)$_2$D$_3$ ↓)
Extravascular deposits
   Osteoblastic metastases
   Acute pancreatitis
   Hyperphosphatemia

Hypocalcemia - ionized Ca^{++} < 1.14 mmol/L.

Symptoms: paresthesia, cramps, diarrhea, headaches, irritability, seizures, tiredness, muscular weakness, confusion, hallucinations…
Signs: Chvostek's sign, Trousseau's sign, tetany, laryngeal stridor, carpopedal spasm …
ECG: ↑ QT interval.

Causes See algorithm	1. ↓ intake or absorption: vitamin D deficiency (malnutrition, malabsorption). 2. ↑ losses: alcohol, chronic kidney disease, diuretics. 3. Endocrine disorders: idiopathic hypoparathyroidism (rule out polyglandular autoimmune syndrome) or post-op, pseudohypoparathyroidism, calcitonin (medullary thyroid neoplasia). 4. Vitamin D conversion disorders: vitamin D resistant rickets. 5. Other: sepsis, hyperphosphatemia (chronic kidney disease, rhabdomyolysis), alkalosis, drugs (aminoglycoside, foscarnet, diuretics, bisphosphonates), hungry bone syndrome , hypomagnesemia, some cancers (breast, prostate), acute pancreatitis, etc.

Management	Rule out ↓ Mg^{++}, ↓ albumin.
	Corrected Ca^{++} = [measured Ca^{++}] + 0.025 (40 - albumin [g/L]).
	
	Work-up: Ca^{++}, PO$_4$$^{3-}$, albumin, Mg^{++}, PTH, serum calcidiol (25-OHD) or calcitriol (1.25(OH)$_2$D$_3$), malabsorption workup if needed, ECG (QT ↑).
	
	Treatment :
	- Severe (tetany, arrhythmia, seizures): calcium gluconate 10 % IV:
	  e.g.: 1 vial (10 mL = 94 mg elementary Ca^{++}) IV over 10-20 min then 10 vial/ 500 mL
	  D5W or NaCl 0.9 % at 50 mL/h over 4-6 h. Adjust according to response.
	
	- Mild: Calcium carbonate 500 mg PO tid between meals, thiazides ± vitamin D.
	
	- If there is concomitant hypocalcemia and vitamin D deficiency, repletion of vitamin D is required.
	
	Note: always correct hypocalcemia before correcting acidosis (because of risk of seizures).
	
	Administering calcium to a patient taking digoxin can enhance digoxin toxicity and cause death.

Disorders of Serum Magnesium

Hypermagnesemia - Mg^{++} > 1.0 mmol/L
Clinical findings: nausea, vomiting, bradycardia, hypotension, muscle paralysis, respiratory depression, hyporeflexia, confusion, cardiac arrest ...

Causes	Chronic or acute renal failure. Familial hypocalciuric hypercalcemia. Catabolic states (e.g.: tumor lysis syndrome). Endocrine: acromegaly, adrenal failure, primary hyperparathyroidism, diabetic ketoacidosis. Drugs: antacids, laxatives, lithium, theophylline toxicity.
Management	Workup: associated ↓ Ca^{++}. ECG ≈ looks like ↑ K^{+}. Treatment: If chronic kidney disease: hemodialysis > peritoneal dialysis. Calcium gluconate IV (1 or 2 vial [10 mL] over 5 to 10 minutes).

Hypomagnesemia - Mg^{++} < 0.7 mmol/L
Clinical findings: weakness, anorexia, nausea, tetany, muscle cramps, tremor, irritability, seizures, hyperreflexia, hypertension, ventricular arrhythmia (torsades de pointe, especially with sotalol and digoxin), prolonged QT interval.

Causes	*GI losses:* Malabsorption (celiac disease, steatorrhea), NGT suction, vomiting, diarrhea, laxatives, after extensive intestinal surgery, acute pancreatitis, intestinal fistulae, etc. *Renal losses:* Hypercalcemia, osmotic diuresis (with diabetes or other causes), polyuria (post-ATN, post obstruction, post renal transplantation), hypophosphatemia, primary hyperaldosteronism, hyperthyroidism, post-parathyroidectomy, alcohol, drugs (diuretics, ampho B, cisplatin, aminoglycosides, cyclosporine, tacrolimus, foscarnet, pentamidine), Gitelman's syndrome.

Management	Workup: ↓ Ca^{++} (because PTH release is inhibited), ↓ K^{+} (because ↓ Mg^{++} increases K^{+} secretion),
	    ECG: QT ↑, QRS ↑, PR ↑.
	    Measure 24h urinary Mg^{++} or fractional excretion of Mg^{++} as needed.
	
	Usual deficit 75-150 mEq, so you will need 8-12 g of MgSO$_4$ (except if there is CKD)
	
	Treatment: if symptomatic: 2-3 g IV over 1-2 min then 4 g/250 mL over 4 h. Aim for Mg^{++} > 0.4 mmol/L.
	    Asymptomatic: Mg^{++} Rougier® 15-30 mL PO tid or Maglucate® 500 mg tid (side effect = diarrhea).
	    IV Bolus 4g/250 mL over 4 hours as needed.

Disorders of Serum Phosphate

Hyperphosphatemia - PO_4^{3-} > 1.45 mmol/L

Clinical findings: symptoms of the underlying disease ex.: tetany if associated hypocalcemia, ectopic calcifications.

Causes	Rule out pseudohyperphosphatemia: Hemolysis, hypertriglyceridemia, hyperglobulinemia (multiple myeloma), hyperbilirubinemia. **Endocrine:** Hypoparathyroidism, pseudohypoparathyroidism, hyperthyroidism, acromegaly or growth hormone treatment. **Decreased excretion:** Acute or chronic renal failure, Mg^{++} deficiency, bisphosphonates. **Catabolic state:** rhabdomyolysis, tumor lysis syndrome, chemotherapy, malignant hyperthermia, hemolysis, lactic acidosis, ketoacidosis … **Excessive intake or absorption:** Fleet enema or oral PO_4^{3-} laxatives (Fleet phosphosoda), vitamin D excess.
Management	Workup: Ca^{++}, PTH. Treatment: Treat underlying cause. Stop intake if needed. Use chelation therapy (calcium carbonate 500 mg tid at each meal, sevelamer), especially effective for ESRD.

Hypoposphatemia - PO_4^{3-} < 0.84 mmol/L

Clinical findings: If **acute**: acute hemolytic anemia, platelet and leukocyte dysfunction, susceptibility to infections, rhabdomyolysis, encephalopathy, heart failure, respiratory muscle weakness, respiratory failure.
If **chronic**: anorexia, bone and muscle pain, fractures.

Causes	**Low intake or absorption:** fasting, malabsorption, chronic alcohol intake, intestinal bypass, TPN, aluminium or Mg^{++} containing antacids, chronic diarrhea, osteomalacia secondary to vitamin D resistant or deficient states. **Increased losses:** alcohol, vitamin D deficiency, uncontrolled diabetes, renal tubular acidosis, hyperthyroidism, hyperparathyroidism, renal transplant, phosphaturic drugs (diuretics, theophylline, steroids, bronchodilators, acetazolamide, imatinib). **Cellular redistribution:** respiratory alkalosis (with ASA intoxication, pain, anxiety), sepsis, after DKA, hungry bone syndrome, steroids, estrogen, oral contraceptive, etc. **Electrolyte abnormalities:** hypercalcemia, hypomagnesemia, metabolic alkalosis.
Management	Workup: CBC, Ca^{++}, CK, osteomalacia if chronic (X-ray, bone biopsy). Treatment: 2-3 g PO/day in 2-4 dose of $NaHPO_4$ (side effect: diarrhea). IV if severe (< 0.32 mmol/L): 5-10 mL K_2PO_4 or $NaHPO_4$/250 mL NaCl 0.45% IV over 4h. Monitor PO_4^{3-} every 6 h and check for hypocalcemia.

Acid-Base Disorders

Henderson-Hasselbalch equation: $pH = 6.1 + \log \dfrac{[HCO_3]}{0.03 \times pCO_2}$

Adequate compensation:
- In acute respiratory acidosis, ↑ pCO_2 of 10 mmHg will cause a ↑ HCO_3^- of 1 mEq/L (over minutes-hours).
- In chronic respiratory acidosis, ↑ pCO_2 of 10 mmHg will cause a ↑ HCO_3^- of 3.5 mEq/L (days).
- In acute respiratory alkalosis, ↓ pCO_2 of 10 mmHg will cause a ↓ HCO_3^- of 2 mEq/L (over minutes-hours).
- In chronic respiratory alkalosis, ↓ pCO_2 of 10 mmHg will cause a ↓ HCO_3^- of 4 mEq/L (days).
- In metabolic acidosis, ↓ HCO_3^- of 10 mEq/L will cause a ↓ pCO_2 of 12 mmHg (in 12-24 hours).
- In metabolic alkalosis, ↑ HCO_3^- of 10 mEq/L will cause a ↑ pCO_2 of 7 mmHg (in 24-36 hours).

Metabolic	Calculate the anion gap = $Na^+ - (HCO_3^- + Cl^-)$. Normal = 7-16 mEq.

Acidosis	- If anion gap is normal, check the urinary gap (= $UNa^+ + UK^+ - UCl^-$): if ⊕ = renal loss of HCO_3^-. If ⊖ = GI loss of HCO_3^-. - If anion gap is ↑ : → calculate the ratio: $\dfrac{\Delta \text{ anion gap}}{\Delta HCO_3^-}$ [i.e.: actual anion gap - normal anion gap (10)] [i.e.: actual HCO_3^- - normal HCO_3^- (24)] If ≈ 1.6: lactic acidosis. If ≈ 1.1: ketosis. If ≈ ≤ 1.1: normal and high anion gap acidosis. If ≈ ≥ 2.1: added metabolic alkalosis. - If anion gap is ↑: calculate osmolar gap = Posm - calculated osmolality ($2Na^+$ + BUN + glucose + ethanol). Normal =10 mosm/L.
Causes	Anion gap may be ↓ with hypoalbuminemia (↓ 10 g/L albumin = ↓ 2.5 mEq of anion gap), monoclonal gammopathy, ↑ Ca^{++}, ↑ Mg^{++}, ↑ K^+, lithium toxicity, carbenicillin. **Normal** anion gap secondary to either loss of bicarbonate (gastro-intestinal or urinary), or to a decreased renal excretion of hydrogen, or to the administration of an acid. - If K^+ ↓ or normal: diarrhea, fistula, ileal bladder, ureterosigmoidostomy, carbonic anhydrase inhibitor, type I renal tubular acidosis (which may be due to Sjögren's syndrome, hypergammaglobulinemia, sickle cell disease, toluene, amphotericin B, lithium), or type II (which may be secondary to myeloma, cystinosis, lead, tetracycline, acetazolamide), recovery from DKA, posthypocapnia. - If K^+ ↑ or normal: HCl administration, TPN with arginine or lysine, $NH4Cl$, calcium chloride, adrenal insufficiency, renal failure, obstructive uropathy, congenital adrenal hyperplasia, type IV renal tubular acidosis (which may be secondary to diabetes, interstitial nephritis, spironolactone, amiloride, cyclosporine). Anion gap ↑ : **G**lycols (ethylene, propylene). **O**xoproline (with acetaminophen use). **L**-lactate (with cellular hypoxia [shock, mesenteric ischemia...], liver failure, cyanide intoxication, carbon monoxide intoxication, drugs (metformin in renal failure, alcohol, nucleoside reverse transcriptase inhibitors, iron, isoniazid, toluene, etc) **D**-lactate (with short bowel syndrome). **M**ethanol. **A**spirin. **R**enal failure. **K**etoacidosis (diabetes, alcohol, fasting). Acidosis with ↑ anion gap and ↑ osmolar gap (> 10 mosm/L) : **M**ethanol. **C**hronic kidney disease. **T**oluene. **E**thylene glycol.
Treatment	According to cause. Acute: $NaHCO_3$ if HCO_3^- < 10 mmHg. Aim for HCO_3^- 10-12 mmHg or pH > 7.10-7.20 (number of mmol of HCO_3^- necessary = 0.5 x weight x [desired HCO_3^- (10) - measured HCO_3^-]: To correct IV over 4 to 8 h if possible). Takes 30 minutes to reach equilibrium. Note: 1 vial (50 mL) $NaHCO_3$ = 50 mEq HCO_3^-.
Respiratory Acidosis	Secondary to hypoventilation. The alveolo-arterial gradient ($A-aDO_2$) is useful to distinguish between an alveolar hypoventilation (where gradient is normal) and a pulmonary disease (V/Q mismatch, shunt, diffusion problem where gradient is ↑):

	$A\text{-}aDO_2 = PAO_2$ ($150 - [1.25 \times PCO_2])$ - PaO_2 (in room air). Normal < 30 (depending on age: 6-10 at 20 y.o., 26-30 at 70 y.o.).
Cause	**Acute:** airway obstruction (asthma, aspiration, laryngospasm), depression of respiratory control centers (drugs [opiate, sedatives], oxygen therapy in COPD, central sleep apnea), gas exchange problems (ARDS, cardiogenic pulmonary edema, pneumonia, pneumothorax), neuromuscular disease (myasthenic crisis, periodic paralysis, Guillain-Barré, bolutism), hypokalemia or severe hypophosphatemia, mechanical hypoventilation, post cardiopulmonary arrest, etc. **Chronic:** COPD, depression of respiratory control centers, neuromuscular disease (polymyositis, amyotrophic lateral sclerosis, myxoedema), restrictive disease, kyphoscoliosis, morbid obesity, sleep apnea.
Treatment	Depending on cause. Naloxone for overdose.
Metabolic Alkalosis	Hypovolemic state or hypervolemia (can be differentiated with urinary chloride). If $pCO_2 > 55$ mmHg: mixed metabolic alkalosis/respiratory acidosis.

Cause	**If urinary Cl⁻ < 20 mmol/L :**
	– H⁺ losses:
	    o GI losses: vomiting, nasogastric suction, antacids, especially with kayexalate, laxative abuse.
	    o Renal losses: Thiazide or loop diuretics, penicillin or high dose carbenicillin, sulfate, phosphate, post-hypercapnia, hypercalcemia with milk-alkali syndrome, hypermineralocorticoid state, Bartter's syndrome.
	– Gain of HCO_3^-: massive transfusions (citrate), $NaHCO_3$ administration, use of Ringer's lactate, TPN.
	– Shift of intracellular hydrogen: hypokalemia.
	– "Contraction alkalosis" secondary to hypovolemia.
	
	If urinary Cl⁻ > 20 mmol/L: check urinary K⁺ and blood pressure:
	- If UK⁺ < 30 mmol/L: laxative abuse or severe K⁺ depletion.
	- If UK⁺ > 30 mmol/L and low or normal blood pressure: Bartter's syndrome or diuretic abuse.
	- If UK⁺ > 30 mmol/L and hypertension: check renin:
	    – If low renin: primary hyperaldosteronism or licorice abuse.
	    – If high renin: Cushing's disease, juxtaglomerular apparatus tumor, malignant hypertension or renovascular hypertension.

Treatment	Emergency if pH > 7.60. Treatment according to cause : – If hypovolemia: IV NaCl 0.9 %, stop diuretics. – If hypokalemia, give KCl. Rule out hypomagnesemia. – If edematous state, correct hypokalemia first if necessary, can use acetazolamide (250 up to 375 mg daily or bid).
Respiratory Alkalosis	Secondary to hyperventilation. If $pCO_2 < 15$ mmHg: mixed respiratory alkalosis/metabolic acidosis.
Cause	Hypoxemia: Pulmonary disease (edema, PE, pneumonia, asthma, interstitial fibrosis...) heart failure, high altitude, hypotension, severe anemia, etc. Central nervous system disorders: anxiety, neurologic disease (stroke, pontine tumor), fever, pain, encephalopathy, hepatitis, drugs (salicylates, xanthines, nicotines), hormones (progesterone, pregnancy), sepsis, after quick correction of a metabolic acidosis. Mechanical hyperventilation.
Treatment	According to cause.
Mixed Disorders	Two or more disorders often coexist. Use rules of thumb above to determine whether the compensation corresponds to that expected for a pure respiratory or metabolic acidosis or alkalosis. If it doesn't, there is most likely a mixed disorder.

Glomerulonephritis

Nephritic Syndrome

Active sediment (hematuria, RBC casts, proteinuria usually < 3 g/day), hypertension, edema and occasionally oliguria.
Medical emergency!! Quick assessment in order to avoid chronic kidney disease.

Workup: C3, C4, ANA, ANCA, anti-GBM antibodies, antistreptolysin O, hepatitis B and C serology, cryoglobulins, serum and urinary protein electrophoresis, renal biopsy.

Focal involvement:	
Involving some glomeruli (focal) or a portion of the glomeruli (segmental).	
IgA Nephropathy (Berger)	**Clinical**: most frequent cause of idiopathic glomerulonephritis: age < 35 years. Male: female ratio of 1. Occasionally positive family history. History of microscopic or post-URTI recurrent macroscopic hematuria (latency < 5 days). **Causes**: most often idiopathic: occasionally associated with Henoch-Schönlein purpura, cirrhosis, rheumatoid spondylitis, psoriasis, Reiter, enteritis, inflammatory bowel disease, celiac disease, dermatitis herpetiformis, HIV. **Workup**: Renal biopsy : diffuse mesangial deposits of IgA **Treatment**: controversial: if mild renal failure and non nephrotic proteinuria, ACEI ± ARB could be tried before steroids to ↓ proteinuria and ↓ BP; steroids (particularly with mild, non chronic changes on biopsy or if disease progresses despite ACEI or ARB) ± immunosuppressive agents. Fish oil could be tried if non nephrotic proteinuria ± mild renal failure. ACEI ± ARB to ↓ proteinuria and ↓ BP **Prognosis**: variable: 20-30 % ESRD overall; 20 % CKD over 20 years. Recurrence in transplanted kidney may occur but rarely causes graft failure.
Hereditary Nephropathy (Alport)	3 forms of genetic transmission (80 % of cases X- linked). **Clinical**: hearing and ocular defects **Workup**: renal biopsy: thickening of the GBM on electron microscopy. **Treatment**: no specific treatment. ACEI and/or ARB. Dialysis or renal transplant. **Prognosis**: ESRD among males 15-40 years old but variable.
Diffuse involvement	
Infection-Related Glomerulo-nephritis	**Causes**: streptococcus (group A), staphylococcus, pneumococcus, virus, parasites, fungi, endocarditis, infected shunt, abscess, osteomyelitis, severe pneumonia, etc. **Clinical**: hematuria, proteinuria, edema, hypertension abruptly 7-21 days after the infection. **Workup**: culture ⊕ or ASO ⊕, complement ↓. Large subepithelial deposits (humps) on renal biopsy if poststreptococcal. **Treatment** symptomatic therapy and antibiotics for infection (does not alter the nephritis). **Prognosis**: good; hematuria resolved in 6 months. No recurrence. CKD occurs rarely (< 5 %).
Membrano-proliferative	5 % of glomerulonephritis in adults. 3 types on pathology (type 1, 2 or 3) **Cause**: idiopathic (primary) or secondary to SLE, HBV, HCV, cryoglobulinemia, infections (endocarditis), cancer (CLL). **Clinical** mixed nephrotic and nephritic. **Workup**: complement ↓ 50 % (↓ C3 in type II). C3NeF ↑ especially in type II. **Treatment**: controversial: steroids ± immunosuppressive agents if disease progresses. Antiplatelet agent. Treat primary cause. **Prognosis**: frequently leads to CKD.
Rapidly Progressive	**Clinical**: with constant deterioration and active sediment. Biopsy shows crescents in > 50 % of glomeruli. **3 types**: - Type 1: Anti-GBM (10 % cases): young man, pulmonary hemorrhage (Goodpasture's syndrome): linear deposit of IgG + C3: normal complement. - Type 2: immune complex (40 % of cases): secondary (SLE, infection, cryoglobulinemia, cancer …) or primary (glomerulonephritis: membranoproliferative,

	membranous, IgA nephropathy). - Type 3: Pauci-immune (50 % of case): majority ANCA⊕: few or no immune deposits on immunofluorescence or at electron microscopy. **Workup**: ANCA, anti-GBM antibodies, ANA, C3, C4, vasculitis workup, renal biopsy. **Treatment**: steroids + immunosuppressive agents. Plasma exchange for Goodpasture's syndrome. **Prognosis**: depends on cause and treatment: poor if treated with creatinine > 530 µmol/L.
Fibrillary	Pathology similar as amyloidosis. No treatment.

Nephrotic syndrome
Proteinuria > 3.0-3.5 g/day, hypoalbuminemia (< 35 g/L), edema, hyperlipidemia, lipiduria, hypercoagulability.

Workup: C3, C4, ANA, serum and urine protein electrophoresis, hepatitis B and C, HIV, cryoglobulins. Renal biopsy.

Primary	
Membranous	Second most common type of glomerulonephritis in adults (25-30 %): renal vein thrombosis a possible complication. **Cause**: often idiopathic: sometimes secondary to solid tumor (10 %), Hodgkin's lymphoma, SLE, rheumatoid arthritis, thyroiditis, infections (HBV, HCV, syphilis, malaria), drugs (penicillamine, captopril, gold, NSAIDs). **Workup**: on biopsy, thickened GBM and subepithelial IgG + C3 granular deposits on electron microscopy. **Treatment**: immunosuppressive agents ± steroids if risk of progression (man > 50 years old, renal insufficiency, severe nephrotic-range proteinuria (particularly if > 10 g/day).persistent proteinuria, glomerular scarring). **Prognosis**: at 10 years: 5-20 % spontaneous resolution, 25 % to 40 % partial resolution (proteinuria < 2 g/day), 30 % to 40 % progressive CKD to ESRD.
Minimal Change	Most frequent cause in children, 15-25 % of glomerulonephritis in adults. **Causes**: most often idiopathic: sometimes cancer related (Hodgkin's lymphoma, leukemia), diabetes, drugs (NSAIDs, lithium). **Workup**: on biopsy, fusion of foot processes on electron microscopy. **Treatment**: steroids. If inadequate response, steroid dependance or frequent recurrences: immunosuppressive agents. **Prognosis**: Good; no progression to CKD. 30 to 50 % recurrence. If steroid resistance, suspect focal segmental glomerulosclerosis; repeat renal biopsy as needed.
Focal Segmental Glomeruloscle-rosis	The most frequent in adults (25-30 %): most frequent in African Americans. **Clinical features**: hypertension, hematuria, ↑ creatinine in 50 %: nephrotic-range proteinuria in 66 % on presentation: associated tubular dysfunction. **Causes**: most often idiopathic; may be due to heroin, HIV, sickle cell, reflux nephropathy, obesity, cyanotic heart disease, ↓ renal mass. May also be hereditary (treatment differs accordingly). **Workup**: on biopsy, focal zones of sclerosis. **Treatment**: If primary: steroids (40-50 % response). If inadequate response, steroid dependance or frequent recurrence, immunosuppressive agents, ACEI ± ARB. **Prognosis**: poor: < 10 % spontaneous remission: CKD after 1-20 years. Aggressive in HIV (ESRD in 1 year).
Other causes	Membranoproliferative glomerulonephritis 7 %, rapidly progressive glomerulonephritis 2 %, fibrillary 1% (Note: active sediment found in these conditions).

Secondary :	
25 % of nephrotic syndromes are secondary. Causes: diabetes (most frequent cause), SLE, amyloidosis (if > 45 years old), vasculitis, cancer, infection (HBV, HCV, HIV), preeclampsia.	
Treatment	– Water and salt restriction (< 2 g/day), low satured fat and proteins (1 g/kg/d). – Diuretics for edema and hypertension (furosemide ± thiazides). – Lipid-lowering therapy as needed. – Vitamin supplements with vitamin D and iron. – Consider ACEI or ARB to reduce proteinuria. – Risk for infections (vaccines, immunoglobulins as needed) and thrombosis (renal vein, legs, pulmonary embolism). – Adjust drug doses (because of hypoalbuminemia).

Hematuria

Definition: ≥ 3 red blood cells/field (magnification 400 x), on ≥ 2/3 samples.
Look for: history of renal disease, stone or coagulopathy; family history; recent URTI; painful (stone, infection, infarction) vs. painless hematuria (exercise, glomerulonephritis, tumor, polycystic kidney disease, tuberculosis); initial (at initiation of micturition; urethra) - mid-stream vs. terminal hematuria (end of micturition; prostate, bladder); microscopic or macroscopic hematuria ; hematuria with vs. without proteinuria; with vs. without dysuria; with vs. without systemic symptoms : with vs. without obstructive symptoms; with vs. without clots; coloration of urine.

Causes	Glomerular

	Primary or secondary glomerulonephritis (see: glomerulonephritis table).
	    Thin basal membrane disease (benign familial hematuria).
	    Fabry's disease.
	Non glomerular
	    - Renal parenchyma: renal adenocarcinoma, simple cyst, vascular (exercise, malignant hypertension, arteriovenous malformation or shunt, renal infarction, renal vein thrombosis, loin pain hematuria syndrome), metabolic (hypercalciuria, hyperuricosuria, hyperoxaluria, cystinuria), familial (polycystic kidney, medullary sponge kidney), infection (acute pyelonephritis, tuberculosis), papillary necrosis.
	    - Extrarenal: tumor (pelvis, bladder, ureter, prostate), benign prostatic hypertrophy, stone, infection (cystitis, prostatitis, urethritis, schistosomiasis, tuberculosis).
	    - Others: drugs (heparin, warfarin, cyclophosphamide), coagulopathy, trauma (recent urinary catheter, boxing, football, vigorous exercise), fever.
	
	Differential diagnosis: menstruation.
	
	Differential diagnosis of hematuria on dipstick without red cells on microscopy: myoglobinuria, hemoglobinuria, alkaline urine (UpH ≥ 9), proviodine, diluted urine, sperm.
	
	Differential diagnosis of red urine with normal urinalysis: beet ingestion, phenazopyrine, rifampicine, porphyria.

Workup	– Urinalysis and culture, **urinary sediment** (to differentiate between glomerular [casts, dysmorphic red cells...] and non glomerular hematuria). – CBC, electrolytes, Ca^{++}, uric acid, INR, aPTT, urinary **cytology**. – If it doesn't seem to be of glomerular origin: abdominal ultrasonography or spiral CT± cystoscopy (if ≥ 40 years old or smoker) ± IV pyelography. – If needed: mycobacterial urine culture, anti-schistosomiasis antibodies. – Workup for nephrolithiasis: stone analysis if possible: urinalysis and culture: 24 h urine collection for volume, creatinine, Ca^{++}, Na^+, uric acid, oxalate, citrate: ± Mg^{++}, PO_4^{3-}, urea.

Proteinuria	
Definitions: Proteinuria > 150 mg/24 h. Nephrotic > 3.0 to 3.5 g/24 h. Microalbuminuria 30-300 mg/24 h, macroalbuminuria > 300 mg/24 h. Dipstick: trace = 0.1g/L; 1+ = 0.3 g/L; 2+ = 1 g/L; 3+ = 3 g/L; 4+ = 10 g/L. False ⊕ if urine is concentrated, hematuria, pH > 8, antiseptic, contrast agents. False ⊖ if urine is diluted or if the protein in urine is not albumin (e.g.: light chain).	
Causes	Non nephrotic proteinuria: - Functional proteinuria can occur with fever, exercise, seizure or decompensated heart failure or uncontrolled diabetes. - Orthostatic proteinuria. - Urinary infection. - Glomerular diseases (especially at the onset). - Multiple myeloma. - Tubulointerstitial diseases : interstitial nephritis, reflux nephropathy, Wilson's, cystinosis, renal tubular acidosis, Fanconi's, heavy metal toxicity, obstructive uropathy, vitamin D overdose, radiotherapy, etc. - Glomerular sclerosis secondary to hyperfiltration (for example in chronic kidney disease.) - Ischemic nephropathy (nephrotic range rare). Nephrotic proteinuria: see Glomerulonephritis table.
Workup	– Urinalysis and urine culture and sediment. – Protein, albumin, creatinine, lipid, serum and urine protein electrophoresis, serum and urine protein immunoelectrophoresis, ANA, complement, cryoglobulines, HBV serology, HCV and HIV, ASO ... based on the clinical picture. – Protein/creatinine ratio on a random urine sample is a good estimate of the 24h urinary protein excretion. – Supine (8 h) and standing (16 h) proteinuria (diagnosis of orthostatic proteinuria). – Renal ultrasonography. – Renal biopsy if no diagnosis (contraindication if solitary kidney, atrophic kidneys, multiple bilateral renal cysts, hydronephrosis, cancer, active renal or perirenal infection, severe hypertension, coagulopathy): not necessary if proteinuria < 1-2 g/day, normal GFR, no hypertension and no evidence of systemic disease.
Management	– Depending on cause. – Water and salt restriction ± diuretics. – ACEI ± ARB (because a lower proteinuria slows the progression of the chronic kidney disease). – Target BP < 130/80 mm Hg and possibly lower if proteinuria > 1g/day (caution if systolic BP < 110 mmHg). – Avoid nephrotoxic agents. – Lipid lowering therapy as needed.

Acute Renal Failure

Definition:
- Anuria < 50 mL/24 h (differential diagnosis: rapidly progressive glomerulonephritis, cortical necrosis, bilateral renal artery occlusion, single renal artery occlusion, urinary obstruction with stone or other, obstructed bladder catheter).
- Oliguria < 400 mL/24 h.
- ARF without oliguria (particularly with aminoglycosides).
- Polyuria > 3000 mL/24 h (diagnosis: partial obstruction).

Renal clues to differentiate between pre-renal vs renal ARF:

	prerenal	renal (acute tubular necrosis)
Urinary osmolality	> 500 mosm/kg H_2O	< 400 mosm/kg H_2O
Urinary density	> 1.018	< 1.015
Urinary sediment	Normal	Granular casts
Urinary Na^+	< 20 mmol/L	> 40 mmol/L
U creat / P creat	> 40	< 20
P BUN / P creatinine	> 0.1	< 0.05
Fractional excretion of Na^+ (UNa^+/PNa^+)/ (Ucreat/Pcreat)	< 0.01	> 0.02

Differential diagnosis:
↑ creatinine (not related to kidney function): diabetic ketoacidosis, isopropylic acid, antibiotics (trimethoprim, cefoxitin), cimetidine, ASA, amiloride, flucytosine, famotidine, ranitidine, rhabdomyolysis.
↑ BUN (not related to kidney function): catabolism, high-protein diet, GI bleeding, fever, amino acid infusion, steroids, tetracycline.

Causes		Workup
Prerenal	True hypovolemia (shock, bleeding, polyuria, skin and GI losses), decreased effective volume (3rd spacing, low cardiac output, severe nephrotic syndrome, cirrhosis). Hepatorenal syndrome. Drugs: NSAIDs (including Cox-2 specific), ACEI, ARB, diuretics.	Urinary electrolytes
Renal	**Acute tubular necrosis** : Ischemia. Exogenous nephrotoxins: aminoglycosides, amphotericin B, Chinese herbal medicines, vancomycin, pentamidine, contrast agents, cisplatin, etc. Endogenous nephrotoxins: myoglobin (rhabdomyolysis), hemoglobin (hemolysis).	Urinalysis Urinary electrolytes Sediment CK ± myoglobinuria Hemolysis workup
	Glomerulonephritis: see. glomerulonephritis table	Sediment -HIV-etc
	Acute interstitial nephritis: Drugs: NSAIDs, antibiotics (penicillin, quinolones, sulfonamides, rifampicin, cephalosporins), interferon, ACEI, acetaminophen, anticonvulsants, lithium, allopurinol, cyclosporine, tacrolimus, chemotherapy, Chinese herbal medicines, etc. Sarcoidosis, lymphoma, infection, autoimmune diseases.	Sediment (WBC cast) Eosinophilia. Eosinophiluria. Urine culture. Gallium renal scan

	Vascular : Bilateral renal artery or vein thrombosis. Malignant hypertension. Vasculitis. Embolism (cholesterol, cardiogenic). TTP/HUS (± HELLP or postpartum). Cortical necrosis (with pregnancy). Papillary necrosis (especially with diabetes). After CABG or AAA surgery. Aortic dissection. Disseminated intravascular coagulation. Scleroderma. Cyclosporine.	Renal U/S, Doppler Vasculitis workup ECG, Echocardiography Complement Eosinophil count Blood smear Hemolysis workup + DIC workup.
Postrenal	**Intrinsic:** multiple myeloma, crystal nephropathy (uric acid, acyclovir, methotrexate, ethylene glycol, calcium oxalate, sulfonamides, protease inhibitors ...). **Extrinsic:** benign prostate hypertrophy, cancer, retroperitoneal fibrosis, bilateral nephrolithiasis, catheter, lymphadenopathy, clot.	Renal ultrasonography Bladder catheter. Protein electrophoresis, uric acid, etc.
Management	Look for causes on history, physical examination (dry mucous membrane, bladder, prostate...) and workup. Look for consequences (edema, bleeding, encephalopathy [asterixis], pericarditis). Biopsy rarely necessary for diagnosis. Adjustment of drugs doses (because of the ↓ glomerular filtration rate). Treatment : depend on the cause : – Reverse the cause if known. – Optimize blood volume. – Hydration ± forced diuresis (NaCl 0, 9 % vs NaHCO$_3$ ± mannitol) for myoglobinuria. – High dose diuretic for severe acute tubular necrosis in order to control volemia. – Steroids, immunosuppressors for acute interstitial nephritis. Consider trial of Prednisone 1 mg/kg daily for 2-3 months. – Relieve obstruction in postrenal failure. – Dialysis for : 1- ↑ K$^+$, ↑↑ PO$_4$$^{3-}$ 2- Severe metabolic acidosis 3- Pericarditis 4- Encephalopathy 5- Edema 6- BUN > 35 mmol/L (?) Prevention: with the administration of contrast in high risk patients (if creatinine >140 µmol/L or clearance < 50 mL/min) : stop diuretics, ACEI, ARB, NSAIDs the day before – give 3 vials of 50 mL of NaHCO$_3$/1 litre D5W at 3 mL/kg 1 hour before procedure and 1 mL/kg for 6 hours post-procedure or NaCl 0.9 % 1 mL/kg/hour 12 hours before and after the procedure ± N-acetylcysteine 600-1200 mg bid the evening before, and on the day of the procedure (benefit from N-acetylcysteine controversial).

Chronic Kidney Disease

Definition	According to *National Kidney Foundation*, CKD is : 1- kidney damage ≥ 3 months, confirmed by pathologic abnormalities or by markers, with or without fall in glomerular filtration rate (GFR) **or** 2- GFR < 60 mL/min for ≥ 3 months, with or without renal damage.

Stages of severity	Normal glomerular filtration rate (GFR) :
	    Man : 95-145 mL/min.
	    Woman : 75-115 mL/min.
	
	National Kidney Foundation's stages of severity:
	Stage 1: Creatinine clearance ≥ 90 mL/min/1.73 m^2: kidney damage with normal or ↑ GFR.
	Stage 2: Creatinine clearance 60-89 mL/min/1.73 m^2: kidney damage with mild ↓ of GFR.
	Stage 3: Creatinine clearance 30-59 mL/min/1.73 m^2: moderated ↓ of GFR.
	Stage 4: Creatinine clearance 15-29 mL/min/1.73 m^2: severe ↓ of GFR.
	Stage 5: Creatinine clearance < 15 mL/min/1.73 m^2 (or dialysis): kidney failure.

Causes	1- Diabetic nephropathy: causes 37 % of CKD; most often associated with proteinuria > 3.5 g/d and retinopathy: occurs around 25 years after diagnosis of diabetes but quite variable. 2- Hypertension (nephroangiosclerosis, ischemic nephropathy) causes 30 % of CKD (African-American > Caucasian). 3- Glomerulopathy (other than diabetes): causes 12 % of CKD: associated with proteinuria > 3.5 g/d, active sediment or evidence of systemic disease associated with glomerulonephritis. 4- Other causes: polycystic kidney 4 %, chronic interstitial nephritis 4 %, obstructive uropathy, myeloma kidney, transplant disease (severe acute rejection, chronic dysfunction, calcineurin inhibitor nephrotoxicity [cyclosporine, tacrolimus], recurrence of disease), etc.
Complications	Cardiovascular: edema, hypertension, accelerated atherosclerosis, cardiomyopathy, pericarditis, tamponade. Electrolyte and acid-base: metabolic acidosis, hyperkalemia. Endocrine: hyperparathyroidism, defect in vitamin D metabolism, decreased libido, impotence, hyperprolactinemia, insulin resistance. Gastrointestinal: anorexia, nausea and vomiting, stomatitis, pancreatitis, gastritis. Hematologic: anemia, platelet dysfunction (bleeding). Neurologic: encephalopathy, restless leg syndrome, cramps, distal neuropathy, impaired concentration, insomnia. Rheumatologic: amyloidosis (β-2 microglobulin deposits), crystal-induced arthropathy, renal osteodystrophy. Skin: pruritus, delayed wound healing. Acquired polycystic kidney (> 5 cysts: ↑ risk of renal cancer x 5).
Workup	Basic workup : CBC, Na$^+$, K$^+$, Cl$^-$, Ca^{++}, PO$_4^{3-}$, albumin, glucose, creatinine, BUN, uric acid, ferritin and transferrin saturation, PTH, venous blood gas analysis, serum and urine protein electrophoresis, urinalysis ± sediment, chest X-ray , renal ultrasound. If needed: immunologic workup, serology (HBV, HCV, HIV), measurement of glomerular filtration rate, renal Doppler, renal CT-angio or MR-angio, renal arteriography, biopsy, etc. Distinguish between ARF and CKD: for ARF the causal event can often be identified: for CKD anemia is usually present, as well as ↑ PO$_4^3$, ↓ Ca^{++}, small kidneys on U/S. Refer to a nephrologist, at the latest, when creatinine ≥ 300 µmol/L or creatinine clearance < 30 mL/minute, or earlier if creatinine increases rapidly.

Cockcroft-Gault formula : Creatinine clearance (mL/min) = $$\frac{(140\text{-age}) \times \text{weight (kg)} \quad (\times 1.02 \text{ for women} : \times 1.25 \text{ for men})}{\text{serum creatinine } (\mu\text{mol/L})}$$ Simplified MDRD formula (*Modification of Diet in renal Disease*) (available on following website: http://mdrd.com): Creatinine clearance (mL/min/1.73 m²) = 175 x (creatinine/88.4) $^{-1.154}$ x (age) $^{-0.203}$ x (0.742 if female) x (1.210 if African-American).	

Treatment	Identify and correct/avoid reversible causes of the renal deterioration: hypovolemia, heart failure, postrenal obstruction, accelerated hypertension, drugs (NSAIDs [including Cox-2 specific], ACEI, ARB), contrast agents, ischemic nephropathy.
	
	 – Low protein diet (1 g protein/kg if GFR 13-25 mL/min), low potassium and phosphorus diet ± water and salt restriction.
	 – ACEI or ARB for diabetic nephropathy if microalbuminuria ⊕ and for non diabetic nephropathy if proteinuria ⊕ (slows renal deterioration).
	 – Renal angioplasty for renovascular disease (> 50-70 % stenosis and kidney > 8 cm): consider for poor control of BP with ≥ 3 antihypertensives or fibromuscular dysplasia or history of pulmonary edema or unexplained progressive renal failure. Benefits to stabilize renal function at long term are not demonstrated.
	 – Treatment of anemia with erythropoietin or darbopoietin (Eprex® or Aranesp®): indicated if hemoglobin (Hb) < 100 g/L and GFR ≤ 30 mL/min. Target Hb 100-120 g/L (add iron as needed PO or IV for ferritin > 100 µg/L and transferrin saturation > 20 %).
	 – Prevention of renal osteodystrophy:
	   - If ↑ PO_4^{3-} → ↓ in diet.
	   - If ↑ PO_4^{3-} > 1.49 for stages 3 et 4 and > 1.78 mmol/L for stage 5: chelating agents: calcium carbonate with meals max. 1.5 g/d, sevelamer (Renagel®).
	   - If CKD stage 3, 4 or 5 and PTH ↑ : if calcium (corrected) 2.10-2.37 mmol/L **and** PO_4^{3-} 0.87-1.49 mmol/L with chelating agent in stage 3-4 or PO_4^{3-} 0.87-1.78 mmol/L with chelating agent in stage 5, give 1.25(OH)$_2$D$_3$ (Rocaltrol® or One-Alpha®) → follow Ca⁺⁺ and PO_4^{3-} and stop if Ca⁺⁺ x PO_4^{3-} > 4.3.
	   Target PTH normal in stage 3, PTH 8-12 pmol/L in stage 4 and PTH 17-33 pmol/L in stage 5.
	 – Treatment of metabolic acidosis (occurs when GFR < 25 mL/min): NaHCO₃ 0.5-1 mEq/kg/d in 2 doses to titrate for HCO₃⁻ at 22-24 mmol/L (watch for volume overload).
	 – Treatment of hyperkaliemia: see table in "Disorders of Serum Potassium".
	 – Aggressive treatment of cardiac risk factors:
	   - Control BP: target < 130/80 mmHg.
	   - Control dyslipidemia (target LDL < 2 mmol/L and ratio total cholesterol/HDL < 4) and blood glucose.
	   - Stop smoking.
	   - Aspirin
	
	 Adjust all drugs according to GFR and hypoalbuminemia.
	
	 Dialysis: peritoneal or hemodialysis: begin when creatinine clearance 10-15 mL/min, or persistent nausea and vomiting, diuretic resistant volume overload, pericarditis, evidence of undernutrition, uremic encephalopathy.
	 Consider kidney transplantation.
	
	 Note: Preparation for dialysis takes at least one year (this is why it must be addressed as soon as possible, when creatinine clearance < 25-30 mL/min in a patient who is a dialysis candidate).
	 Education - Support group.
	
	 Prevention : with the administration of contrast in high risk patients (if creatinine > 140 µmol/L or clearance < 50 mL/min) : stop diuretics, ACEI, ARB, NSAIDs … the day before – give 3 vials of 50 mL of NaHCO₃/ 1 litre D5W at 3 mL/kg 1 hour before procedure

| | and 1 mL/kg for 6 hours post-procedure or NaCl 0.9 % 1 mL/kg/hour 12 hours before and after the procedure ± N-acetylcysteine 600-1200 mg bid the evening before, and on the day of the procedure (benefit from N-acetylcysteine controversial). |

Useful References: NEPHROLOGY

Acid-Base Disorders: Lancet 1998; 352: 474-79 (review article)
    N Engl J Med 1998; 338: 26-34 & 107-111 (review article)
Acute Interstitial Nephritis: J Am Soc Nephrol 1998; 9: 506-15 (review article)
Acute Renal Failure: Lancet 2005 ; 365 : 417-30 (review article)
    Mayo Clin Proc 2001; 76: 67-74 (review article)
Acute Tubular Necrosis: Ann Intern Med 2002; 137: 744-52 (review article)
Autosomal Dominant Polycystic Kidney Disease: Lancet 2007; 369: 1287-301 (review article)
    N Engl J Med 2008; 359: 1477-85 (review article)
Calcium Disorders: Lancet 1998; 352: 306-11 (review article)
Chronic Kidney Disease: CMAJ 2008; 179: 1154-62 (CSN Guidelines)
    Mayo Clin Proc 2008; 83: 1064-69 (review article)
    CMAJ 2003; 168: 1553-60 (review article)
    Ann Intern Med 2003; 139: 137-47 (NKF American Guidelines)
Contrast Nephropathy: J Am Coll Cardiol 2008; 51: 1419-28 (review article)
    N Engl J Med 2006; 354: 379-86 (review article)
Diabetes Insipidus: Cleve Clin J Med 2006; 73: 65-71 (review article)
Diabetic Nephropathy: Diabetes Care 2005; 28: 164-176 (review article)
    N Engl J Med 2002; 346: 1145-51 (review article)
Dialysis: N Engl J Med 1998; 338: 1428-37 (review article)
Glomerulonephritis: N Engl J Med 1998; 339: 888-99 (review article)
    Diagnostic: Arch Intern Med 2001; 161: 25-34 (review article)
    … Acute: Postgrad Med J 2003; 79: 206-13 (review article)
Graft-Versus-Host Disease: Lancet 2009; 373: 1550-61 (review article)
Hematuria: Med Clin North Am 2004; 88: 329-44 (review article)
    … Microscopic: N Engl J Med 2003; 348: 2330-38 (review article)
    Urology 2001; 57: 599-603 & 604-610 (AUA Guidelines)
Hypercalcemia: N Engl J Med 1992; 326: 1196-203 (review article)
    Treatment: J Am Soc Nephrol 2001; 17: S3-9 (review article)
    … paraneoplastic: N Engl J Med 2005 ; 352 : 373-79 (review article)
Hypernatremia: N Engl J Med 2000; 342: 1493-99 (review article)
Hyperparathyroidism: J Clin Endocrinol Metab 2009; 94: 335-39 (American Guidelines)
    Lancet 2009; 374: 14-58 (review article)
    N Engl J Med 2004; 350: 1746-51 (review article)
Hypokalemia: N Engl J Med 1998; 339: 451-8 (review article)
    Arch Intern Med 2000; 160: 2429-2436 (review article)
Hyponatremia: N Engl J Med 2000; 342: 1581- (review article)
    CMAJ 2002; 166: 1056-62 (review article)
    … Treatment: Am J Med 2007; 120: S1-S21 (review article)
Hypophosphatemia: Am J Med 2005; 118: 1094-1101 (review article)
IgA Nephropathy: Clev Clin J Med 2008; 75: 569-76 (review article)
    N Engl J Med 2002; 347: 738-48 (review article)
Magnesium and Phorphorus Disorders: Lancet 1998; 352: 391-96 (review article)
Metabolic Alkalosis: J Am Soc Nephrol 2000; 11: 369-75 (review article)
Milk-Alkali Syndrome: Mayo Clin Proc 2009; 84: 261-67 (review article)
Nephrolithiasis: N Engl J Med 2004; 350: 684-93 (review article)
    Lancet 2001; 358: 651-6 (review article)
    … Recurrent: CMAJ 2002; 166: 213-8 (review article)
Nephrotic Syndrome: N Engl J Med 1998; 338: 1202-11 (review article)
Parathyroid Disorders: N Engl J Med 2000; 343: 1863-75 (review article)
Potassium Disorders: Lancet 1998; 352: 135-40 (review article)
Proteinuria: Am J Med Sci 2000; 320: 188-94 (review article)
Renal Angioplasty: Circulation 2006; 113; 1464-1473 (review article)
Renovascular Disease: Ann Intern Med 2006; 145: 901-912 (review article)
    Circulation 2005; 112: 1362-1374 (review article)
    N Engl J Med 2001; 344: 431-42 (review article)
Rhabdomyolysis: N Engl J Med 2009; 361: 62-72 (review article)
Sodium Disorders: Lancet 1998; 352: 220-28 (review article)
SIADH: N Engl J Med 2007; 356: 2064-72 (review article)

Chapter 8

Neurology

Coma	
– History: time course of altered consciousness, recent medical history, initial symptoms, psychiatric and surgical history, medication, drug abuse. Check with family, neighbours, witnesses and ambulance personnel, as needed. – Physical examination: vital signs, respiratory pattern, response to painful stimuli, pupillary response, eye movements, fundi by direct ophthalmoscopy, meningismus, brainstem reflexes (gag, palpebral, pupillary, corneal, oculocephalic, oculovestibular), limb movements, deep tendon reflexes, muscle tone … – General physical examination (odors, skin lesions, mouth, signs of trauma, cardio-pulmonary and abdominal examination). Look for Medic-Alert® bracelet.	

Causes	In general, if focal signs on physical examination = underlying structural lesion. If not = metabolic cause. Mnemonic: **DASSAMI**: **D**rugs intoxication (including toxins and medications). **A**lcohol intoxication. **S**troke: brainstem (reticular activating system), or both cerebral hemispheres. **S**eizures: postictal state. **A**noxia: post-cardiac arrest, massive hemorrhage. **M**etabolic: secondary to electrolyte disturbance (Ca^{++}, Na^{++}), hypoxia, hypo/hyperglycemia, severe hypo/hyperthyroidism, thiamine deficiency. **I**nfectious: meningitis, encephalitis, etc. **Other rarer causes:** Trauma, mass lesion (tumor, abscess, hydrocephalus), basilar migraine, neuroleptic malignant syndrome, psychiatric (conversion disorder) … Note: 2/3 of all comas have a metabolic cause (usually without lateralizing signs).
Glasgow Coma Scale (GCS)	Especially useful for coma of traumatic etiology: – Eye opening: spontaneous = 4; to verbal stimuli = 3; to painful stimuli = 2; none, even with painful stimuli = 1. – Speech: oriented and converses = 5; disoriented but converses = 4; inappropriate words = 3; incomprehensible sounds = 2; no verbalization, even with painful stimulus = 1. – Motor: follows commands = 6; localizes painful stimuli = 5; withdraws from painful stimuli = 4; flexor posturing with central pain = 3; extensor posturing with central pain = 2; no response to painful stimuli = 1. Maximum score, 15; minimum score, 3. If asymmetrical motor or eye opening, the highest score is used.
Workup	– Laboratory studies: CBC, Na^+, K^+, glucose, Ca^{++}, Mg^{++}, creatinine. – As needed: PO_4^{3-}, CK, blood gas, INR, aPTT, BUN, hepatic enzymes, TSH, plasma osmolality, urinalysis, toxicology screen, plasma ethanol. Blood cultures and infectious workup if clinically indicated. – ECG, Chest X-ray. – Brain imaging (CT, MRI) stat if structural lesion suspected or diagnosis unclear. – EEG and lumbar puncture if clinically indicated.
Management	A-B-C-D as usual: 2 large-bore venous catheters, vital signs (temperature, O_2 sat.), glycemia. STAT lab studies. Give Naloxone - Thiamine - Glucose (if documented hypoglycemia). Flumazenil if benzodiazepine overdose (and no past history of seizure or tricyclic antidepressant use). Endotracheal intubation if gag reflex absent or GCS < 8. Further treatment according to diagnosis.

Dementia

- Impairment of cognitive function without alteration of level of consciousness.
- Differential diagnosis: delirium, depression.
- Prevalence: 8 % > 65 years, 29 % > 85 years, 58 % > 95 years in Canada (1991).
- Cortical vs subcortical (where motor impairment is more pronounced than language impairment, e.g..: Huntington, Parkinson, dementia with Lewy bodies).
- Irreversible (Alzheimer, vascular, alcoholic, Parkinson, Huntington, head trauma, anoxia) vs. reversible (rare < 1 %: depression, normotensive hydrocephalus, cancer, metabolic, infection, subdural hematoma, medication-induced).

Note: Patients scoring < 24/30 on MMSE are ineligible to hold a driver licence of any class pending complete neurological assessment.

Diagnostic criteria (DSM-IV)	Memory impairment *and* alteration of one or more of the following cognitive spheres: aphasia, apraxia, agnosia, executive function (planning, organising, abstract thinking ...). Decline of social and professional functioning compared to former level.
	Patients with complaints of subjective memory loss with or without objective deficits, but with preservation of other spheres and no decline of functioning are classified as having Mild Cognitive Impairment (MCI). Annual risk of conversion to Alzheimer's Disease : 10-15 %.
Workup	Head CT or MRI for all patients (2001 American Guidelines).
	Minimal lab works for all patients: CBC, electrolytes, fasting glucose, Ca^{++}, vitamin B12 level, TSH.
	If needed: liver function tests, renal workup, ammonia, Mg^{++}, urinalysis, folate, sedimentation rate, cortisol, FAN, syphilis serology, toxicology screen, HIV, blood gas, urinary porphobilinogen, Chest X-ray, ECG, EEG, lumbar puncture, neuropsychological testing, cerebral PET scan.
	Genetic testing for Apo E genotype not recommended for AD. CSF protein 14-3-3: If Creutzfeld-Jacob disease suspected.
Alzheimer's Disease (AD)	70 % of all dementias. Predominant temporo-parietal involvement. Risk factors: positive family history, age, Down syndrome, female sex, head trauma, genetic mutations, lower educational status.
	"Definite" diagnosis through confirmation by biopsy or autopsy, "probable" if all other causes excluded and "possible" if atypical elements present.
Stages of severity (Reisberg scale)	I: Normal. II: Subjective memory loss, but normal examination. III: Difficulty at work, in unfamiliar places, language disturbance, slight alteration of memory on examination. IV: Decreased capacity to travel, calculate. Memory deficits for recent events. V: Disorientation in time and space. Needs help to choose clothes. VI: Disorientation in time, space and person. Needs help to get dressed, to eat and for hygiene, incontinence. VII: Severe language disturbance. Loss of most cognitive functions, incontinence, motor rigidity.

Treatment	• Non-pharmacological: caregiver education, support groups, discuss power of attorney, will, driving licence, Medic-Alert® bracelet. Stop unnecessary medication. • Pharmacological: - Acetylcholinesterase Inhibitors: Donepezil (Aricept®), rivastigmine (Exelon®) or galantamine (Reminyl®) indicated for moderate disease (stade 3-5, MMSE 10-26), except donezepil indicated for mild to severe disease (MMSE 1-26): treat for 6 months with serial cognitive evaluation. Side effects: nausea, vomiting, diarrhea, insomnia, anorexia, weight loss, sinus bradycardia, high-degree AV block (contraindicated with LBBB or high degree AV-block). - Memantine (Ebixa®): NMDA-antagonist, indicated for moderate-severe disease (stade 5-6, MMSE 3-14). Few side effects. Additive effect with cholinesterase-inhibitors. Treatment of associated diseases: depression, agitation, psychosis, sleep disturbance (Risperidone sometimes helpful, small doses, short duration of therapy). Prognosis: variable, usually progressive deterioration over 8-10 years.

Vascular Dementia (VD)	30 % of dementias, 20 % mixed with AD. Overdiagnosed?
	Risk factors: Hypertension and other stroke risk factors.
	Causes: multiple symptomatic or asymptomatic cortical or lacunar infarcts, or Binswanger's disease (subcortical arteriosclerotic encephalopathy).
	
	Clinical presentation: Modified Hachinski scale
	   - abrupt presentation (2 points)
	   - stepwise deterioration (1)
	   - somatic complaints (1)
	   - emotional lability (1)
	   - history or presence of hypertension (1)
	   - history of stroke (2)
	   - focal neurological symptoms (2)
	   - focal neurological findings (2)
	   ⇒ If score > 6 points = diagnosis of vascular dementia.
	
	Sometimes progressive course as AD.
	Treatment: ASA, anticoagulation (if embolic etiology demonstrated), control (if risk factors, consider cholinesterase-inhibitors if elements of AD.

Dementia with Lewy Bodies (LBD)	5 % of dementias. 3 % mixed with Alzheimer. Clinically: dementia with at least one of the following: visual hallucinations (sometimes well-formed), extrapyramidal symptoms (rigidity, bradykinesia ...), fluctuations in cognitive function. Treatment: difficult, may benefit from cholinesterase-inhibitors (rivastigmine?), risperidone, clozapine or olanzapine for hallucinations. Avoid haloperidol and other traditional neuroleptics. Dopaminergic agonists or L-Dopa at low doses for rigidity, but risk of aggravating hallucinations.
Frontotemporal Dementia (FTD)	7 % of dementias. 2 % mixed with Alzheimer. Disproportionate disturbance of reasoning and judgement relative to memory function. Pick's disease constitutes one subtype of FTD. Differential diagnosis: behavioural disorders, mania, depression. Sometimes difficult to distinguish. Diagnosis: neuropsychology. CT/MRI may show predominant frontotemporal atrophy. Supportive treatment.

Normal Pressure Hydrocephalus (NPH)	Enlarged lateral ventricles with normal CSF opening pressure. Incidence: ~ 2 % of dementias. Clinical findings: classical triad of gait apraxia (early), dementia, and urinary incontinence (late). Miller-Fisher test + if improved gait after removal of 30-50 mL CSF. Treatment: ventriculoatrial or ventriculoperitoneal shunting. Partial and limited reversibility if cognitive function is severely impaired.
Pseudomentia	Also known as cognitive dysfunction linked to depression. Incidence ~ 5 % of dementias. Clinical findings: prominent depressive symptoms, history of depression, recent onset, rapid progression, answers "I don't know" to questions, cognitive complaints exceed objective findings, preserved language and motor skills …
Other Causes	Secondary to alcohol abuse (± 5 % of dementias). Other causes, < 2 % of dementias respectively: drug side effects (sedatives, hypnotics, anxiolytics, drugs inhaling, others), neurodegenerative (Parkinson, Huntington), head trauma, cerebral anoxia, neoplasm, metabolic (thyroid dysfunction, electrolytes, hypoglycemia, hyperglycemia, renal failure, liver failure, vitamin B 12, folate, B1, B6, C deficiency), infectious (HIV, CJD, syphilis …), sleep apnea, subdural hematoma, arteritis, connective tissue disease.

Delirium

- Disturbance of level of consciousness (sudden, fluctuating, rapidly improving with treatment of underlying cause): disturbance in behavior, mood, perception, altered sleep-wake cycle; trembling or tremor, flapping tremor / asterixis, nystagmus, incoordination, associated urinary incontinence.
- Risk factors: age (> 65), organic cerebral syndrome, alcohol abuse, diabetes, neoplasia, sensory impairment, malnutrition.
- Mortality at 3 months 23-33 %, at 1 year 50 %.
- Differential diagnosis: dementia (chronic, non fluctuating), psychosis, depression, Wernicke's aphasia …

Causes	– Intracerebral: trauma, epilepsy and postictal state, infection (bacterial, viral, abscess), cancer, vascular.
	– Extracerebral:
	   - Drugs (anticholinergics, lithium, sedatives, opioids, etc), intoxication (carbon monoxide).
	   - Endocrine: glucose, hypopituitary, pancreas, adrenal glands, parathyroid, thyroid.
	   - Systemic: hepatic, renal, pulmonary, cardiovascular (arrhythmia, heart failure, hyperviscosity syndrome).
	   - Thiamine, folate, B12, nicotinic acid deficiencies, systemic infections (sepsis, malaria, endocarditis).
	   - Electrolyte disturbances.
	   - Postoperative, fecaloma, urinary retention, sleep deprivation, etc.
	
	20 % of all acute confusional states remain unexplained after extensive work-up.

Workup	– Complete physical + neurological examination – Basic labs: CBC, Na$^+$, K$^+$, Cl$^-$, Ca^{++}, hepatic + renal function, glucose, TSH, urinalysis, ECG, Chest X-ray. – As needed: EEG, toxicology screen, VDRL/RPR, HIV, B12, folate, CK, troponin, blood cultures, urine culture, lumbar puncture, head CT/MRI.
Treatment	According to underlying cause. **Environmental support** (family, close friends, decoration, clock, calendar, regular orientation), sensory support, physical restraints if needed only. **Pharmacological treatment** : if agitation: 1st line treatment: haloperidol 0.5-1 mg PO bid

± same dose every 6 h as needed or 0.5-1 mg IM, can be repeated 60 min later if needed. Avoid use if withdrawal, Parkinson's disease or neuroleptic malignant syndrome. Alternatives: risperidone 0.5 PO bid, olanzapine 2.5-5 mg PO HS or quetiapine 25 mg PO bid. Also Lorazepam 0.5-1 mg PO/IV every 4-6 h (recommended if withdrawal or neuroleptic malignant syndrome).

Note: Atypical antipsychotics have been shown to increase mortality in patients with dementia.

Stroke

Etiology	**Hemorrhagic 15%:** subarachnoid hemorrhage or intracerebral hemorrhage, sub-dural or epidural hematomas, hemorrhagic transformation of an ischemic stoke.
	
	Ischemic 85%:
	    Atherosclerosis (20 %): Artery-to-artery embolism, atherothrombosis, diffuse hypoperfusion.
	    Lacunar infarct (25 %).
	    Cardiogenic embolism (20 %): atrial fibrillation, valvular disease, paradoxical embolism, bacterial or marantic endocarditis.
	    Cryptogenic (30 %).
	    Other causes (5 %): vasculitis (primary central nervous system vasculitis, temporal arteritis, Behçet, Takayasu, infectious), arterial dissection, vasospasm, hypercoagulable state, drugs (oral contraceptives…), central venous thrombosis, hyperviscosity syndrome, trauma, fibromuscular dysplasia, Moyamoya, CADASIL, etc.
	
	Differential diagnosis: hypoglycemia, seizures, migraine, trauma, cataplexy, demyelinating diseases, encephalopathy, cerebral tumor, conversion disorder, malingering.

Ischemic TIA- Stroke	Transient ischemic attack: a transient episode of neurological dysfunction caused by focal brain, spinal cord, or retinal ischemia, without acute infarction.
Clinical findings	*Left hemisphere (dominant):* Aphasia, right hemiparesis, right hemisensory deficit, right hemianopsia, dysarthria, dysgraphia, dyslexia, dyscalculia. *Right hemisphere (non-dominant):* left hemianopsia, negligence of the left visual field, left-sided extinction on simultaneous stimulation, left hemiparesis, dysarthria, left hemisensory deficit, spatial disorientation, anosognosia (no awareness of the deficit). *Bilateral occipito-temporal and posterior fossa regions:* quadriplegia, sensory deficit of the four limbs, Ataxia, dysarthria, nystagmus, dizziness/vertigo, nausea, vomiting, amnesia, and bilateral cortical visual deficit. *Lacunar strokes:* Pure motor hemiparesis, pure sensory stroke, sensory-motor stroke, ataxic hemiparesis, dysarthria-clumsy hand among others. *Brainstem stroke:* 18 different syndromes including ipsilateral cranial nerve involvement, contralateral hemiparesis or hypoesthesia and ipsilateral or contralateral or bilateral ataxia, according to location of the lesion.
Workup	− CBC, INR, aPTT, electrolytes, renal function, glucose, lipids, ECG, head CT scan, carotid Doppler (if anterior circulation involved), MRI (if posterior circulation involved, arteriovenous malformation, aneurysm or central venous thrombosis suspected) − If needed: Echocardiography (if there is a known cardiac pathology or an abnormal ECG), Holter, VDRL or RPR, liver and renal function tests, arterial blood gas, ESR, thrombophilia workup (if < 50 years or history of thrombo-embolism), lumbar puncture, chest X-ray, EEG, CT-Angiography, MR-Angiography, digital subtraction angiography.

Management	Hospitalisation: every stroke or TIA (except TIA dating > 2 weeks or amaurosis fugax if the workup can be done in < 1 week). Note: A patient with TIA should be considered as an equivalent to "brain's unstable angina". Short term risk of a stroke is around 9-12 % at 30 days, 10-20 % at 90 days (See ABCD2 rule below). Every patient should be treated in an interdisciplinary stroke unit. Nutritional and hydration status should be screened within the first 48 hours of admission. Every patient should be screened for swallowing disorders; if abnormal, evaluation by a speech therapist. NPO if bulbar involvement. Bed rest for 24 h depending on the neurological deficit. Rehabilitation (physiotherapy, occupational therapy). Oxygen as needed. Keep an IV line open. Thiamine if needed. Keep body temperature normal, blood pressure < 220/120 mmHg and blood glucose < 11 mmol/L. **ABCD2 Rule** evaluating risk of stroke within 7 days after TIA: **A: A**ge > 60 years old: 1 point. **B:** Initial **B**lood pressure > 140/90 mmHg: 1 point. **C: C**linical factors: unilateral weakness (2 points); speech impairment without weakness (1 point). **D: D**uration: symptoms > 60 minutes (2 points); between 10-60 minutes (1 point). **D: D**iabetes (1 point). If < 4 points: 1.2 % stroke risk within 7 days post-TIA. If 4-5 points: 6 %. If > 5 points: 12 %.

Treatment	**Pharmacological:**
	 – *Antiplatelet*: for non-cardioembolic stroke:
	   - ASA initial dose 160-325 mg, followed by 80-325 mg daily (but ASA 75-325 mg/d in cardioembolic stroke who have contraindications to anticoagulant therapy) **or**
	   - ASA 50 mg-dipyridamole 200 mg (Aggrenox®) bid, contraindication: CAD with stable or unstable angina; side effects: headaches **or**
	   - Clopidogrel (Plavix) 75 mg daily.
	   Note: avoid long term use of the aspirin/clopidogrel combination because of increased risk of bleeding.
	 – *Anticoagulation (warfarin)*: indications:
	   - Cardioembolic stroke: except if massive cerebral infarct, uncontrolled high blood pressure or high bleeding risk.
	   - Stroke and antiphospholipid syndrome (target INR 2-3).
	   - Stroke after myocardial infarct (if anterior infarct, severe right ventricular dysfunction, congestive heart failure, atrial fibrillation, intra-cardiac thrombus, past history of embolus).
	   - Stroke and deep vein thrombosis.
	 – *Heparin*: If severe carotid stenosis while waiting for surgery, arterial dissection, or venous thrombosis. Prophylactic subcutaneous heparin if prolonged immobilisation to prevent thromboembolic complications.
	 – *Thrombolysis*: tPA if can be given < 4.5 hours after the onset of symptoms. Improves slightly but significantly the long-term functional deficit. Side effects: 6.5% hemorrhage (NINDS study). Intra-arterial tPA is an option for middle cerebral artery occlusion (without major early infarct signs) in specialised centers for strokes during first 6 hours if tPA IV cannot be administered (4.5 hours delay expired or recent surgery). Start ASA 24h after thrombolysis.
	 – *Statins*: to consider as secondary prevention targeting LDL < 2 mmol/L in all patients with TIA/Stroke of atherosclerotic origin.
	 – *Antihypertensive medication*: ACEI and/or thiazide diuretics (combination often necessary to lower BP < 140/90 mmHg): hypertension treatment in acute phase of a stroke is controversial: avoid treating except if systolic BP > 220 and/or diastolic BP > 120 mmHg, aiming a ↓ of 15-25 % over 24 hours. If thrombolysis with tPA, treat with

	labetalol 10-20 mg IV if BP > 185/110 mmHg. For patient previously on antihypertensive treatment, restart medication after 24 hours in most cases of stroke.
	Surgical: – Carotid endarcterectomy indicated if carotid stenosis 70-99% and symptoms for < 6 months and < 6 % surgical risk and life expectancy at 5 years > 50% (26% vs 9% of ipsilateral stroke after 2 years - NASCET study 1991 medical vs surgical group). Ideally within 2 weeks of the incident TIA/stroke. – If stenosis 50-69% symptomatic and 2% surgical risk, *controversial*: 22% vs 16% of ipsilateral stroke after 5 years (NASCET study 1998); should be evaluated by a physician with expertise in stroke management. – If asymptomatic stenosis and surgical risk < 3%, < 75 y.o.; *controversial*: ipsilateral stroke 10.6% vs 4.8% at 5 years (ACAS study); should be evaluated by a physician with expertise in stroke management.
Prognosis	Complications: – Neurologic: brain edema (peaks at 3-5 days: treatment; water restriction, raise head at 30°, hyperventilation, mannitol + furosemide, shunt), hydrocephalus, intracranial hypertension, hemorrhagic transformation, and seizures. – Medical: hypoventilation, pneumonia, myocardial infarction, arrhythmia, thrombophlebitis, pulmonary embolism, urinary tract infection, urinary and fecal incontinence, pressure sores, malnutrition, dysphagia and aspiration, contractures, immobilisation syndrome, falls, depression (10-30 % after a stroke). 10-15% death (mainly secondary to myocardial infarction). 20 % recurrence at 2 years. 1/3-1/2 of patients recover with residual deficits.
Arterial Dissection	Frequent cause of stroke in young adults. Spontaneous, due to trauma, or in patients with connective tissue disease. Most often implies extra-cranial internal carotid artery. Causes unilateral periorbital pain (carotid), or occipital pain (vertebral), Horner syndrome, amaurosis, hemispheric or posterior ischemia, nerve palsies, subarachnoid hemorrhage, cerebral infarction. Diagnosis with MR-Angiography or arteriography. Treatment controversial: empirical heparin + anticoagulation 3-6 months (except if hemorrhage is present).
Intracerebral Hemorrhage	Most often due to hypertension (most often involved: basal ganglia [putamen, caudate nucleus], pons, thalamus, cerebellum, white matter). Also secondary to amyloid angiopathy, hematologic diseases, anticoagulation, tumor, aneurysm, arteriovenous malformation, trauma, vasculitis, cerebral venous thrombosis, or hemorrhagic transformation of ischemic stroke. Suspect venous thrombosis if hemorrhage spreads beyond usual arterial vascular territories.
Clinical findings	Often declares during activity. Loss of consciousness, vomiting, headache, focal neurologic symptoms and signs, often progressive (depending on location), seizures.
Workup	See ischemic stroke workup above. MRI superior to CT scan in the first 48 hours. Rule out underlying tumor.
Treatment	ICU admission. Endotracheal intubation if Glasgow < 8 or loss of airway protection reflexes. Reversal of anticoagulation STAT if patient is anticoagulated (with prothrombic complex concentrates or with recombinant factor VIIa + vitamin K).

	Supportive therapy: hyperventilation + mannitol if herniation. Control blood pressure (maintain mean blood pressure >70 mmHg but <130 mmHg). Antiepileptics if seizures occur (stop after 30 days if no recurrence). Intra-ventricular shunt if hydrocephalus develops. Surgery if needed: strongly recommended for cerebellar hemorrhage (especially if hematoma > 3 cm), to consider if the hemorrhage is lobar, or if basal ganglia hemorrhage > 30 mL, if there is expansion or neurological deterioration. Intermittent pneumatic compression devices for thromboprophylaxis, and heparin s/c as soon as the patient is stable.
Prognosis	30-40 % mortality. Functional prognosis better than ischemic stroke. Relapse of hemorrhage secondary to an arteriovenous malformation = 2 %/year. *ICH* Score in order to evaluate prognosis: Glasgow scale: 3-4/15: 2 points; 5-12/15; 1 point. Age ≥ 80 years old; 1 point. Hematoma volume ≥ 30 mL; 1 point Intraventricular hemorrhage; 1 point. Sub-tentorial hemorrhage; 1 point. If < 2 points: 0-13 % mortality in 30 days. If 2-4 points: variable prognosis. If ≥ 5 points: 100 % death.
Subarachnoid Hemorrage (SAH)	Most often due to ruptured aneurysms, arteriovenous malformation or perimesencephalic bleed; no cause identified in 20%. Sometimes familial or congenital (polycystic kidney disease, Marfan).
Clinical findings	Violent sudden severe headache often upon straining ± nausea, vomiting ± altered level of consciousness. Up to 40% have a sentinel bleed (transient and less severe headache).

Severity scale	Glasgow Coma Scale. Hunt and Hess scale: Grade 0 is asymptomatic.
	    Grade 1: Mild headache, no neurological deficit.
	    Grade 2: Moderate to severe headache or meningismus but no neurological deficit other than cranial nerve palsy.
	    Grade 3: Drowsiness and mild focal neurologic deficit.
	    Grade 4: Stupor, moderate to severe hemiparesis.
	    Grade 5: Coma.

Workup	Head CT scan: 90 % sensitivity. If negative perform lumbar puncture and repeat if needed after 6-12 hours. Negative cerebral angiography in 10-30% of cases. 20% have more than one aneurysm.
Treatment	Bed rest, analgesics, laxatives. Aim for BP 170-180/100 mmHg during acute phase. Nimodipine 60 mg every 4 hours PO or via Levine for 21 days (vasospasm prophylaxis); not recommended if perimesencephalic bleed. Early intracranial surgery < 3 days. Triple "H" therapy (hypertension, hypervolemia, hemodilution) postoperatively to prevent vasospasm.
Complications	Hemorrhage recurrence. Vasospasm 3-10 days after the event. Hydrocephalus. Others: cardio-vascular, respiratory, gastrointestinal bleeding, cerebral salt wasting, SIADH, etc.
Prognosis	Death in 25-45 %. Persistent neurological deficit in about 50 %.
Venous Thrombosis	Clinical findings: headaches, seizures, confusion, ↑ intracranial pressure, focal neurologic deficit, menigismus sometimes. Can be a complication of maxillofacial or intracranial infection or associated with thrombophilia, polycythemia vera, sickle cell anemia, cyanotic heart disease or pregnancy/post-partum and oral contraceptives.

Diagnosis	Brain CT or MRI.
	CT-Angio or MR-Angio or cerebral arteriography as needed.
	Consider lumbar puncture to rule out infectious cause.
	Thrombophilia workup according to clinical findings.
Treatment	IV heparin or LMWH during acute phase, even in the presence of hemorrhagic infarction.
	Anticoagulation for up to 12 months, INR 2-3.
	Anticonvulsivants or treatment of intracranial hypertension as needed.

Stroke: Diagnostic and Therapeutic Approach

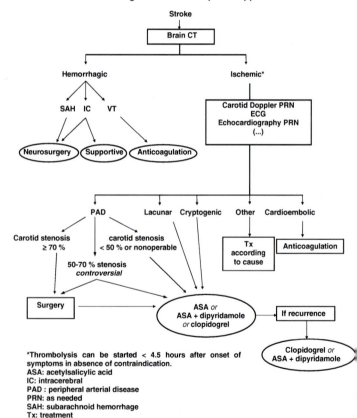

*Thrombolysis can be started < 4.5 hours after onset of symptoms in absence of contraindication.
ASA: acetylsalicylic acid
IC: intracerebral
PAD : peripheral arterial disease
PRN: as needed
SAH: subarachnoid hemorrhage
Tx: treatment
VT: veinous thrombosis

Headache

History:
Age, circumstances of headache onset (menstruation, at rest, stress-induced, ...), localisation, duration, frequency, aura, paresthesia, paresis, paralysis, photo-/osmo-/phonophobia, nausea, vomiting, precipitating factors, attempted medication, head trauma, dental/sinus/temporo-mandibular disease, family history.

Red flags:
First or worst headache of life, change in frequency, severity or character of pain, new-onset headache in middle-aged or elderly patient, new-onset of slowly progressive headache over several days, caused by cough, Valsalva or exercise, nocturnal or early-morning headache, systemic symptoms (fever, myalgia, weight loss), jaw claudication, scalp tenderness.
Elements indicating neoplasm, infection, systemic or vascular disease, trauma: focal neurological signs, confusion, seizures, alteration of level of consciousness.

Physical + neurological examination:
Neck stiffness, fundi, pupils, visual fields, cranial nerves, deep tendon reflexes, muscle strength, gait, etc, vascular examination, temporal artery, temporomandibular joint, teeth, sinus, cervical spine and paraspinal muscles.

Always rule out Giant Cell Arteritis if new-onset headache in a patient > 50 years old (see Vasculitis table).

Migraine	Migraine with and without aura, familial or sporadic hemiplegic migraine, basilar migraine, retinal migraine.

Diagnostic criteria	Migraine **without aura**:
	At least 5 attacks fulfilling criteria 1-3:
	    1. Headache attack lasting 4-72 hours (untreated or unsuccessfully treated).
	    2. > 2/4 of the following characteristics: unilateral localisation *or* pulsatile quality *or* moderate to severe pain intensity *or* aggravation by or causing avoidance of routine physical activity (walking, climbing stairs).
	    3. During headache, at least one of the following: nausea, vomiting, photophobia, phonophobia.
	
	Migraine **with aura**:
	At least 2 attacks fulfilling criteria 1-3:
	    1. Aura consisting of at least one of the following, but no motor weakness:
	        (1) fully reversible visual symptoms including positive (spots, lines) and/or negative features (loss of vision) *or*
	        (2) fully reversible sensory symptoms including positive (pins and needles) or negative features (numbness) *or*
	        (3) fully reversible dysphasic speech disturbances.
	    2. > 2/4 of the following: homonymous visual symptoms and/or unilateral sensory symptoms *or* an aura developing gradually over ≥ 5 min and/or a different aura in succession over ≥ 5 min *or* each aura lasting 5-60 min.
	    3. Headache fulfilling criteria for migraine without aura begins during the aura or follows aura within 60 minutes.
	
	Chronic migraine if > 15 attacks/ month for > 3 months.
	Status migrainosus if attack lasts > 72 h.
	Probable migraine if one diagnostic criteria missing.

Treatment of acute attack	**Mild attacks:** Acetaminophen (1000 mg), ASA (900 mg), Ibuprofen (400-800 mg), Naproxen (500-1000 mg). *Adjuvant*: Dimenhydrinate (50-100 mg), Domperidone (10-20 mg), Metoclopramide (10 mg). **Moderate attacks:** NSAIDs (Ibuprofen, Naproxen, mefenamic acid (250-500 mg).

	5-HT1-agonists: sumatriptan (50-100 mg PO, or 20 mg inh. or 6 mg s/c), rizatriptan (5-10 mg), almotriptan (12.5 mg), naratriptan (2.5 mg), eletriptan (20-40 mg), zolmitriptan (2.5-5 mg), frovatriptan (2.5 mg). Contraindication: coronary heart disease, pregnancy, DHE or ergotamine use within previous 24 hrs. Avoid narcotics alone or in combination (risk of medication-induced headache). Limit intake to 2-3 days/week. **Severe attacks:** 5-HT1-agonists, butorphanol 1 mg intranasal every 3-4 h (see ER treatment below).
ER treatment	Prochlorperazine 10 mg IV + DHE 0.5-1 mg IV every 8 h until complete pain relief. Contraindication: coronary heart disease, peripheral vascular disease, pregnancy, uremia, liver failure, severe hypertension. Droperidol 2.5 mg + Diphenhydramine 25 mg IV or IM (after ECG, rule out long QTc). Contraindication: past history of acute dystonia with neuroleptics or malignant arrhythmia. 2nd line alternative: Prochlorperazine 10 mg IV + Diphenhydramine 10 mg IV every 4-6 h until pain relief. Chlorpromazine 10-12.5 mg (0.1 mg/kg) IV, followed by bolus 500 mL NaCl 0.9 %. Dexamethasone 8-20 mg IM or IV, Methylprednisolone 100-250 mg IV. Dexamethasone 8 mg IM + Meperidine 75-100 mg + Promethazine 50 mg IM.

Prophylactic treatment	Indicated if severe attacks, with > 3-4 days/ month, without adequate response to acute treatment.
	– Beta-blockers: (Propranolol 40-120 mg PO bid, Metoprolol 100-200 mg PO daily)
	    Contraindication: asthma. Side effects: fatigue, bradycardia, sleep disturbance.
	– Amitriptyline 10-75 mg HS. Side effects: dry mouth, weight gain, sedation.
	– Valproic acid 250-500 mg PO bid. Side effects: weight gain, nausea, tremor, teratogenic.
	– Calcium channel blockers (Verapamil 160-320 mg daily, Flunarizine 5-15 mg PO daily). Side effects: fatigue, weight gain, depression (Flunarizine), extrapyramidal side effects (Flunarizine), constipation, edema.
	– Topiramate 25-100 mg PO bid. Side effects: confusion, weight loss, language disorder, paresthesias.
	– Methysergide 1-6 mg daily. Side effects: fatigue, muscle cramps, alopecia, retroperitoneal fibrosis (stop for 1 month every 6 months).
	        Contraindication: CAD, hypertension, connective tissue disease, pregnancy.
	
	Non-pharmacological treatment:
	Education, sleep hygiene, avoid precipitating agents, relaxation.

Tension-Type Headache	Pressing/tightening headache, mild to moderate intensity, bilateral, often occipital, non-pulsating and not aggravated by routine physical activity. Classification: Infrequent episodic if headache < 1 day / month. Frequent episodic if 1-14 days/month and chronic if ≥ 15 days/month. Treatment: relaxation, massages, usual analgesia, Amitriptyline 25-75 mg PO HS. Avoid regular analgesic medication (> 2-3 x / week) because of risk for medication-withdrawal headache.
Cluster Headache (Horton's)	Unilateral, periorbital, very intense, with tearing, nasal stuffiness and discharge, diaphoresis of affected hemicranium, conjunctival injection, miosis, ptosis, agitation. Often at night or early morning. Duration 150-180 min 1-2 days, up to 8/day. Often daily headache for several weeks or months, then spontaneous remission for 6-24 months on average. Provoked by alcohol or nitroglycerine. Male preponderance (8:1). Age 20-40. Acute treatment: oxygen 100 % for 10 min, Sumatriptan 6 mg s/c.

	Prophylactic treatment: Prednisone 40-80 mg daily for 7 days, then taper over 5 days and combine with Verapamil SR 120-360 mg/daily or Lithium 300 mg tid for the duration of the cluster period. Alternative treatment: methysergide, valproic acid, surgery …
Chronic Paroxysmal Hemicrania	Similar to cluster headache in intensity and localization, but shorter (2-30 min) and more frequent (5-30/day). Rare in men. Complete remission with indomethacine.
Vascular Headache (see Stroke Table)	Subarachnoid hemorrhage or sentinel bleed: classically, worst headache of life, diagnosis by CT or lumbar puncture. Cerebral venous thrombosis: subacute headache ± focal signs ± precipitating factors: diagnosis by CT/MRI or angiography. Other causes: stroke, intracranial hematoma, arteriovenous malformation, arteritis, malignant hypertension, arterial dissection …
Rebound Headache or Medication-Induced Headache	Possible with every drug, particularly with ergotamine, NSAIDs, acetaminophen (especially if combined with opioids), barbiturates or caffeine. Develops if use of ergotamine > 2 days /week, combined analgesics > 3 x/week, or simple analgesia > 5 x/week. Treatment: discontinue analgesic drug (slow tapering, especially if barbiturate or opioid) Non-pharmacological approach (treat depression, anxiety, insomnia, often present). DHE, triptans, NSAIDs. Start prophylactic treatment quickly.
Tumoral Headache (see CNS Cancer table)	Classically, change in frequency, severity, or character of headache or headache precipitated by Valsalva or associated with weight loss or focal signs. (see CNS Cancer able)
Pseudotumor Cerebri	Also idiopathic intracranial hypertension: increased intracranial pressure without evidence of hydrocephalus. Headache, visual disturbances, diplopia, tinnitus and other non specific symptoms. Associated with obesity, dysmenorrhea, dysthyroidism, hypoparathyroidism, adrenal insufficiency, iron deficiency anemia, drugs (vitamin A, tetracycline, oral contraceptives, indomethacine …) Papilledema, visual field deficits, 6th cranial nerve paralysis. Diagnosis: MRI and MR-Angio, to rule out fistula and venous sinus thrombosis. Lumbar puncture with ↑ opening pressure > 25 cm H_2O.
Other Forms of Headache	Primary stabbing headache, primary thunderclap headache, hypnic headache (in older patient, nocturnal, 30 minutes, bilateral, mild to moderate), hemicrania continua, new daily-persistent headache. Primary cough or exertional headache, primary headache associated with sexual activity Secondary headaches : attributed to head and/or neck trama, to cranial or cervical vascular disorder, to intracranial disorder, to infection, to disorder of cranium, neck, eye, ears, nose, sinuses, teeth, mouth, etc. Cranial neuralgias, central and primary facial pain, and other headaches: trigeminal neuralgia, glossopharyngeal neuralgia, etc. Sleep-apnea related headaches: morning headache, associated with other OSA findings.

Neurological Weakness (Frequent Diseases)
Multiple Sclerosis

Definition: ≥ 2 separate attacks caused by 2 or more objective clinical CNS lesions **or** 1 attack with one or more objective clinical lesions and dissemination in time and space, supported by paraclinical investigation (McDonald criteria, 2001).

Usual age < 55 years. Female preponderance (2:1).
Factors aggravating symptoms: infection, hyperthermia (Uhthoff's sign), trauma: relapses ↑ 2-3 months post-partum.
Clinical findings: optic neuritis (presenting symptom in 17 %), transverse myelitis (Lhermitte's sign), weakness, paresthesias, diplopia, internuclear ophthalmoplegia, impaired balance, vertigo, muscle spasms, urinary disturbance, constipation, sexual dysfunction, cerebellar syndrome, encephalomyelitis, trigeminal neuralgia, cognitive disturbance, depression, anxiety, fatigue, etc.

Evolution: 4 types:
Relapsing-remitting (66 %), primary progressive (~ 10 %), secondary progressive (20 %), progressive-relapsing (15 %). 10 % show a benign course over > 20 years.

Differential diagnosis:
Autoimmune (SLE, polyarteritis nodosa, Behçet, Sjögren, chronic inflammatory demyelinating polyneuropathy), infectious (post-encephalomyelitis, Lyme, HIV, HTLV-1, syphilis, progressive multifocal leucoencephalopathy), granulomatoses (sarcoidosis, Wegener's, lymphomatous granulomatosis), metabolic (↓ B12), vascular (vasculitis, hemangioma, stroke), posterior fossa or spinal lesions (Arnold-Chiari malformation, cervical spinal stenosis, myelopathy, etc), neoplastic or paraneoplastic disorders, psychiatric, genetic, acute disseminating encephalomyelitis (3-6 weeks post-viral infection or vaccine, monophasic).

Workup	– CSF: normal proteins or mild ↑ (< 2 x normal) in 20-30 %, leukocytes (lymphocytes) normal (66 %) or ↑ to 20-50 x 10^6/L, oligoclonal bands. – Evoked potentials: visual, auditory, somatosensory, brainstem. – Cerebral + spinal imaging (MRI + gadolinium > CT); white matter lesions. – Laboratory studies: CBC, VDRL/RPR, ANA …according to clinical findings.
Treatment	**Acute:** - If functional impairment (or optic neuritis) → Methylprednisolone 1g IV daily for 3-5 days, followed by Prednisone 60 mg PO daily, tapered over 2-3 weeks (no consensus on dose and duration). If no response and severe episode, plasmapheresis? - If no functional impairment: no treatment, steroids hasten remission but do not modify long-term outcome. **Long-term:** Relapsing-remitting type: - Interferon β-1a or β-1b s/c: ↓ frequency of relapses by 30 %. - Glatiramer s/c (Copaxone®). - Other treatments: Natalizumab, immunoglobulins IV, immunosuppression under investigation, plasmapheresis. Secondary progressive type: Interferon β-1b, mitoxantrone IV. Primary progressive type and progressive relapses: methotrexate, cyclophosphamide?, cyclosporine ?, trial of steroids if acute and fast deterioration. Try to refer to specialist for clinical study participation. Treat a first demyelinating episode (and MRI +) with Interferon β-1a (especially if multiple lesions on MRI). Treatment of complications (amantadine for fatigue, meclizine for vertigo, baclofen for spasticity, carbamazepine, phenytoin, gabapentin, amitryptiline cannabinol [Sativex®] or valproic acid for pain, anticholinergics for spastic bladder, catheterization if atonic

	bladder).
	Evaluate for depression and suicide risk.
	Physiotherapy, occupational therapy.
	Avoid hyperthermia (vaccination if needed, but avoid hepatitis B vaccine if risk > benefit).
	Support groups.
Prognosis	Unfavourable if progressive disease, motor and cerebellar signs, multiple lesions on T2-weighed MRI at presentation, short intervals between relapses, male, late onset (> 40), frequent relapses, incomplete remissions.
	Favourable if female, young at onset, complete remission between relapses, sensory symptoms.
	50 % without significant handicap after 10 years. 10 % in wheelchair after 10 years.
	Causes of death: aspiration pneumonia, urosepsis, suicide …

Myasthenia Gravis

Autoimmune disease where auto-antibodies react against acetylcholine receptors of neuro-muscular junction and stop normal muscle contraction. .
Associated with thymoma, hypo-hyperthyroidism, rheumatoid arthritis, SLE and other autoimmune diseases. ↑ frequency with age.

Clinical findings: fluctuating muscle weakness, with diplopia, ptosis or secondary dysphagia: cranial and ocular muscles, respiratory and limb muscles particularly affected.
Nasal voice secondary to facial muscles weakness. Acute or sub-acute symptomatology. Often asymmetrical weakness.

Classification	Modified Osserman scale:
	Stage 1: Focal disease, ocular involvement.
	Stage 2: Mild generalized weakness, usually with ocular muscle weakness.
	Stage 3: Predominantly bulbar involvement, usually with mild generalized weakness.
	Stage 4: Moderate generalized weakness.
	Stage 5: Severe generalized weakness.
Diagnosis	– Edrophonium (Tensilon®) test: 10 mg IV (2 mg IV stat, wait 1 min, then 3 mg IV, wait 1 min, then 5 mg IV, stop if objective response): short-acting cholinesterase-inhibitor with ↑ muscle strength for 5 minutes.
	– EMG/nerve conduction study may show muscle fatigability with repetitive stimulation.
	– Antibodies to muscle nicotinic acetylcholine receptor ⊕ in 80-90 % (50 % in ocular form).
	– Chest X-ray, thoracic CT or MRI to rule out thymoma (present in 10-15 % of cases).
	– Biochemistry: ANA, rheumatoid factor, anti-thyroid antibodies, TSH, PPD (if immunosuppression planned), glucose.
	Differential diagnosis:
	– *Myasthenic syndrome* (Eaton-Lambert): autoimmune, paraneoplastic (SCLC), antibodies against tumor antigens cross-react with voltage-gated calcium channels: muscle weakness *decreases* with repetitive contractions, hyporeflexia, dysautonomia. Diagnosis: response to repetitive nerve stimulation. Treatment: plasmapheresis, immunosuppression, treat underlying neoplasm.
	– *Botulism*: Occurs following ingestion of canned food contaminated with toxin of *Clostridium botulinum,* fulminating weakness 12-72 hours after ingestion, severe and fluctuating: diplopia, facial weakness, dysphagia, mydriasis, respiratory difficulty and limb weakness: orthostatic hypotension, ileus, dry mouth. Diagnosis: electrophysiology. Treatment: antitoxin + laxatives + support.
	– *Aminoglycoside antibiotics*: rarely produce a "botulism-like" syndrome, preventing release of acetylcholine from nerve endings, avoid in patients with preexisting conditions (MG).
	– *Other*: stroke or brain-stem lesions, multiple sclerosis, thyroid ophtalmopathy, leptomenigitis involvement, (carcinomatosis, tuberculosis, fungal), oculopharyngeal dystrophy, amyotrophic lateral sclerosis, etc.

Treatment	– Avoid aminoglycosides. Careful with tetracycline, class I antiarrhythmics and beta-blockers.
	– Cholinesterase-inhibitors as symptomatic treatment: neostigmine or pyridostigmine qid; overmedication may increase weakness.
	– Thymectomy: if < 60 years, except recent onset or slow progression (spontaneous remission possible).
	– Corticosteroids if weak response to cholinesterase-inhibitors or surgery: start in hospital as weakness may worsen, progressive tapering until minimal effective dose.
	– Azathioprine and mycophenolate may be helpful in second line to allow steroids tapering.
	– Plasmapheresis or IV immunoglobulins if major handicap despite therapy, myasthenic crisis or pre-operative.
	– Intubation if FVC < 15 mL/kg.

Amyotrophic Lateral Sclerosis

Peak 55-65 years, but may occur after age 10, sometimes positive family history. Associated with Parkinson's and fronto-temporal dementia.
Weakness and muscle atrophy without sensory changes, upper and lower motoneuron signs, dysphagia, dysarthria, dyspnea, weak cough, fasciculations of tongue and limbs, depressive attitude ...

Diagnosis	EMG (must be ⊕ in 3 of 4 segments (bulbar, cervical, thoracic or lumbar), normal or slightly ↓ conduction velocity, sensory nerve conduction study normal, CK normal or slightly ↑.
	Differential diagnosis: Pure motor syndrome with monoclonal gammopathy, multifocal motor neuropathy.
Treatment	Riluzole slows progression by several months. Symptomatic treatment: anticholinergics for hypersalivation, baclofen or diazepam for spasticity, physiotherapy, liquid or puree diet if dysphagia (speech therapy evaluation, fluoroscopic swallowing studies), tracheostomy if respiratory failure.
Prognosis	Progressive and fatal within 2-5 years. 25 % survival at 5 years, 8-16 % at 10 years.

Guillain-Barré Syndrome

Acute inflammatory demyelinating polyneuropathy, occurring 5 days-3 weeks after respiratory or gastrointestinal viral syndrome (autoimmune process likely).
↑ incidence with ↑ age, Hodgkin's lymphoma, pregnancy, postoperative.

Clinical findings	1st symptom: symmetric weakness of limbs with paresthesias, legs > arms and ascending progression. Sometimes beginning with cranial nerve weakness. Loss of deep tendon reflexes after a few days, dysautonomia, dyspnea.
	Variant: Miller-Fisher syndrome: gait ataxia, areflexia, ophthalmoparesis, pupillary abnormalities.
	Progression of symptoms up to 4 weeks and stabilization and improvement (until nearly complete recuperation).
Differential diagnosis	Spinal pathology (compression, myelitis), diphtheria, poliomyelitis, AIDS, acute porphyria, hypophosphatemia, toxic neuropathies (thallium, arsenic), botulism, CIDP if progression > 4 weeks.
Workup	EMG diagnostic. Lumbar puncture: characteristic abnormality with ↑ protein and normal cell counts. Serial vital capacities. Natremia (SIADH frequent). ↑ liver function test in 1/3.

Treatment	ICU if rapid decrease of VC or < 18 mL/kg or cardiovascular dysautonomia. Plasmapheresis vs immunoglobulins IV (may be equivalent) if moderate to severe disease (unable to walk w/o help). Respiratory physiotherapy, antithrombotic prophylaxis. Pressure sores. Intubate if FVC < 15 mL/kg. Treat SIADH. Mortality 15-30 % if intubated.
Myopathy	See Connective Tissue Disease Table.

Parkinson's Disease

Degenerative pathology of the basal ganglia, most often idiopathic.
Prevalence 2-3/1000, 1 % > 50 years, 2 % > 65 years. 20 % of cases < 50 years.
Mean age at onset 60 years.

Clinical findings	Classic tetrade:
	    - resting tremor (unilateral → bilateral).
	    - rigidity.
	    - bradykinesia.
	    - postural instability (minimal at onset).
	
	Dysautonomia, subcortical cognitive disturbance (20 % dementia), decreased facial expression, hypophonia, hypersalivation, seborrhea, ↓ frequency of blinking, ↓ arms movement, micrographia, cog wheel, ↓ quick alternate movements, erectile dysfunction, hallucinations, depression, anxiety.
	
	Wait at least 3 years before diagnosing possible → probable Parkinson's disease.

Differential diagnosis	– Parkinsonism secondary to medication or drug-induced: antipsychotic drugs, metoclopramide, reserpine, methyldopa, calcium channel blockers, MPTP (methylphenyl-tetrahydropyridine), etc. – Postencephalitic. – Lacunar. – Bifrontal cortical disease. – Metabolic: hypothyroidism, Wilson's, hypercalcemia, liver disease. – Creutzfeld-Jacob disease. – Degenerative: Progressive supranuclear palsy (initially, vertical eye movements limited), Huntington's disease, cortico-basal degeneration (alien hand phenomenon), multi-system atrophy (Shy-Drager syndrome [prominent orthostatic hypotension], nigro-striatal degeneration [predominant rigidity + bradykinesia], sporadic olivo-ponto-cerebellar atrophy [predominant ataxia]). – Posttraumatic (*dementia pugilistica*). – Depression.
Severity of disease	Modified Hoehn and Yahr Staging: Stage 0 = No signs of disease. Stage I = Unilateral disease. Stage I.5 = Unilateral disease plus axial involvement. Stage II = Bilateral disease, without impairment of balance. Stage II.5 = Mild bilateral disease, with recovery on pull test. Stage III = Mild to moderate bilateral disease; some postural instability; physically independent. Stage IV = Severe disability; still able to walk or stand unassisted. Stage V = Wheelchair bound or bedridden unless aided.

Treatment	Individual approach with each patient (consider age, functional capacity, patient's expectations). **General measures:** Patient education, support groups, physiotherapy, occupational therapy, speech therapy, nutritionist. Treatment of complications: dysautonomia, depression, falls, cognitive symptoms (cholinesterase inhibitors) … **Pharmacotherapy:** – Levodopa: most effective treatment of Parkinson's disease; if no response, reconsider diagnosis. Start Sinemet® 100/25 mg tid (or Sinemet® CR 100/25 bid) and ↑ every week up to 200/50 tid. Side effects: nausea (to ↓: take with food, domperidone 10 mg PO tid), orthostatism (to ↓: ↑ diet Na^+, Florinef ®), hallucinations (clozapine, quetiapine), dyskinesias, fluctuations (see below). – Dopamine agonists: (bromocriptine [Parlodel®], ropinirol [Requip®], pramipexole [Mirapex®]): monotherapy in early phase (stage1-2), mostly if young patient (slows development of long-term motor complications) or in combination if need for Levodopa > 800 mg/day. Side effects: orthostatic hypotension, hallucinations, dyskinesias, compulsive behavior, nausea, somnolence. No driving with pramipexole, ropinirol for 3 months (risk of sleep attacks documented, but remains controversial). – *Anticholinergics* (Cogentin®, Artane®, Kemadrin®): especially effective for tremor. Anticholinergic side effects: contraindicated in elderly patients or with cognitive deficits. – Amantadine (Symmetrel®): anticholinergic effect and ↑ dopamine release: fast effect but lasts only a few months. 1st line if mild disease? – Selegiline (Eldepryl®) and rasagiline (Azilect®): MAO-B inhibitor. Side effects: Insomnia, hallucinations, arterial hypertension. Indicated in monotherapy for an early disease or in adjuvant treatment for a moderate to severe disease (but neuroprotective effect not clearly documented). – Entacapone (Comtan®): COMT-inhibitor. Side effects: dyskinesias, nausea, vomiting, hypotension, diarrhea, urine discoloration. Dose: 200 mg PO with each dose of Levodopa. **Surgery:** For selected cases: bilateral deep stimulation, thalamotomy, pallidotomy if side effects of medical treatment intolerable or poor response to treatment. Fetal tissue grafts experimental. **Management:** - In younger patient (< 50 years) + mild disease: start with amantadine or anticholinergics (if tremor) → when onset of disturbing symptoms: dopamine agonists (1st choice) and/or Levodopa (Sinemet CR). - In older patients (> 70 years): start with Levodopa; add dopamine agonists or amantadine as needed.
Motor complications of treatment	– Peak-dose dyskinesia: choreiform movements at the peak of therapeutic response. Treatment: give Levodopa CR, stop selegiline, ↓ dose Levodopa, add or ↑ dopamine agonists, amantadine, consider surgery. – Diphasic dyskinesias: violent, large-amplitude dyskinetic movements of the lower body during the time of increasing and decreasing L-dopa levels. 15-30 minutes post-dose: in young patients. Treatment: difficult, regular Levodopa. ↑ dose Levodopa or dopamine agonist, entacapone, surgery. – Akathisia: treatment difficult; ↑ Levodopa, add entacapone, dopamine agonist. – Off-period dystonia: usually in the more severely affected foot in the morning. Treatment: Sinemet CR HS, dopamine agonist, entacapone, regular Levodopa early in the morning. – Motor fluctuations: 2 types: *Wearing-off*, most common type of motor fluctuation. Return of parkinsonism before next dose. *On-off*, unpredictable reappearance of parkinsonism. Treatment: Sinemet CR, increase frequency of drug administration, dopamine agonist, entacapone, surgery.

Epilepsy	
Overview	One seizure is not epilepsy. Epilepsy = 2 or more seizures (except if the seizures are explained by transient triggering factor, e.g.: hyponatremia). Status epilepticus: ongoing seizure > 5 minutes or 2 or more seizures without complete return of awareness in between. Differential diagnosis: psychogenic non-epileptic attack, syncope (post-event confusion < 5 minutes), migraine, hypoglycemia, TIA-stroke, periodic paralysis, drug toxicity.
Causes	Idiopathic vs secondary to underlying cause: alcohol, drug (theophylline, isoniazid, antipsychotics, xylocaine, beta-lactam antibiotics, acyclovir, beta-blockers, tricyclic antidepressants, antihistaminics), street drugs, trauma, infection, central nervous system tumor or malformation, systemic disease (electrolytes disturbances, cancer, SLE), genetic, etc. In patients > 65 years: idiopathic 51%, cerebrovascular 33%, degenerative 12%, trauma 3%, tumor 3%, infection 1%.
Classification	– Provoked seizure vs unprovoked seizure. – Partial seizure: first clinical and electroencephalographic changes indicate initial activation of a system of neurons limited to part of one cerebral hemisphere: sub-divided in simple partial (without impairment of consciousness) or complex partial (with impairment of consciousness). An aura is a simple partial seizure. – Secondarily generalized partial seizure: begins as partial seizure and evolves to a secondarily generalized seizure. – Generalized seizure (primarily generalized): generalized movements at the beginning of the seizure: sub-divided in absence, myoclonic, tonic, clonic, tonic-clonic and atonic seizures.
Workup	EEG. Video-EEG. Brain imaging (MRI is better). **If acute new onset seizure:** Vital signs (rectal temperature, oxymetry), cardiac monitoring, IV lines Blood tests : serum or capillary glucose, CBC, INR, aPTT, electrolytes, creatinine, BUN, Mg^{++}, Ca^{++}, PO_4^{3-}, CK, liver function tests, arterial blood gas, serum ethanol, toxicologic screening, serum anticonvulsant levels, urinalysis. Immediate prolactine dosage to distinguish seizures from pseudoseizures (transient elevation of prolactine with convulsive seizures). Emergent brain imaging. EEG ± EEG monitoring Lumbar puncture if clinically indicated.
Management	**Driving** (for private drivers): No driving for 12 months after a seizure except if: 1- Single unprovoked seizure with normal workup (including EEG +brain imaging) = no driving for 3 months. 2- If toxic, alcoholic or drug induced origin identified + abstinence from the agent during this time = no driving for 6 months. The patient can drive after 12 months without seizures or if during 12 months the seizures were only simple partial or occured only during sleep. After 12 months without seizures, if the seizures relapses because of a drug switch prescribed by a physician = 3 months without driving: if relapse occur under exceptional circumstances = 3 months without driving. **Women:** Drug interaction with contraceptive pill (reduction of the efficacy of the contraceptive pill with phenytoin, carbamazepine, oxcarbazepine, phenobarbital and topiramate): malformations associated with epilepsy and its treatment (especially valproate - 10%), changes in serum concentration of the drugs during pregnancy.

	First seizure: usually: no treatment if seizure is provoked: treat if CT scan, MRI or EEG is abnormal. If the workup is normal : no treatment (after discussing the issue with the patient) but treatment can be sometimes initiated on an individual basis, depending on the risk of relapse and the risks associated with the event (work, social setting).
Treatment	Choosing treatment: – Partial seizures ± secondary generalization: 1st choice: carbamazepine, oxcarbazepine, phenytoin, lamotrigine. Can also be used: gabapentin, clobazam (combined with another anticonvulsant), valproic acid, topiramate, levetiracetam… – Generalized tonic-clonic seizures or myoclonic epilepsy: 1st choice: valproic acid, lamotrigine (1st choice for young women). Can also be used: topiramate, levetiracetam. – Absence seizures: 1st choice: valproic acid: 2nd choice: lamotrigine, ethosuximide. "Classical" antiepileptic drugs: – Phenytoin (Dilantin®): starting dose 300 mg daily in one or two divided doses (200 mg if > 65 years old): maintenance 300-400 mg daily. Side effects at therapeutic levels: confusion, lethargy… at toxic levels (120 µmol/L): nystagmus, ataxia, diplopia. With chronic use: acne, hirsutism, gingival hyperplasia, osteoporosis, rash, neuropathy, lymphadenopathy, hepatitis, nephritis, lupus-like syndrome, cerebellar degeneration, etc. – Carbamazepine (Tegretol®): starting dose 100 mg twice a day or 200 mg daily: progessive increments over 3 weeks: usual dose 800-1200 mg daily. Side effects: ataxia, vertigo, headache, nausea, chronic diarrhea, constipation, rash, leucopenia, aplasic anemia, hepatitis, hyponatremia, etc. – Valproic acid (Depaken®, Epival®): starting dose 15 mg/kg/day in one or two divided doses (400 mg if > 65 years old) increase by 5-10 mg/kg/day/week: usual dose range 1000-1500 mg/day: maximum dose 60 mg/kg/day. Side effects: few at non-toxic level: tremor, nausea, weight gain (50%), transient hair loss, rash, mentrual disorders, toxic hepatitis, pancreatitis, nephritis, hyperammonemia … – Phenobarbital, Primidone (Mysoline®): rarely used because of side effects. – Benzodiazepines: Clobazam: used as adjunct therapy. "New" antiepileptics (similar efficacy, better tolerated, less drug interactions, no hematologic or hepatic follow-up necessary): – Lamotrigine (Lamictal®): starting dose 25 mg/day and raise by 25 mg every two weeks until 100-400 mg/day in two divided doses. Side effects: rash (5 %) that can be severe (<1%) but there is low risk with slow titration, fatigue, diplopia. – Topiramate (Topamax®): starting dose 25 mg/day and raise by 25 mg every two weeks until 100-400mg/day in two divided doses. Side effects: dizziness, fatigue, weight loss (10-20%), paresthesias, cognitive decline, nephrolithiasis (< 1%). – Oxcarbazepine (Trileptal®): alike carbamazepine, starting dose 150 mg twice daily and increase by 300 mg every 2-3 days up to 1200-1800 mg/day in two divided doses (usual). Side effects: fatigue, dizziness, hyponatremia (2-5 %). – Gabapentin (Neurontin®): starting dose 300 mg daily raise every 1-2 days up to 900-3600 mg/day in 3 divided doses. Side effects: sleepiness (dose-dependent), ataxia, weight gain. Exclusive renal elimination. – Levetiracetam (Keppra®): starting dose 500 mg at bedtime and raise by 500 mg every week until 1000-3000 mg/day in two divided doses. Side effects: sleepiness, irritability (5%), psychosis (< 1%). Exclusive renal elimination. Note: drug interactions are frequent; always verify before prescribing.

| *Status epilepticus* treatment | Stabilisation: A-B-C-D, ECG, nasogastric tube if needed.
- Thiamine 100 mg IV.
- Dextrose if hypoglycemia.
- Lorazepam: 0.1 mg/kg at 2 mg/min: if seizure stops and definite cause established, no other therapy necessary; if not:
- Phenytoin: 20 mg/kg IV in NaCl 0.9% at 50 mg/min. If the seizure does not stop add 5-10 mg/kg.
- If *status epilepticus* occurs in the ICU or there is known severe systemic disorders (e.g. : extreme hyperthermia) or the seizure goes on for more than 60-90 minutes : procede immediately to general anesthesia with midazolam;
if not:
- Phenobarbital: 10-20 mg/kg IV at 50-75 mg/min (patient must be intubated).
- If ineffective: additional 5-10 mg/kg of phenobarbital IV.
- If ineffective: midazolam anesthesia (bolus 0.2 mg/kg, maintain 0.75-10 µg/kg/min) or propofol (bolus 1-2 mg/kg, maintain 2-10 mg/kg/h) depending on the appropriate protocol.
- EEG monitoring. |

Dizziness	
1- True Vertigo (50 %)	
Peripheral	
Benign Positional Vertigo (BPV)	Most frequent cause: mean age > 50 years, due to canalolithiasis (precipitated by infection, trauma, etc). Duration 10-20 seconds, maximum 1 minute. With change of head position, getting up, extension of cervical spine, lying down or while turning around in bed. Rapidly decreasing at rest. Recurrent. Diagnosis: Dix Hallpike testing (with vertical/rotatory nystagmus, delayed in onset by 1-10 seconds, duration 30-30 seconds, attenuated response with repeated manoeuvres). Electronystagmography not helpful. Treatment: repositioning maneuver (Epley). Possibly surgery if refractory.
Vestibular Neuronitis and Labyrinthitis	Viral etiology? Often recent febrile or viral episode. Acute, severe with nausea, vomiting: (if ↓ hearing = labyrinthitis). Duration 2 days-6 weeks. No severe trunk ataxia (relative to brainstem stroke), but gait can be very unsteady and lateralizing to affected side. Positive head thrust. **No recurrence**. Treatment: symptomatic (Dimenhydrinate, Meclizine, Betahistine, Clonazepam). Steroids (Prednisone 50-60 mg daily for 10 days and tapering over 10 days), if onset < 72 hours.
Ménière's Syndrome	Thought to be due to increased volume of labyrinthine endolymph spaces (endolymphatic hydrops). Rare > 70 years. Acute, fluctuating hearing loss (low frequencies), tinnitus, vertigo, sensation of fullness in the ear, nausea, vomiting. Duration 5 minutes - 20 hours. Exacerbating-remitting course. *Recurrent neuronitis* if = Ménière's disease but no tinnitus, no hearing loss. Diagnosis by audiometry as needed. Treatment: spontaneous ↓ frequent, reassurance. Avoid caffeine. Antivertiginous medication (Dimenhydrinate, Meclizine, Betahistine, Clonazepam), diuretics (hydrochlorothiazide, triamterene), ↓ NaCl, ototoxic therapy, surgery (endolymphatic shunting) as needed.
Acoustic Neuroma	Asymmetric hypoacousis, progressive, unilateral, high frequencies, tinnitus, vertigo (rare), cranial neuropathy (V, VII), brainstem, cerebellum. Diagnosis: audiometry, MRI. Treatment: surgery.

Other peripheral causes	Drug toxicity, trauma (perilymphatic fistula), cervicogenic (turning the head), otitis media, cholesteatoma, otosclerosis, Ramsay-Hunt syndrome (otoscopic examination), meningeal carcinomatosis.
Central	Associated with other neurological signs and symptoms (diplopia, dysarthria, ataxia, dysmetria, paresis). Suggested by unidirectional or vertical nystagmus. Causes: stroke, epilepsy, vertebrobasilar insufficiency, tumor, multiple sclerosis, basilar migraine.
2- Presyncope and Lipothymia (17 %)	Same causes as syncope (see Syncope table). - Cardiovascular: ↓ intravascular volume, obstruction, arrhythmia (bradycardia, tachycardia), neurocardiogenic (vagal). Classically, sudden onset and quick recovery. - Neurologic: stroke (usually with other neurologic symptoms), migraine, subclavian steal, seizures … Classically, sudden onset - slow recovery. - Metabolic: hypo-/hyperglycaemia, hypo-/hypercalcemia … Classically, slow onset - slow recovery. Measure orthostatic blood pressure, carotid sinus massage. Diagnosis and treatment: according to cause (See Syncope table).
3- Gait Disorder (17 %)	Due to intracerebral pathology, intramedullary, peripheral lesion (nerve or muscular) or multifactorial (decreased eye sight …) Neurologic examination: gait, Romberg, cerebellar testing, visual acuity, fundus examination. Treatment according to underlying cause.
4- Light-headedness (17 %)	Hyperventilation test (reproducing symptoms) may prove diagnosis. Treatment: Breaking the vicious circle by helping patients recognize symptoms caused by hyperventilation during the provocation test. Teach symptom control by respiratory control. Reassurance. Anxiolytics as needed.

Useful References: NEUROLOGY

Alzheimer's Disease: Lancet 2006; 368: 387-403 (review article)
    Treatment: Am J Med 2007; 120: 388-97 (review article)
    N Engl J Med 2004; 351: 56-67 (review article)
Amyotrophic Lateral Sclerosis: Lancet 2007; 369: 2031-41 (review article)
    N Engl J Med 2001; 344: 1688-1700 (review article)
Arterio-Venous Malformation: N Engl J Med 2007; 356: 2704-12 (review article)
Bell's Palsy: N Engl J Med 2004; 351: 1323-31 (review article)
Brain Tumor: N Engl J Med 2001; 344: 114-123 (review article)
    Meningioma: Lancet 2004; 363: 1535-43 (review article)
Carotid Stenosis: Mayo Clin Proc 2007; 82: 851-858 (review article)
    N Engl J Med 2001; 345: 1113-18 (review article)
    Treatment: Mayo Clin Proc 2009; 84: 362-368 (review article)
    J Am Coll Cardiol 2008; 51: 979-85 (review article)
Cerebral Aneurysms: N Engl J Med 2006; 355: 928-39 (review article)
Cerebral Venous Thrombosis: N Engl J Med 2005; 352: 1791-8 (review article)
Cerebrovascular Disease: Med Clin N Am 2009; 93: 353-69 (review article)
Cervical Radiculopathy: N Engl J Med 2005; 353: 392-9 (review article)
Coma: Crit Care Med 2006; 34: 31-41 (review article)
Delirium: N Engl J Med 2006; 354: 1157-65 (review article).
    BMJ 2001; 322: 144-9 (review article)
    Am J Psychiatry 1999; 156 (5 suppl): 1-20 (American Guidelines).
Dementia: Alzheimers Dement 2007; 3: 262-440 (Canadian Guidelines)
    Neurology 2001; 56: 1143-53 (American Guidelines)
    Dementia: Diagnosis: CMAJ 2008; 178: 825-36 (review article)
    Dementia, Mild to Moderate - Treatment: CMAJ 2008; 179: 1019-26 (review article)
    Dementia, Mild to Moderate - Management: CMAJ 2008; 179: 787-93 (review article)
    Dementia, Severe - Management: CMAJ 2008; 179: 1279-87 (review article)
Diabetic Neuropathy: Diabetes Care 2005; 28: 956-62 (Guidelines)
Dizziness: Med Clin N Am 2009; 93: 263-271 (review article)
Dystonia: N Engl J Med 2006; 355: 818-29 (review article)
Epilepsy: Neurology 1998; 51 (suppl 4): S1-43 (American Guidelines)
    CMAJ 2003; 168: 441-8 (review article)
    Med Clin N Am 2009; 93: 343-51 (review article)
    Initial Management: N Engl J Med 2008; 359: 166-76 (review article)
    Refractory E.: N Engl J Med 1999; 340: 1565-70 (review article)
    Status Epilepticus: Chest 2004; 126: 582-591 (review article)
    N Engl J Med 1998; 338: 970-76 (review article)
Guillain-Barré Syndrome: Lancet 2005; 366: 1653–66 (review article)
Headache: Med Clin N Am 2006; 90: 275-290 (review article)
    … Chronic: N Engl J Med 2006; 354: 158-65 (review article)
Herpes Zoster and Postherpetic Neuralgia: Mayo Clin Proc 2009; 84: 274-280 (review article)
Horton Headache: Lancet 2005; 366: 843-55 (review article)
Huntington's Disease: Lancet 2007; 369: 218-28 (review article)
Intra-Cerebral Hemorrhage: Mayo Clin Proc 2007; 82: 987-990 (review article)
    Lancet 2009 ; 373 : 1632-44 (review article)
    Stroke 2007; 38: 2001-23 (American Guidelines)
Ischemic Stroke: Stroke 2007; 38: 1655-1711 (AHA/ASA Guidelines)
    CMAJ 2008; 179 (12 suppl): S1-S25 (Canadian Guidelines)
    Lancet 2008; 371: 1612-23 (review article)
    …Acute: N Engl J Med 2007; 357: 572-9 (review article)
    …Secondary Prevention: Stroke 2008; 39: 1647-1652 (AHA/ASA Guidelines)
Lumbar Spinal Stenosis: N Engl J Med 2008; 358: 818-25 (review article)
Ménière's Disease: Lancet 2008; 372: 406-14 (review article)
Migraine: Lancet 2004; 363: 381-91 (review article)
    CMAJ 1997; 156: 1273- (Canadian Guidelines)
    Neurology 2000; 55: 754-63 (American Guidelines)
    N Engl J Med 2002; 346: 257-70 (review article on treatment)
Mild Cognitive Impairment: CMAJ 2008; 178: 1273-85 (review article)
Multiple Sclerosis: Med Clin N Am 2009; 93: 451-476 (review article)
    Lancet 2008; 372: 1502-17 (review article)
Myasthenia Gravis: Lancet 2001; 357: 2122-28 (review article)
    Treatment: Neurology 2003; 61: 1652-61 (review article)
Optic Neuritis: N Engl J Med 2006; 354: 1273-80 (review article)
Parkinson's Disease: N Engl J Med 2005; 353: 1021-7 (review article)
    Lancet 2009; 373: 2055-66 (review article)

Neurology 2001; 56 (Suppl 5): S1-88 (American Guidelines)
Neurology 2002; 58: 11-17.
Can J Neurol Sc 2003; 30 (Suppl 1): S27-33.
Levodopa: N Engl J Med 2008; 359: 2468-76 (review article)
Treatment: Cleve Clin J Med 2007; 74: 313-28 (review article)
Peripheral neuropathy: Med Clin N Am 2009; 93: 317-342 (review article)
Subarachnoid Hemorrhage: Stroke 2009; 40: 994-1025 (AHA-ASA Guidelines)
N Engl J Med 2006; 354: 387-96 (review article)
Lancet 2007; 369: 306-18 (review article)
Transient Cerebral Ischemia: Stroke 2009; 40: 2276-93 (AHA-ASA Guidelines)
N Engl J Med 2002; 347: 1687-1692 (review article)
Tremors: Arch Intern Med 2000; 160: 2438-44 (review article)
Essential: Neurology 2005; 64: 2008-20 (American Guidelines)
Trigeminal Neuralgia: Neurology 2008; 71: 1183-90 (AAN Guidelines)
Vertigo: Lancet 1998; 352: 1841-46 (review article)
Acute Vestibular Syndrome: N Engl J Med 1998; 339: 680-85 (review article)
Benign Positional Vertigo: N Engl J Med 1999; 341: 1590-96 (review article)
Treatment: Neurology 2008; 70; 2067-74 (review article)

Chapter 9

Pneumology

Dyspnea

Dyspnea is a term used to characterize a subjective experience of breathing discomfort that consists of qualitatively distinct sensations that vary in intensity.

Orthopnea: dyspnea exacerbated in a lying position and improved in a standing position: e.g.: in heart failure, bilateral diaphragmatic paralysis, severe COPD.

Paroxysmal nocturnal dyspnea: nocturnal dyspnea, relieved by the sitting position: e.g.: in heart failure, asthma or COPD.

Trepopnea: dyspnea occurring only in right or left lateral decubitus: e.g.: with left main bronchus tumor, unilateral pleural effusion, or unilateral diaphragmatic paralysis.

Platypnea: Dyspnea occurring only in standing position: e.g.: with hepatic disease (hepatopulmonary syndrome), severe pulmonary fibrosis, pulmonary arteriovenous disease, or post-pneumonectomy.

Causes	**Cardiac:**
	1 - Ischemia.
	2 - Cardiomyopathy (heart failure).
	3 - Arrhythmia: tachycardia, bradycardia.
	4 – Valvular heart disease.
	5 – Pericardial disease: constrictive pericarditis, tamponade.
	6 – Congenital heart disease.
	Pulmonary:
	1- Airway disorders: asthma, COPD, obstruction of the pharynx, larynx, trachea, bronchus, etc.
	2- Parenchymal or interstitial diseases: pneumonia (infectious, eosinophilic), pneumoconiosis, aspiration, diffuse alveolar hemorrhage, atelectasia, pneumonitis (hypersensitivity, radiation-induced, etc), drug induced (amiodarone, methotrexate …), adult respiratory distress syndrome, etc.
	3- Pulmonary vascular diseases: embolism, primary pulmonary hypertension, veno-occlusive disease, etc.
	4- Disorders of the pleura or chest wall: pleural effusion, pneumothorax, obesity, kyphoscoliosis, etc.
	5- Neuromuscular disorders: Guillain-Barré, amyotrophic lateral sclerosis, spinal cord lesion, myasthenia gravis, poliomyelitis, stroke, diaphragmatic paralysis (idiopathic, post-op), etc.
	Other causes (where O_2 saturation is usually normal):
	Hyperventilation - anxiety - panic attack - malingering.
	Anemia.
	Acidosis.
	Shock.
	Sepsis.
	Hypermetabolic states (hyperthyroidism).
	Abdominal distension.
	Deconditioning.
	Clinical approach to dyspnea in relation with its mode of presentation:
	- **Acute** dyspnea (< 2 weeks): asthma or COPD exacerbation, aspiration, pneumonia, pulmonary embolism, alveolar hemorrhage, pneumothorax, ARDS, acute hypersensitivity pneumonitis, cardiac ischemia, heart failure, arrhythmia, pericardial disease, sepsis.
	- **Subacute** dyspnea (2-8 weeks): pulmonary embolism, hypersensitivity pneumonitis, pleural effusion, cardiac ischemia, heart failure, pericardial disease, *Pneumocystis jiroveci*.
	- **Chronic** dyspnea (> 2 months): asthma, COPD, interstitial lung disease, pulmonary

	hypertension, neuromuscular disorders, hyperventilation, chest wall disorders, cardiac ischemia, heart failure, valvular heart disease, pericardial disease, congenital heart disease, anemia, deconditioning, pulmonary embolism, pleural effusion. Note: COPD, asthma, interstitial lung disease and heart diseases account for 2/3 of investigations for dyspnea. In 1/3 of cases, there is more than one explanation to dyspnea; deconditioning is often a contributing factor in patients with a chronic pulmonary disease.
Stage of dyspnea severity	According to the classification of the *Medical Research Council*: 1: Not troubled by breathlessness except with strenuous exercise. 2: Troubled by shortness of breath when hurrying or walking up a slight hill. 3: Walks slower than people of the same age due to breathlessness or has to stop to catch breath when walking at own pace on the level. 4: Stops after about 100 m or after a few minutes on the level. 5: Too breathless to leave the house or breathless when dressing or undressing. Note: Dyspnea can be graded from 0 to 4 or from 1 to 5. A dyspnea of 1/4 is equal to a dyspnea of 2/5.
Management	**Workup**: CBC, renal workup, arterial blood gas or oximetry, pulmonary function tests, Chest X-ray, ECG. **As needed** : CK, troponin, D-dimers, INR, aPTT, *Brain Natriuretic Peptide* (BNP) (if available), cardiopulmonary exercise testing, ventilation-perfusion scan, chest CT (± high-resolution), bronchoscopy, methacholine challenge test, echocardiogram, cardiac stress test, isotopic ventriculography … according to clinical findings. Dyspnea with **normal** chest X-ray: asthma, COPD (occasionally), pulmonary embolism, hyperventilation, deconditioning, cardiac ischemia, bradycardia, valvular heart disease, sepsis, neuromuscular disorders, anemia, etc. **Treatment** according to cause.

Cough	
Overview	On history, look for: duration, symptoms suggestive of infection, post nasal drip, gastroesophageal reflux, associated wheezing, specific risk factors (smoking, HIV), use of angiotensin converting enzyme inhibitors (ACEI). On physical examination, look for: oropharynx exam , cardiac and lung exam, signs of cancer …
Causes	**Acute cough** (< 3 weeks): bronchitis, pneumonia, sinusitis, abscess, upper respiratory tract infection (URTI),allergic rhinitis, whooping cough (*Bordetella pertussis* infection), COPD exacerbation, foreign body aspiration, heart failure, asthma, pulmonary embolism, etc. **Subacute cough** (3-8 weeks): post-infectious, *Bordetella pertussis* infection, sinusitis, asthma, etc. **Chronic cough** (> 8 weeks): – Pulmonary: asthma, COPD (chronic bronchitis), benign or malignant pulmonary or extrapulmonary tumor, bronchiectasis, abscess, granulomatous disease (sarcoidosis, tuberculosis), interstitial lung disease, medication (ACEI), eosinophilic bronchitis, aspiration, etc. – Non pulmonary: upper airway cough syndrome (UACS) (or "postnasal drip syndrome" with sinusitis, rhinitis: most frequent cause), gastroesophageal reflux disease, heart failure, etc. Note: 90 % of chronic cough, excluding smoking and ACEI-induced is due to asthma, an upper airway cough syndrome, or gastroesophageal reflux disease. Up to 50 % of persistent cough may have more than one cause.
Management	If history and physical examination are suggestive of etiology: treat accordingly. If no etiology: withdraw irritants and suspected medications. Chest X-ray and spirometry. As needed, depending on initial evaluation and clinical suspicion: complete pulmonary function tests, methacholine challenge testing, bronchoscopy (if cancer or foreign body suspected), high-resolution chest CT (if suspicion of bronchiectasis or interstitial disease), sinus imaging (if upper respiratory tract infection and no response to initial treatment), ENT evaluation, pH monitoring, barium swallow, empiric treatment of gastroesophageal reflux, sputum culture, cardiac evaluation, etc. Treatment depending on the cause : – If active smoker: stop tobacco (partial effect generally in 4-8 weeks). – Cough caused by angiotensin converting enzyme inhibitors (ACEI): stop medication. May take 4-12 weeks to resolve. – URTI: dexbrompheniramine plus pseudoephedrine (Drixoral®) x 1 week (or nasal ipratropium, another option). – Allergic rhinitis: avoid allergens. Loratadine 10 mg every day or intra-nasal steroids ± long term desensitization. – Vasomotor rhinitis: Drixoral®. Second option: intranasal ipratropium. – Acute sinusitis: intra-nasal oxymetazoline 2 inh. bid x 5 days + antibiotic therapy x 2 weeks + intranasal steroids. If chronic sinusitis, give dexbrompheniramine, pseudoephedrine + antibiotics x 3 weeks + bid nasal decongestant x 5 days. Afterwards, if effective: intra-nasal steroids x 3 months ± ENT consultation. – Whooping cough (*Bordetella pertussis* infection): Macrolide or TMP/SMX x 14 days. – Post-infectious: dexbrompheniramine plus pseudoephedrine. If no response and severe, systemic steroids x 2-3 weeks. If cough is very severe, dextromethorphan, hydrocodone or codeine. If bronchial hyperreactivity, treat like asthma. – Upper airway cough syndrome: treat according to cause (allergic or non-allergic rhinitis, vasomotor rhinitis, chronic sinusitis?). If non-allergic or vasomotor rhinitis,

	treat as post-URTI (Drixoral). – Eosinophilic bronchitis: Inhaled steroids (± systemic) x 2-3 weeks. – Gastroesophageal reflux: Diet, change living habits, proton pump inhibitors for 3 months, minimum. Resolution of cough can take up to 6 months of treatment! – Cough caused by angiotensin converting enzyme inhibitors (ACEI): stop the medication. Can take 4 weeks to resolve. – Asthma and COPD: see respective tables. Note: A systematic approach should resolve 85 % of chronic coughs. If the cause remains unknown, consider empiric treatment; first, treat as upper airway cough syndrome; if failure, treat as gastroesophageal reflux.

Hemoptysis	
Overview	Expectoration of blood originating below the vocal cords. Distinguish from upper GI bleeding or epistaxis ("pseudohemoptysis"). There are 2 arterial circulations in the lung: bronchial (low flow, high pressure) vs. pulmonary (high flow, low pressure). Massive hemoptysis if > 200 mL/24 hours.

Causes	– Pulmonary :
	   o Tracheobronchial origin: cancer, bronchitis or bronchiectasis, trauma, foreign body, aspiration, broncholithiasis, etc.
	   o Parenchymal origin: pneumonia, abscess, tuberculosis, mycetoma or aspergilloma, lung contusion, inhaled cocaine, etc.
	   o Vascular origin: pulmonary embolism, pulmonary infarction, arteriovenous malformation, venous pulmonary hypertension, Goodpasture's syndrome, vasculitis (Wegener's, microscopic polyangiitis, etc), connective tissue disease (SLE or other), idiopathic pulmonary hemosiderosis, etc.
	– Cardiac: mitral stenosis, heart failure.
	– Iatrogenic: Swan-Ganz catheter, pulmonary biopsy, oral anticoagulants or antiplatelet agent.
	– Other causes: coagulopathy, pulmonary endometriosis, etc.
	
	Up to 30 % of hemoptysis remains of unknown etiology despite an adequate investigation.

Workup	– Chest X-ray, CBC. – According to clinical findings: INR, aPTT, urinalysis, renal workup, Gram and culture of sputum, Ziehl + mycobacterial cultures, sputum cytology, ANCA, ANA, complements, anti-GBM antibodies, chest CT, bronchoscopy, echocardiogram, ventilation-perfusion scan, etc. Note: Evaluation to be done according to individual risk of underlying disease, i.e. more extensive in a smoker over age 40.
Treatment	Depends on the cause and emergency : Oxygen. If massive hemorrhage: avoid asphyxia ± intubation if continuous bleeding or hypoxemia despite oxygen: may be selective or double lumen intubation to isolate both lungs: keep sitting position or lateral decubitus on side of bleeding. Bronchial arterial embolization, surgical resection or endobronchial tamponade.
Prognosis	60 % mortality if loss of > 1 liter/24 hours. Otherwise, < 10 % mortality.

Acute Respiratory Distress Syndrome (ARDS)

Acute hypoxemic respiratory failure secondary to a pulmonary or systemic insult without evidence of heart failure. Bilateral pulmonary infiltrates are present.
Occurs rapidly: 12-48 hours after insult.

Definition of acute lung injury:
1. PaO_2/FIO_2 ratio ≤ 300.
2. Bilateral pulmonary infiltrates.
3. Absence of clinical evidence of left atrial hypertension (or pulmonary-artery wedge pressure < 18 mmHg if measured).
4. Acute onset (< 7 days).

Definition of acute respiratory distress syndrome:
1. PaO_2/FIO_2 ratio ≤ 200.
2. Bilateral pulmonary infiltrates.
3. Absence of clinical evidence of left atrial hypertension (or pulmonary-artery wedge pressure < 18 mmHg if measured).
4. Acute onset (< 7 days).

Causes	– Indirect: sepsis, shock, trauma, transfusions, extracorporeal circulation, pancreatitis, burns, drug overdose (opiates, aspirin, antidepressants, amiodarone, nitrofurantoin, some chemotherapy…), thrombotic thrombocytopenic purpura, etc. – Direct: diffuse pneumonia (viral, bacterial, mycoplasma, Pneumocystis, Legionella, severe acute respiratory syndrome, blastomycosis, miliary tuberculosis, hantavirus), aspiration, embolism (fat, gas, thrombus, amniotic fluid), near-drowning, pulmonary contusion, toxic inhalation (smoke, nitrogen dioxide, chlorine, ammonia…), post pulmonary reperfusion (transplantation, embolectomy), high-altitude, etc. Differential diagnosis: Cardiogenic pulmonary edema (pulmonary-artery wedge pressure > 18 mmHg), diffuse alveolar hemorrhage, COP/BOOP, acute eosinophilic pneumonia, hypersensitivity pneumonitis, acute interstitial pneumonitis, etc.

Treatment	Treat the primary cause or the underlying infection as required.
	
	Mechanical ventilation as needed if acute respiratory failure :
	    Assist/control mode with tidal volumes of 6 mL/kg of ideal body weight: rate up to 30-35/min: minimal PEEP for adequate oxygenation (5-7 cm H_2O up to 15-20 max.)
	    Aim for: O_2 saturation 88-95 % with minimal FIO_2 and plateau pressure < 30 mmHg. Heavy sedation according to standardized protocol ± paralysis + many possible ventilation strategies: ↑ PEEP, permissive hypercapnia (by ↓ tidal volume).
	
	Steroids: not routinely because no proven benefits on mortality: to use accordingly to ARDS cause and clinical evolution.
	
	Other treatments to consider:
	  - Keep the head of the bed at 30° for intubated patient, except if contraindication (for ventilator-associated pneumonia prevention).
	  - Diuretics as needed (keeping minimal capillary pressure).
	  - Nutritional support.
	  - Glycemic control.
	  - Thromboembolic and stress ulcer prophylaxis.
	
	If refractory hypoxemia:
	    Prone positioning as needed (improves O_2 saturation without lowering mortality).
	  - Nitric oxide (NO) (especially useful for refractory hypoxemia: but no proven benefit on mortality).
	  - Recruiting maneuvers if needed.
	
	No effective prevention.

Prognosis	≈ 30-40 % mortality.
	Mortality due to the initial cause, to a multiple organ failure, or to sepsis.
	Poor prognostic factors: older age, chronic liver disease, extrapulmonary multiple organ failure, sepsis.
	Return to near baseline lung condition after 6-12 months in most survivors.
	In cases of severe ARDS, can have permanent sequelae, especially for gas exchange and diffusion capacity.

Asthma

Disease characterized by an inflammatory reaction of the airway resulting in persistent or paroxysmal symptoms (dyspnea, chest tightness, wheezing, cough), associated with a variable airflow limitation and a bronchial hyperreactivity to endogenous or exogenous stimuli.

Prevalence: ≥ 5 % of the population.

Asthma can be induced and/or exacerbated by exercise, work (occupational asthma with isocyanates - spray paint, plastic manufacture -, dyes, wood dust, acrylate - resin and glue - metals, cereals, flour, latex), medications (ASA, NSAIDs, beta-blockers), drugs (heroin, cocaine), allergens (cats, dogs, acarina), cold, infections, rhinitis, gastroesophageal reflux …

A triad of asthma - nasal polyps - aspirin sensitivity (and NSAIDs) exists.

Differential diagnosis: vocal cords dysfunction or paralysis, foreign body aspiration, laryngotracheal mass, tracheal obstruction, tracheomalacia, airway edema with angioedema or toxic inhalation, COPD (age > 40, smoking of > 10-20 pack-years), bronchiectasis, allergic bronchopulmonary aspergillosis, cystic fibrosis, chronic eosinophilic pneumonia, parasitic infection, bronchiolitis obliterans, Churg-Strauss syndrome, left heart failure (cardiac asthma), pulmonary embolism, hyperventilation, malingering, etc.

Evaluation	Workup: perform objective measurement to confirm the diagnosis and evaluate gravity in all patients with suggestive symptoms: demonstration of reversibility with FEV_1 (spontaneous variability or with steroid trial for 10-14 days [variation of ≥ 20 % and ≥ 250 mL] or post bronchodilator [if ≥ 12 % and ≥ 180 mL]) or with peak expiratory flow (PEF: variability of ≥ 20 % over many weeks) or of bronchial hyperreactivity (methacholine challenge testing).
	Perform cutaneous allergy tests at least once. Occasionally, associated eosinophilia.
	Environmental control: avoid tobacco exposure, pollution, allergens, acarina, animals, and respiratory irritants, maintain humidity < 50%. Evaluate the possibility of occupational asthma in all adults with a diagnosis of asthma.
	Patient education: *essential:* educational program ("asthma education centers") and establish an action plan to be used when control is lost.
	Ensure periodically treatment compliance and adequate technique for inhalers use. Self-monitoring of PEF as needed.
	Refer patients who constantly need > 1000 µg of beclomethasone/day or equivalent for adequate control or patients with severe or poorly controlled asthma to a specialist.
	Rule out, among others, gastroesophageal reflux, chronic rhino-sinusitis or allergic bronchopulmonary aspergillosis in cases of refractory asthma.

Treatment	In accordance with the Canadian Guidelines updated in 2003 :
	Evaluate control with acceptable control as being defined by :

Evaluate control with acceptable control as being defined by :
- Daytime symptoms < 4 days/week.
- Night-time symptoms < 1 night/week.
- Mild, infrequent exacerbations.
- No absenteeism due to asthma.
- Normal physical activity.
- Fewer than 4 doses/week of short-acting β-2 agonist needed.
- FEV1/ PEF > 90 % of personal best.
- PEF diurnal variation of less than 10-15 %.

If adequate control, after a few months → reduce dosage of inhaled steroids.
If a better result is possible or inadequate control despite a dose of beclomethasone ≥ 500 µg/day or equivalent → start additional therapy (usually a long-acting β-2 agonist). If control is lost → start oral steroids.

Concept of continuum in asthma management.

Two types of asthma treatment exist: medications used for rapid relief of symptoms (β-2 agonists) and medications that treat inflammation (steroids, leukotriene receptor antagonists, cromoglycate, nedocromil) :

- Short-acting β-2 agonists: symptomatic treatment as needed, not regularly. Adequate as only therapy in exercise induced asthma *or* if isolated use 4 times a week: if not, inhaled steroids are *essential*.
- Steroids: Inhaled corticosteroids (ICS): the basis of anti-inflammatory treatment: indicated in all patients except those with benign symptoms (need for short-acting β-2 agonist < 4 times/week): initial dose 400-1000 µg/day of beclomethasone or equivalent. If exacerbation: double inhalation therapy from 2 to 4 or give PO steroids (e.g.: Prednisone 30-60 mg) usually for > 10-14 days depending on the severity of exacerbation. Rinse mouth after inhalation. Bone density suggested if chronic requirement of > 1000µg of beclomethasone/day or multiple risk factors for osteoporosis. In patients with personal or familial history of glaucoma, measure ocular pressure a few days after starting therapy and periodically afterwards.

  Note: 1000 µg of beclomethasone = 800 µg of budesonide = 500 µg of fluticasone = 400 µg of ciclesonide.

- Long-acting β-2 agonists (LABA): additional therapy added to low doses inhaled steroids (equivalent to ≥ 500 µg of beclomethasone/day) if inadequate control. **Do not use** without anti-inflammatory treatment. Combination therapy with ICS is available (Advair® and Symbicort®). Option of one inhaler (Symbicort®) as maintenance and emergency treatment if already under ICS and not controlled.
- Leukotriene receptor antagonists: additional therapy that can be added to low doses inhaled steroids (equivalent to ≥ 500 µg of beclomethasone/day) if inadequate control or presence of mild asthma and fear of ICS toxicity or as an alternative if exercise induced asthma.
- Anti-allergic agents: cromoglycate: few indications at the moment: possible alternative to steroids but less effective.
- Theophylline and derivatives: rarely used. Therapeutic trial necessary to identify responders. Monitor for drug interactions. Frequent side effects.
- Anticholinergic agents: few indications except if concomitant COPD or β-2 agonists intolerance.
- Omalizumab: if allergic severe asthma with continuous or frequent Prednisone treatment.
- Non-steroidal immunosuppressive agents (e.g.: methotrexate, cyclosporine, gold salts): to consider only in severe asthma with long term steroid dependence (but few clinical data available).

	→ To summarize: 1) Short-acting β-2 agonists alone if used ≤ 3 x/week. 2) Add ICS if β-2 agonists > 3x/week or 1x/week at night. 3) Add long-acting β-2 agonists if usage of mild dose ICS (equivalent to 500 μg of beclomethasone/day) and inadequate control. 4) Consider adding leukotriene receptor antagonists or increasing ICS dose to equivalent dose of 1000 to 2000 μg of beclomethasone/day. 5) Consider theophylline as 3rd option for treatment. 6) Consider Prednisone if severe asthma not responding to previous treatment. 7) Consider omalizumab.
Emergency	Asthma gravity criteria: near-fatal previous episode (intubation, loss of consciousness), recent hospitalization or emergency room visit, nocturnal symptoms, limitation of daily activities, need for short acting β-2 agonist many times a day or nightly, steroid dependence, abnormal physical examination (↓ level of consciousness, difficulty to talk, cyanosis, respiratory rate > 30/min, pulse > 120/min, pulsus paradoxicus > 20 mmHg, use of accessory muscles, silent chest), abnormal laboratory values (FEV1 or PEF < 60 %, FEV1 < 1L, pCO$_2$ normal or ↑, pO$_2$ ↓, pneumothorax or pneumomediastinum). Status asthmaticus if impending respiratory failure.
Management	**Workup:** FEV1, oximetry, arterial blood gas (if saturation < 90 %, suspected hypercapnia, critical asthma or FEV1 < 25 % or PEF < 120 L/min), Chest X-ray. ECG if older patient or CAD. **Hospitalize if:** pre-treatment FEV1 < 25 % (or < 1L), post-treatment FEV1 < 40 % (or < 1.6 L): Hospitalization as needed for FEV1 40-60 % (grey zone). **Intensive care if** severe obstruction with little improvement despite treatment (↑ pCO$_2$, FEV1 < 25 %, altered level of consciousness). **Treatment :** 1st line : - *Oxygen*: aim for SaO$_2$ > 92 %. - *β-2 agonists*: salbutamol 100 μg/puff: via metered-dose inhalers: 4-8 inh. (100 μg) every 15-20 min x 3 generally: ↑ to 1 inh. every 30-60 s. as needed: via nebulizer if unable to use metered-dose inhaler 2,5 mg every 15-20 min x 3 : continuously as needed. - *Anticholinergics*: for 24-48 hours in moderate to severe crisis: ipratropium 20 μg/puff: via metered-dose inhalers: 4-8 inh. (20μg) every 15-20 min x 3 in general: ↑ to 1 inh. every 30-60 s. as needed: via nebulizer : 0.5 mg every 15 - 20 min x 3: continuously as needed. - *Steroids*: PO or IV **and** inhaled (e.g.: prednisone 40-60 mg daily or methylprednisolone 40 mg IV every 6 hours when acute). Effective dose probably equivalent. To give for 7-14 days. - Antibiotic if evidence of infection. Note: most patients improve within 1-3 hours. 2nd line : - *Magnesium sulfate* IV 2 g. in 20 minutes. - *Aminophylline*: loading dose 6 mg/kg IV in 30 min (no loading dose if the patient already uses it): IV infusion 0.05 mg/kg/h: monitor blood levels. 3rd Line : - *Salbutamol IV*: loading dose 4 μg/kg (in 2-5 min): IV infusion 0.1-0.2 μg/kg/min. - *Epinephrine*: 1:1000 s/c 0.3-0.5 mL every 15-20 min PRN: IV infusion (1:1000 in 250 mL D5W = 4 μg/mL) IV 4-8 μg/min. -**Intubation** *by an expert* if: exhaustion, altered level of consciousness, ↑ pCO$_2$ progressive, impending cardio-respiratory arrest. If intubation: options of midazolam, propofol, ketamine + succinylcholine. Heliox or

	inhaled anesthetics if refractory. Consider transfer in specialized center since ventilation is often difficult.
	Refer to a specialist if severe asthma (FEV1/PEF < 40 % or frequent attacks) during hospitalization or on an outpatient basis.
	Discharge when FEV1/PEF > 60-70 %, adequate medication, adequate inhaler technique, and written action plan for exacerbations. Medication on discharge: β-2 agonists as needed. Prednisone 30-60 mg/day PO (initial dosage) for 7-14 days **and** inhaled steroids ± long-acting ß2 agonists.
	Education at discharge is mandatory: review mode of administration and adherence to treatment, role of medication (acute phase vs. anti-inflammatory), explain exacerbations (symptoms), consult the "asthma education center", smoking cessation, environmental control.
	Ensure adequate medical follow-up.

Chronic Obstructive Pulmonary Disease

Overview	Respiratory disorder characterized by a progressive, partially reversible airway obstruction and lung hyperinflation, systemic manifestations, and increasing frequency and severity of exacerbations, caused by persistent inflammation of the airway and lung parenchyma (largely caused by smoking).
	Chronic bronchitis: daily productive cough ≥ 3 months for ≥ 2 consecutive years without any other disease that could explain symptoms (clinical definition). *Emphysema*: abnormal and permanent enlargement of the airways distal to the terminal bronchioles accompanied by destruction of the walls without obvious fibrosis (pathologic definition).
	- Fourth cause of mortality in Canada. - About 15 % of smokers will develop COPD.
	Risk factors: tobacco smoke (usually > 10-20 packs/year), asthma, α1-antitrypsin deficiency (1-3 % of patients), air pollution, respiratory infections during infancy.
	Differential diagnosis: asthma, heart failure, bronchiectasis, tuberculosis, bronchiolitis, cystic fibrosis, allergic bronchopulmonary aspergillosis, bronchial obstruction, etc.
Stages of severity	In accordance with the 2007 Canadian Guidelines, classification of COPD must take into consideration symptoms and disability, as well as impairment of pulmonary function.

Stages of severity	According to symptoms and disability:	According to impairment of pulmonary function:
	- Mild if dyspnea of Medical research Council (MRC) 2/5*. - Moderate if dyspnea MRC 3-4/5 - Severe if dyspnea MRC 5/5 or presence of chronic respiratory failure or clinical signs of right heart failure. * See dyspnea table for details on The *Medical Research Council* Dyspnea Scale.	- Mild: FEV1 ≥ 80 % †, FEV1/FVC < 70 % †. - Moderate: FEV1 50-80 %, FEV1/FVC < 70 % - Severe: FEV1 30-50 %, FEV1/FVC < 70 % - Very severe: FEV1 < 30 %, FEV1/FVC < 70 % † Postbronchodilator.

Workup	Pulmonary function tests in all patients (assess bronchodilator response).
	Arterial blood gas if FEV1 < 40-50 % or suspicion of respiratory failure.
	CBC: polycythemia with severe COPD.
	Chest X-ray in order to evaluate differential diagnosis.
	As needed: α1-antitrypsin measurement if early disease (< 45 years old), family history, basal involvement, bronchiectasis.
	High-resolution chest CT (rarely necessary but more sensitive): hyperinflation, bullous disease.
	Echocardiogram and ECG if suspected co-morbidity (pulmonary hypertension, heart failure).
Management	Patient education
	Smoking cessation: nicotine replacement, bupropion, varenicline.
	Vaccination (influenza yearly, Pneumovax®).
	Adequate diet (avoid malnutrition and weight loss, except if obesity).
	Polysomnography if concomitant sleep apnea suspected.
	Air travel: patient at risk if PaO_2 < 70 mmHg: aim at PaO_2 > 50 mmHg during air flight, for example in ↑ O_2 by 2L/min if already treated with supplemental O_2.
	Consider referral to a specialist if: uncertain diagnosis, severe symptoms or out of proportion to the gravity of disease, or before 45 years of age.
	Follow-up with a specialist suggested if FEV1 < 50 %.
Treatment of stable COPD	**Pharmacologic**
	Continuum concept of treatment according to gravity and response
	- For patients with symptoms that are only noticeable on exertion and who have relatively little disability, initiation of a short-acting bronchodilator treatment (ß2 agonists or anti-cholinergics) as needed is acceptable (salbutamol 100 µg/puff 2-4 inh. qid, ipratropium 20 µg/puff 3-4 inh. qid). Choice of treatment should be based on clinical response and side effects. Some patients can benefit from a long acting bronchodilator.
	- For patients with more persisting symptoms and moderate to severe airflow obstruction, a long-acting bronchodilator such as tiotropium (18 µg daily) (1st choice) or salmeterol is recommended. Short-acting ß-2 agonists for immediate symptom relief can be used, as needed.
	- For patients with moderate to severe COPD and persistent symptoms but infrequent exacerbations (< 1/year average on 2 consecutive years), a combination of tiotropium and ß-2 agonist long acting (BALA) (salmeterol 50 µg bid) is recommended. A salmeterol/fluticasone combination, small dose (50/250 µg bid) could replace salmeterol in patients with persisting dyspnea despite the long acting bronchodilator combination (salmeterol + tiotropium). Short-acting ß-2 agonists will be used, as needed, for immediate symptom relief.
	- For patients with moderate to severe COPD and persistent symptoms and a history of exacerbations (≥ 1/year average on 2 consecutives years) a tiotropium combination plus BALA and inhaled corticosteroid (CSI) (salmeterol/fluticasone 50/500 µg or formoterol/budesonide 12/400 µg bid) is recommended. Short-acting ß-2 agonists, as needed, may be used for immediate symptom relief.
	- For patients with severe symptoms despite the use of tiotropium and a BALA/CSI, a long-acting preparation of oral theophylline (SR 200 mg bid or 400 mg HS) may be tried, although monitoring of blood levels, side effects and potential drug interactions is necessary.
	- Use of CSI as monotherapy or long-term treatment with oral corticosteroids is not recommended.

	- Other possible treatments : In severe disease: narcotics – benzodiazepines to ↓ dyspnea (palliative treatment). Supplemental α1-antitrypsin to consider if deficiency with blood level < 11 μmol/L and other gravity criteria (but effectiveness is controversial, costly). **Oxygen therapy** (minimum 15 h/day) : lowers mortality : *indications* : – If pO_2 ≤ 55 mmHg at rest, sitting, with optimal therapy. – If pO_2 55-59 mmHg and bilateral ankle edema, *cor pulmonale* or polycythemia (hematocrit > 56 %) – If pO_2 ≥ 60 mmHg in certain particular states, exercise desaturation: controversial but could be considered in the context of a pulmonary rehabilitation program). **Pulmonary rehabilitation**: program of education, exercise and physical therapy that can ↑ functional capacity and quality of life and ↓ dyspnea and hospitalizations in COPD patients. Indicated for dyspneic patients with limited functional capacities despite optimal treatment. **Surgery**: bullectomy or lung volume reduction sometimes indicated. Requires extensive preoperative evaluation. Pulmonary transplantation (but no survival benefit).
Complications	Acute exacerbation (see below). *Cor pulmonale* (right heart failure), spontaneous pneumothorax, ↑ risk of lung cancer. ↑ risk of cardiovascular diseases. Survival prognosis = 4 years if FEV1 ≤ 1L/min but variable. Prognosis also depend on dyspnea exacerbation, exercise capacity and ↓ BMI (BODE index).

Acute Exacerbations of COPD

Definition	Acute exacerbations of COPD (AECOPD) is defined as a sustained (lasting 48 hours or more) worsening of dyspnea, cough or sputum production leading to an increase in the use of maintenance medications and/or supplementation with additional medications. Should be defined as either purulent or nonpurulent exacerbations.
Causes	Infection (viral, pneumococcus, *Haemophilus*, *Moraxella*) in about 50 %. Ventricular failure, pulmonary embolism, concomitant disease that ↑ metabolic needs, noncompliance to medication, abdominal surgery, pneumothorax, irritant or allergen inhalation, aspiration, medication (beta-blockers, sedatives), myocardial infarction, arrhythmia, etc.
Stratification of AECOPD	In accordance with the 2007 Canadian Guidelines: "Simple" exacerbation if COPD without risk factors. Probable pathogens: *Haemophilus influenzae*, *Haemophilus* sp., *Moraxella catarrhalis*, *Stretococcus pneumoniae*. "Complicated" exacerbation if COPD with risk factors: FEV1 < 50 % predicted, ≥ 4 exacerbations/year, ischemic heart disease, use of home oxygen, chronic oral steroids or use of antibiotic within 3 months. Probable pathogens: as in simple + *Klebsiella* sp. and other Gram neg., ↑ probability of beta-lactamases resistance.

Management	Workup: CBC, creatinine, infectious workup (sputum culture if frequent exacerbations), arterial blood gas, ECG, chest X-ray (in the emergency room) … according to clinical findings. No spirometry in emergency room! (except to conduct diagnosis if there wasn't any before). Hospitalization : - if acute exacerbation and inadequate response to initial treatment, severe baseline COPD, significant comorbidity, new arrhythmia, uncertain diagnosis, advanced age, hypoxemia, inadequate home support … - *In ICU if*: severe dyspnea not responding to initial treatment, confusion, lethargy, coma, hypoxemia (< 40 mmHg), hypercapnia (> 60 mmHg) or acidosis (pH < 7.25) despite oxygen and assisted invasive or noninvasive ventilation (see below).
Treatment	According to exacerbation cause : **Pharmacological :** - Bronchodilators: Ipratropium (20 µg/puff) 4 inh. every 4 h or nebulized 0.5 mg every 4 h + salbutamol (100 µg/puff) 4 inh. every 2-4 h, or nebulized 2.5 mg every 2-4 h. Role for long acting bronchodilators hasn't been studied. - Steroids: for moderate to severe exacerbation: dosage and duration controversial (recommended for 7 to 14 days): e.g.: methylprednisone 40 mg IV every 6 h for 24-48 hours, then taper off or Prednisone 30-40 mg every day depending on the gravity of the exacerbation. - Antibiotics: beneficial for **purulent** exacerbations. - If "simple" exacerbation: use amoxicillin, doxycycline, TMP/SMX, 2nd - 3rd gen-cephalosporins, wide-spectrum macrolides. - If "complicated" exacerbation: use ß-lactam/ß-lactamase inhibitor, fluoroquinolone (antibiotics for uncomplicated patients when combined with oral steroids may suffice). For frequent exacerbations (recurrence within 3 months), consider changing antibiotic class to avoid resistance. Note: Avoid sedatives! **Non pharmacological**: - Oxygen therapy: aim for SaO_2 90 % (Beware of CO_2 retention). - Noninvasive positive pressure ventilation ("Bi-PAP®", e.g.: expiratory pressure 4-8 cm H_2O and inspiratory pressure 10-15 cm H_2O) as needed, especially if dyspnea with use of accessory muscles, pH 7.25-7.35 and pCO_2 > 45 mmHg, respiratory rate 25/min, **but** without altered level of consciousness or impending respiratory failure or hemodynamic instability. - Mechanical ventilation, as needed (if ↓ sensorium, severe acidosis < 7.20 and hypercapnia or refractory hypoxemia or if noninvasive ventilation failure). - Consider intensity of treatment (ventilatory support to be discussed with the patient prior to acute exacerbation). - Follow-up in 4-6 weeks after hospital discharge.

Interstitial Lung Disease

Heterogeneous group of diseases characterized by inflammation (alveolitis) and fibrosis of the inter-lobular septa.
Clinical findings: exertional dyspnea of insidious onset, dry cough, clubbing, inspiratory crackles.
On pulmonary function tests: restrictive syndrome in general, but more rarely obstructive syndrome with some diseases.

Causes	More than 180 identified causes :
	 – Idiopathic interstitial pneumonitis: the most frequent cause: subdivided in clinically and histologically distinct entities (by order of frequency):
	    1 - Usual interstitial pneumonitis (UIP) (synonym of idiopathic pulmonary fibrosis): chronic presentation: > 50 years old, bi-basal predominance.
	    2 - Nonspecific interstitial pneumonia (NSIP): sometimes associated with connective tissue disease or drugs, younger patients in general: Sub-acute to chronic presentation.
	    3 - Respiratory bronchiolitis associated-interstitial lung disease (RB-ILD)/Desquamative interstitial pneumonia (DIP): Subacute or chronic presentation, smoker.
	    4 - Cryptogenic organizing pneumonia (COP): idiopathic form of bronchiolitis obliterans organizing pneumonia (BOOP): subacute presentation, BOOP may be secondary to connective tissue disease, infections, drugs, radiotherapy.
	    5 - Acute interstitial pneumonia (AIP): abrupt presentation (< 3 weeks).
	    6 - Lymphocytic interstitial pneumonia (LIP): associated with Sjögren, HIV, lymphoma, inflammatory bowel disease: chronic presentation.
	 – Connective tissue disease/vasculitis.
	 – Granulomatous diseases: unknown (sarcoidosis) or known causes.
	 – Inhalation: occupational: secondary to organic dust (hypersensivity pneumonitis: see below) or inorganic dust – pneumoconiosis (e.g.: asbestosis, silicosis).
	 – Hereditary: neurofibromatosis, tuberous sclerosis.
	 – Iatrogenic: medication, irradiation.
	 – Certain specific entities: eosinophilic pneumonia, Langherhans cell histiocytosis (see below), lymphangioleiomyomatosis (especially in pre-menopause woman, with recurrent pneumothorax, uterine leiomyomas, renal angiomyolipomas, pulmonary cysts on CT), alveolar proteinosis (alveolar accumulation of lipoprotein derived from surfactant, especially among smokers < 50 years old; broncho-alveolar lavage usually diagnostic; lymphangitic carcinomatosis, amyloidosis, diffuse alveolar hemorrhage.
	
	 Rule out any other diagnosis that could present with similar symptoms (e.g.: heart failure, Pneumocystis infection).

Diagnosis	Initial evaluation : history, physical examination, occupational and expositional history, medication, pulmonary function tests, laboratory studies, review previous chest X-rays: – If occupational/environmental (medication, inhalation, antigen): evaluate work/home: confirm with withdrawal test. – If systemic disease (multisystemic involvement, aspiration, neoplasm, infection): do serologies, endoscopy, and biopsy as needed, according to clinical evaluation: evaluate response to treatment. – If unknown cause: if high-resolution chest CT is diagnostic, treat; if Θ, consider: bronchoscopy with transbronchial biopsy + bronchoalveolar lavage: if diagnostic, treat; if Θ, consider or lung biopsy either by thoracoscopy or open (especially if < 65 years old, if not, evaluate risk/benefit). Note: Chest CT can show patterns suggestive of Langherhans cells histiocytosis, asbestosis, silicosis, lymphangioleiomyomatosis, idiopathic pulmonary fibrosis, lymphangitic carcinomatosis and, occasionally, sarcoidosis, BOOP, alveolar proteinosis, eosinophilic pneumonia and mycobacteria. Bronchoalveolar lavage is diagnostic for infections, alveolar proteinosis, and alveolar hemorrhage and may suggest eosinophilic pneumonia, hypersensivity pneumonitis and

	sarcoidosis. Transbronchial biopsy may help to make a diagnosis of sarcoidosis, hypersensitivity pneumonitis, lymphangitic carcinomatosis, alveolar proteinosis, or miliary tuberculosis. Lung biopsy via thoracoscopy remains necessary to bring precision to the diagnosis of UIP, although not always essential, diagnosis may be made in absence of biopsy if presentation is typical.
Treatment	General measures: education, exercise, nutrition, smoking cessation, immunization, O_2 as needed. - for granulomatous disease or connective tissue disease/vasculitis: treat accordingly. - for idiopathic interstitial pneumonitis: DIP/RB-ILD, NSIP and BOOP frequently respond to corticosteroids (prednisone 1 mg/kg/day). No effective treatment for UIP (steroids + azathioprine ± N-acetylcysteine often tried, but no evidence of survival benefit) and for AIP (support + steroids). Consider lung transplantation if < 65 years old. Follow-up with chest X-rays and serial pulmonary function tests ± high-resolution chest CT.
Prognosis	Poor for UIP: mortality 50-80 %, 5 years after diagnosis. Poor for AIP: mortality 50-80 %, short term. NSIP: mortality < 10 % at 5 years. DIP/RB-ILD: mortality 5 % at 5 years. Very good prognosis for COP-BOOP.
Hypersensitivity Pneumonitis	Synonyms: Extrinsic allergic alveolitis, farmer's lung disease, bird breeder's disease, hot tub lung, etc. Caused by a hypersensitivity allergic reaction to different organic antigens, including grain dust and mold (farmer's lung), birds (bird breeder's lung), certain animals, nontuberculous mycobacteria (spa), etc. Can present with an acute inflammatory disease (4-8 hours after exposure), a sub-acute or chronic presentation. In acute presentation: dyspnea, cough, chest pain, fever, headaches, discomfort, fatigue. In chronic presentation, the findings may be identical to usual interstitial pneumonitis. **Diagnosis:** Chest X-ray may be normal or almost normal: sometimes interstitial involvement. In general, pulmonary function tests show a restrictive pattern (with DLCO) ± hypoxemia (sometimes severe). High-resolution chest CT: non specific lung micronodules and ground-glass opacities; radiologic pattern sometimes identical to usual interstitial pneumonitis if chronic. Bronchoscopy: bronchoalveolar lavage: most often lymphocytosis; if biopsy: non-caseating granulomas. Serous precipitins: occasional false ⊕ and false ⊖. Leukocytosis, sedimentation rate ↑. ANA or rheumatoid factor sometimes ⊕. **Treatment:** Remove exposure to antigen. Steroids sometimes necessary, according to severity.

Langerhans Cell Histiocytosis	Rare pulmonary disease among young smokers (especially Caucasians). 25 % asymptomatic; otherwise: dyspnea, cough, recurrent spontaneous pneumothorax. Possibly, central diabetes insipidus and hypopituitarism, bone involvement. **Diagnosis:** Chest X-ray: cysts and interstitial infiltrate. High-resolution chest CT: nodules, micronodules and cysts, especially in upper lobes. Fibrosis if chronic. Obstructive, restrictive or mixed pattern in pulmonary function tests with possible hypoxemia and ↓ DLCO. **Treatment:** Stop tobacco smoking (stabilization/improvement in 2/3 of patients). Steroids according to severity: chemotherapy? Lung transplantion if needed.

Sarcoidosis

Multisystemic granulomatous disease of unknown etiology, for which the characteristic lesion is a noncaseating granuloma made of epithelioid cells.

Age of onset: especially between 20-40 years old.
Prevalence 1-3/10 000, variable according to ethnic background, sex and country.

Differential diagnosis: hypersensitivity pneumonitis, lymphoma, mycobacteria (tuberculosis, avium), fungi (histoplasmosis, blastomycosis, aspergillosis), berylliosis (positive occupational exposure), granulomatous vasculitis (Wegener's), granulomatous reaction due to cancer.

Clinical findings	- Asymptomatic in 20-40 %. - Non-specific symptoms: malaise, fatigue, fever, weight loss. - Pulmonary symptoms: dry cough, dyspnea, chest tightness; hemoptysis and clubbing are rare. Possible airway involvement (bronchiectasis, obstruction, bronchial hyperreactivity). Rarely: pleural effusion, chylothorax, pneumothorax, pachypleuritis, calcification, cavity formation. - Ocular (anterior uveitis, keratoconjonctivitis), cutaneous (erythema nodosum, lupus pernio, nodules), nose involvement, enlargement of parotid, salivary or lacrymal glands. - Lymphadenopathy, hepato or splenomegaly, arthritis. - Central or peripheral nervous system involvement (meningeal, hypothalamus, pituitary involvement …myelopathy, cranial nerve VII, peripheral nerves). - Myocardial involvement: arrhythmia, cardiomyopathy, pericarditis. - Hypercalcemia, nephrocalcinosis, kidney stones, interstitial nephritis. - GI tract involvement … Löfgren's syndrome: fever, hilar lymphadenopathy, erythema nodosum, periarthritis. Heerfordt's syndrome: fever, parotid enlargement, facial palsy and anterior uveitis.
Staging	Stage 0: normal chest X-ray. Stage 1: bilateral hilar lymphadenopathy. Stage 2: bilateral hilar lymphadenopathy with diffuse pulmonary involvement. Stage 3: parenchymal infiltrates without lymphadenopathy. Stage 4: irreversible pulmonary fibrosis.
Diagnosis	If Löfgren's syndrome or stage 1 and asymptomatic without asymmetric or massive lymphadenopathy: observation with close follow-up: (X-ray every 3-6 months until clear evolution): if non-classical presentation → rule out lymphoma (by mediastinoscopy or transbronchial biopsy, or biopsy of other sites). If stage 2 or 3: bronchoscopy with transbronchial biopsy (75-90 % of sensitivity): if no diagnosis, mediastinoscopy or pulmonary biopsy or biopsy of other involved sites. Rule out other causes of granuloma (tuberculosis). Avoid to biopsy erythema nodosum since there is no granuloma in these lesions.

	– Testing on initial evaluation: Chest X-ray, pulmonary function tests (spirometry and CO diffusion capacity), CBC, calcium, creatinine, BUN, liver enzymes (AST, ALT, alkaline phosphatase), PPD, urinalysis, ECG, ophthalmologic evaluation ± high-resolution chest CT ± bronchoscopy. – Other tests as needed: angiotensin converting-enzyme (for follow-up, mostly helpful if ↑ > 2 x normal), protein electrophoresis, urinary calcium, biopsy of other involved sites, CT or MRI (lung, cerebral), cardiac tests (echocardiogram, thallium scan, Holter), positron emission tomography, etc.
Treatment	Stage 1: watchful waiting in general. Stages 2-3: symptomatic: prednisone 20-40 mg PO daily for 1-3 months: if improvement, taper down to 7.5-10 mg daily: for a total of 12-24 months then completely withdraw and follow-up to detect recurrence. In case of deterioration, ↑ Prednisone. If asymptomatic but deterioration after 6-12 months: consider treatment. Stage 4: treatment not effective in general; consider transplantation. For Löfgren: NSAIDs. Prednisone if ineffective. For uveitis, hypercalcemia, hepatitis, myocardial neurological involvement or renal persistent: prednisone 40-80 mg daily, according to severity. If no response to steroids: consider immunosuppressive agents: methotrexate, azathioprine, hydroxychloroquine: cyclophosphamide, infliximab or mycophenolate if refractory disease ? Topical corticosteroids effective for mild cutaneous involvement.
Prognosis	Spontaneous remission in 60-80 % of stage 1, 50-60 % of stage 2, < 30 % of stage 3, 0 % in stage 4. > 85 % of remissions occur in the 2 years following initial presentation; if not, chronic evolution is frequent. More aggressive disease in African-Americans or if disease occurred after age 40. Mortality 1-5% with pulmonary, central nervous system or cardiac involvement. Löfgren's syndrome = good prognosis. Minimal follow-up of 3 years recommended after stopping treatment: beware of patients who responded to corticosteroids since recurrence is more frequent. If steroids are not indicated at diagnosis, only 10 % require treatment in the future.

Pulmonary Hypertension	
Overview	Symptoms of progressive dyspnea on exertion leading to right-sided heart failure, chest pain, fatigue, syncope, palpitations, hoarseness (Ortner's syndrome), sudden death.
	Diagnostic criteria for pulmonary hypertension: *systolic* pulmonary artery pressure > 40 mmHg (World Health Organization) or *mean* pulmonary artery pressure > 25 mmHg (or > 30 mmHg during exercise) by cardiac catheterization (National Institutes of Health).
	When present, pulmonary hypertension is associated with structural damage to pulmonary vessels and *in situ* thrombosis. The measured pulmonary hypertension does not reflect the clinical severity of the disease. Measurement of pulmonary vascular resistance is required to evaluate severity.
Causes	Revised classification of pulmonary hypertension (Venice 2003):

	1. Pulmonary arterial hypertension:
	  – Idiopathic: if no secondary cause found: mean age 36 years old, 62% are women.
	  – Familial (rare).
	  – Associated with: connective tissue disease, congenital systemic-to-pulmonic shunt, portal hypertension, HIV, drugs and toxins, other (thyroid disorders, glycogen storage disease, Gaucher's disease, hereditary hemorrhagic telangiectasia, hemoglobinopathies, myeloproliferative disorders, splenectomy).
	  – Associated with significant venous or capillary involvement: pulmonary veno-occlusive disease, pulmonary capillary hemangiomatosis.
	  – Persistent pulmonary hypertension of the newborn.

	2. Pulmonary hypertension with left heart disease (left-sided ventricular or atrial disease, left-sided valvular disease).

	3. Pulmonary hypertension associated with lung disease and/or hypoxemia:
	  – COPD.
	  – Interstitial lung disease.
	  – Sleep-disordered breathing (obesity-hypoventilation ± sleep apnea).
	  – Alveolar hypoventilation disorders.
	  – Chronic exposure to high altitude.
	  – Developmental abnormalities.

	4. Pulmonary hypertension due to chronic thrombotic and/or embolic disease:
	  – Thromboembolic obstruction of proximal or distal pulmonary arteries.
	  – Non-thrombotic pulmonary embolism (tumor, parasites, foreign bodies).

	5. Miscellaneous: sarcoidosis, Langerhans cell histiocytosis, lymphangiomyomatosis, compression of pulmonary vessel (lymphadenopathy, tumor, fibrosing mediastinitis).
Workup	– Laboratory studies: basic + CBC + connective tissue disease workup, HIV and blood gas + according to clinical findings: liver workup, TSH, etc. – Echocardiography: with measurement of tricuspid regurgitant flow and determination of right ventricular systolic pressure, an approximation of the systolic pulmonary artery pressure. Transesophageal echocardiography to rule out shunt as needed. – Chest X-ray, pulmonary function tests including CO diffusion capacity; as needed, high-resolution chest CT. – Nocturnal oximetry or polysomnography if suspected sleep apnea. – ECG: right atrial distension, right ventricular hypertrophy, right axis deviation, non-specific repolarization abnormalities. – Exercise stress test (prognostic). Six-minute walk test. – Ventilation-perfusion scan essential. CT-Angiography or pulmonary angiography as needed (caution is warranted since risk of complication is ↑ with conventional angiography). – Right heart catheterization: gold standard essential to diagnosis (pulmonary vascular

	resistance measurement) and hemodynamic testing (performed with epoprostenol IV, adenosine IV, or inhaled nitric oxide). – Lung biopsy rarely needed. – Genetic counseling for familial pulmonary arterial hypertension.

Treatment	- According to cause.
	
	- If functional class ≥ II/IV:
	– Refer to a specialist.
	– Avoid strenuous activities and high altitude, sodium restriction, vaccination.
	– Oxygen therapy if hypoxemia < 60 mmHg.
	– Anticoagulation: mortality ↓ proven in idiopathic form. Also to be considered in other causes of significant pulmonary hypertension. Aim for INR 2-2.5.
	– Vasodilators: efficacy proven for idiopathic or scleroderma-related pulmonary hypertension:
	  - Calcium channel blockers: useful if ⊕ response to hemodynamic testing : nifedipine, amlodipine and diltiazem: Only 10 % responders (i.e.: mean pulmonary artery pressure ↓ of ≥ 10 % to ≤ 40 mmHg with elevation of or stable cardiac output).
	  - IV prostacyclin (epoprostenol): effective for idiopathic pulmonary hypertension and in some forms of secondary hypertension: to be used if functional class III-IV/IV and no response to hemodynamic testing or if clinical worsening: continuous infusion via pump but costly!
	  - Oral endothelin antagonist (bosentan): indicated for idiopathic pulmonary hypertension and secondary to scleroderma or to congenital heart diseases; to be used if functional class II-III/IV, no response to hemodynamic testing or if clinical worsening: hepatic side effects.
	  - Phosphodiesterase inhibitor: sildenafil PO: indicated for primary pulmonary hypertension: to use if functional class II-III/IV and no response or not candidate to calcium blockers.
	  - Other vasodilators: treprostinil, sitaxsentan.
	
	In summary: If ⊕ response to hemodynamic testing, use a calcium channel blocker (if functional class ≥ II/IV): if negative response to hemodynamic testing and functional class III/IV, use an endothelin antagonist, IV eoprostenol or other prostanoid analogs: if functional class IV/IV, use epoprostenol. Combination therapy under investigation.
	
	– Digoxin if refractory right heart failure.
	– Diuretics if edema (beware of hypovolemia).
	– Avoid oral contraceptives, pregnancy, negative inotropic drugs (e.g.: verapamil).
	
	– Surgery: mostly for patients with a functional class III-IV/IV and refractory to medical treatment.
	  ○ Atrial septostomy: via catheterization, creation of a right-to-left shunt as a "bridge" while awaiting lung transplantation.
	  ○ Pulmonary transplantation: definitive treatment. No reported recurrence of pulmonary hypertension.
	
	- If chronic pulmonary embolism: pulmonary thromboendarterectomy possible for proximal embolism not responding to anticoagulation.
	- If associated to a connective tissue disease, treat as above: immunosuppressive agents to be considered.
	- Treatment of sleep-related respiratory disorders, if needed.

Prognosis	Depends of the cause. In idiopathic pulmonary hypertension, the median survival is 2.8 years if untreated. With epoprostenol, 5 year survival is 55 %. With transplantation, 5 year survival is 37-44 % in selected patients.

Disorders of the Pleura	

Pleural Effusion	Abnormal fluid accumulation in the pleural space (normally = 5-15 mL).
	
	Pleural effusion is visible on antero-posterior chest X-ray with > 175-200 mL of pleural fluid (or > 50 mL on lateral chest X-ray).
	
	Distinguish exudate from transudate with the Light criteria:
	It is an exudate if :
	    1- pleural-fluid protein to serum protein ratio > 0.5 *or*
	    2- pleural-fluid LDH to serum LDH ratio > 0.6 *or*
	    3- pleural-fluid LDH > 2/3 upper limit of normal for serum:
	    $\rightarrow$ if not = transudate.
	
	Note: excellent sensitivity but specificity $\approx$ 85 %, especially if heart failure under diuretics.
	
	Hemothorax if pleural/serum hematocrit > 0.5.
	Chylothorax if triglycerides > 1.24 mmol/L or chylomicrons present.
	Pseudochylothorax if pleural cholesterol > 5.2 mmol/L, triglycerides < 1.24 mmol/L and absence of chylomicrons.
	
	Low pleural-fluid glucose (< 3.3 mmol/L) or pH < 7.3 with rheumatoid or lupus effusion, cancer, empyema, esophageal rupture or tuberculosis.
	
	Pleural-fluid lymphocytosis (> 80 % of lymphocytes) with: tuberculosis, chylothorax, lymphoma, rheumatoid arthritis (often with pulmonary entrapment), yellow nail syndrome, sarcoidosis, acute pulmonary graft rejection, post-CABG ($\pm$ pulmonary entrapment).
	
	Pleural-fluid eosinophilia (> 10 % of eosinophils) with: pneumothorax, hemothorax (after 10-14 days), benign asbestos effusion, pulmonary embolism, parasites or fungi, drugs, lymphoma, carcinoma, Churg-Strauss syndrome, etc.
	
	Parapneumonic effusion: **simple** if pH > 7.2 or **complicated** if pH < 7.2, if LDH > 1000 UI/L, if glucose < 2.2 mmol/L or if Gram or culture $\oplus$ or if radiologic evidence of loculations. Empyema if pus present.

Causes	– Transudates:
	    Heart failure ($\approx$ 90 % of transudates: bilateral in 80%), cirrhosis (hepatic hydrothorax), nephrotic syndrome, peritoneal dialysis, acute atelectasis, myxedema, pulmonary embolism, severe hypoalbuminemia, urinothorax, constrictive pericarditis, superior vena cava obstruction ...
	
	– Exudates:
	    - Cancer: lung, lymphoma, mesothelioma, metastasis.
	    - Infection: parapneumonic, tuberculosis, viral, parasites, abdominal abscess, etc.
	    - Gastro-intestinal: pancreatitis, esophageal rupture, abdominal surgery, sclerotherapy for esophageal varices, etc.
	    - Connective tissue disease: rheumatoid arthritis, SLE, Sjögren, etc.
	    - Drugs: drug-induced lupus, nitrofurantoin, amiodarone, phenytoin, methysergide, bromocriptine, methotrexate, bleomycin, etc.
	    - Lymphatic disease: lymphangioleiomyomatosis, yellow nail syndrome.
	    - Other inflammatory diseases: pulmonary embolism, Dressler's syndrome, benign asbestos effusion, uremia, radiotherapy, Wegener's, Familial Mediterranean fever, Churg-Strauss, sarcoidosis, etc.
	    - Transudate can transform into an exudate from induced diuresis (calculate the gradient of serum minus pleural protein: if > 31 g/L, probable transudate).
	
	– Transudates or exudates with pulmonary embolism (usually exudates), Meigs' syndrome (benign ovarian tumor).
	– Hemothorax: trauma, cancer, pulmonary embolism, uremic pleuritis, benign asbestos effusion, post-cardiac surgery.
	– Chylothorax: thoracic duct trauma, tumor (lymphoma, solid), tuberculosis,

	lymphangioleiomyomatosis, cirrhosis, nephrotic syndrome, rheumatoid arthritis, amyloidosis. – Pseudochylothorax: past tuberculosis, rheumatoid arthritis, empyema. Note: May be secondary to supra or infra-diaphragmatic disease.

Management	- Decubitus chest-X ray or ultrasonography can help see if effusion is present (layering of the pleural effusion).
	- Diagnostic thoracentesis etiology (ultrasonographic guidance as needed, but normally can be done blindly if > 1 cm at lateral decubitus chest X-ray):
	  Workup to do on pleural fluid :
	    - **Basic**: cell count, protein, glucose, LDH, pH, Gram stain + culture of fluid, cytology.
	    - **As needed**: triglycerides (chylothorax), amylase (pancreatitis, pseudocyst, cancer, esophageal rupture), Ziehl + mycobacterial culture ± PCR (especially if lymphocytic effusion), cholesterol (for pseudochylothorax), hematocrit (hemothorax), creatinine (urinothorax), complement (rheumatoid arthritis).
	
	Therapeutic trial of diuretics can be attempted if bilateral pleural effusion and suspected heart failure: if effusion persists after 3 days, perform thoracentesis.
	
	- If etiology remains ?: rule out pulmonary embolism. Thoracoscopic pleural biopsy (if tuberculosis or cancer suspected); bronchoscopy if abnormal X-ray: Chest or abdominal CT as needed (contrast enhanced CT scan ⊕ suggestive of empyema).
	
	Note: 10-20 % of effusions remain of unexplained etiology despite an extensive evaluation.

Treatment	– Transudates: treat underlying cause.
	– Exudates :
	    - For malignant effusion: therapeutic thoracentesis and if reaccumulation, consider pleurodesis or cancer treatment (chemotherapy).
	    - For parapneumonic and uncomplicated effusion: treat pneumonia: if complicated (pus, positive Gram stain or culture, pH < 7.2-7.3 or LDH > 1000 U/L or glucose < 2.2 mmol/L or loculations) → chest tube + appropriate antibiotic therapy: if no improvement in 24 h → rule out loculation by ultrasonography and/or chest CT; if present, drainage ± intrapleural streptokinase (but controversial; especially for poor surgical candidate) or decortication.
	– Hemothorax: chest tube.

Pneumothorax	Symptoms of acute dyspnea and chest pain. Respiratory distress + tracheal deviation in cases of tension pneumothorax. Causes: spontaneous (primary or secondary) or traumatic (iatrogenic). *Primary spontaneous* in thin young male: family history, smoking ⊕. *Secondary spontaneous* with COPD, asthma, cystic fibrosis, tuberculosis, interstitial lung disease (*Pneumocystis* pneumonia, lymphangioleiomyomatosis, Langerhans cells histiocytosis, sarcoidosis, idiopathic pulmonary fibrosis), lung cancer, Marfan syndrome, menstruations (catamenial). Expiratory chest X-ray diagnostic. Chest CT sometimes useful to rule out emphysematous bullae or other cause. Complications: pneumomediastinum, subcutaneous emphysema, bronchopleural fistula. Treatment: if small (< 15 %) → observation alone. If > 15 % or symptomatic or secondary cause or while under mechanical ventilation → drainage. Thoracoscopy or thoracotomy indicated for recurrence, bilateral pneumothorax, or for ineffective drainage or secondary cause; with pleurodesis or bullae resection in mind. Recurrence 30 % after 1 episode, if spontaneous; 60 % if more than 1 episode. Smoking cessation (↑ recurrence with tobacco smoking).

	Scuba-diving contraindicated.
Malignant Mesothelioma	See Lung cancer Table.

Sleep-Related Respiratory Disorders

Obstructive Sleep Apnea (OSA)	Periodic cessation of breathing (≥ 10 seconds) during sleep as a result of intermittent obstruction of the upper respiratory tract. These obstructive episodes may be terminated by micro-awakening of the patient.
	Apnea: cessation of breathing lasting ≥ 10 seconds despite persistant or increased respiratory effort.
	Hypopnea: transient reduction in breathing lasting ≥ 10 seconds with at least a 30 % reduction in thoracoabdominal movement or airflow, as compared to baseline, and with ≥ 4 % desaturation.
	Obstructive sleep apnea-hypopnea syndrome: implies presence of obstructive sleep apnea with symptoms, especially excessive daytime spleepiness.
	Present in 2-4 % of middle-aged population. 80-85 % not diagnosed. Risk factors: mainly men, ↑ age, obesity, but also tobacco smoking, alcohol drinking, arterial hypertension, acromegaly, anatomic abnormalities, post-menopause, family history.
Clinical findings	Symptoms: - Excessive daytime spleepiness. - Choking or gasping during night, recurrent awakenings, unrefreshing sleep, daytime fatigue, impaired concentration, morning headaches, nocturia, enuresis, night sweats. On physical examination: hypertension, obesity (70-80 % of patients), craniofacial abnormalities (macroglossia, retrognathy), ↑ adjusted neck circumference (= measured neck circumference + 3 cm for history of snoring, + 3 cm for history of withnessed apneas, + 4 cm for history of hypertension; ≥ 43 cm ↑ risk). The **STOP** questionnaire (**S**nore loudly, feel **T**ired, **O**bserved apnea, ↑ **B**lood **P**ressure) can also help to identify patient with OSA. The Epworth scale (see appendix) can also be useful when evaluating these patients. Differential diagnosis of ↑ spleepiness: narcolepsia, restless legs syndrome, central apnea, non-adherence to treatment (C-PAP), lack of sleep, depression, medication side effects, etc.
Associated diseases	- Cardiovascular: hypertension, myocardial infarction, arrhythmia, heart failure, accelerated atherosclerosis, pulmonary hypertension (if COPD or obesity-hypoventilation syndrome). - Neurological: stroke, cognitive impairment, chronic headaches. - Endocrine: insulinoresistance. - Other diseases: ↑ anesthesic/analgesic sensitivity and benzodiazepine, ↑ post-operative complications, ↑ frequency of road accidents (relative risk 2-3).

Workup	Polysomnography in laboratory or home-based with measurement of apnea/hypopnea index (AHI)/hour. C-PAP titration in a second time when diagnosis is established. Nocturnal oximetry may suggest OSA, but it is not sensitive enough and specific in general to confirm diagnosis.

Severity	The severity of OSA has 2 components: severity of daytime spleepiness and severity of overnight monitoring (severity rating should be based on the most severe component):
	
	<table><tr><td>Sleepiness:
	- Mild: unwanted sleepiness occurs during activities requiring little attention (ex.: television).
	- Moderate: unwanted sleepiness occurs during activities requiring some attention (ex.: concerts).
	- Severe: unwanted sleepiness occurs during activities requiring more active attention (ex.; while driving a car, conversation, eating).</td><td>Apnea-Hypopnea index:
	  < 5: normal.
	  5-15: mild.
	  15-30: moderate.
	  > 30: severe.</td></tr></table>

Treatment	Patient education, ↓ weight (± bariatric surgery), positional treatment (in certain cases), stop tobacco, avoid alcohol, sedatives or narcotics before sleep. C-PAP if symptomatic, especially if AHI moderate – severe; consider treatment if AHI severe even in absence of symptoms, if co-morbidity important or if high-risk job. Secondary effects: nasal congestion or obstruction, xerostomia, leaks, aerophagia, claustrophobia … Use a minimum of 5-6 hours each night. If C-PAP not tolerated: oral appliance treatment (especially if retrognathia) or surgery (uvulopalatopharyngoplasty - UPPP - but less effective than oral appliance, in general not recommended - or maxillomandibular surgery – available in ultra-specialized centers - tracheotomy to be considered if severe and refractory). If persistent sleepiness on C-PAP without any other cause: modafinil ? Car driving: Patients with moderate to severe OSA, documented by sleep study, who are *not* compliant with treatment and are considered at increased risk for motor vehicle accident by the treating physician, should not drive any type of motor vehicle.
Central Sleep Apnea	A periodical cessation of breathing (≥ 10 seconds) during sleep, with absent or reduced respiratory effort. Normocapnia: $PaCO_2$ < 45 mmHg at awakening. Idiopathic or due to neurological diseases (post-stroke), heart failure, high altitude … Treatment according to etiology: Treatment of heart failure, otherwise treatment controversial: C-PAP? Oxygen?

Sleep Hypoventilation Syndrome	Associated with obesity (obesity-hypoventilation syndrome or Pickwick's), neuromuscular diseases (amyotrophic lateral sclerosis, Duchenne muscular dystrophy), restrictive disease (scoliosis), brainstem diseases or idiopathic.
	Hypoventilation provoking hypercapnia at awakening ($PaCO_2$ > 45 mmHg) and nocturnal hypoxemia, especially during REM sleep. May be associated with sleep apnea (especially if obesity-hypoventilation syndrome).
	Symptoms: sleepiness, right heart failure and pulmonary hypertension. Secondary polycythemia can occur.
	Diagnosis: Polysomnography which demonstrates desaturation not explained by apnea/hypopnea. CBC, TSH (rule out hypothyroidism), arterial blood gas. Chest X-ray and pulmonary function tests (to rule out lung disease).
	Treatment: according to cause. Avoid alcohol, sedatives, and opiates. Weight loss if obesity. C-PAP (especially if apnea associated) or Bi-PAP ± oxygen if persistent hypoxemia despite treatment. Tracheostomy if refractory.

Pulmonary Nodule and Mass

Pulmonary nodule if lesion < 3 cm. Pulmonary mass if > 3 cm.
Benign lesions 60 %: malignant 40 % (varies in different case series).
Pulmonary masses are often malignant.

Malignant lesions more frequent in older men, > 60 years old, superior lobe involvement, active smoking or cessation within 7 years, nodule > 2 cm (where 80 % are neoplastic, vs 1 % if 1-5 mm and 33 % if 11-20 mm), irregular margins (*corona radiata* or spiculated), doubling time of the lesion (i.e.: ↑ 30 % of diameter) between 30-500 days, absence of calcifications or satellite lesion.

On history, look for: age, prior chest X-ray, smoking, previous cancer, contact with tuberculosis, travel, recent infection, trauma, asthma, immunodeficiency, ENT symptoms, systemic diseases, family history of arteriovenous malformation ...

Causes	– Benign lesions: hamartoma ("pop-corn" calcifications), tuberculosis, histoplasmosis, Coccidioidomycosis, undifferentiated granuloma, rheumatoid nodule, fibroma, lipoma, leiomyoma, hemangioma, papilloma, abscess, Wegener's granulomatosis, arteriovenous malformation, resolving pneumonia, etc.
	– Malignant lesions: primary 70 %, metastasis 30 %: carcinoid, sarcoma, lymphoma, mesenchymal, etc.
Workup	– Basic workup (CBC, Na^+, K^+, creatinine, Ca^{++}, alkaline phosphatase, liver enzymes) ± sputum cytology x 5 (specific but not very sensitive).
	– Look for nodule on old chest X-ray: check nodule appearance or progression.
	– Chest CT with imaging of adrenals.
	– Bronchoscopy ± bronchial biopsy (especially if proximal nodule).
	– If non-diagnostic bronchoscopy, transthoracic biopsy (but 20 % false Θ and pneumothorax in up to 25 % of cases) or surgery, depending on the lesion.
	– Complete pulmonary function test before any diagnostic or therapeutic procedure.
	– Pleural-fluid cytology if effusion present.
	– Positron emission tomography (PET scan) if available, especially if nodule ≥ 1 cm; allows a better diagnosis and staging for cancer. False ⊕ with infection or inflammation, false Θ possible with bronchioloalveolar carcinoma or carcinoid.
	– Abdominal ultrasonography, bone scan or cerebral CT or MRI depending on symptoms and other tests results.
	– Investigation for other distant primary tumor elsewhere is rarely useful except if symptoms, signs or laboratory evidences suggesting an extra-pulmonary tumor.

The approach to pulmonary nodules depends on the probability of underlying cancer, which is mainly related to the size of the nodule, history of smoking, patient's age, and CT characteristics of the nodule :
- If the probability of cancer is low (< 10 %) may follow-up with serial CT scans (every 3 months for 1 year, then every 6 months).
- If the probability of cancer is high and operative risk is low, proceed with surgery right away.
- If the risk of cancer is intermediate (10-60 %): PET scan or transthoracic biopsy is possible, depending on the characteristics of the nodule and patient's wishes. If PET is negative, follow with serial CT scan (e.g.: repeat at 3-6-12-24 months).

Note: If the lesion didn't progress in 2 years, it is probably benign (but exceptions are possible, for example, bronchioloalveolar carcinoma or carcinoid).

Useful References: RESPIRATORY MEDICINE

Acute Bronchitis: N Engl J Med 2006; 355: 2125-30 (review article)
Acute Respiratory Distress Syndrome: Lancet 2007; 369: 1553-65 (review article)
   … Treatment: Chest 2007; 131: 921-29 (review article on mechanical ventilation)
Allergic Bronchopulmonary Aspergillosis: Chest 2009; 135: 805-826 (review article)
Alpha-1 Antitrypsin Deficiency: N Engl J Med 2009; 360: 2749-57 (review article)
   Am J Med 2008; 121: 3-9 (review article)
Aspergillosis: N Engl J Med 2009; 360: 1870-84 (review article)
Asthma: Can Respir J 2001; 8 (Suppl A): 1A-26A & 2004; 11 (Suppl A) (Canadian Guidelines)
   Eur Respir J 2008; 31: 143-178 (GINA Guidelines)
   Chest 2004; 125: 1081-1102 (review article)
   Am J Respir Crit Care Med 2003; 168: 740-59 (review article on acute severe asthma)
   … in Pregnancy: N Engl J Med 2009; 360: 1862-9 (review article)
   … Occupational Asthma: Am J Respir Crit Care Med 2005; 172: 280-305 (review article)
   … Resistant Asthma: Am J Med 2007; 120: 760-763 (review article)
   … Treatment: N Engl J Med 2009; 360: 1002-14 (review article)
Bronchiectasis : N Engl J Med 2002; 346: 1383-93 (review article)
   Chest 2008; 134: 815-23 (review article)
Bronchiolar Disorders: Am J Respir Crit Care Med 2003; 168: 1277-92 (review article)
Chronic Obstructive Pulmonary Disease:
         Can Respir J 2007; 14 (Suppl B): 5B-32B (Canadian Guidelines)
         Eur Respir J 2004; 23: 932-46 (ATS-ERS Guidelines)
         Am J Respir Crit Care Med 2007; 176: 532-555 (GOLD Guidelines)
         N Engl J Med 2004; 350: 2689-97 (review article)
         Lancet 2003; 362: 1053-61 (review article)
   … Exacerbation: Can Respir J 2003; 10 (Suppl B): 3B-32B (Canadian Guidelines)
         Ann Intern Med 2001; 134: 595-620 (American Guidelines)
         Eur Respir J 2007; 29: 1224-38 (review article)
         N Engl J Med 2002; 346: 988-994 (review article)
   … Stable: Ann Intern Med 2007; 147: 633-638 (ACP Guidelines)
   … Severe: Lancet 2004; 364: 883-95 (review article)
Cough: Chest 2006; 129 (Suppl); 1S-23S (consensus américain)
   N Engl J Med 2000; 343: 1715-21 (review article)
   … Chronic Cough - Management: Lancet 2008; 371: 1375-84 (review article)
   … Chronic Cough - Prevalence - Causes: Lancet 2008; 371: 1364-74 (review article)
Cystic Fibrosis in Adults: Lancet 2009; 373: 1891-1904 (review article)
   JAMA 2007; 298: 1787-93 (review article)
Diffuse Alveolar Hemorrhage - Diagnosis: Cleve Clin J Med 2008; 75: 258-80 (review article)
Dyspnea: Med Clin N Am 2006; 90: 453-479 (review article)
   Chronic: J Respir Dis 2001; 22: 79- (review article)
Hemoptysis: Postgrad Med 2002; 112: 101- (review article)
   … Massive: Crit Care Med 2000; 28: 1642-47 (review article)
Hypersensitivity Pneumonitis: Clin Chest Med 2004; 25: 531-47 (review article)
Idiopathic Pulmonary Fibrosis: CMAJ 2004; 171: 153-60 (review article)
   Respir Med 2006; 100: 1871-85 (review article)
Interstitial Lung Disease: Am J Respir Crit Care Med 2005; 172: 268-79 (review article)
   Am J Respir Crit Care Med 2002; 165: 277-304 (ATS-ERS Guidelines on classification)
   Mayo Clin Proc 2007; 82: 976-986 (review article)

Langherhans Cell Histiocytosis: Eur Respir J 2006; 27: 1272-85 (review article)

Lymphangioleiomyomatosis: Chest 2008; 133: 507-16 (review article)

Malignant Effusion: Mayo Clin Proc 2008; 83: 235-250 (review article)
    Thorax 2003; 58 Suppl 2: ii29-38 (BTS Guidelines)

Malignant Mesothelioma: Chest 2004; 126: 1318-29 (2004 review article)

Mechanical Ventilation: Tobin MJ. *Principles and Practice of Mechanical Ventilation*, 2nd Edition. McGraw Hill, New York, 2006.
    ... Weaning from Mechanical Ventilation: Eur Respir J 2007; 29: 1033-56 (review article)
        Chest 2001; 120 (Suppl): 375S-484S (review article)

Noninvasive positive pressure ventilation: CMAJ 2007; 177: 1211-8 (review article)

Obesity-Hypoventilation Syndrome: Am J Med 2005; 118: 948-956 (review article)

Obstructive Sleep Apnea: N Engl J Med 2002; 347: 498-504 (review article)
    Lancet 2002; 360: 237-45 (review article)
    Can Respir J 2006; 13: 387-92 (Canadian Guidelines)
    ... Diagnostic: Chest 2007; 132: 325-337 (review article)
    ... and C-PAP : N Engl J Med 2007; 356: 1751-8 (review article)

Parapneumonic Effusion: Thorax 2003; 58 Suppl 2: ii18-28 (BTS Guidelines)
    Clin Infect Dis 2007; 45: 1480-6 (review article)
    Chest 2000; 118: 1158-71 (Guidelines)

Pleural Effusion: Thorax 2003; 58 Suppl 2: ii8-17 (BTS Guidelines)
    N Engl J Med 2002; 346: 1971-7 (review article)

Pleural Infection: Thorax 2003; 58 Suppl 2: ii18-28 (Guidelines)

Pulmonary Function Test: Eur Respir J 2005; 26: 948-68 (ATS-ERS Guidelines)
    Mayo Clin Proc 2003; 78: 758-63 (review article)

Pulmonary Hypertension: Chest 2004; 126: 1S-92S (ACCP Guidelines)
    Mayo Clin Proc 2009; 84: 191-207 (review article)
    J Am Coll Cardiol 2008; 51: 1527-38 (review article)
    J Am Coll Cardiol 2009; 53: 1573-1619 (ACCF-AHA Guidelines)
    ... Treatment: Chest 2007; 131:1917-1928 (updated ACCP Guidelines)
    ... Secondary Pulmonary Hypertension: Circulation 2008; 118: 2190-99 (review article)

Pulmonary Nodule: N Engl J Med 2003; 348: 2535-42 (review article)
    Chest 2007; 132 (Suppl): 108S-130S (ACCP Guidelines).
    Am J Respir Crit Care Med 2000; 162: 782- (review article)
    ...Small Pulmonary Nodules on CT: Radiology 2005; 237: 395-400 (Guidelines)

Pulmonary Rehabilitation in COPD: N Engl J Med 2009; 360: 1329-35 (review article)

Sarcoidosis: Am J Respir Crit Care Med 1999; 160: 736-55 (American Guidelines)
    N Engl J Med 2007; 357: 2153-65 (review article)
    Am J Med 2007; 120: 403-07 (review article)

Sleep-Related Respiratory Disorders in Adults:
    Can Respir J 2006; 13: 387-92 (Canadian Guidelines)

Spontaneous Pneumothorax: N Engl J Med 2000; 342: 868-74 (review article)
    Thorax 2003; 58(suppl II): ii32-ii52 (BTS Guidelines)

Varenicline: N Engl J Med 2008; 359: 2018-24 (review article)

Chapter 10

Rheumatology

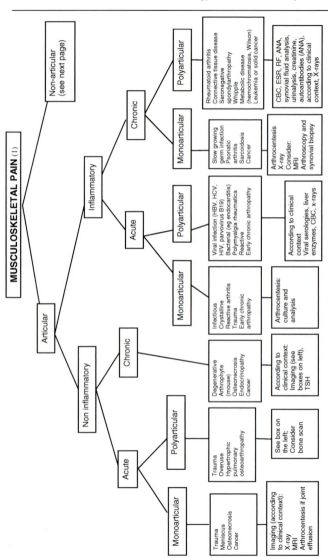

MUSCULOSKELETAL PAIN (1)

- Articular
  - Non inflammatory
    - Acute
      - Monoarticular
        - Trauma
        - Meniscus
        - Osteonecrosis
        - Cancer

        Imaging (according to clinical context): X-ray MRI Arthrocentesis if joint effusion
      - Polyarticular
        - Trauma
        - Overuse
        - Hypertrophic pulmonary osteoarthropathy

        See box on the left; Consider bone scan
    - Chronic
      - Degenerative
      - Arthrophyte (mouse)
      - Osteonecrosis
      - Endocrinopathy
      - Cancer

      According to clinical context: Imaging (see boxes on left), TSH
  - Inflammatory
    - Acute
      - Monoarticular
        - Infectious
        - Crystalline
        - Reactive arthritis
        - Trauma
        - Early chronic arthropathy

        Arthrocentesis: culture and analysis
      - Polyarticular
        - Viral infection (HBV, HCV, HIV, parvovirus B19)
        - Bacterial (eg endocarditis)
        - Polymyalgia rheumatica
        - Reactive
        - Early chronic arthropathy

        According to clinical context Viral serologies, liver enzymes, CBC, X-rays
    - Chronic
      - Monoarticular
        - Slow growing germ infection
        - Psoriatic arthritis
        - Sarcoidosis
        - Cancer

        Arthrocentesis X-ray Consider: MRI Arthroscopy and synovial biopsy
      - Polyarticular
        - Rheumatoid arthritis
        - Connective tissue disease
        - Seronegative spondylarthropathy
        - Whipple
        - Metabolic disease (hemochromatosis, Wilson)
        - Leukemia or solid cancer

        CBC, ESR, RF, ANA, synovial fluid analysis, urinalysis, creatinine, autoantibodies (ANA), according to clinical context, X-rays
- Non-articular (see next page)

Musculoskeletal Pain (2), Continued :

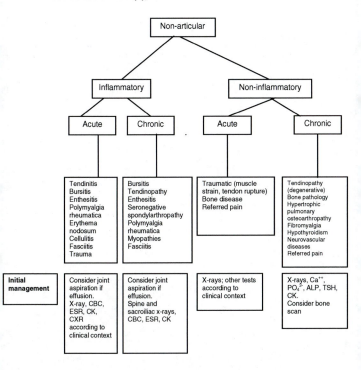

ANA: antinuclear antibody. Ca⁺⁺: calcium. CBC: complete blood count. CK: creatine kinase. CXR: chest x-ray. ESR: erythrocyte sedimentation rate. HBV: hepatitis B virus. HCV: hepatitis C virus. MRI: magnetic resonance imaging. ALP: alkaline phosphatase. PO$_4^{3-}$: phosphate. RF: rheumatoid factor. TSH: thyroid-stimulating hormone.

Osteoarthritis

Most common arthropathy. Degeneration of articular cartilage with concomitant damage to subchondral bone (osteophytes, sclerosis), synovial membrane, ligaments and muscles.
Between 55 and 74 years, prevalence of osteoarthritis is: 70 % in hands, 40 % in feet, 20 % in knees, 3 % in hips. Approximately 10 % symptomatic.
Multifactorial etiology (aging, sex, genetics, mechanical forces, nutrition, overweight, etc).

Clinical findings	Begins later than inflammatory pathologies: > 40 years. Insidious pain with gradual progression. **Mechanical pain**: worse at the end of the day and with activity, alleviated with rest. Morning stiffness < 30 minutes. On physical exam: Heberden's and Bouchard's nodes. Crepitus. Decreased range of motion. Hallux valgus, hallus rigidus, moderate inflammation occurring periodically with joint effusion. Distribution: proximal and distal interphalangeal joints, thumb (carpometacarpal joint), hips, knees, feet (first metatarsophalangeal, tarsus), neck, lumbar spine.
Differential diagnosis	– Secondary osteoarthritis (posttraumatic, microtrauma, lower limb anomalies, obesity, congenital anomalies, hemochromatosis, Paget's disease, aseptic necrosis, acromegaly, neuroarthropathy, hemophilia, Wilson's disease, etc). - When to think about it: clinical context, early onset osteoarthritis, osteoarthritis in unusual sites: metacarpophalangeal joint, wrists, elbows, shoulders, ankles. – Inflammatory diseases (such as rheumatoid arthritis, SLE, polymyalgia rheumatica, pseudogout).
Workup	Depends on clinical findings. If necessary: CBC, electrolytes, liver function tests, alkaline phosphatase, creatinine, urinalysis. If doubt about diagnosis or if suspicion of secondary cause: ESR, C-reactive protein, calcium, phosphate, serum protein electrophoresis, rheumatoid factor, ANA, synovial fluid analysis (< 2 x 10^9 leukocytes/L), joint X-rays (standing X-rays for knees) : joint space narrowing, osteophytes, cysts (geodes) and subchondral sclerosis.
Treatment	Step-wise approach: 1. Nonpharmacologic: education, weight loss as needed (BMI > 25 increases risk of hip and knee OA, physiotherapy, exercise programs, occupational therapy, orthoses, cane, walker. The Arthritis Society education program. 2. Simple analgesic therapy: acetaminophen up to 4 g/day (be careful if hepatic disease, alcoholism or warfarin use). 3. Nonsteroidal anti-inflammatory drugs (see appendix on NSAIDs): Nonselective NSAIDs if no risk factor for ulcer: combine with cytoprotective agent (misoprostol or proton pump inhibitor) or use selective COX-2 inhibitor for patients with risk factors (age > 65 years, uncomplicated ulcer, steroids, cardio-pulmonary diseases) or COX-2 inhibitor + gastroprotection if history of complicated ulcer or anticoagulation or age > 75 years). Nonsalicylated salicylates may be useful for patients at risk (no renal and platelet toxicity) but CNS and ocular toxicity can occur. Note: Selective COX-2 inhibitors have the same renal toxicity as non-selective NSAIDs: be careful in patients with chronic renal failure, age ≥ 65 years, hypertension, cardiac failure, diuretic, ACEI or ARB use. Celecoxib contraindicated if allergy to sulfa. Note: Selective COX-2 inhibitors may slightly increase the risk of cardiovascular events: be careful in patients with risk factors (evaluate risk/benefit ratio). 4. Intra-articular steroid injections for monoarticular knee involvement with effusion or inflammation, or other accessible joint (max 3-4 times /year/joint). Intra-articular hyaluronic acid injection for mild to moderate monoarticular knee involvement without effusion. Consider isotopic synoviorthesis for recurrent hydrarthrosis.

	5. Local approach: local friction with capsaicin cream 0.025 % qid for > 2 weeks (side effect: burning sensation), diclofenac 1.5% (drops) applicable up to qid. Acupuncture.
	6. When preceding measures ineffective or contraindicated: reconsider differential diagnosis; consider surgery or opiates.
	Natural products: glucosamine or chondroitin may be tried for 3 months and continued when effective.

Seronegative Spondyloarthropathies

Group of diseases having in common the following characteristics:
– Sacroiliitis.
– Peripheral arthritis involving predominantly the joints of the lower limbs asymmetrically
– Negative rheumatoid factor, absence of rheumatoid nodules.
– Associated with HLA-B27.

Ankylosing Spondylitis

– HLA-B27 ⊕ in > 90 %.
– In general population, HLA-B27 ⊕ in 8 %, but 2 % of the latter will develop the disease: risk up to 20 % for those with family history and HLA-B27 ⊕.
– Age < 40 years. Prevalence 0.2 %. Male > female. May be more indolent in females.

Clinical findings	– Insidious inflammatory axial pain: morning > evening, < with exercise.
	– Alternating pseudosciatica (right and left alternately).
	– Local tenderness, decreased lumbar lordosis, cephalic progression, costochondritis.
	– Asymmetrical large joint peripheral arthritis, 50 % transient and 25 % chronic (hip, shoulder especially). Other articulations rarely involved). Enthesopathy, plantar fasciitis, heel pain
	– ↓ chest expansion first (< 5 cm at T4), positive Schober test (< 5 cm), painful sacroiliac joints, ↑ occiput-wall distance (> 0 cm).
	– Spinal fracture (transverse, similar to fractures in long bones, therefore risk of spinal cord involvement, *cauda equina* syndrome and spinal stenosis).
	– Systemic symptoms possible: fever, weakness, weight loss.
	– Extra-articular manifestations: acute anterior uveitis 20-25% (usually unilateral, recurrent) scleritis, episcleritis rare.
	– Cardiac: conduction defects (AV block 1st to 3rd), aortic regurgitation (up to 10 % after 30 years).
	– Lung: apical fibrocavitary lesions (similar to tuberculosis), possible superinfection with Aspergillus sp., mycobacteria… Restrictive lung disease.
	– Gastrointestinal: bowel ulcerations similar to Crohn's disease 30-50 % (subclinical).
	– Renal: secondary amyloidosis, drug toxicity (NSAIDs), IgA nephropathy.
	– Osteoporosis.
	– Rarely: polychondritis, retroperitoneal fibrosis.
Diagnosis	– ESR ↑ 70 %. Mild normocytic anemia (15 %).
	– Spinal x-rays: squaring of edges of vertebral bodies, shiny corners, syndesmophytes, "bamboo spine". Sacroiliac joints: if X-rays negative, MRI first choice; if not available: perform sacroiliac CT or bone scan.
	– Differential diagnosis of sacroiliitis: bilateral (symmetrical or not): other seronegative arthropathy (psoriasis, Reiter's), condensing osteitis, DISH (diffuse idiopathic skeletal hyperostosis); usually unilateral: cancer, Paget's, infections (Brucellosis, *Serratia* sp., *Staphylococcus* sp.).
	– See algorithm on page 10-8.

Treatment and prognosis	Physiotherapy. Postural training, joint range of motion exercises, aerobics.
	Pharmacologic:
	– Axial involvement: NSAIDs: usually high doses ($\downarrow$ risk of uveitis). If failure after 3 months, change anti-inflammatory; if repeated failure after 3 months, start anti-TNF (etanercept, infliximab, adalimumab or golimumab).
	– Sulfasalazine and methotrexate can be useful if peripheral involvement; not very effective for axial involvement.
	– Infiltrations: for local involvement: enthesitis, arthritis, sacroiliitis.
	– Other: IV pamidronate (60 mg every month x 6) sometimes effective.
	Very slow progression in 50 %. Relapsing and remitting course. 10 % cannot work after 10 years.
	Higher risk for osteoporosis: screen with BMD (bone mineral density) testing.

Reiter's Syndrome (Reactive Arthritis)

HLA-B27 $\oplus$ in 75 %. Male = female. 20-40 years.
Aseptic inflammatory syndrome onset 1-4 weeks after an infectious diarrhea (Salmonella, Shigella, *Yersinia, Campylobacter, Clostridium*) or a sexually transmitted disease (Chlamydia, Ureaplasma) or respiratory infection (streptococcus ß haemolytic group A, C. *pneumoniae*).
Association with HIV (incomplete Reiter's: no conjunctivitis or urethritis).

Clinical findings	Reiter: Triad of arthritis-urethritis-conjunctivitis with or without muco-cutaneous involvement.
	Sterile arthritis, asymmetric large joints most often of the lower limbs, "additive" onset (one adding to the other), dactylitis, sacroiliitis 20 %, lasts > 1 month.
	Enthesopathy: Achilles tendonitis, plantar fasciitis
	Fever or weight loss at presentation: occasionally.
	Cutaneous findings: palatal ulcers (asymptomatic), balanitis circinata, keratoderma blennorrhagica ($\approx$ palmoplantar psoriasis).
	Acute anterior uveitis.
	Cardiac involvement (5-10 %): $\uparrow$ PR interval, AV block, bundle branch bloc, non-specific ST segment anomalies, aortic regurgitation.
	Rule out HIV in every patient with Chlamydia-associated Reiter's syndrome.
Diagnosis	Clinical.
	CBC, ESR, CRP, creatinine, urinalysis (to detect pyuria), ECG if needed, joint aspiration for cultures (rule out septic arthritis), joint x-rays.
	Look for signs and symptoms of acute anterior uveitis.
Treatment and prognosis	NSAIDs.
	Antibiotics (tetracycline or derivatives) for 3 months may $\downarrow$ duration of symptoms if associated with Chlamydia (?).
	Intra-articular steroids.
	Sulfasalazine if no response, methotrexate for chronic disease?
	Spontaneous recovery in 1 to 12 months, but 15% of cases relapse and 15 % become chronic. 10 % develop a clinical picture similar to ankylosing spondylitis.

Psoriatic Arthritis

Occurs in 5-30 % of patients with psoriasis.
70 % of patients have psoriasis before arthritis, 15 % develop both concomitantly and 15 % develop arthritis first. HLA-27 ⊕ in 50 % if axial involvement, 20 % if peripheral involvement only.

Clinical findings	Five patterns: 1- Rheumatoid arthritis-like (rheumatoid factor ⊖: 20-60 %) 2- Asymmetric mono/oligoarthritis (20-40 %: frequent mode of presentation, but that can evolve into oligo or polyarticular involvement). 3- Arthritis mutilans with osteolysis (less than 5 %; late appearance of the disease). 4- Spondylitis (30 %), with or without sacroiliitis. 5- Monoarthritis or asymmetric arthritis of distal interphalangeal joints of feet or hands, ± pitting or onycholysis (10-15 %) Enthesopathy: plantar fasciitis, Achilles tendonitis, pelvic ligament insertions. Dactylitis: "sausage digits". Acute anterior uveitis.
Workup	↑ ESR. X-rays of affected joints: hands, feet, (involvement of wrists, MCP, PIP, DIP; bone destruction: erosions, acro-osteolysis, pencil in cup deformity; bone production (ankylosis, periosteal reaction), spine (syndesmophytes, ankylosis), sacroiliac joints: less symmetric than ankylosing spondylitis.
Treatment	Axial involvement: see ankylosing spondylitis. Peripheral involvement: - Mono or oligoarticular: infiltrations, NSAIDs. Methotrexate, sulfasalazine if failure. Anti-TNF as third line. - Polyarticular forms: NSAIDs + anti-rheumatic drugs: Methotrexate, salazopyrine. Leflunomide, azathioprine, mycophenolate (MMF). Anti-TNF for refractory disease.

Arthritis Associated with Inflammatory Bowel Disease

Inflammatory bowel diseases are associated with arthritis in 20 %.
Usually, the bowel disease precedes the arthritis, but the reverse may occur or the arthritis may dominate the clinical picture.
HLA-B27 ⊕ in 50 % if axial involvement; 10 % if peripheral involvement only.
Whipple's procedure and jejunoileal bypass could cause arthritis by the same mechanism.

Clinical findings	Two patterns: 1- Spondyloarthropathy: independent of inflammatory bowel disease activity: indistinguishable from ankylosing spondylitis. 2- Peripheral asymmetric non-erosive oligoarthritis, mostly affecting large joints, lower limbs: activity tends to parallel activity of inflammatory bowel disease. Extra-articular manifestations: acute anterior uveitis, conjunctivitis, erythema nodosum, pyoderma gangrenosum, amyloidosis.
Treatment	Controlling the bowel disease controls the peripheral arthritis (steroids, immunosuppressants). For spondylitis: physical therapy + NSAIDs ± anti-TNF (= ankylosing spondylitis) (Note: etanercept not effective for intestinal disease). Note: NSAIDs may exacerbate the inflammatory bowel disease: do not begin during active bowel disease. Intra-articular steroids.

Investigation for Ankylosing Spondylitis

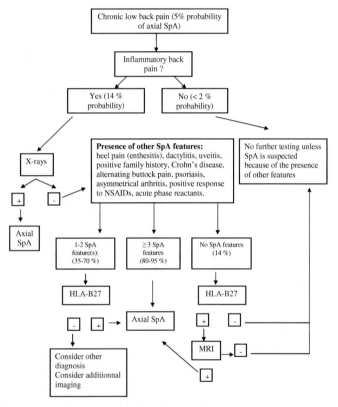

From: M Rudwaleit M, van der Heijde D, Khan MA, Braun J, Sieper J. How to diagnose axial spondyloarthritis early. Ann Rheum Dis 2004 ; 63 : 535-543.

Crystal-Induced Arthropathies	
Gout	Risk factor = hyperuricemia. Caused by : – 90 % underexcretion (< 600 mg/day): idiopathic, chronic renal failure, endocrine disorders (diabetic ketoacidosis, hypo-hyperparathyroidism, adrenal insufficiency), drugs (diuretics, low-dose aspirin, niacin, cyclosporine, ethanol, ethambutol, L-dopa, pyrazinamide). – 10 % Overproduction: cancer, psoriasis, chronic hemolytic anemia, drugs (chemotherapy), alcohol, hereditary (rare). Attacks precipitated by trauma (iatrogenic: surgery), severe illness, fasting, infection, acidosis, transfusions, alcohol. < 25 % of hyperuricemic patients will develop gout.
Clinical findings	Prevalence: up to 1-2 % of adult population, increase with aging. Male:female ratio = 5:1. Rare in premenopausal women. Family history in 6-18% – Acute gout attack = monarticular (polyarticular in < 30%). – Localization: First metatarsophalangeal (50% at onset, 90% later in disease), ankle, tarsus, knee, elbow, finger. – Other clinical manifestations: intercritical gout, chronic tophaceous gout (common sites for tophi: ear helix, hands, olecranon bursae, Achilles tendons, feet), gouty nephropathy, urolithiasis.
Workup	– Presumptive clinical diagnosis (acute attacks, in particular podagra, hyperuricemia, complete response to treatment, asymptomatic between attacks) or definitive diagnosis (presence of crystals in synovial fluid). – Hyperuricemia (normal in 20 % during an attack), 24 hour urinary uric acid excretion, creatinine. – Synovial fluid analysis: inflammatory liquid (leukocytes > 2 x 10^9/L up to 40): intracellular urate crystals present (negative birefringence). – Tophi: aspiration or biopsy if necessary. – X-rays: punched-out erosions with overhanging edges, soft tissue edema, normal interarticular space, little or no osteopenia.
Treatment	Strong association of gout with metabolic syndrome: look for and treat if necessary. Non-pharmacologic: Education: weight loss if obesity, avoid alcohol (especially beer), avoid purine-rich food: chicken, turkey, sardines, red meat, giblets, shellfish Asymptomatic hyperuricemia: do not treat. Acute gout attack: 1. Nonsteroidal anti-inflammatory drugs (NSAIDs). 2. If NSAIDs contraindicated: steroids (intra-articular 20-80 mg methylprednisolone acetate or triamcinolone acetonide or oral or IV if > 1 joint: e.g.: 30-40 mg for 3 days followed by a two week weaning). 3. Option: oral colchicine: 1.2 mg loading dose, followed by 0.6 mg every 2 hours until resolution or maximum of 3 mg. Maintenance therapy: if ≥ 2 attacks/year and no response to alcohol and diuretic cessation, weight loss, etc. Or if bone erosions, tophi, urolithiasis, gouty nephropathy, urinary uric acid > 800-1000 mg/day. Only 25% of patients experience more than 1 attack over 12 years (according to Framingham): so maintenance therapy is not always necessary.

	If maintenance therapy necessary: – Allopurinol is the preferred agent (indicated for tophaceous gout, urolithiasis, creatinine clearance < 65 mL/min, urinary uric acid > 800-1000 mg/24 h, use of cytotoxic agents). – If toxicity or contraindication to allopurinol: desensitization (if mild reaction, i.e.: rash; otherwise: avoid); uricosuric agent (sulfinpyrazone, probenecid): indicated for renal undersecretion, no urolithiasis, no aspirin, creatinine clearance > 60 mL/min, no cardiac failure (increased hydration needed (1-2 L/day) if these agents are taken). – Other agents: mildly uricosuric agents to consider according to clinical context: losartan, fenofibrate, vitamine C (500 mg daily). – Colchicine alone: if contraindication to formerly mentioned drugs or inability to reach uric acid targets, or if persistent attacks. Note: if use of colchicine for many months, it is recommended to proceed with CK assay and CBC every 6 months (screening of colchicine bone marrow and muscle toxicity). Sudden changes in uric acid concentration may precipitate acute attacks → give colchicine 0.6 mg daily or bid concomitantly with uric acid lowering treatment for 2-4 months (to prevent further attacks) or begin low dose allopurinol (50-100 mg/day and ↑ over 3-4 weeks). Adjust dose in renal failure. Look out for drug interactions (azathioprine, mercaptopurine, warfarine). Therapeutic target: < 360 µmol/L. Sometimes necessary to increase allopurinol to 600-800 mg/day or more in order to reach target; adjust according to plasma uric acid.
Pseudogout	Calcium pyrophosphate deposition disease can take different forms: 1. Asymptomatic chondrocalcinosis. 2. Pseudogout: acute inflammatory arthropathy, mono or oligoarticular. 3. Pseudo rheumatoid arthritis: polyarticular presentation with distribution similar to rheumatoid arthritis. 4. Osteoarthritis: degenerative arthropathy which can affect unusual sites: shoulders, wrists, MCPs, ankles. 5. Neuroarthropathy-like presentation. Causes: idiopathic, genetic (rare) and the 4 "H": **h**emochromatosis, **h**ypothyroidism, **h**ypomagnesemia, **h**yperparathyroidism. Other causes: gout, chronic renal failure, amyloidosis, Wilson's, acromegaly, hypophosphatasia. Precipitated by trauma (iatrogenic: surgery), severe illness, fasting, infection, acidosis, transfusions, alcohol.
Clinical findings	Age > 60 years. Prevalence < 0.1 %. Acute recurrent arthritis, rarely chronic. Mostly large joints (knee, wrist, ankle). Knees > first metatarsophalangeal joint.
Workup	Synovial fluid analysis: inflammatory: calcium pyrophosphate crystals ⊕ (rhomboid-shaped, positively birefringent). Workup: rule out associated conditions: check: Ca^{++}, PO_4^{3-}, Mg^{++}, alkaline phosphatase, ferritin, transferrin saturation, glucose, TSH, uric acid. X-rays: punctate or linear radiodensities (chondrocalcinosis). X-ray hands/wrists, shoulders, pelvis, knees.

Treatment	Treat primary cause. Acute attack : 1- NSAIDs, 2- If NSAIDs contraindicated: steroids (intra-articular or systemic if > 1 joint) or colchicine. Maintenance therapy : if ≥ 2 attacks/year : 1- Colchicine 0.6 mg bid, 2- If colchicine contraindicated: long-term NSAIDs and gastroprotection. Note: If colchicine is used for many months, it is recommended to proceed with CK dosage and CBC every 6 months (screening for bone marrow and muscle toxicity of colchicine).
Other crystals	– Hydroxyapatite (calcium phosphate): calcific periarthritis, synovitis, subcutaneous calcinosis, destructive arthropathy ("Milwaukee's shoulder"). Most often idiopathic; therapeutic approach similar to that of pseudogout. – With dialysis: calcium oxalate, hydoxyapatite, monosodium urate, calcium pyrophosphate. – Cholesterol, cryoglobulin, corticosteroids, xanthine, cystine, aluminium, etc. – Diagnosis by synovial fluid analysis.

Osteoporosis

Definition: bone fragility caused by qualitative and quantitative deterioration of bone tissue: ↓ bone density (T-score < -2.5).
Prevalence: after 50 years, 25 % of women and 12.5 % of men.

Causes	Primary osteoporosis or Secondary to: hyperthyroidism, hyperparathyroidism, Cushing's, hypogonadism, prolactinoma, multiple myeloma, mastocytosis, pernicious anemia, rheumatoid arthritis, SLE, chronic renal failure, renal tubular acidosis, hypercalciuria, ankylosing spondylitis, malabsorption (celiac disease), inflammatory bowel disease, chronic liver disease (primary biliary cirrhosis), drugs (steroids - even inhaled [very high doses], anticonvulsants, heparin, cyclosporine, anti-androgens, aromatase inhibitors, GNRH agonists).
Screening	Screen postmenopausal women and men > 50 years according to risk factors : – Major risk factors: age > 65 years, vertebral compression fracture, fragility fracture after 40 years, family history of osteoporotic fractures, steroids (≥ 7.5 mg/day for > 3 months), malabsorption (celiac disease), primary hyperparathyroidism, risk of falling, osteopenia on plain film, hypogonadism, early menopause (< 45 years). – Minor risk factors: rheumatoid arthritis, history of hyperthyroidism, anticonvulsants, poor calcium intake, smoking, chronic alcoholism, heavy caffeine use, weight < 57 kg, weight loss > 10% of body weight at 25 years of age, chronic heparin use. ⇒ In presence of 1 major factor or 2 minor factors: perform bone densitometry. ⇒ If history of osteoporotic fracture or patient ≥ 65 years: perform bone densitometry.
Diagnosis	Workup: CBC, Ca++, alkaline phosphatase, creatinine, serum protein electrophoresis. If needed: TSH, ESR, phosphorus, estradiol, 24 hour urinary calcium, according to clinical findings. FSH, LH, testosterone in men < 65 years. Bone mineral density results (for Caucasian post-menopausal woman): - Normal if T-score > -1. - Osteopenia if T-score between - 1 to - 2.5 (relative risk (RR) for fracture x 2). - Osteoporosis if T-score < -2.5 (RR x 4-5). - Severe osteoporosis if T-score < -2.5 with evidence of a fragility fracture (RR x

	20). X-rays have poor sensitivity for the diagnosis, but are useful to show fractures and to look for secondary causes.			

10-year fracture risk for women	Âge	Low risk (< 10 %)	Moderate risk (10-20 %)	High risk (> 20 %)
	Lowest T-score (lumbar spine, total hip, femoral neck, trochanter)			
	50	> - 2.3	- 2.3 to - 3.9	< - 3.9
	55	> - 1.9	- 1.9 to - 3.4	< - 3.4
	60	> - 1.4	- 1.4 to - 3.0	< - 3.0
	65	> - 1.0	- 1.0 to - 2.6	< - 2.6
	70	> - 0.8	- 0.8 to - 2.2	< - 2.2
	75	> - 0.7	- 0.7 to - 2.1	< - 2.1
	80	> - 0.6	- 0.6 to - 2.0	< - 2.0
	85	> - 0.7	- 0.7 to - 2.2	< - 2.2

Note: Fragility fracture after age 40 or glucocorticoid use increase risk categorization to the next level (e.g.: from low to moderate, etc).

For the fracture risk for men, see appendix.

| Treatment | Nonpharmacologic: physical activity (≥ 30 minutes ≥ 3 times per week), stop smoking, high calcium intake.

Pharmacologic :
– Calcium: calcium carbonate or citrate with food: 1000 mg/day (total recommended daily dose: 1500 mg).
– Vitamin D: every patient > 65 years or with osteoporosis: 800 IU/day. Give 1.25-$(OH)_2D_3$ (activated vitamin D - Rocaltrol®) or $1\alpha OHD_3$ in chronic renal failure.
– Bisphosphonates: renal elimination.
  - Alendronate (Fosamax®): 70 mg weekly (or 10 mg daily). Side effects: abdominal pain, nausea, diarrhea, bone pain (rare). Contraindications: oesophageal abnormality, creatinine clearance < 35 mL/min, inability to remain seated or in standing position for 30 minutes. Indicated for osteoporosis prophylaxis: 5 mg daily.
  - Risedronate (Actonel®): 35 mg weekly, 150 mg once a month or 75 mg for 2 consecutive days every month (or 5 mg daily). Side effects: abdominal pain, hypertension, joint pain, bone pain, Contraindications: same as for alendronate. Note: if creatinine clearance between 15-30 mL/min, half dose (35 mg every 2 weeks) may be used (little evidence however) although full dose has been used in clinical trials and found to be effective and safe.
  - Etidronate (Didronel - Didrocal®): cyclic therapy 14 days /90. Contraindication: osteomalacia, creatinine clearance < 35 mL/minute, etc. Efficacy has only been demonstrated in ↓ vertebral fractures.
  - Zoledronic acid (Aclasta®): 5 mg IV once a year.

– Hormone replacement therapy (HRT). Contraindications: undiagnosed vaginal bleeding, active liver disease, breast cancer, acute vascular thrombosis. Be careful in presence of migraine, previous thromboembolism, hypertriglyceridemia, uterine fibroids, endometriosis, uterine cancer, gallbladder disease, family history of breast cancer, chronic hepatic dysfunction. Caution: increased risk of breast cancer when used > 5 years, increased risk of coronary heart disease and stroke. Use for as short a time as possible. Some women (10%) do not respond to HRT and decrease bone density.
– Selective estrogen receptor modulators: raloxifene (Evista®). May decrease risk of breast cancer. Side effects: vasomotor flushes, leg cramps, Contraindications: history of thromboembolic disease.
– Calcitonin (Miacalcin NS®): 200 IU daily intranasally. Second line therapy. Side effect: rhinitis, epistaxis, abdominal pain. Useful analgesic for pain related to acute vertebral fractures.
– Teriparatide (Forteo®): for severe osteoporosis: 20 μg s/c daily for 18 months. Side |

	effects: nausea, dizziness, leg cramps. Contraindications: hypercalcemia, severe renal failure, bone metastasis, history of bone cancer or bone radiotherapy, Paget's, ↑ alkaline phosphatase of unknown cause.
	– Other treatments: testosterone in men with hypogonadism
	– Combination therapy with HRT or raloxifene + bisphosphonates not recommended due to lack of evidence. If bone density decreases (> 5% in 2 years) despite Ca++, vitamin D and antiresorption agent, consider combination therapy and referral to a specialist.
	
	⇒ Treatment Algorithm :
	– If low risk (< 10%) of fracture on 10 years: adequate calcium and vitamin D intake. No other pharmacological treatment.
	– If moderate risk (10-20 %): pharmacological treatment on a case by case basis.
	– If high risk (> 20 % or taking steroids):
	    1st line treatment: alendronate or risedronate.
	    → If vasomotor symptoms: hormone replacement therapy.
	    → If bisphosphonate failure (confirmed new vertebral fracture): teriparatide x 18 months, followed by alendronate or risedronate.
	    → If major digestive intolerance to bisphosphonates (despite PPI bid x 2 months): teriparatide x 18 months or IV bisphosphanates (pamidronate, zoledronic acid).
	    → If risk of vertebral fractures > non vertebral: raloxifene.
	        → If raloxifene contraindicated: calcitonin may be an alternative.
	
	If steroids (≥ 5-7.5 mg prednisone or equivalent for ≥ 3 months): bone densitometry before beginning treatment, and then every 6 months to 1 year. Stop smoking and ↓ alcohol if excessive. Regular physical activity. Correct hormonal deficit as needed. Calcium 1-1.5 g/day + vitamin D 400-800 IU daily. Bisphosphonates. Calcitonin as 2nd line. Thiazide as needed if ↑ calciuria.
	
	If vertebral fractures: NSAIDs, acetaminophen. Corset as needed.
	If severe pain: hospital admission. Rest with progressive weight bearing. Opioids if needed. Calcitonin s/c as needed. Epidural injection with anesthetics or steroids. Physical therapy. Refer to a pain clinic, as needed.
	Resolution in 6-12 weeks.
	
	Hip fracture: determine circumstances of the fall (reversible factors?). Requires emergency surgery within 48 hours. Post-op antithrombotic and pressure ulcer prophylaxis. Caution with opioids!
	Rehabilitation with physical and occupational therapy. Investigation and treatment for osteoporosis as above when appropriate. ≈ 20 % mortality at 1 year. 2/3 never regain their prior functional status.

Follow-up	Repeat bone densitometry at one year if risk of rapid bone loss (e.g.: steroids, hypogonadism, hyperparathyroidism), at 1-2 years after beginning bisphosphonates and every 2 to 3 years afterwards in a treated patient whose bone mineral density is stable.
	
	What change of bone mineral density is considered significant?
	– To calculate, use density in g/cm2, and not T score.
	    - According to site and precision of measurement: Confidence interval 95 % implies 2.77 x precision of measurement.
	      Lumbar spine: precision = 2 %. So, 2 % x 2.77 = 5.5 %.
	      Femoral neck (precision = 3.2 %): 8.9 %.
	      Hip (precision = 2.4 %): 6.6 %.
	– Changes inferior to these threshold values are unlikely to be significant.

Osteomalacia

Definition: diffuse bone disease, characterized by inadequate bone mineralization.

Causes:
- Secondary to abnormality of vitamin D metabolism or vitamin D deficiency (most frequent cause): diet, malabsorption, inadequate sun exposure, liver disease such as cirrhosis (25-hydroxylation) or severe renal disease (1 α-hydroxylation: renal failure: loss of vitamin D binding protein: nephrotic syndrome), anticonvulsivant therapy, abnormality of vitamin D receptor response
- ↓ PO_4^{3-}: decreased intake (such as use of antacids), disorder of renal phosphorus reabsorption: vitamin D-resistant rickets, Fanconi, multiple myeloma, hyperparathyroidism, oncogenic osteomalacia (with benign mesenchymal tumor, prostate cancer).
- Inhibition of mineralization: fluoride, aluminium, etidronate, tetracycline; hypophosphatasia; abnormal matrix (e.g.: osteogenesis imperfecta).
- Other causes: metabolic acidosis.

Clinical findings	Often asymptomatic. Skeletal pain with or without fracture, proximal myopathy, hypotonia, myalgias, muscular wasting. Pseudofracture.
Diagnosis	Initial workup: calcium, phosphorus, alkaline phosphatase, 25(OH)D, venous blood gas, x-rays. As needed: PTH assay, urinary collection for calcium and phosphorus. Interpretation: *table below* N: normal. ↑ 1.25 $(OH)_2D_3$ in vitamin D resistance. X-ray : pseudofractures ("Looser's zones"): fissures perpendicular to the cortical margins of bone; common sites: pubic and ischial rami, femoral neck, proximal femoral diaphysis under lesser trochanter, scapula, humerus, ribs, clavicle; biconcave aspect of vertebrae, demineralization Definitive diagnosis by biopsy: usually not required.
Treatment	According to cause: - Vitamin D deficiency: vitamin D 1000-7000 IU daily or more according to the specific cause. - 1.25 $(OH)_2D_3$ if absence of vitamin D hydroxylation. - Phosphates if deficiency or renal loss. - Prophylactic vitamin D recommended with prescription of anticonvulsants. - Calcium supply: 1000 mg daily. - Monitor for hypercalciuria, hypercalcemia, and renal failure during treatment.

	Calcium	PO_4^{3-}	Alkaline phosphatase	Vitamin D 25(OH)/1.25 $(OH)_2D$
Vitamin D deficiency/abnormality (PTH ↑)	N or ↓	↓	↑	↓ / N or ↓
Hepatic disease Malabsorption	N or ↓	↓	↑	↓ / ↓
Renal failure	N or ↓	↑	↑	N / ↓
Phosphorus renal loss	N	↓	N	N
Metabolic acidosis	N	N	N	N
Hypophosphatasia	N	N	↓	N
Inhibition of mineralization	N	N	N	N

Paget's Disease of Bone

Metabolic bone disease of unknown cause characterized by focal (17 %) or multifocal (83 %) areas of increased bone turnover: viral or genetic cause suspected.
Rare before age 40.
Family history in 12 %. Significant geographical variation.
Bones most frequently involved: skull, thoracic or lumbar spine, sacrum, pelvis, femur, tibia, humerus.

Clinical findings	– Usually asymptomatic: only 5-30 % have symptoms.
	– Depending on involved sites:
	   • All sites: bone pain in 25-30 %, local warmth, pathologic fractures.
	   • Skull: neurologic complications (cranial nerve compression VIII= deafness], hydrocephalus, vertebro-basilar insufficiency, subdural hematoma, platybasia).
	   • Spine: spinal stenosis, compressive radiculopathy, spinal cord ischemia by vascular steal.
	   • Articular complications when disease near a joint (secondary osteoarthritis), sarcomatous change (< 1 %).

Workup	– ↑ alkaline phosphatase (reflecting osteoblastic activity), ↑ urinary pyridinolines and hydroxyprolines (reflecting osteoclastic activity). Follow-up with alkaline phophatase levels q 6-12 months. – X-ray: localized osteoporosis (skull), abnormal bone structure (thickened cortex and disorganized trabeculae, bone thickening, "cotton-wool" appearance, "picture frame" appearance (enhanced vertebral outline), ivory vertebra – Bone scan to evaluate the extent of disease : increased uptake in one or many bones

Treatment	Indications for treatment: pain, skull involvement, neurological complications, disease of lower limbs or spine, pathologic fractures, bone deformity, young patient, high output congestive heart failure, hypercalcemia, ↑ alkaline phosphatase > 2 x normal level, preparation for orthopedic surgery, lesions close to a joint.
	
	Goal: pain relief, normalization of biochemical tests of bone remodelling, restoration of normal bone, prevention of complications.
	
	Therapeutic agents:
	– Bisphosphonates: ↓ osteoclastic activity. Take on empty stomach. Renal elimination (contraindicated if creatinine clearance < 35 mL/min).
	   - Alendronate: 40 mg daily x 6 months. Follow-up with biochemical tests.
	   - Risedronate: 30 mg daily x 2 months.
	   - Pamidronate: IV: indicated as preparation for elective surgery (with calcitonin).
	   - Zoledronic acid: IV: 5 mg, single dose.
	   Calcium and vitamin D supplements during treatment.
	– Calcitonin: subcutaneous or intranasal (but less effective), plateau in efficacy, antibodies, side effects. Analgesic effect.
	– Other possible treatments (gallium nitrate, mithramycine) are rarely used.
	– Repeat alkaline phosphatase 6 months after end of treatment (nadir).
	– X-rays may be repeated 6-12 months after end of treatment to evaluate improvement of bone architecture.

Fibromyalgia	
Overview	Prevalence 3-10 % in general outpatient population. More common in women between 20-50 years old. Shares many features with chronic fatigue syndrome (see Fatigue table). Unknown etiology. May complicate hypothyroidism, rheumatoid arthritis or other chronic rheumatic disorders, sleep apnea
Clinical findings	The 1990 American College of Rheumatology criteria: widespread pain (bilateral, including axial and upper and lower limb involvement) for > 3 months. At least 11 of 18 specific tender points (palpation with a force of 4 kg/cm): see figure. Associated with fatigue, non-refreshing sleep, morning stiffness. Associated with irritable bowel syndrome, Raynaud's phenomenon, headaches, subjective edema, paresthesias, psychological distress Differential diagnosis: chronic fatigue syndrome, polymyalgia rheumatica, polymyositis (if predominant weakness), connective tissue disease, seronegative spondyloarthropathies, depression, hypothyroidism, adrenal insufficiency, sleep apnea, cancer.
Workup	Clinical diagnosis. Not a diagnosis of exclusion. CBC, ESR, CRP, CK, calcium, phosphate, alkaline phosphatase, TSH: all should be normal.

Treatment	Nonpharmacological: education and progressive aerobic exercises, ideally under supervision (walking, swimming, aqua-aerobics) are the bases of treatment.
	Biofeedback, hypnosis, acupuncture, behavioural therapy: poorly studied
	
	Pharmacological:
	  – Antidepressants: amitriptyline (10-50 mg HS, more frequently prescribed) with significant response in 25-30%. Duloxetine (60-120 mg/day). Cyclobenzaprine (10-30 mg HS), venlafaxine are effective but less well studied. Selective serotonin reuptake inhibitors (SSRIs) only if depression or in association with tricyclics.
	  – Anti-epileptics: gabapentin (300-2400 mg/day) or pregabalin (75-450 mg/day): results beneficial and superior to placebo.
	  – Analgesics: acetaminophen.Tramadol, NSAIDs poorly effective. Steroids are not effective. Opioids on a case by case basis, but generally not recommended.
	  – Others: S-adenosyl-L-methionine (SAMe), 5-hydroxytryptophan, ondansetron effectiveness suggested in small studies.
	  – Benzodiazepines: not effective and not recommended.
	
	Symptomatic approach:
	  – Pain: tricyclics, cyclobenzaprine, venlafaxine, gabapentine, pregabalin, pramipexole, opioids, cannabinol (Sativex®).
	  – Sleep: tricyclics, gabapentin, pregabalin, 5-hydroxytryptophan, cyclobenzaprine, sleep hygiene.
	  – Fatigue: bupropion, venlafaxine.
	  – Anxiety: SSRIs.
	  – Depressive symptoms: duloxetine, SSRIs, tricyclics.

Prognosis	Significant symptoms improvement in less than 50 % of patients, despite treatment. Resolution in 3 % after 3 years in one study!

Fibromyalgia Tender Points

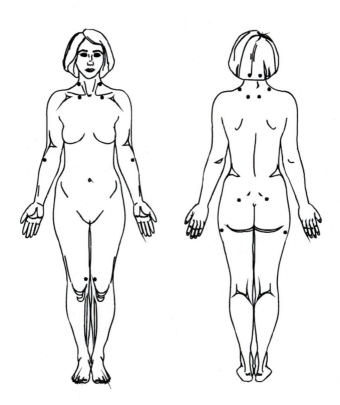

Low Back Pain	
Overview	70 % of adults will suffer from low back pain at some point in their life. Second most common reason to seek medical care. Male = female. Peak prevalence 30-50 years. Acute if < 4 weeks, subacute if 4-12 weeks or chronic if > 12 weeks (5 %).

Causes	Mobile segments (disks, facets, ligaments, spinal muscles).
	    – Mechanical pain (97%): usually during the day, relief with rest; worse with
	        exercise.
	      - Lumbar strain, sprain 70 %.
	      - Degenerative process (disk or facet) 10 %.
	      - Spondylolisthesis 2 %.
	      - Congenital disease < 1 %.
	      - Osteochondrosis.
	    – Inflammatory :
	      - Inflammatory arthritis (3 %): ankylosing spondylitis, psoriatic, Reiter,
	         inflammatory bowel disease: early morning awakening, morning stiffness,
	         improved with physical activity.
	
	Neurologic:
	    – Herniated disk 4 %: sciatica, crural pain.
	    – Spinal stenosis 3 %: look for neurogenic claudication.
	
	Bone disorders (1 %): diurnal and nocturnal pain.
	    – Cancer (0.7 %): multiple myeloma, metastases, lymphoma, leukemia, spinal
	        cord tumors, primary vertebral tumors
	    – Infection (0.01 %): osteomyelitis, discitis, paraspinal or epidural abscess,
	        tuberculosis, endocarditis.
	    – Paget's disease (may produce mechanical pain).
	    – Fracture: osteoporotic or traumatic.
	
	Visceral pain (2 %):
	    – Pelvic disease: prostatitis, endometriosis, pelvic inflammatory disease,
	        pregnancy and others
	    – Renal diseases: urolithiasis, pyelonephritis, perirenal abscess
	    – Abdominal aortic aneurysm.
	    – Gastrointestinal disease: pancreatitis, cholecystitis, perforated ulcer
	    – Retroperitoneal fibrosis (periaortitis)
	
	85 % of patients with isolated low back pain have no specific diagnosis.
	
	If > 65 years, cancer, compression fracture, spinal stenosis and aortic aneurysm
	become more frequent.

Evaluation	See algorithm (next page).
	Look for red flags:
	    - Bone pathology (e.g.: cancer, infection, fracture).
	    - Major neurological involvement (e.g.: severe paresis, plegia, incontinence, *cauda
	       equina*).
	    - Evidence of inflammatory arthropathy.
	    - Visceral disease.
	
	History: age (> 50 years), history of cancer, weight loss, injection-drug use, chronic
	infection. Characteristics of pain: location, radiation (sciatica? abdominal or pelvic
	pain?), duration (morning stiffness, effect of exercise on pain), nocturnal pain, position
	causing pain, change with Valsalva or effort, response to treatment. Sciatica,
	pseudoclaudication, paresthesias, paresis, fecal or urinary incontinence or retention.
	Psychological or social factors aggravating or prolonging low back pain.

	On physical exam: fever, spinal tenderness, ↓ chest expansion, straight-leg raising test, Schober test, neurologic exam (sensory, motor, reflexes). Hip and sacroiliac joint exam. Abdominal exam. Rectal exam. – Involvement of the L4 nerve root: ↓ knee jerk, sensory loss in medial leg, ↓ knee extension and ankle dorsiflexion (↓ capacity to walk on heels). – Involvement of the L5 nerve root: normal reflexes, sensory loss in lateral leg and dorsal foot (mostly between 1st and 2nd toes), ↓ great toe dorsiflexion and ↓ foot eversion. – Involvement of the S1 nerve root: ↓ ankle jerk, sensory loss in lateral foot and ↓ plantar flexion of the foot (↓ capacity to tiptoe).
Workup	– No workup necessary for low back pain < 4 weeks in absence of red flags. – According to clinical findings: CBC, ESR, CRP, serum protein electrophoresis, prostate specific antigen. – Lumbar spine X-ray if infection, cancer, fracture or spondylarthropathy are suspected or for patients with neurologic deficits, age > 50 years, fever, weight loss, immunosuppression, recent bacterial infection, injection-drug use, steroids, nocturnal pain, osteoporosis, recent trauma, sustained morning stiffness. Also perform X-rays if no improvement after 4-6 weeks. – Reserve CT scans and MRI if high suspicion of infection or cancer, progressive neurologic deficit, *cauda equina* syndrome or persisting neurologic deficit after 4-6 weeks. – Bone scan for infection, metastasis, fracture or Paget's disease. Refer to surgeon if: *cauda equina* syndrome, progressive or severe neurological deficit, persistent motor deficit after 4-6 weeks of supportive treatment, persistent sciatica after 4-6 weeks, with consistent clinical and neurologic involvement, persistent and incapacitating spinal stenosis provoking sciatica or claudication (not effective if only lumbar pain), segmental instability consistent with clinical involvement.
Treatment	Patient education is primordial. Postural education, strengthening exercises for stabilizing muscles. Nonspecific low back pain: NSAIDs, physical therapy, rapid return to normal activities (avoid heavy lifting, torsion, vibration), avoid bed rest > 48 hours, muscle relaxants for 1-2 weeks. Chiropractic? Massotherapy? Disc herniation: treatment as above. May require opioids for 1-2 weeks, if needed. Short-term relief with epidural infiltration. Chronic low back pain: aerobic exercises, physical therapy, antidepressants, gabapentin/pregabalin, tramadol, NSAIDs, acetaminophen often not effective. Facet joint injection may provide short-term relief. Consider referral to pain clinic.
Prognosis	For nonspecific low back pain, up to 95 % of spontaneous resolution after 6-8 weeks. Frequent relapses. For disc herniation, only 10 % experience persistent pain after 6 weeks, requiring surgical evaluation. Spinal stenosis remains stable in 70%, deteriorates in 15 %.

Diagnostic Algorithm for Recent Low Back Pain

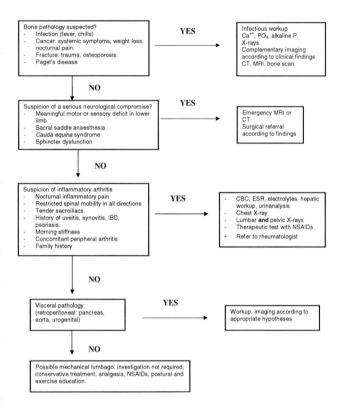

Adapted from Dudler J, Balagué F. What is the rational diagnostic approach to spinal disorders? Best Pract Res Clin Rheumatol 2002 ; 16 : 43-57.

Rheumatoid Arthritis	
Overview	A systemic inflammatory disease mainly involving joints. Affects 1 % of adults: 3 women for 1 man (50% men after age 60). Irreversible joint destruction (erosions) may develop as early as the first year. ↓ severity during pregnancy.
Diagnosis	Diagnostic criteria (American College of Rheumatology, 1987): 　1. Morning stiffness ≥ 1 hour .[1] 　2. Arthritis of ≥ 3 joint areas simultaneously.[1,2] 　3. Arthritis of hand joints : wrists, MCPs, PIPs.[1] 　4. Symmetric arthritis.[1] 　5. Rheumatoid nodules. 　6. Positive rheumatoid factor. 　7. Radiographic changes (erosions and periarticular osteopenia in hands, wrists and feet). [1] Present for ≥ 6 weeks. [2] 14 possible areas: PIP, MCP, wrist, elbow, knee, ankle, MTP bilaterally. ⇒ ≥ 4/7 criteria for diagnosis. Note: Only 50 % of patients with rheumatoid arthritis meet these criteria during the first year of their disease. Consequently, it is not necessary to meet all of the required criteria to make a clinical diagnosis and begin treatment! 20-25 % of patients with ≥ 4/7 criteria initially progress to another type of arthritis.
Differential diagnosis	Systemic lupus erythematosus and other connective tissue diseases and systemic vasculitides (look for extraarticular involvement), psoriatic arthritis (search for IPD involvement, asymmetry, axial involvement), palindromic rheumatism (lasts a few days), pseudogout (X-rays : chondrocalcinosis, crystals in synovial fluid analysis), cryoglobulinemia (purpura, neuropathy, glomerulonephritis), acute rheumatic fever (post-infectious, migrating arthritis), viral infection or reactive arthritis (HCV, HBV, measles, parvovirus B19, Whipple's, HIV : usually lasts < 1-2 months), adult-onset Still's disease (fever, rash, ferritin ↑↑↑), arthritis of systemic diseases (cancer – solid (rare, explosive beginning, especially larger joints, asymmetric), leukemia, hemochromatosis, thyroid disorder, inflammatory bowel disease, sarcoidosis, amyloidosis, Behçet's), etc. Differential diagnosis of synovitis of the hands: gout, inflammatory osteoarthritis, pseudogout, viral arthritis, connective tissue diseases, psoriatic arthritis, sarcoidosis, multicentric reticulohistiocytosis, etc.
Clinical findings	– Insidious onset in 50-70%, acute onset in 15-20 %. 50 % seropositive at presentation (80% in the long term). – Early (< 6 months), medium term (6-24 months), late (> 24 months). – Systemic symptoms (fatigue, stiffness, fever). – Cervical spine involvement (C1-C2) common: subluxation in up to 30% of severe erosive arthritis. – Other joints: rarely distal interphalangeal. Temporomandibular joints. Popliteal cyst. Extraarticular manifestations: – Skin: rheumatoid nodules (20 % of seropositive patients), purpura, skin ulcerations. Rheumatoid vasculitis. – Ocular: scleritis, scleromalacia perforans, keratoconjunctivitis sicca (10-35 %), episcleritis. – Renal: rarely clinically significant. Amyloidosis, drug toxicity. – Respiratory (up to 33 % of patients): cricoarytenoid joint (dysphonia, laryngeal pain, odynophagia), pleural, interstitial, nodules, bronchiolitis obliterans, BOOP, Caplan's

	syndrome, drug-induced pneumopathy (methotrexate, leflunomide, anti-TNF)
	– Cardiac: pericarditis, effusion, cardiomyopathy, conduction defects, valvular lesions.
	– Hematologic: anemia (chronic disease or drug-induced - NSAIDs, immunosuppressants), Felty's syndrome (triad arthritis, leukopenia (neutropenia, sometimes lymphopenia), splenomegaly), LGLS (*large granular lymphocyte syndrome* : severe neutropenia with recurring serious infections, *lymphocytosis* → diagnosis on blood smear + lymphocyte phenotyping), lymphoma (caused by immunosuppressants or by rheumatoid arthritis itself).
	– Neurological: entrapment neuropathy (carpal tunnel, Guyon's canal, C1-C2 instability) or secondary to rheumatoid vasculitis.
Functional capacity	I: Able to perform usual activities of daily living (self-care, vocational and avocational). II: Able to perform self-care and vocational activities, but limited in avocational activities. III: Able to perform usual self-care activities, but limited otherwise. IV: Limited in ability to perform usual self-care, vocational and avocational activities.
Workup	CBC, electrolytes, creatinine, sedimentation rate, hepatic enzymes, calcium, phosphate, protein, albumin, urinalysis, rheumatoid factor, ANA, X-rays of hands and feet, ECG, chest X-ray If necessary: viral serology (for differential diagnosis, or prior to beginning methotrexate therapy), C-spine X-ray, anti-CCP (anti-cyclic citrullinated peptide).
Treatment	Early treatment is primordial (irreversible damages in <2 years). Goals of treatment: alleviate pain, regression of synovitis and induction of remission, prevent joint erosions, articular and extraarticular complications, preserve functional autonomy. In practice, if persistent polyarthritis for more than 6 weeks, without evidence of alternate diagnosis, and even if all required diagnostic criteria not met, start treatment. – NSAIDs ± gastroprotection or selective COX-2 inhibitors if ≥ 65 years, cardio-pulmonary disease, history of ulcer, steroids or anticoagulation (give COX-2 inhibitors + gastroprotection if history of complicated ulcer or anticoagulation). Caution because COX-2 inhibitors increase risk of cardiovascular events (evaluate the global risk/benefit ratio). – Methotrexate (MTX): cornerstone of treatment. In monotherapy or combined therapy. 7.5 mg /week → 15 mg / week (up to 20-25 mg if tolerated). (Effective doses are usually between 15 and 25 mg/week) Folic acid 1 mg 24 hours after MTX. Give s/c or IM if PO ineffective. Control liver function tests + albumin + CBC + creatinine every 4-8 weeks. Avoid folate antagonists such as TMP/SMX. – Hydroxychloroquine: for mild arthritis, older patients: 200 mg bid (max 6.5 mg/kg). Ophtalmological exam yearly. – Steroids PO 2-15 mg/day in 1 or 2 doses or intra-articular if persistent symptoms despite NSAIDs. Mostly used in early disease as a bridge therapy until disease-modifying drugs take effect (see above). Consider osteoporosis prophylaxis. – According to disease course: sulfasalazine, azathioprine, leflunomide. – Anti-TNF α (etanercept, infliximab, adalimumab, golimumab): To consider after failure of two conventional anti-rheumatismals. Anti-TNF is more effective when combined with methotrexate. – Selective costimulation modulators: Abatacept: consider after failure of two conventional anti-rheumatic drugs. – Rituximab: consider after failure of ≥ 1 anti-TNF. More effective if used with methotrexate – Gold salts, cyclosporine less commonly used. – Combination therapy (add hydroxychloroquine and sulfasalazine to methotrexate if ineffective alone). Other combination therapies (MTX + leflunomide, MTX + etanercept or infliximab, MTX + cyclosporine) are possible if usual treatment remains ineffective. – Monitor patient for drug toxicity. Wait at least 6 months before concluding treatment failure. Caution in young women because some drugs are teratogenic. – Surgery: if pain is refractory to optimal treatment, for functional limitation or C1-C2

	instability.
	– Physical and occupational therapy.
	– Vaccination for influenza and pneumococcus. Watch for infections +++.
	– Support groups.
	– Avoid alcohol and smoking. Control cardiovascular risk factors.
	Evaluation of treatment effectiveness (aim for remission!):
	– Quantify painful joints, swollen joints, inflammatory indices (sedimentation rate, and/or C-reactive protein) and compare from one visit to another.
Prognosis	– 20 % of patients experience 1 flare of disease that resolves in 2 years. Most patients suffer from a polycyclic disease course and 10 % suffer from a progressive and refractory disease.
	– 50 % present disabilities after 5 years. Loss of 7-10 years of life expectancy if onset before age 50.
	– Markers of persistence and severity:
	- Erosions.
	- Seropositivity for rheumatoid factor and/or anti-CCP.
	- Persistence of CRP elevation and polysynovitis.
	- Tobacco use.
	– 10 % mortality caused by drug toxicity (NSAIDs, steroids).
	– ↑ risk of cardiovascular mortality
	– Remission if 5/6 of the following criteria for ≥ 2 consecutive months:
	1. Stiffness < 15 minutes.
	2. No fatigue.
	3. No joint pain.
	4. No tenderness to palpation or pain on movement.
	5. No joint or tendon sheath edema.
	6. Sedimentation rate (by Westergren method) < 30 mm/h (in women) or < 20 mm/h (in men).

Connective Tissue Diseases

Systemic Lupus Erythematosus (SLE)

Prevalence 1/1000: female > male (but same ratio during childhood and after age 50): black > white.
Associated with decreased complement (C1-C2-C4) levels.
Association with antiphospholipid syndrome: see Hypercoagulability table.

Differential diagnosis:

Drug-Induced Lupus: procainamide, hydralazine, isoniazide, methyldopa, carbamazepine, quinidine, D-penicillamine, lovastatine, interferon, ß-blockers, sulfasalazine, 5-ASA.
Antihistone antibodies ⊕ in almost all patients (However, also present in ≥ 50 % of SLE, therefore not very useful clinically); renal involvement, anti- DS-DNA and decreased complement deficit are rare.
Subacute Cutaneous Lupus Erythematous: skin involvement with some systemic manifestations (up to 50 %).
Anti-Ro and anti-La antibodies ⊕, low C2 levels.
Chronic Discoid Lupus Erythematosus: isolated skin involvement: → 1-5 % progress to SLE.

Diagnostic Criteria (ACR 1997)	1- Malar rash. 2- Discoid rash. 3- Photosensitivity. 4- Oral ulcers (usually painless). 5- Non erosive arthritis. 6- Pleuritis or pericarditis. 7- Renal disorder: proteinuria (> 0.5 g/day or 3+) or cellular casts. 8- Neurologic disorder: seizures or psychosis. 9- Hematologic disorder: hemolytic anemia or leukopenia (< 4 x 10^9/L) or lymphopenia (< 1.5 x 10^9/L) or thrombocytopenia (< 100 x 10^9/L) on ≥ 2 occasions. 10- Immunologic disorder: anti-DNA or anti-SM antibodies or antiphospholipid antibodies (anticardiolipin antibodies or lupus anticoagulant or false-positive VDRL). 11- ANA ⊕. Diagnosis if ≥ 4/11 criteria present serially or simultaneously. Note: These criteria may be inadequate for a diagnosis, especially during early stages of the disease. Examples of other possible manifestations, which do not appear among the diagnostic criteria: - General: fatigue, fever, weight loss. - Skin: subacute lupus, bullous lupus, Chilblain, skin vasculitis. - Neurological: central: alteration of cognitive functions, chorea, demyelinating disease, aseptic meningitis, ischemic events, myelopathy; Peripheral: demyelinating disease, peripheral or cranial neuropathy, mononeuritis multiplex. - Musculoskeletal: myopathy, avascular bone necrosis. - Pulmonary: parenchymal involvement: acute lupic pneumopathy, BOOP, chronic interstitial pneumopathy, shrinking lung syndrome, pulmonary hypertension, pulmonary capillaritis (presents with alveolar hemorrhage), pulmonary embolism - Cardiac: myocarditis, pericarditis, endocarditis, coronary vasculitis - Gastro-intestinal: peritonitis (serositis), vasculitis, pancreatitis, hepatitis - Lymphadenopathy: hepato/splenomegaly.

Workup	Goal: Evaluate activity and extent of the disease.
	• Baseline:
	  – CBC, creatinine, aPTT, ESR, CRP, AST, ALT, CK, C3, C4, CH50 (↓ with ↓ hereditary low C2 or ↓ hereditary C1), urinalysis, urinary sediment, search for proteinuria (protein/creatinine ratio) anticardiolipin antibodies, lupus anticoagulant, chest X-ray, ECG.
	  – Antibodies: DS-DNA associated with nephritis; SM = specific for SLE; anti-Ro with neonatal lupus, congenital cardiac block and photosensitivity; antihistone if drug-induced (in 95 % of cases and in up to ≥ 50 % of SLE).
	  – Lipid workup, glycemia: consider lupus patients at high risk of cardiovascular diseases.
	• During follow-up: CBC, sedimentation rate, C3, C4, urinalysis, protein/creatinine ratio, electrolytes, creatinine.
	• Other: according to clinical circumstances:
	  – Renal biopsy if renal involvement.
	  – Test for anti-Ro and anti-La in pregnant women (neonatal lupus).
	  – Imaging: echocardiography, cerebral MRI.
	  – Screening for osteoporosis (bone densitometry), especially if corticosteroids.

Treatment	According to clinical findings: – Musculoskeletal: NSAIDs: antimalarial drugs if no response. Methotrexate; Physical therapy. – Photosensitivity: sunscreens, antimalarial drugs, mechanical photoprotection. – Dermatitis: topical steroids: antimalarial drugs if no response → prednisone 20 mg/day, tapering dose→ methotrexate. Also retinoids, dapsone, thalidomide, topical cyclosporine/ tacrolimus. – Serositis: NSAIDs or prednisone 20-40 mg/day → steroids + antimalarial drugs → steroids ± immunosuppressants. – Severe complications (cerebral vasculitis, hemolytic anemia, thrombocytopenia): steroids ± immunosuppressants. – IV immunoglobulins ± steroids for thrombocytopenia or hemolytic anemia. Splenectomy if unresponsive. – Glomerulonephritis: treatment depends on kidney biopsy (WHO classification). – Central nervous system: depends on the etiology: inflammatory: steroids ± immunosuppressants. – Hypercoagulability: anticoagulants. Note: In case of CNS manifestations, always rule out infection, drug side effects or neurological manifestations secondary to metabolic disorders associated with systemic involvement of the disease.
Prognosis	Prognosis: 10 year survival 90%; 20 year 70%. Relapsing-remitting course. Causes of death: bimodal; first 5 years of disease: infection, active disease; thereafter: infection and CAD. Pregnancy: possible if inactive disease: 25 % neonatal lupus and 2 % bundle branch block if anti-Ro ± La antibodies present: abortion 1.5-3 x normal.

Sjögren's Syndrome

Autoimmune exocrinopathy involving the salivary *and* lacrimal glands.
90% females: primary or secondary (associated with rheumatoid arthritis, SLE, scleroderma, polymyositis, primary biliary cirrhosis).
Alternative causes of sicca syndromes: anticholinergics, diuretics, opiates, antihistamines, benzodiazepines, tobacco, infiltrating disease, radiotherapy.

Clinical findings	– Sicca: xerostomia and keratoconjunctivitis sicca. – Parotid gland enlargement. – Vaginal and vulvar dryness, upper airway dryness. – Systemic manifestations : fatigue, arthralgias, myalgias, Raynaud's, cutaneous vasculitis. – Interstitial pulmonary disease, lymphadenopathy, interstitial nephritis, distal renal tubular acidosis, peripheral polyneuropathy. – ↑ incidence of B-cell lymphoma and Waldenström's macroglobulinemia: risk factors: parotid gland enlargement, lymphadenopathy, purpura, peripheral neuropathy, low complement, anemia/lymphopenia, cryoglobulinemia. Otherwise: very low risk.
Management	– Diagnostic workup: ESR ↑, hypergammaglobulinemia, anemia, leukopenia, hyperamylasemia. Autoantibodies: ANA (80%), rheumatoid factor, anti-Ro (50-80%), anti-La (30-50%), cryoglobulins, ↓ C3-C4 if vasculitis or SLE. – Diagnosis (American-European consensus): Subjective criteria: 1- Xerostomia. 2- Keratoconjunctivitis sicca. Objective criteria: 3- Schirmer's test or rose Bengal stain. 4- Sialography, salivary gland scan. 5- Minor salivary gland biopsy: useful for ruling out other diseases (sarcoidosis) or for an atypical presentation (an HIV ⊕ male for example). 6- Anti-Ro/La antibodies. Diagnosis if ≥ 4 criteria including 5) or 6) and exclusion of diseases associated with

	sicca syndrome (neck radiation, HIV, hepatitis C, lymphoma, sarcoidosis, graft-versus-host, anticholinergic drugs, diuretics)
	– Treatment: artificial tears, ocular gel, lacrimal duct occlusion, artificial saliva, sugar-free candy, dental care, oral pilocarpine; for arthralgias: NSAIDs, antimalarial drugs.

Scleroderma
Prevalence 1/10 000. Female preponderance (5:1): 30-50 years.
± overlap syndromes (with anti-RNP antibodies).

Clinical findings	Raynaud's phenomenon is an early manifestation in virtually all patients (otherwise the diagnosis is in question).
	5 disease patterns:
	Generalized :
	1- Limited systemic scleroderma: CREST (**C**alcinosis, **R**aynaud's, **E**sophageal dysmotility, **S**clerodactyly, **T**elangiectasia): 80 %: skin involvement limited to hands + feet up to elbows and knees: face may be involved too: less systemic involvement except GERD: frequent; symptomatic pulmonary hypertension: up to 20 % (late complication).
	2- Diffuse scleroderma: 20 %: gastrointestinal involvement (GERD, dysphagia, malabsorption caused by bacterial overgrowth, wide mouth diverticula, constipation), lungs (interstitial disease, pulmonary hypertension), pericardium, pleura, heart (conduction defects, cardiomyopathy, pericarditis), kidneys (hypertensive crisis in up to 20%), etc.
	3- Scleroderma sine scleroderma (no skin involvement): only visceral disease.
	Localized :
	4- Morphea (plaques) } usually in patients < 30 years;
	5- Linear scleroderma (*en coup de sabre*) } visceral involvement rare (< 5 %).
	Differential diagnosis: eosinophilic fasciitis, vinyl chloride exposure, L-tryptophan, solvents, medication (bleomycin), etc.
	Differential Diagnosis of sclerodactyly: diabetes, trauma, bleomycin, amyloidosis, toxins.
Management	Workup: ANA ⊕ in 90 % (CREST = anticentromere antibodies ⊕ in 50 %: diffuse scleroderma = anti-Scl-70 ⊕ in 40 %), hypergammaglobulinemia, eosinophilia 5-10 %. Anemia by GI spoliation or malabsorption. Urinalysis, creatinine. ECG, echocardiography: evaluate pulmonary hypertension. Chest x-ray: basilar fibrosis. Pulmonary function tests: restrictive pattern and ↓ diffusing capacity. High-resolution thoracic CT for suspected fibrosis. GI evaluation: according to symptoms.
	Treatment: Supportive, according to involved organs:
	- Raynaud's: avoid smoking and cold exposure, calcium channel blockers, topical nitrates, stellate ganglion block, ARB, alpha blockers, fluoxetine, sildenafil, bosentan if severe.
	- Myositis: Prednisone.
	- Esophagitis: anti-reflux lifestyle modifications + proton pump inhibitors ± prokinetic agent.
	- Bacterial overgrowth: antibiotics.
	- Alveolitis: cyclophosphamide + steroids.
	- Pulmonary hypertension: anticoagulation ± calcium channel blockers or endothelin receptor antagonists, prostaglandins, sildenafil.
	- Hypertensive reno-vascular crisis = high-dose ACEI.
	- Skin disease: no specific treatment. Methotrexate?
	Warning: high-dose steroids ↑ risk of renal hypertensive crisis.
Prognosis	Better with CREST than diffuse scleroderma. More complications during first five years, except for isolated pulmonary hypertension: late complication (≥ 10-15 years). ↑ risk of cancer, particularly lung cancer (controversial).

Idiopathic Inflammatory Myopathies

Polymyositis

Dermatomyositis: association with malignancies < 10%: carcinoma of the lungs, ovaries, stomach: following age-specific prevalence.

Clinical findings	Polymyositis: proximal, symmetric weakness of the neck and trunk. Myalgia, fever, dysphagia, hypoventilation, laryngeal weakness and aspiration.
	Dermatomyositis: skin disease may precede muscle disease: heliotrope rash, Gottron's papules, papular dermatitis with scaling on the face, trunk, extremities, scalp, thorax (V-neck sign), periungual erythema, "mechanic's hands" (peeled palms), cutaneous vasculitis (with cancer).
	Pulmonary involvement (interstitial disease), cardiac involvement (arrhythmias, bundle branch block, cardiomyopathy).
	Differential diagnosis : − Inclusion body myositis: male > 50 years, slowly progressive more distal myopathy, mildly elevated CK: diagnosis on biopsy: unresponsive to treatment. − Inflammatory myopathy associated with cancer or connective tissue disease. − Toxic (colchicine, statins, steroids, zidovudine…), traumatic, endocrine (hypothyroidism, hypo-hyperparathyroidism, acromegaly), neuromuscular (myasthenia gravis), infectious (influenza, HIV…), rheumatologic (vasculitis…), metabolic (McArdle, carnitine, purines, mitochondrial diseases, etc) myopathies, muscular dystrophy.
Management	− Workup: CK ↑, ESR ↑, ANA ⊕ (80-90 %), anti-Jo-1 antibodies ⊕ (25 %), EMG, muscle biopsy, chest X-ray. − Search for malignancy if dermatomyositis: screening according to general age-specific recommendations. − Treatment: steroids ± immunosuppressants (↓ CK). IV immunoglobulins for refractory dermatomyositis.

Mixed Connective Tissue Disease

Features of scleroderma ± SLE ± polymyositis ± rheumatoid arthritis: high-titer anti-RNP antibodies in almost all patients (99 %). Absence of other autoantibodies. Female preponderance (9:1).

Clinical findings	Frequent early symptoms: Raynaud's phenomenon, peripheral symmetrical joint pain/arthritis, myalgias/myositis, edema of fingers (sausage shaped digits), acrosclerosis. Symptoms of overlapped connective tissue diseases may appear late during follow-up. - Arthritis: 60 %, usually non erosive; rheumatoid distribution. - Heart: pericarditis: 10-30 %; other: myocarditis, conduction disturbances. - Lungs (25 %): interstitial infiltrates, pleural effusion, pulmonary. - Kidneys (up to 25 %): membranous GN most often; Hypertensive renal crisis: rare. - Digestive (60-80 %): Most often: Motility disorder of upper digestive tube. Other: as in scleroderma. - Neurologic: most often: trigeminal neuralgia.
Diagnostic criteria (Alarcon-Segovia)	- High anti-RNP titers (practically, anti-RNP in the presence of high ANA titer: ≥ 1600) and - 3 of the following criteria: hands swelling, Raynaud's, acrosclerosis, myositis, synovitis.
Prognosis	Usually good: 10 year survival: 82 %, depending on the involved organs. Causes of mortality: pulmonary hypertension, CNS complications (rare). Can differentiate into SLE or scleroderma.
Treatment	According to involved organs (see SLE and scleroderma).

Undifferentiated Connective Tissue Disease (UCTD)

Not corresponding to any specific connective tissue disease (for now).

Appendix: Some Serologic Tests in Rheumatology.

None of the following laboratory tests is in itself entirely specific or diagnostic of an autoimmune disease. Consequently, ordering tests must be based on **a reasonable clinical suspicion**.

ANA (anti-nuclear antibody):

When to order: Clinical suspicion of connective tissue disease.

Remember:	Titer	Prevalence in normal population
	1 : 40	30 %
	1 : 80	10 - 12 %
	1 : 160	5 – 7 %
	1 : 320	3 %
	1 : 640	≤ 1 %

    So, interpretation must be based on clinical findings.

Clinical associations (sensitivity):
- Useful for diagnosis: SLE: ≥ 95 %; drug-induced lupus: 100 %; mixed connective tissue disease: 95-100 %; scleroderma: 90-95 %; Sjögren: 75 %; Poly/dermatomyositis 40-80 %.
- Less useful for diagnosis: Discoid lupus: 15 %; autoimmune hepatitis: 50-100 %; other autoimmune diseases: Hashimoto/Graves' disease thyroiditis: 45-50 %; rheumatoid arthritis: 40 %.

False positive: technical error (repeat test if needed); age (prevalence increases with age); infectious diseases, cancers.

False negative: anti-Ro/SSa antibodies (SLE, Sjögren), and anti Jo-1 (polymyositis) sometimes yield negative ANA; technical error (repeat test if needed).

Specific auto-antibodies:
- Anti ds-DNA: SLE: 70 %.
- Anti-Sm: SLE: 15-30 %.
- Anti U_1 –RNP: SLE: 45 %; mixed connective tissue disease: 95-100 %; Scleroderma 20 %; Sjögren 5-60 %.
- Anti Ro: SLE: 40 %; Sjögren: 60-80 %; neonatal lupus, congenital heart block; sub-acute cutaneous lupus, photosensitivity.
- Anti La: SLE: 15 %; Sjögren: 40-60 % (congenital heart block (in association with anti Ro)
- Anti topoisomerase I: Diffuse scleroderma: 15-40 %
- Anticentromere: Limited scleroderma: 20-50 %.
- Anti Jo-1: autoimmune myositis: 20-30 %.
- Anti histones: more or less useful clinically. Positive in >= 95 % of drug-induced lupus. Also present in ≥ 50 % of SLE, thus cannot discriminate between the two.

ANCA:

When to order: suspicion of ANCA associated vasculitis (Wegener, microscopic polyangiitis (MPA), Churg-Strauss syndrome (CSS), glomerulonephritis (GN).
- **First step:** immunofluorescence: peripheral pattern (pANCA) or cytoplasmic (cANCA).
- **2nd step:** Search for antigenic target: myeloperoxidase (MPO) or proteinase 3 (PR3) (usually be ELISA).

cANCA/anti-PR3: suggesting Wegener's; pANCA/anti-MPO: suggesting MPA, CSS, GN, or Wegener's:
- Double positivity of ANCA and its corresponding antigenic target confers a specificity of around 98 % for the diagnosis of ANCA associated vasculitis, **in an appropriate clinical context.**

ANCA present in up to 90 % Wegener's, 70 % PAM, 30-50 % CSS, 80 % pauci-immune GN.

Note: Poor correlation between antibody titer and disease activity.

Rheumatoid factor:

When to order: suspicion of rheumatoid arthritis (RA), Sjögren, cryoglobulinemia.

Positive; if titer ≥ 40 UI/mL.

Note: Only 50-75 % of RA are seropositive during the first year.

False positive: age, infections, cancer.

Anti-CCP:

Rheumatoid arthritis: specificity: > 95 %; sensitivity: 40-50 % for recent onset RA.

When to order: clinical suspicion of rheumatoid arthritis. Prognostic utility?

Vasculitis

Large-Vessel Vasculitis (Aorta and Its Major Branches)

Giant Cell (Temporal) Arteritis

Pathology	Granulomatous arteritis of large and medium-sized vessels (aorta, its major branches and arteries of the head, mostly extracranial.
Clinical findings	Age > 50. Average age = 74 years old. Associated polymyalgia rheumatica in 40 % (see below). Scalp tenderness, headache (frontal, temporal or occipital), ocular symptoms (partial or complete loss of vision, amaurosis fugax, diplopia, visual hallucinations,), jaw or tongue claudication, fever of unknown origin, weight loss, limb claudication, mono or polyneuropathy, TIA, CVA, respiratory symptoms (cough, hoarseness, sore throat) Aortitis or aneurysm ± dissection in up to 20 % in the long term. Rare: brachial plexus neuralgia secondary to ischemic radiculopathy. On physical examination: temporal arteries: tenderness, redness, nodularity swelling, weak pulse, bruit. In up to 35 %, temporal arteries are normal on examination. Ophthalmoscopy: search for papilloedema, papillary pallor, cottonwool spots, exudates; Asymmetry of peripheral pulses and blood pressure, listen for murmur of aortic regurgitation. Differential diagnosis: tension headache and other types of headache, atherosclerosis, retinal embolism, amyloidosis, other systemic vasculitides, thyroid disorder, cancer (renal cell carcinoma, multiple myeloma)
Diagnostic criteria	American College of Rheumatology criteria: Diagnosis if ≥ 3 criteria (sensitivity 93 %, specificity 91 %): - Age of onset ≥ 50 years - New headache - Temporal artery signs - Increased erythrocyte sedimentation rate (≥ 50 mm/h) by Westergren method - Abnormal temporal artery biopsy. Note: These criteria are only guidelines. Temporal artery biopsy MUST be done if there is a clinical suspicion.
Workup	ESR (normal in 20 %). C-reactive protein, CBC, electrolytes, creatinine, AST, ALT, alkaline phosphatase, ECG. Temporal artery biopsy (3 to 5 cm on symptomatic side). Contralateral biopsy as needed (usually not necessary although controversial). Temporal artery Doppler ultrasound may show a "halo": diagnostic value is operator-dependant, and, thus, more or less sensitive and specific in most centres. Angiography of major vessels: if needed. Chest X-ray every year for 10 years, to rule out thoracic aortic aneurysm.
Treatment	Prednisone 40-60 mg daily for 1 month. If clinical improvement ± ↓ ESR → ↓ 10 % every 2-4 weeks down to 10 mg daily (maintenance dose), then ↓ 1 mg each month. If clinical relapse ↑ 10 mg for 2-4 weeks; then, weaning resumes. Methylprednisolone 1g IV daily x 3 days if recent or imminent loss of vision. Average duration of treatment ≈ 2 years. Then follow-up after 6 months-1 year. Relapses are common (50 %). If steroid tapering is difficult or if there are complications of steroids: consider Methotrexate (7.5-20 mg/week). ASA 80 mg daily for all (less ischemic complications reported). Osteoporosis prophylaxis.

Polymyalgia Rheumatica

Pathology	Inflammatory disease often associated with temporal arteritis. Polymyalgia rheumatica occurs in 40% of temporal arteritis. 15% of patients with polymyalgia rheumatica develop temporal arteritis. Symptoms caused by bursitis, tenosynovitis and/or synovitis of proximal joints.
Clinical findings	Symmetric bilateral aching in the shoulder and hip girdles > 4 weeks. Morning stiffness, systemic symptoms and rapid response to steroids (almost diagnostic). Occasionally distal symptoms (asymmetric non erosive arthritis, carpal tunnel syndrome, edema over the hands and wrists). Look for symptoms of temporal arteritis. Differential diagnosis: rheumatoid arthritis (more peripheral manifestations), SLE (look for systemic manifestations), RS3PE (remitting seronegative symmetric synovitis with pitting edema) (mainly upper limbs), seronegative spondyloarthropathy (look for axial manifestations, younger patients), fibromyalgia, bacterial endocarditis, solid or hematologic (myeloma) cancer, toxic or infectious myositis, systemic amyloidosis
Workup	Routine workup. ESR (may be normal in 7-20 %), C-reactive protein, CK, TSH. Ultrasound or MRI may show subacromial or deltoid bursitis. Temporal artery biopsy only if temporal arteritis is suspected on clinical grounds. Chest X-ray on initial evaluation.
Treatment	Prednisone 15-20 mg daily, ↓ by 2.5 mg every 3-4 weeks down to 10 mg (maintenance dose), then ↓ 1 mg q 1 month. Treat for 1 year or more, according to clinical response. Follow-up 6 months to 1 year post treatment. Classically rapid response to steroids in 3-7 days. Osteoporosis prophylaxis. Frequent relapses.

Takayasu's Arteritis

Pathology	Granulomatous inflammation of the aorta and its major branches. May also affect pulmonary arteries.
Clinical findings	Female preponderance (4:1 ratio). Age < 50. Systemic symptoms, heart failure (hypertension, aortic regurgitation), mesenteric ischemia, limb claudication, stroke. 20 % monophasic course, without relapse; 80 % progressive course, with relapses and remissions.
Workup	Blood pressure in 4 limbs. Routine workup. ESR, C-reactive protein. Evaluate extension (systemic and pulmonary circulation): MRI/MR-Angio or CT/CT-Angio. Evaluate disease activity with MRI/angio or CT/angio or PET scan preferably if available. Angiography (for stenosis and aneurysms): if revascularization procedures needed or to evaluate central BP if peripheral BP not reliable.
Treatment	Prednisone ± immunosuppressants if no improvement or if steroid dependance. Revascularization procedures (surgical or endovascular) for symptomatic stenosis/occlusions or progressive aneurysms. Osteoporosis prophylaxis.

Medium-Sized-Vessel Vasculitis (Small and Medium-Sized Arteries)	
Polyarteritis Nodosa	
Pathology	Necrotizing inflammation of small and medium-sized arteries. Idiopathic or secondary (to HBV, HCV, HIV, hairy cell leukemia). Prevalence: ≈ 30/1 000 000.
Clinical findings	Constitutional symptoms (fever, weight loss, myalgia, arthritis). Skin involvement (livedo reticularis, digital ischemia, ulcerations, subcutaneous nodules). Renal (hypertension, renal failure, proteinuria). Gastrointestinal (pain, bleeding, pancreatitis, bowel ischemia/infarction/perforation). Neurological (mononeuritis multiplex, stroke). Cardiac (coronary vasculitis). Scleritis, testicular infarction Note: significant negatives: no pulmonary involvement, no glomerulonephritis, ANCA negative.
Workup	Routine workup. ANCA. Fundi. Biopsy of muscle, nerve, testicle, liver, kidney, skin…depending on involvement. Serology for HBV, HCV, HIV. Abdominal angiography: mesenteric, renal, celiac trunk: aneurysms.
Treatment	Prednisone 1 mg/kg/day, taper over 6-12 months. Add cyclophosphamide: if ≥ 1 factor of the five factor score (FFS): heart, CNS, severe gastro-intestinal involvement, renal involvement (with proteinuria > 1 g/day or creatinine > 140 µmol/L) or no response. For HBV-related PAN: plasma exchange and anti-HBV agents (interferon α or lamivudine); steroids for severe manifestations of vasculitis.
Kawasaki's Syndrome	

Clinical findings	Childhood disease: 80 % < 4 years.
	Criteria :
	  1) Fever lasting ≥ 5 days
	  2) Bilateral conjunctival injection
	  3) Lips and mouth : redness, "strawberry" tongue, erythema of mucous membranes
	  4) Hands and feet : first redness and edema, then desquamation of fingers tips
	  5) Rash
	  6) Cervical lymphadenopathy (usually unique and ≥ 1.5 cm)
	Diagnosis if 5 of 6 criteria including fever.
	Mucocutaneous symptoms + lymphadenopathy. Associated with coronary vasculitis that may progress to aneurysms.

Treatment	ASA 100 mg/kg/day until fever resolves followed by 3-5 mg/kg/day for 6-8 weeks. Intravenous immunoglobulins 2g/kg x 1 (repeat if necessary).
Small-Vessel Vasculitis (Arterioles, Capillaries, Post-Capillary Venules)	
Wegener's Granulomatosis	
Pathology	Granulomatous inflammation involving the respiratory tract and systemic necrotizing vasculitis.
Clinical findings	Begins at any age. Involves upper respiratory tract in 90 % (sinusitis, otitis media, subglottic stenosis), eyes (anterior uveitis, scleritis), lungs in 80 % (cough, hemoptysis, dyspnea, granuloma), kidneys (80 % will develop glomerulonephritis), arthritis, mononeuritis multiplex, purpuric rash.

Workup	Routine workup. C-ANCA (anti-PR3) ⊕ > 90 % with diffuse disease; less frequent if limited disease. Chest X-ray, thoracic CT scan, urinary sediment. Sinus and orbit CT scans for all patients at presentation. Biopsy of involved tissue (upper airways, lungs, kidneys).
Treatment	Prednisone (1 mg/kg) for 1 month and taper over 6-12 months + cyclophosphamide PO (2 mg/kg: take into account renal function) or IV pulse 0.6 g/m^2 on day 0, 15, 30 then every 3 weeks for 3-6 months, for life-threatening disease, until clinical remission. Switch to methotrexate (MTX) or azathioprine after the acute episode. Prednisone + MTX if not initially life-threatening. TMP-SMX to prevent Pneumocystis infection. Only indication as monotherapy: ENT manifestations (controversial). For refractory disease: consider rituximab. Plasmapheresis: for patients with creatinine ≥ 500 μmol/L or dialysis-dependent at initial presentation. Relapses: 50 %. Need for lifelong follow-up.

Churg-Strauss Syndrome

Pathology	Eosinophil-rich granulomatous inflammation with necrotizing vasculitis.
Clinical findings	Asthma, hypereosinophilia, vasculitis. Constitutional manifestations, involves skin, gastrointestinal tract, kidneys, prostate, lungs, mononeuritis multiplex, heart (#1 cause of mortality).
Workup	Eosinophilia > 1.5 x 10^9/L. Routine workup + ECG, echocardiography. Urinary sediment, chest X-ray ± thoracic CT scan. Biopsy of involved tissue. P-ANCA/anti-MPO ⊕ 30-70 %.
Treatment	Stop leukotriene receptor antagonists if previously used. Prednisone: 1 mg/kg, taper over several months. Immunosuppressants (cyclophosphamide) for severe disease; see FFS for polyarteritis nodosa above. Relapses: 25%.

Microscopic Polyangiitis

Pathology	Necrotizing vasculitis affecting small vessels, and sometimes small and medium-sized arteries.
Clinical findings	Pulmonary and renal disease. Palpable purpura, mononeuritis multiplex, peripheral neuropathy. Focal segmental necrotizing glomerulonephritis.
Workup	P-ANCA (anti-MPO) ⊕ > 80 %. Urinalysis and urinary sediment, chest X-ray. Thoracic CT-scan, biopsy of involved organs.
Treatment	Similar to Wegener's. Plasmapheresis: for patients with creatinine ≥ 500 μmol/L or dialysis-dependant at initial presentation. Plasmapheresis may also be an option for pulmonary hemorrhage, if severe presentation. Relapse: 35-40 %.

Henoch-Schölein Purpura	
Pathology	Vasculitis with IgA deposits affecting small vessels.
Clinical findings	Mostly childhood disease. Arthralgias, arthritis, purpura of lower limbs, gastrointestinal involvement (abdominal pain, bleeding), renal disease (hematuria, acute renal failure rare)
Workup	Routine workup. Normal complement. Urinary sediment. Biopsy + immunofluorescence of affected organs.
Treatment	No specific treatment besides stopping the offending drug or treating the associated infection. Prednisone for severe disease. IV immunoglobulins ?
Cryoglobulinemic Vasculitis	
Pathology	Vasculitis associated with cryoglobulin immune deposits involving small vessels.
Clinical findings	Essential mixed cryoglobulinemia if no underlying disease (Brouet type 2). Association with HCV, HBV, endocarditis, lymphoproliferative disease (lymphoma, Waldenström, rare with myeloma), connective tissue diseases. Lower extremity rash, arthralgias/arthritis, weakness, glomerulonephritis in 50 %, polyneuropathies, secondary Sjögren's or Raynaud's.
Workup	Cryoglobulins, CBC, AST, ALT, serum and urinary protein electrophoresis. Search for HCV, HBV, rheumatoid factor ⊕ 70-80 %. Low complement (mostly C4). Biopsy and immunofluorescence of affected tissues. Search for cancer, connective tissue diseases, infections.
Treatment	Steroids ± immunosuppressants ± plasma exchange. Interferon/ribavirin if hepatitis C.
Cutaneous Leukocytoclastic Angiitis (Leukocytoclastic Vasculitis)	
Clinical findings	Isolated cutaneous vasculitis. Drug-induced +++ (antibiotics, NSAIDs, allopurinol, propylthiouracil, thiazides, anticonvulsants), infection, systemic diseases (connective tissues diseases, paraproteinemia, cancer). If palpable purpura: look for possible gastrointestinal, renal and systemic involvement.
Workup	CBC, ESR, CRP, creatinine, urinalysis and urinary sediment, complement, ANA, rheumatoid factor, ANCA, cryoglobulins, chest X-ray, liver enzymes, viral serologies (HBV, HCV, HIV). Search for cancer (serum and urinary protein electrophoresis, serum immunoelectrophoresis).
Treatment	According to etiology. Stop offending drug. Usually no other treatment except if recurrence or chronic: hydroxychloroquine, colchicine, dapsone, pentoxifylline, steroids.

Others	
Behçet's syndrome	Recurrent oral ulcers (essential for diagnosis), genital ulcers, uveitis, skin lesions (pathergy, erythema nodosum, folliculitis), CNS involvement, arthritis, arteritis (any sized vessels), thrombophlebitis Poor prognostic factors: male, young age Treatment: according to the affected organ: – Mucocutaneous: topical steroids, colchicine, dapsone, thalidomide, methotrexate. – Articular: colchicine, NSAIDs, methotrexate, azathioprine. – Eye: azathioprine, cyclosporine, cyclophosphamide, chlorambucil. For refractory cases: infliximab, interferon alpha. – CNS (vasculitis): steroids and (cyclophosphamide or chlorambucil). – Venous thrombosis: steroids ± immunosuppressants.
Isolated vasculitis of central nervous system	Diverse clinical presentations: Granulomatous angiitis of the CNS: 20 % of cases. Subacute to chronic presentation, with headache, confusion, altered level of consciousness, multifocal strokes. Benign angiopathy of the CNS (more appropriately renamed: Reversible Cererebral Vasoconstrictive Syndrome [RCVS]): 20 %: Women > Men, mean age 40 y.o., acute onset, headache, focal neurological event, arteriography ⊕. Other: presentations not corresponding to the above: presentation as cerebral mass lesion: majority of cases. Differential diagnosis: systemic vasculitides, infections, neoplasms, intravascular lymphoma, atherosclerotic disease, cocaine, malignant hypertension, preeclampsia. Diagnosis: – Arteriography (if RCVS: ⊕ in 100 %; if granulomatous angiitis: ⊕ in only 20-40 %). – MRI: multifocal ischemic areas, white and gray matter. – Lumbar puncture – Brain biopsy. Treatment: granulomatous angiitis = steroids + cyclophosphamide; RCVS = short course steroids + calcium channel blockers.
Thromboangiitis obliterans (Buerger's disease)	Not a true vasculitis: rather an inflammatory thrombotic condition. Affects male smokers < 50 years: claudication, digital ischemia, migratory superficial thrombophlebitis 40%. Arterial and venous involvement (mostly distal). Allen test sometimes ⊕. Diagnosis: arteriography of involved limbs: 100% have > 1 limb involvement; if non-diagnostic, study unaffected limbs. ESR normal. Characteristic histology (inflammatory thrombus). Rule out autoimmune diseases, polyarteritis nodosa, diabetes, hypercoagulable states and embolic disease. Treatment : stop smoking
Pseudovasculitis	Always consider in the differential diagnosis of systemic vasculitis. Embolism: cholesterol, myxoma, endocarditis Meningococcemia, gonococcemia, antiphospholipid syndrome and other prothrombotic disorders, Trousseau's syndrome, thrombotic thrombocytopenic purpura, intravascular lymphoma, Goodpasture's syndrome, drugs

Useful References: RHEUMATOLOGY

Introduction to rheumatology: CMAJ 2000; 162: 1011-6: 1157-63: 1318-25: 1577-83: 1833-8.
            CMAJ 2000; 163: 176-83: 417-23: 721-8: 999-1005: 1285-91.
            CMAJ 2001; 164: 223-227: 1182-7: 1459-68: 1595-1601.
            CMAJ 2001; 165: 45-50.
            Arthritis Rheum 1996; 39: 1-8.

Acute Monoarthritis: CMAJ 2009; 180: 59-65 (review article)
ANCA: Arthritis Rheum 1998; 41: 1521-37 (review article)
Ankylosing Spondylitis: Lancet 2007; 369: 1379-90 (review article)
         Ann Rheum Dis 2006; 65: 423-32 (consensus)
Antinuclear Antibody (ANA):
         Arthritis Rheum (Arthritis Care Research) 2004; 47: 128-139 (review article)
Behçet's Disease: N Engl J Med 1999; 341: 1284-91 (review article)
         Best Pract Res Clin Rheumatol 2004; 18: 291-311 (review article)
Cryoglobulinemic Vasculitis: Arthritis Rheum 1999; 42: 2507-16 (review article)
      … and Hepatitis C : Arthritis Rheum 2002; 46: 585-97 (review article)
Fibromyalgia: JAMA 2004; 292: 2388-95 (review article)
         Curr Opin Rheumatol 2007; 19: 111-117 (review article)
      … Treatment: Am J Med 2008; 121: 555-61 (review article)
Giant Cell Arteritis: N Engl J Med 2002; 347: 261-71 (review article)
         Ann Intern Med 2003; 139: 505-15 (review article)
         Arthritis Rheum (Arthritis Care Research) 2004; 51: 128-139 (review article)
Gout: N Engl J Med 2003; 349: 1647-55 (review article)
         Am J Med 2007; 120: 221-24 (review article)
         Ann Rheum Dis 2006; 65: 1301-11 & 1312-24 (Guidelines)
Immunosuppressants and Pregnancy: Arthritis Rheum 1995; 38: 1722-32 (review article)
Laboratory tests in rhumatology: Am J Med 1996; 100 (suppl 2a): 16-23 (review article)
         CMAJ 2000; 162: 1157-63 (review article)
Low Back Pain: N Engl J Med 2001; 344: 363-370 (review article)
         Med Clin N Am 2009; 93: 477-501 (review article)
      … Diagnosis and Treatment : Ann Intern Med 2007; 147: 478-491 (ACP Guidelines)
      … Nonpharmacological Treatment : Ann Intern Med 2007; 147: 492-504 (review article)
      … Pharmacologic Treatment : Ann Intern Med 2007; 147: 505-514 (review article)
Marfan Syndrome: Circulation 2008; 117: 2802-13 (review article)
Microscopic Polyangiitis: Arthritis Rheum 2001; 44: 666-75 (review article)
Neck Pain: Med Clin N Am 2009; 93: 273-284 (review article)
Osteoarthrosis : Ann Intern Med 2000; 133: 635-46 & 726-37 (review article)
         Arthritis Rheum 2000; 43: 1905-15 (American Guidelines on medical treatment of osteoarthritis of the hip
            and knee)
         Lancet 1997; 35: 503-8 (review article)
         Ann Rheum Dis 2004; 63: 117-122 (review article)
         Ann Rheum Dis 2000; 59: 936-44 (European Guidelines on knee osteoarthritis treatment)
      … Hip: N Engl J Med 2007; 357: 1413-21 (review article)
Osteopenia: N Engl J Med 2007; 356: 2293-300 (review article)
Osteoporosis: J Obstet Gynaecol Can 2006; 28: S111-S132 (Canadian Guidelines)
         JAMA 2001; 285: 785-95 (American consensus)
         Mayo Clin Proc 2006; 81: 662-72 (review article)
         N Engl J Med 2005; 353: 595-603 (review article)
         Can Assoc Radiol J 2005; 56: 178-88 (Bone Densitometry Interpretation Guidelines)
            Screening: Ann Intern Med 2002; 137: 526-41 (American Guidelines)
                      N Engl J Med 2005; 353: 164-71 (review article)
      … Glucocorticoid-Induced Osteoporosis:
            Arthritis Rheum 2001; 44: 1496-503 (American Guidelines)
            Curr Opin Rheum 2007; 19: 370-75 (review article)
      … Osteoporosis in Men: N Engl J Med 2008; 358: 1474-82 (review article)
      … Treatment: Ann Intern Med 2008; 149: 404-15 (ACP Guidelines)
Paget's Disease of Bone: Lancet 2008; 372: 155-63 (review article)
Polyarteritis Nodosa: JAMA 2002; 288: 1632-39 (review article)
Polymyalgia Rheumatica: N Engl J Med 2002; 347: 261-71 (review article)
         Ann Intern Med 2003; 139: 505-15 (review article)
Polymyalgia Rheumatica and Temporal Arteritis: Lancet 2008; 372: 234-45 (review article)
Polymyositis and Dermatomyositis: Lancet 2003; 362: 971-82 (review article)
Pregnancy and Rheumatology: Ann Rheum Dis 2006; 65 (Suppl III): iii58-60 (review article)
Psoriasis Arthritis: Arthritis Rheum 2007; 56: 1051-66 (review article)

Rheumatoid Arthritis: Arthritis Rheum 2002; 46: 328-46 (American Guidelines)
        Lancet 2009; 373: 659-72 (review article)
        Treatment: Arthritis Rheum 2008; 59: 762-84 (American Guidelines)
                Lancet 2007; 370:1861-74 (review article)
Scleroderma: Rheum Dis Clin N Am 2003; 29: 211-439 (review article)
Systemic Lupus Erythematosus: Lancet 2007; 369: 587-96 (review article)
        Arthritis Rheum 1999; 42: 1785-96 (Guidelines)
Thromboangeitis obliterans (Buerger's disease): N Engl J Med 2000; 343: 864-69 (review article)
Vasculitis: Lancet 1997; 349: 553-58 (review article)
        N Engl J Med 1997; 337: 1512-23 (review article)
        Rheum Dis Clin N Am 2001; 27: 677- (review article)
    ... ANCA-Associated - Treatment: JAMA 2007; 298: 655-669 (review article)
    ... Diagnostic Approach:
                Best Practice Research Clin Rheum 2001; 15: 203-33 (review article)
                Curr Opinion Rheumatol 2001; 13: 23-34 (review article)

Chapter 11

Appendix

Non-Steroidal Anti-inflammatory Drugs

Agent	Commercial Name (exemple)	Caplet	Initial dose	Usual dose (ad max)	Comments
Celecoxib	Celebrex	100 mg 200 mg	100 mg bid or 200 mg od	200 mg bid.	Cox 2 specific. Indicated for OA et RA (bid for RA). Contraindicated if allergies to sulfas. Precautions if CAD
Diclofenac	Voltaren	Regular ; 25-50 mg SR 75-100 mg.	75 mg/day	150 mg/day.	Regular, long-action.
	Arthrotec (combined with misoprostol) Arthrotec 50; 50mg diclofenac + 200mg misoprostol. Arthrotec 75; 75 mg diclofenac + 200mg misoprostol.			Arthrotec 50 1 co tid. Arthrotec 75 1 co bid.	Suppositories available (50-100 mg).
	Pennsaid (topic)	Drops 1.5%	40 drops qid		Indicated for osteoarthritis of the knee Also used for treatment of superficial musculoskeletal pain.
	Voltaren emulgel	1.16% gel	2 to 4 g (covers 400-800 cm^2)		Indicated for treatment of superficial musculoskeletal pain
Diflunisal		250 mg 500 mg	250 mg bid	500 mg bid.	
Etodolac	Apo-E	200 mg 300 mg	200 mg bid	1000 mg/day.	
Flurbiprofen	Ansaid Froben	50 mg 100 mg	50 mg qid	300 mg/day in fractionated doses	
Ibuprofen	Motrin Advil	200 mg (Advil) 300 mg 400 mg 600 mg (Motrin)	1200 mg in 3-4 doses	2400 mg/day.	Suspension Advil.
Indomethacin	Indocid	25 mg 50 mg	25 mg bid-tid	150-200 mg/day.	Suppositories available (50-100 mg).
Ketoprofen		50 mg 100 mg SR 200 mg/day 150 mg 200 mg	100 mg bid	150-200 mg/day.	Suppositories available (50-100 mg).

Ketorolac	Toradol	10 mg		40 mg/day PO. 120 mg IM.	Intramuscular route.
Mefenamic acid	Apo-Mefenamic	250 mg	Start with 500 mg, then 250 mg q 6 h.	1000 mg/day	Formely Ponstan
Meloxicam	Mobicox	7.5 and 15 mg	7.5-15 mg od	7.5-15 mg od	Indicated in OA and RA. Precautions if CAD
Nabumetone	Relafen	500 mg 750 mg	1000 mg	2000 mg/day.	
Naproxen	Naprosyn	125 mg 250 mg 375 mg 500 mg SR 750 mg (Naprosyn)	500 mg	1000 mg/day.	Suppositories available (500 mg). Suspension
Oxaprozine	Daypro	600 mg	600-1200 mg/day	1800 mg/day in 2 doses.	
Piroxicam		10 mg 20 mg	10 mg bid or 20 mg od	10 mg bid or 20 mg od.	Suppositories available (20 mg).
Salsalate		500 mg 750 mg		750 mg 2 co bid.	
Sulindac	Clinoril	150 mg 200 mg			
Tenoxicam		20 mg	20 mg od	20 mg/day.	
Tiaprofenic acid	Surgam	300 mg SR 300 mg	300 mg	600 mg/day in 2 doses.	

Inhaled Bronchodilators

Agent	Commercial name	Concentration	Forms	Initial dose ad max. chronic treatment	Comments
β_2-agonists :					
Side effects: tachycardia, hypokalemia, tremors.					
Fenoterol	Berotec	100 mcg/inh.	Metered-dose inhaler	1-2 inh. PRN	
Formoterol	Foradil	12 mcg/capsule	Dry-powder inhaler	12 mcg bid	Long-action β_2-agonist with quick onset
	Oxeze Turbuhaler	6 et 12 mcg/inh.			
Salbutamol	Ventolin	100 mcg/inh.	Metered-dose inhaler	2 inh. PRN	HFA: without CFC
	Airomir (salbutamol HFA)	100 mcg/inh.	Metered-dose inhaler		
	Ventodisk Diskus	200 and 400 mcg per blister	Dry-powder inhaler	1-2 blisters or rotacaps PRN	
Salmeterol	Serevent Diskus	50 mcg/inh.	Dry-powder inhaler	1 inh. bid	Long-action β_2-agonist
Terbutaline	Bricanyl Turbuhaler	0.5 mg/inh.	Dry-powder inhaler	1 inh. PRN	

Anti-allergic agent					
Side effects: dryness of the throat, dysgeusia.					
Cromoglycate	Apo-Cromolyn	10 mg/mL	Nebulisation	20 mg tid-qid	Before an effort or an allergic contact. Rarely used.
Anticholinergics					
Side effects: dryness of the throat, constipation, tachycardia, atrial fibrillation, blurred vision, glaucoma, urinary retention, headache, dysgeusia.					
Ipratropium	Atrovent HFA	20 mcg/inh.	Metered-dose inhaler	2-4 inh. qid	Rarely used.
Tiotropium	Spiriva	18 mcg/inh.	Dry-powder inhaler	1 inh. od	Not indicated for asthma

Inhaled Corticosteroids

Agent	Commercial name	Concentration per inhalation	Forms	Initial dose ad max.	Equivalent dose
Side effects : Oral candidiasis, hoarseness, inhibition of the hypothalamic-pituitary axis, osteoporosis					
Interaction between fluticasone and ritonavir.					
Beclomethasone	Qvar (without CFC)	50 and 100 mcg	Metered-dose inhaler	100-500 mcg/day bid	500 mcg
Budesonide	Pulmicort Turbuhaler	100, 200 and 400 mcg	Dry-powder inhaler	200-800 mcg bid	400 mcg
Ciclesonide	Alvesco	100 and 200 mcg	Metered-dose inhaler	100-800 mcg in 1-2 takes	160 mcg
Fluticasone	Flovent	50, 125 and 250 mcg	Metered-dose inhaler	125-500 mcg/day bid	250 mcg
	Flovent Diskus	50, 100, 250 et 500 mcg	Dry-powder inhaler		

Combinations

Agent	Commercial name	Concentration per inhalation	Forms	Initial dose ad max.
Budenoside + formoterol	Symbicort turbuhaler	100 / 6 mcg (budenoside + formoterol) 200 / 6 mcg	Dry-powder inhaler	1-2 inh. bid
Salmeterol + fluticasone	Advair Diskus	100 / 50 mcg (salmeterol / fluticasone) 250 / 50 mcg 500 / 50 mcg	Dry-powder inhaler	1 inh. bid

Systemic Anticoagulants

Agent	Commer-cial name	Prophylactic dose	Treatment dose	T1/2 (h)	Comments
Heparin	Hepalean	5000 U s/c q 8-12 h.	60-80 U/kg bolus and 12-18 U/kg/h IV depending on the indication (or fixed-dose s/c).	0.5-3	Adjust according to aPTT or heparinemia.

Low-molecular-weight heparin					
Dalteparin	Fragmin	5000 U s/c q 24h.	100 U/kg q 12h 200 U/kg q 24h Unstable angina 120 U/kg q 24h	2-5	Can accumulate in renal failure with treatment doses. Prophylactic dosing appears safe.
Enoxaparin	Lovenox	40 mg s/c q 24h. 30 mg s/c q 12h.	1 mg /kg q 12h 1.5 mg/kg q 24h	2.2-6	Can accumulate in renal failure
Nadroparin	Fraxiparin	2850 U q 24h.	171 U/kg q 24h Unstable angina 86 U/kg q12h	2.2-3.5	Can accumulate in renal failure
Tinzaparin	Innohep	3500 U q 24h. 50 U/kg q 24h.	175 U/kg q 24h	1.4-1.9	Can accumulate in renal failure
Direct thrombin inhibitor					
Argatroban	Argatroban	N/A	2 mcg/kg/min	39-51 minutes	Reduce dose to 0.5 mcg/kg/min with hepatic dysfunction. Reduce dose to 0.5-1.2 mg/kg in patients with heart failure, multiple organ system failure, or severe anasarca or who are postcardiac surgery. Monitoring via aPTT.
Bivalirudin	Angiomax	N/A	0.1 mcg/kg bolus, puis 0.25 mcg/kg/h	25 minutes	Approved for patients with acute coronary syndrome undergoing PCI. Monitoring via aPTT.
Dabigatran	Pradax	220 mg od	N/A	8-17	Indication: elective hip or knee replacement surgery Renal elimination. Dose adjustments: 150 mg od if age > 75 or CrCl 30-50 mL/min. Contraindicated in renal failure (CrCl < 30 mL/min).
Lepirudin	Refludan	N/A	0.1 mg/kg/h	1.3	Reduce dose in renal failure. Monitoring via aPTT. Bolus dose of 0.2 mg/kg can be considered in life threatening situations.
Direct factor Xa inhibitor					
Rivaroxaban	Xarelto	10 mg od	N/A	9	Indication: elective hip or knee replacement surgery. Contraindicated in renal failure (CrCl < 30 mL/min).
Other agents					
Danaparoid	Orgaran	If < 90 kg : 750 U s/c bid-tid If > 90 kg 1250 U s/c bid or 750 U tid	1250-3750 U bolus, depending on weight, then 400 U/h X 4h, then 300 U/h X 4h, then 150-200 U/h	25	Can accumulate in renal failure Monitoring via anti-Xa levels.
Fondaparinux	Arixtra	2.5 mg od		17-21	Contraindicated in renal failure (CrCl < 30 mL/min).

N/A : not applicable

Anticonvulsants

Agent	Commercial name	Adult dose / day (mg)	Posology	T½ (h)	Indications				
					TC	Abs	M	Ato	P
Carbamazepin	Tegretol	200-1200	bid-qid	11-17	√				√
Clobazam	Frisium	5-80			√	√	√	√	√
Ethosuximide	Zarontin	500-1500	od-tid	15-68		√			
Gabapentin	Neurontin	900-1800	tid	5-7					√
Lamotrigine	Lamictal	25-700	bid	18-30					√
Levetiracetam	Keppra	500-1500	bid	6-8					√
Oxcarbamazepin	Trileptal	600-2400	bid-tid	8-10					√
Phenobarbital		60-250	od-bid	30-50	√				√
Phenytoin	Dilantin	300-600	od-tid	15-30					
Primidone	Mysolin	100-2000	od-tid	11-19	√				√
Topiramate	Topamax	50-1600	bid	18-23					√
Valproate	Epival	5-60 mg/kg/day	bid-tid	6-8	√	√	√	√	√
Vigabatrin	Sabril	1000-4000	od-bid	5-8					√

TC: Generalized tonic-clonic
Abs: Generalized absence
M: Generalized myoclonic
Ato: Generalized atonic
P: Partials, including simples, complexes and secondary generalized.

Oral Antihyperglycemic Agents

Agent	Commercial Name	Caplet	Initial dose	Maximum dose	Renal elimination
Sulfonylureas					
Side effects: hypoglycemia, weight gain. Less hypoglycemia with gliclazide and glimepiride.					
Glimepiride	Amaryl	1, 2 and 4 mg	1 mg od	8 mg od	Yes
Chlorpropamide	Diabenese	100 mg and 250 mg	100 mg od	500 mg od	Yes
Glyburide	Diabeta / Euglucon	2.5 mg and 5 mg	2.5 mg od	10 mg bid	Yes
Gliclazide	Diamicron Diamicron MR	80 mg 30 mg	80 mg od 30 mg od	160 mg bid 120 mg od	Yes
Tolbutamide	Orinase	500 mg	500 mg od	500 mg qid	No
Meglitinides					
Side effects: hypoglycemia, weight gain. Prolonged hypoglycemia with repaglinide + gemfibrozil combination. To take 0-30 minutes before meal					
Repaglinide	GlucoNorm	0.5, 1 and 2 mg	0,5 mg tid	4 mg qid	No
Nateglinide	Starlix	60, 120 and 180 mg	120 mg od	180 mg od	No
Biguanides					
Side effects: abdominal pain, diarrhea, nausea, metallic taste, lactic acidosis. Doesn't cause hypoglycemia. First choice in obese type 2 diabetic patients. Contraindicated in renal, hepatic or heart failure.					
Metformin	Glucophage	500 mg and 850 mg	500 mg od	850 mg tid	Yes
	Glumetza	500 mg	1000 mg od (at supper)	2000 mg od	Yes
Alpha-glucosidase inhibitors					
Side effects : feeling bloated, gas, diarrhea					
Acarbose	Prandase	50 mg and 100 mg	25 mg tid	100 mg tid	No

Digestive lipase inhibitors

Side effects: flatulence, gas, diarrhea. Possible interaction with digoxine.

Orlistat	Xenical	120 mg	120 mg tid	120 mg tid	No

Thiazolidinediones

Side effects: water retention with weight gain, edema or hemodilution (anemia).

↑ incidence of fractures.

Contraindicated in patients with any stage of heart failure.

TZD is not approved for use with metformin and a sulfonylurea.

When associated with insulin, can increase the risk or edema or heart failure. The combination of TZD and insulin is not recommended in Canada.

Rosiglitazone is no longer approved: A) in monotherapy, except when use of metformin is contraindicated or not tolerated, B) in association with a sulfonylurea except when use of metformin is contraindicated or not tolerated.

Pioglitazone	Actos	15 mg, 30 mg and 45 mg	15 mg od	45 mg od	No
Rosiglitazone	Avandia	2 mg, 4 mg and 8 mg	4 mg od	4 mg bid or 8 mg od	No

Incretins

Side effects: ↑ risk of nasopharyngitis, and infections of the upper respiratory tracts. Indicated: in association with metformin.

Sitagliptine	Januvia	100 mg	100 mg od		Yes

Combination

Metformin / Rosiglitazone	Avandamet	500 mg / 1 mg 500 mg / 2 mg 500 mg / 4 mg 1000 mg / 2 mg 1000 mg / 4 mg		2000 mg / 8 mg	Yes
Rosiglitazone/ glimepiride	Avandaryl	4 mg/ 1 mg 4 mg/ 2 mg 4 mg/ 4mg		8 mg/ 4 mg 4 mg/ 4 mg	Yes

Anti-Hypertensive/Anti-Anginal Agents

Agent	Commercial name	Caplet	Initial dose	Usual dose (ad max)	Comments
Nitrates					
Side effects: headaches. Contraindicated with phosphodiesterase type 5 inhibitors.					
	Imdur	60 mg	60 mg od	120 mg/d ad 240 mg/d	od posology should be respected to avoid tolerance
	Isorbide	5,10 and 30 mg	5 mg qid	30 mg qid	Duration of the effect: 4 to 6 hours. 12 hours periods without nitrates are needed to avoid tolerance
	Minitran	0.2, 0.4 and 0.6 mg/h	0.2 mg TO	0.8 mg TO	Application 12 hours per 24 hours to avoid tolerance.
	Nitro-Dur	0.2, 0.4, 0.6 and 0.8 mg/h	0.2 mg TO	0.8 mg TO	
	Transderm-Nitro	0.2, 0.4 and 0.6 mg/h	0.2 mg TO	0.8 mg TO	

β-blockers

Side effects: atrioventricular block, bradycardia, bronchospasm, heart failure, vasospasm, impotence, ↓ HDL, ↑ triglycerides, hypoglycemia unawareness, rebound hypertension.
Contraindicated if anaphylaxis, bronchospasm, high-degree atrioventricular block.

Agent	Commercial name	Caplet	Initial dose	Usual dose (ad max)	Comments
Acebutolol	Sectral Monitan Rhotral	100, 200 and 400 mg	100-200 mg bid	200-600 mg/day ad 800 mg/day < 400 mg/day =1 dose > 400 mg/day = 2 doses	β1-selective (< 800 mg) Intrinsic sympathomimetic activity Liposoluble Renal and hepatic elimination Adjust if CrCl < 50 mL/min
Atenolol	Tenormin	50 and 100 mg	25 mg od	100 ad 200 mg/day	β1-selective Renal elimination Adjust if CrCl < 35 mL/min
Bisoprolol	Monocor	5 and 10 mg	5 mg qod	10-20 mg od	β1-selective Renal and hepatic elimination Used in heart failure
Carvedilol	Coreg	3.125, 6.25, 12.5 and 25 mg	3.25 mg bid	double q 2 weeks ad 25 mg bid (> 85 kg ad 50 mg bid)	Hepatic elimination Indicated in heart failure
Labetalol	Trandate	100 and 200 mg	100 mg bid	200-400 mg bid ad 1200 mg bid	ratio α:β = 1 : 3 Liposoluble Hepatic elimination
Metoprolol	Metoprolol Lopresor Betaloc	25, 50 and 100 mg	25-100 mg bid	400 mg/day	β1-selective Hepatic elimination Liposoluble
	Lopresor SR Betaloc	100 mg and 200 mg	100 mg od	200 mg od	Used in heart failure
Nadolol	Corgard	40, 80 and 160 mg	40 mg od	ad 240-320 mg/day	Renal elimination Adjust if CrCl < 40 mL/min
Oxprenolol	Trasicor	40 mg	20 mg bid	120-320 mg/day ad 480 mg/day (bid when stable)	Intrinsic sympathomimetic activity Hepatic elimination
Pindolol	Visken	5,10 and 15 mg	2.5mg bid (HTN)	ad 40-45 mg/day (in 3 doses if > 30 mg/day)	Intrinsic sympathomimetic activity Hepatic > renal elimination Liposoluble
Propranolol	Propranolol	10, 20, 40 and 80 mg	10-40 mg bid	160-300 mg/day ad 320 mg/day in 3-4 doses	Hepatic elimination Liposoluble
	Inderal-LA	60, 80, 120 and 160 mg	60 mg od	320 mg od	
Sotalol	Sotacor	80 and 160 mg	40 mg bid	240-320 mg/day	Renal elimination Adjust if CrCl < 60 mL/min
Timolol	Blocadren	5, 10 and 20 mg	2.5-10 mg bid	ad 45-60 mg/day	Hepatic > renal elimination Liposoluble

Calcium Channel Blockers

Side effects: atrioventricular block, edema, headache, heart failure. Constipation associated with verapamil et diltiazem.

Hepatic elimination.

Agent	Commercial name	Caplet	Initial dose	Usual dose (ad max)	Comments
Non-dihydropyridine					
Diltiazem	Cardizem reg.	30 and 60 mg	30 mg qid	ad 240 mg/day	Bioavailability of Tiazac is 124 % that of Cardizem CD
	Diltiazem SR	60, 90 and 120 mg	60 mg bid	ad 360 mg/day	
	Cardizem CD Tiazac Tiazac XC	120, 180, 240, 300 and 360 mg	120 mg od	240 mg ad 360 mg/day	
Verapamil	Isoptin Isoptin-SR	80 and 120 mg	80 mg tid-qid	ad 480 mg/day	Contraindicated with lithium.
		120, 180 and 240 mg	120-240 mg od	ad 240 mg bid	
	Covera-HS	180 and 240 mg			
Dihydropyridine					
Amlodipine	Norvasc	5 and 10 mg	5 mg od (2.5 mg if hepatic dysfunction)	10 mg od	Safe in heart failure
Felodipine	Plendil Renedil	2.5, 5 and 10 mg	5 mg od (2.5 mg if hepatic dysfunction)	5-10 mg od ad 20 mg od	Safe in heart failure
Nifedipine	Adalat XL	20, 30 and 60 mg	30 mg	120 mg/day	Available with ASA 81 mg (Adalat XL PLUS)
	Apo-Nifed PA	10 and 20 mg			
	Apo-Nifed	5 and 10 mg			

Angiotensin II Receptor Blockers

Side effects: dizziness, acute renal failure, hyperkalemia.

Contraindicated in pregnancy.

Agent	Commercial name	Caplet	Initial dose	Usual dose (ad max)	Comments
Candesartan	Atacand	8, 16 and 32 mg	8 mg od	32 mg od	Renal elimination 60%
Eprosartan	Teveten	400 and 600 mg	600 mg od	800 mg od	Hepatic elimination 90%
Irbesartan	Avapro	75,150 and 300 mg	150 mg od	150-300 mg od	Hepatic elimination 80%
Losartan	Cozaar	25, 50 and 100 mg	50 mg od	100 mg od	Hepatic elimination 60%
Olmesartan	Olmetec	20 and 40 mg	20 mg od	40 mg od	Renal elimination 30-50%
Telmisartan	Micardis	40 and 80 mg	80 mg od	80 mg od	Stool elimination
Valsartan	Diovan	40, 80, 160 and 320 mg	80 mg od	160 mg od	Hepatic elimination 70%

Angiotensin-Converting Enzyme Inhibitors

Side effects: cough, acute renal failure, ↑ K^+, angioedema, dysgueusia, cutaneous eruptions, proteinuria, cytopenias.

Contraindicated in pregnancy.

Agent	Commercial name	Caplet	Initial dose	Usual dose (ad max)	Comments
Benazepril	Lotensin	5, 10 and 20 mg	10 mg od	20 mg od ad 40 mg od	Renal elimination 88 %
Captopril	Capoten	6.25, 12.5, 25, 50 and 100 mg	6.25-12.5 mg tid	25-50 mg tid ad 450 mg/day	Renal elimination
Cilazapril	Inhibace	1, 2.5 and 5 mg	N = 2.5 mg od > 65 years : 1.25 mg/day	2.5-5 mg/day ad 10 mg/day	Renal elimination
Enalapril	Vasotec	2.5, 5, 10 and 20 mg	5 mg od 2.5 mg od if CHF	ad 40 mg/day (1 or 2 doses) ad 20 mg/day if CHF	Renal elimination
Fosinopril	Monopril	10 and 20 mg	10 mg od	ad 40 mg/day (1 or 2 doses)	Renal 50 % and Hepatic 50 % elimination
Lisinopril	Prinivil Zestril	5, 10 and 20 mg	10 mg od 2,5 mg od if CHF	10-80 mg od ad 20 mg od if CHF	Renal elimination
Perindopril	Coversyl	2, 4 and 8 mg	2-4 mg od	4-8 mg od	Renal elimination
Quinapril	Accupril	5, 10, 20 and 40 mg	10 mg (1 or 2 doses)	10-20 ad 40 mg/day	Renal 60 % and Hepatic 40 % elimination
Ramipril	Altace	1.25, 2.5, 5 10 and 15 mg	2.5 mg od	2.5-10 mg od ad 20 mg od	Renal 60 % and Hepatic 40 % elimination
Trandolapril	Mavik	1, 2 and 4 mg	1 mg od	1-2 mg od ad 4 mg od	Hepatic 97 % Renal 33 % elimination

Diuretics

Side effects: electrolytic disturbances, ↑ LDL, ↑ triglycerides, ↑ uric acid, ↑ glucose.

Agent	Commercial name	Caplet	Initial dose	Usual dose (ad max)	Comments
Ethacrynic acid	Edecrin	25 mg	25 mg od	ad 200 mg/day	
Amiloride	Midamor	5 mg	2.5 mg od	5 mg	
Bumetanide	Burinex	1, 2 and 5 mg	0.5-2 mg/day	ad 10 mg/day	Hepatic and renal elimination
Chlortalidone	Hygroton	50 mg	HTN : 12.5 mg /day	50 mg/day	
Eplerenone	Inspra	25 et 50 mg	25 mg od	50 mg od	Renal elimination
Furosemide	Lasix	20, 40, 80 and 500 mg	20 mg bid	40 mg bid	Renal elimination
Hydrochlorothiazide	HydroDiuril	12.5, 25, and 50 mg	HTN : 12.5 mg od	50 mg/day	Renal elimination
Indapamide	Lozide	1.25 and 2.5 mg	1.25 mg od	2.5 mg od	Hepatic elimination
Metolazone	Zaroxolyn	2.5 mg	2.5-5 mg/day		Renal elimination
Spironolactone	Aldactone	25 and 100 mg	25 mg/day	500 mg/day	Renal elimination
Triamterene	Dyrenium	50 and 100 mg	100 mg bid	ad 300 mg/day	

Renin Inhibitor
Side effects: acute renal failure, hyperkalemia.
Contraindicated in pregnancy.

Agent	Commercial name	Caplet	Initial dose	Usual dose (ad max)	Comments
Aliskirene	Rasilez	150 and 300 mg	150 mg od	300 mg od	Renal elimination

α-blockers
Side effects: orthostatism, hypotension with 1st dose, headache, anticholinergic, ↓ prostatism, ↓ LDL, ↑ HDL.

Agent	Commercial name	Caplet	Initial dose	Usual dose (ad max)	Comments
Doxazocin	Cardura-1 Cardura-2 Cardura-4	1, 2 and 4 mg	1mg od	8 mg/day ad 16 mg/day	
Prazocin		1, 2 and 5 mg	0.5mg bid-tid	1 mg bid-tid ad 20 mg/day	
Terazocin	Hytrin	1, 2 and 5 mg	1 mg HS	↑ q weeks ad 1-5 mg od ad 20 mg od	

Endothelin Inhibitor
Side effects: Peripheral edema, dilutional anemia and hepatitis.
Contraindicated in pregnancy.

Agent	Commercial name	Caplet	Initial dose	Usual dose (ad max)	Comments
Ambrisentan	Volibris	5 and 10 mg	5 mg od	10 mg	Hepatic elimination.

Central Sympatholytics
Side effects : sedation, xerostomia, headache, rebound HTN

Agent	Commercial name	Caplet	Initial dose	Usual dose (ad max)	Comments
Clonidine	Catapress	0.1 and 0.2 mg	0.1 mg bid	ad 1.2 mg/day	
Methyldopa	Apo-Methyldopa	125, 250 and 500 mg	250 mg bid-tid x 48 h.	500 mg-2 g in 2-4x/day ad 3 g/day	1st choice for hypertension in pregnancy. Associated with hepatitis, fever and hemolytic anemia.

Central Vasodilators

Agent	Commercial name	Caplet	Initial dose	Usual dose (ad max)	Comments
Hydralazine		10, 25 and 50 mg	10 mg qid x 2-4 days, then 25 mg qid x 1 week, then 50 mg qid	50-200 mg/day	Drug-induced lupus.
Minoxidil	Loniten	2.5 and 10 mg	5mg bid	10-40 mg/day ad 100 mg/day	Hirsutism.

Combination			
Quinalapril / HCTZ	Accuretic (10/12.5 or 20/12,5 or 20/25 mg)	1 caplet od	2 caplets od
Spirololactone / HCTZ	Aldactazide (25/25 mg) Aldactazide 50 (50/50 mg)	25 mg/day	100 mg/day
Ramipril / HCTZ	Altace-HCT (2.5/12.5, 5/12.5, 10/12.5, 5/25, 10/25 mg)	2.5/12.5 mg od	20 mg ramipril and 50 mg HCTZ.
Methyldopa / HCTZ	Apo-Methazide (250/15 or 250/25 mg)	1 caplet od	ad 3 g methyldopa
Candesartan / HCTZ	Atacand plus (16/12.5 mg)	1 caplet od	1 caplet od
Irbesartan / HCTZ	Avalide (150/12.5, 300/12.5 mg or 300/25 mg)	1 caplet od (150/12.5)	1 caplet od (300/25)
Amlopidine /atorvastatine*	Caduet (5/10, 5/20, 5/40, 5/80, 10/10, 10/20, 10/40, 10/80 mg)	1 caplet 5/10 mg od	1 caplet 10/80 mg od
Perindopril / indapamide	Coversyl-plus (4/1.25 or 8/2.5 mg)	1 caplet od	1 caplet od
Valsartan / HCTZ	Diovan-HCT (80/12.5, 160/12.5 and 160/25 mg)	1 caplet od (80/12.5)	1 caplet od (160/25)
Triamterene / HCTZ	Apo-Triazide (50/25 mg)	½ caplet od	4 caplets od
HCTZ / losartan	Hyzaar (50/12.5 mg) or 100/12.5 mg) Hyzaar DS (100/25 mg)	1 caplet od	2 caplets bid
Cilazapril / HCTZ	Inhibace plus (5/12.5 mg)	1 caplet od	2 caplets od
Telmisartan / HCTZ	Micardis plus (80/12.5 mg or 80/25 mg)	1 caplet od	1 caplet od
Amiloride / HCTZ	Moduret (5/50 mg)	½ caplet od	4 caplet od or more
Olmesartan / HCTZ	Olmetec plus (20/12.5 mg or 40/12.5 mg or 40/25 mg)	1 caplet od	1 caplet od (40/25 mg)
Lisinopril / HCTZ	Prinzide or Zestoretic (10/12.5 or 20/12.5 or 20/25 mg)	1 caplet 10/12.5	ad 1 caplet 20/12.5 or 20/25
Verapamil / Trandolapril	Tarka (2/180 or 1/240 or 2/240 or 4/240 mg)	1 1/180 mg caplet	4 mg od of trandolapril or 240 mg bid of verapamil
Atenolol / Chlortalidone	Tenoretic (50/25 or 100/25 mg)	½ caplet od	1 caplet (100/25) od
Eprosartan / HCTZ	Teveten plus (600/12.5 mg)	1 caplet od (600/12.5)	
Timolol + HCTZ	Timolide (10/25 mg)	1 caplet od	2 caplets od
Enalapril / HCTZ	Vaseretic (5/12.5 or 10/25 mg)	1 caplet od (10/25)	2 caplets od
Pindolol / HCTZ	Viskazide (10/25 mg)	1 caplet (10/25)	ad 20/100
Lisinopril / HCTZ	Zestoretic (10/12.5 or 20/12.5 or 20/25 mg)	1 caplet (10/12.5 or 20/12.5 or 20/25)	

* Combination of anti-hypertensive and statin.

Benzodiazepines

Agent	Commer-cial name	Caplet	Usual dose (ad max.)	Equiva-lent dose	Half-life	Active metabo-lism	Half life metabol.
Alprazolam	Xanax	0.25, 0.5 and 1 mg	0.25 mg bid-tid ad 4 mg/day	0.5 mg	12-15 h.	No	-
Bromazepam	Lectopam	1.5, 3 and 6 mg	6-30 mg/day 1.5-6 mg HS	6 mg	20 h.	Yes	-
Chlordiazepoxide	Librium	5, 10 and 25 mg	15-100 tid-qid	10 mg	5-30 h.	Yes	24-96 h.
Clonazepam	Rivotril	0.25, 0.5, 1 and 2 mg	0.5-2 mg tid ad : 20 mg/day	1 mg	18-50 h.	No	-
Clorazepate	Tranxene	3.75, 7.5 and 15 mg	7.5 mg-15 mg bid-qid	7.5 mg	-	Yes	50-100 h.
Diazepam	Valium	2, 5 and 10 mg	2-10 mg bid-qid	5 mg	20-80 h.	Yes	50-100 h.
Flurazepam	Dalmane	15 and 30 mg	15-30 hs	15 mg	-	Yes	40-115 h.
Lorazepam	Ativan	0.5, 1 and 2 mg	0.5-2 mg bid-tid ad max 10 mg	1 mg	10-20 h.	No	-
Nitrazepam	Mogadon	5 and 10 mg	5-10 mg HS	5 mg	30-40 h.	No	-
Oxazepam	Serax	10, 15 and 30 mg	10-30 mg tid-qid 15-30 mg hs	15 mg	5-20 h.	No	-
Temazepam	Restoril	15 and 30 mg	15-30 mg hs	15 mg	10-40 h.	No	-
Triazolam	Halcion	0.125 and 0.25 mg	0.125-0.25 mg hs	0.25 mg	2-5 h.	No	-

Non-depolarizing Neuromuscular Blockers

Agent	Commer-cial name	Initial dose (mg/Kg)	Dura-tion (min)	Elimination	Active meta-bolites	Hepatic insuffi-ciency	Renal failure	Hypo-tension	Tachy-cardia
Cisatracurium	Nimbex	0.1-0.2	45-60	Hofmann	No	No	No	No	No
Atracurium	Tracurium	0.4-0.5	25-35	Hofmann	No but accumu-lates laudano-sine	No	No	+	No
Pancuronium	Pavulon	0.06-0.1	90-100	Hepatic/renal	Yes	↑	↑	No	+/++
Vecuronium	Norcuron	0.08-0.1	35-45	Hepatic/renal	Yes	↑	↑	No	No
Rocuronium	Zemuron	0.6-1	30	Hepatic	No	↑	Min	No	+

Hypolipidemic Agents

HMG-CoA reductase inhibitors (statins)

Clinical effects: Preferential lowering of LDL.
Side effects: gastrointestinal, headache, muscle aches. Rhabdomyolysis, mostly with combination with fibrates or with P450 cytochrome inhibitors.
Pravastatin and ASA combination available (PravASA 10-81, 20-81 and 40-81 mg).

Agent	Commercial name	Caplet	Initial dose	Maximal dose	Equivalent dose
Rosuvastatin	Crestor®	5, 10, 20, 40 mg	10 mg od	40 mg	2.5 mg
Atrovastatin	Lipitor®	10, 20, 40 and 80 mg	10 mg od	80 mg	5 mg
Fluvastatin	Lescol®	20, 40 and 80 mg	20 mg od	80 mg	40 mg
Lovastatin	Mevacor®	20 and 40 mg	20 mg od	80 mg	20 mg
Pravastatin	Pravachol®	10, 20 and 40 mg	10 mg od	40 mg	20 mg
Simvastatin	Zocor®	5, 10, 20, 40 and 80 mg	10 mg od	80 mg	10 mg

Fibrates

Effects: Preferential lowering of triglycerides and increase of HDL.
Gastrointestinal side effects. ↑ INR possible. Adjustment with CKD.

Agent	Commercial name	Caplet	Initial dose	Maximal dose
Bezafibrate	Bezalip®	200 mg (reg) and 400 mg SR	200 mg tid or 400 mg od SR	600 mg od
Fenofibrate	Lipidil Micro®	67 and 200 mg	67-267 mg od	267 mg od
	Lipidil Supra®	100 and 160 mg	160 mg	200 mg od
	Lipidil EZ®	48 and 145 mg	145 mg od / 48 mg od if CrCl < 30 mL/min.	145 mg od
Gemfibrozil	Lopid®	300 and 600 mg	600 mg bid	1500 mg od

Cholesterol Absorption Inhibitors

Effects: Preferential lowering of LDL (additive effect with statins).
Side effects: comparable with placebo.

Agent	Commercial name	Caplet	Initial dose	Maximal dose
Ezetimibe	Ezetrol®	10 mg	10 mg od	10 mg od
Niacin		Effects: Lowering of triglycerides and LDL, and increase of HDL. Important side effects: vasomotor bursts (reduced with ASA), cutaneous dryness, gastrointestinal, hyperglycemia, orthostatism... Careful with diabetics. Start with 50 mg HS (± ASA 325 mg 1 hour before), increase 50 mg every 7 days up to 100 mg tid. Take with food. Slow-releasing formula available (Niaspan®): start 500 mg od, increase 500 mg/day every 4 weeks up to 2000 mg/day.		
Biliary acid sequestering agents (resins)		Effects: Preferential lowering of LDL, but increase of triglycerides. Side effects: constipation. Decreases absorption of certain drugs. Not recommended with hypertriglyceridemia. – Cholestyramine: 4 g (1 package) 1-6/day. – Colestipol (Colestid®): posology in caplets 2-16 g/day: posology in granules 5-30 g/day. Start with minimal dose bid, and double q months ad required posology.		

Combination

Niacin / Lovastatin	Advicor®	500/20, 1000/20 and 1000/40 mg	500/20 mg od	1000/40 mg od

Insulins

Products	Type	Onset of action (hours)	Peak effect	Duration
Modified insulin				
NovoRapid (aspart)	Ultra fast	0.2	0.5-1.5	3-5
Humalog (lispro)	Ultra fast	0.5-0.75	0.75-2.5	3.5-4.75
Apidra (insulin glulisine)	Ultra fast	0.2-0.5	1.6-2.8	3-4
Lantus (insulin glargine)	ultra lente	1.5		24
Levemir (insulin determir)	ultra lente	3-4	6-8	24
Humalog Mix 25	mixture	0.5-0.75	0.75-2.5	18-24
Humalog Mix 50	mixture	0.5-0.75	0.75-2.5	18-24
MovoMix 30 (insulin asparte biphasic)	mixture	0.2	1-4	24
Human insulin				
Humulin R	fast	0.5-1	2-4	5-8
Novolin GE Toronto	fast	0.5-1	2-4	5-8
Humulin N	lente	3-4	6-12	18-28
Novolin NPH	lente	3-4	6-12	18-28
Novolin GE lente	lente	1-3	8-12	18-28
Novolin GE Ultra lente	ultra lente	3-4	8-15	22-26
Humulin 10/90	Mixture	0.5-1	4-8	24
Humulin 20/80	Mixture	0.5-1	4-8	24
Humulin 30/70	Mixture	0.5-1	4-8	24
Humulin 40/60	Mixture	0.5-1	4-8	24
Humulin 50/50	Mixture	0.5-1	4-8	24
Novolin GE 30/70	Mixture	0.5-1	4-8	24
Novolin GE 40/60	Mixture	0.5-1	4-8	24
Novolin GE 50/50	Mixture	0.5-1	4-8	24

Proton Pump Inhibitors and H2 Antihistamines

Product	Commercial name	Dose/day (mg)	Times per day	Equivalent dose (mg)
Proton Pump Inhibitors				
Esomeprazole	Nexium	20-40	1	20
Lansoprazole	Prevacid	15-30	1-2	30
Omeprazole	Losec	20-40	1-2	20
Pantoprazole	Pantoloc	20-40	1-2	40
Pantoprazole magnesium	Tecta	40	1-2	40
Rabeprazole	Pariet	10-20	1-2	20
H2 Antihistamines				
Cimetidine	Tagamet	800-1200	1-4	400
Famotidine	Pepcid	20-80	1-2	20
Nizatidine	Axid	150-300	1-2	150
Ranitidine	Zantac	75-300	1-2	150

Narcotics

Agent	Commercial name	Route	Source	Duration of action (h)	Equivalent dose		Adjustment in renal failure
					IM	PO	
Narcotic agonists							
Codeine		PO, IM s/c	nat.	3-4	120 mg	200 mg	Yes
	Codeine contin	PO		12			
Fentanyl	Sublimaze	IV	syn.	1-2	50 mcg	-	Yes
	Duragesic	patch		72*			
Hydro-morphone	Dilaudid	PO, IM, s/c, IV	s-syn.	3-4	2	4-6	No
	Hydromorph contin	PO		12			
Meperidine	Demerol	PO, IM, IV, s/c	syn.	2-4	75	300	Yes
Methadone		PO	syn.	4-6	dose-dependant ratio		Yes
Morphine		PO, IM IV, s/c IR	nat.	3-4	10 mg	20-30 mg	Yes
	MS contin	PO		12			
Oxycodone	Supeudol	PO	s-syn.	3-4	–	10-15	No
	Oxy-IR	PO		4-6			
	OxyContin	PO		12**			
Tramadol	Tridural	PO	syn	12		50-100 mg	Yes
Agonist-antagonist narcotics							
Nalbuphine	Nubain	s/c, IV, IM	s-syn	3-6	10	-	No
Pentazocine	Talwin	PO, IM, s/c, IV	s-syn	3-4	60	180	Yes

* Onset of action in 24 hours.
** Onset of action in 45 minutes.

Amines

Dopamine : i.e.: 400 mg / 250 mL D5W.
      Renal effect : 1-2 µg/kg/min (5-8 mL/h).
      predominant β effect: 2-10 µg/kg/min
      α > β effect: > 20 µg/kg/min

Dobutamine (Dobutrex®) : i.e.: 500 mg / 250 mL D5W.
    Dose: 5-15 µg/kg/min.

Epinephrine (Adrenalin®): i.e.: 1 mg / 250 mL D5W or NaCl 0.9%
    Dose: 0.1-1 µg/kg/min.

Norepinephrine (Levophed®) : i.e.: 4 mg / 250 mL D5W
    β dose: < 0.02 µg/kg/min
    α dose: > 0.02 µg/kg/min
    Maximal dose = 8 mg solution / 250 mL at 56 mL/h.

Phenylephrine (Neosynephrine®) : i.e.: 10 mg/100 mL D5W or NaCl 0.9%
    0.5-15 µg/kg/min dose

Important P450 Cytochrome Drug Interactions

Enzymes	Drugs metabolized by the enzymes	Inhibitors	Inducers
CYP1A2	Antipsychotics (i.e.: haloperidol, clozapine, olanzapine), benzodiazepines, caffeine, fluvoxamine, naproxen, theophylline, tricyclic antidepressants, and R-warfarin.	Anastrozole, Antifungal azoles, cimetidine, fluoroquinolones, fluvoxamine, interferon α 2-b, grapefruit juice, isoniazide, macrolides.	BBQ cooking, caffeine, carbamazepine, omeprazole, phenytoin, phenobarbital, primidone, rifampin, ritonavir, tobacco.
CYP2C9/19	Celebrex, clopidogrel, diazepam, fluvastatin, meloxicam, phenytoin, proton pump inhibitors, tricyclic antidepressants, voriconazole, S-warfarin.	Amiodarone (2C9), antifungal azoles (2C9/19), capecitabine (2C9), chloramphenicol, cimetidine (2C9), cotrimoxazole (2C9), efavirenz (2C9/19), felbamate, fluconazole (2C9), fluoxetine, fluvastatin, fluvoxamine, indomethacin, interferon α 2-b, isoniazide (2C9), ketoconazole, lansoprazole, metronidazole (2C9), modafinil, omeprazole (2C9/19), oxcarbazepine, probenecid, rabeprazole, rosuvastatine (2C9), ticlodipine, topiramate (2C9) zafirlukast (2C9).	Bosentan, carbamazepine, glipizide, norethindrone, phenobarbital, phenytoin, prednisone, primidone, rifampin.
CYP2D6	Antipsychotics, tricyclic antidepressants and others, bisoprolol, carvedilol, codeine, flecainide, metoclopramide, metoprolol, opioids, propafenone, propanolol, risperidone, tamoxifene, venlafaxine.	Amiodarone, tricyclic antidepressants, bupropion, chloroquine, cimetidine, cinacalcet, citalopram, duloxetine, escitalopram, fluoxetine, haloperidol, imatinib, methadone, methotrimeprazine, moclobemide, paroxetine, propafenone, quinidine, ritonavir, sertraline, terbinafine.	Carbamazepine, phenobarbital, phenytoin, primidone, rifampin, ritonavir.
CYP3A4	Antifungals, non-sedative antihistaminics, benzodiazepines, calcium-channel blockers, carbamazepine, chemotherapy, cyclosporin, disopyramide, HMG-CoA reductase inhibitors (except fluvastatin, cerivastatin and pravastatin), imatinib, protease inhibitors, quetiapine, quinidine, rivaroxaban, R-warfarin, sildenafil, sibutramine, tacrolimus, telithromycin.	Amiodarone, antifungal azoles, aprepitant, cimetidine, delavirdine, diltiazem, fluoxetine, fluvoxamine, grapefruit juice, imatinib, isoniazide, macrolides, meronidazole, nefazodone, norfloxacin, protease inhibitors, quinidine, verapamil, zafirlukast.	Bosentan, carbamazepine, dexamethasone, efavirenz, nevirapine, phenobarbital, phenytoin, pioglitazone, primidone, rifabutin, rifampin, St. John's wort, topiramate.

Principal Drug Interactions with Digoxin

Drug or class	Mechanism	Suggested management
Amiodarone	Decreases renal and non-renal clearance. Increases digoxin level by 70-100 %.	Follow digoxinemia and symptoms and signs of intoxication. Anticipate necessity to reduce dose by 50%.
Antiacids, cholestyramine, colestipol, phenytoin	Concomitant administration reduces bioavailability by 20-35 %.	Separate doses by at least 2 hours.
Clarithromycin, erythromycin, tetracycline	Alteration of the intestinal flora resulting in increased bioavailability by 40-100 % in about 10 %. Inhibition of P glycoproteins (PGP).	Follow digoxinemia and symptoms and signs of intoxication. Anticipate necessity to reduce dose. Avoid associations.
Cyclosporine	Decreases renal clearance and/or function. Inhibition of P glycoproteins (PGP) is also postulated.	Follow digoxinemia and symptoms and signs of intoxication. Anticipate necessity to reduce dose by 50%.
Diltiazem	Decreases renal and non-renal clearance. Increases digoxin level by 20-30 %.	Follow digoxinemia and symptoms and signs of intoxication. Anticipate necessity to reduce dose.
Diuretics	Thiazides and loop diuretics cause hypokalemia and hypomagnesemia, increasing toxicity risk.	Follow and supplement electrolytes if necessary.
Propafenone	Decreases renal clearance. Increases digoxinemia by 30-40 %.	Follow digoxinemia and symptoms and signs of intoxication. Anticipate necessity to reduce dose.
Quinidine	Decreases renal and non-renal clearance. Reduction in distribution volume and displacement of the tissue binding sites. Increases digoxin level by 100 %.	Follow digoxinemia and symptoms and signs of intoxication. Anticipate necessity to reduce dose by 50 %.
Verapamil	Decreases renal and non-renal clearance. Increases digoxin level by 70-100 %.	Follow digoxinemia and symptoms and signs of intoxication. Anticipate necessity to reduce dose by 50 %.

Principal Drug Interactions with Warfarin

Drug or class	Effect on prothrombin time	Mechanism
Alcohol (acute ingestion), allopurinol, amiodarone, cimetidine, fluconazole, fluvoxamine, grapefruit juice, itraconazole, ketoconazole, macrolides, metronidazole, omeprazole*, phenytoin, propafenone, quinidine, quinolones, sulfamethoxazole	Increase	Inhibition of warfarin metabolism
Thyroid hormones	Increase	Increase in coagulation factors catabolism
Cefamandole, cefoperazone, cefotetan	Increase	Decrease in coagulation factors production
Wide spectrum antibiotics	Increase	Decrease in vitamin K production by the intestinal flora
Acetaminophen, fibrates, lovastatin	Increase	Unknown mechanism
Estrogens and vitamin K	Decrease	Increase in coagulation factors production
Methimazole et proplythiouracile	Decrease	Decrease in coagulation factors catabolism
Barbiturates, carbamazepine, alcohol (chronic ingestion), phenytoin, primidone, rifampin	Decrease	Induction of warfarin metabolism
Cholestyramine, colestipol and sucralfate	Decrease	Decreases absorption
Azathioprine, cyclophosphamide, cyclosporin and mesalamine	Decrease	Unknown mechanism
ASA and other salicylates, NSAIDs, clopidogrel, heparins, ticlopidine	No effect	Increase in bleeding risks

* With omeprazole, interaction of R isomer (less powerful). According to CPS 2002, p. 1040 : "Concomitant treatment with Omeprazole 20 mg/ day did not modify coagulation time in patients receiving a continuous treatment with Warfarin".

SCORE Canada

Assessment of 10-year risk of fatal vascular disease

The evaluation of the global risk of death in a 10 year period from coronary vascular disease is indicated in asymptomatic adult individuals.

The SCORE Canada chart is an evaluation chart to estimate and stratify the cardiovascular risk (cerebral and coronary) in asymptomatic adult individuals.

Several risk factors increase the risk of developing atherosclerosis and vascular disease. These factors interact and sometimes multiply themselves. SCORE Canada takes into account variables such as age, sex, smoking, systolic blood pressure and the total cholesterol to HDL-C ratio.

This risk assessment chart can be used upon request and for any middle age adult presenting at least one cardiovascular risk factor or a family history of premature cardiovascular disease.

Do not use this chart for people with cardiovascular disease, diabetics with target organ damage, those with a very abnormal risk factor requiring a medical intervention or those aged 70 or older.

Using the SCORE table

1. Pick up the case corresponding to the following factors:
- Age (for people under 40 y. o., the relative risk chart must be used).
- Sex.
- Smoking.
- Systolic blood pressure.
- Total cholesterol to HDL-C ratio.

2. The following will give you an estimate of the mortal risk for each cardiovascular disease:
<blockquote>
High ≥ 5 %
Medium: 2 to 4 %
Low: ≤ 1 %
</blockquote>

3. The global risk of death from heart failure may be higher than indicated on the table if:
- The person approaches the next age category.
- Preclinical atherosclerosis is already demonstrated (tomodensitometry, ultrasonography).
- Strong family history of premature vascular disease at an early age (**x 1.4**).
- Obesity, BMI ≥ 30 kg/m^2, waist circumference: ≥ 102 cm (men) and ≥ 88 cm (women).
- Sedentarity.
- Diabetes: multiply the risk by **2** for a man and **4** for a woman.
- High level of triglycerides.
- High level of C-Reactive Protein, fibrinogen, homocystein or B-apolipoprotein or Lp(a).

Note: The SCORE chart should be used to help and not to replace clinical judgment.

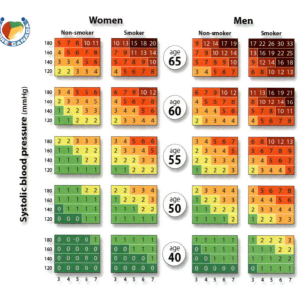

Women   Men

Systolic blood pressure (mmHg)

Total cholesterol to HDL-C ratio

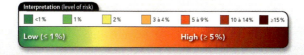

Interpretation (level of risk)

| <1% | 1% | 2% | 3 à 4% | 5 à 9% | 10 à 14% | ≥15% |

Low (≤ 1%)   High (≥ 5%)

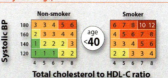

Relative risk assessment (for individuals under 40 years of age)

For individuals under 40 years of age, use the relative risk assessment chart.

The number in the cell means that the person have a *n* times higher cardiovascular risk than another person being the same age for whom all risk factors are minimals.

Systolic BP

Total cholesterol to HDL-C ratio

Estimation of 10-year fracture risk for men

Âge	Low risk (< 10 %)	Moderate risk (10-20 %)	High risk (> 20 %)
	Lowest T-score (lumbar spine, total hip, femoral neck, trochanter)		
50	> - 3.4	≤ - 3.4	
55	> - 3.1	≤ - 3.1	
60	> - 3.0	≤ - 3.0	
65	> - 2.7	≤ - 2.7	
70	> - 2.1	- 2.1 to - 3.9	< - 3.9
75	> - 1.5	- 1.5 to 3.2	< - 3.2
80	> - 1.2	- 1.2 to - 3.0	< - 3.0
85	> - 1.3	- 1.3 to 3.3	< - 3.3
Note: Fragility fracture after age 40 or glucocorticoid use increase risk categorization to the next level (i.e.: from low to moderate, etc.).			

ECOG Grading of Performance Status

Grade	Description
0	Fully active, able to carry on all pre-disease performance without restriction.
1	Restricted in physically strenuous activity but ambulatory and able to carry out work of a light or sedentary nature, e.g., light house work, office work.
2	Ambulatory and capable of all self-care but unable to carry out any work activities. Up and about more than 50% of waking hours.
3	Capable of only limited self-care, confined to bed or chair more than 50% of waking hours.
4	Completely disabled. Cannot carry on any self-care. Totally confined to bed or chair.
5	Dead.

Reference: Oken MM, Creech RH, Tormey DC, Horton J, Davis TE, McFadden ET, Carbone PP.Toxicity And Response Criteria Of The Eastern Cooperative Oncology Group. Am J Clin Oncol 1982; 5: 649-655.

Epworth Sleepiness Scale

How likely are you to doze off or fall asleep in the situations described below,
in contrast to feeling just tired?

This refers to your usual way of life in recent times.

Even if you haven't done some of these things recently try to work out
how they would have affected you.

Use the following scale to choose the <u>most appropriate number</u> for each situation:

> 0 = would <u>never</u> doze
> 1 = <u>Slight</u> chance of dozing
> 2 = <u>Moderate</u> chance of dozing
> 3 = <u>High</u> chance of dozing

Chance of dozing

1. Sitting and reading: _____

2. Watching TV: _____

3. Sitting, inactive in a public place (e.g. a theatre or a meeting):   _____

4. As a passenger in a car for an hour without a break: _____

5. Lying down to rest in the afternoon when circumstances permit: _____

6. Sitting and talking to someone: _____

7. Sitting quietly after an lunch without alcohol: _____

8. In a car, while stopped for a few minutes in the traffic: _____

Total (0-24) _____

Excessive sleepiness if score ≥10, severe sleepiness if ≥ 18

Reference: Johns MW. A new method for measuring daytime sleepiness: the Epworth sleepiness scale. Sleep 1991 ; 14: 540-5.

Associations, foundations,
support groups for patients

Associations, fondations, support group for patients

General information on health: Canadian Health Network
Web site: www.canadian-health-network.ca

Alzheimer's disease: Alzheimer Society of Canada: 1-800-616-8816
Web site: www.alzheimer.ca

Amyotrophic lateral sclerosis: ALS Society of Canada: 1-800-267-4257
Web site: www.als.ca

Arthritis: Arthritis Society of Canada: 1-800-321-1433
Web site: www.arthritis.ca

Asthma: Asthma Society of Canada: 1-866-787-4050
Web site: www.asthma.ca
Québec Lung Association: 1-800-295-8111
Web site: www.pq.poumon.ca

Breast cancer: Canadian Breast Cancer Foundation: 1-800-387-9816
Web site: www.cbcf.org

Cancer: Canadian Cancer Society: 1-888-939-3333
Web site: www.cancer.ca

Celiac disease: Canadian Celiac Association : 1-800-363-7296
Web site: www.celiac.ca

Diabetes: Canadian Diabetes Association : 1-800-226-8464
Web site: www.diabetes.ca
Diabetes Québec : (514) 259-3422, 1-800-361-3504
Web site: www.diabete.qc.ca

Epilepsy : Epilepsy Canada: 1-877-734-0873
Web site: www.epilepsy.ca

Fibromyalgia: National Education Network : (613) 829-6667
Web site: www.mefmaction.net

Headaches: Help for headaches: 1-519-434-0008
Web site: www.headache-help.org

Heart disease: Heart and Stroke Foundation of Canada: 1-613-569-4361
Web site: www.heartandstroke.ca

Hemochromatosis: Canadian Hemochromatosis Society: 1-877- BAD-IRON
Web site: www.cdnhemochromatosis.ca
L'institut québécois de l'hémochromatose : (819) 643-2096

Associations, fondations, support group for patients

Hemophilia: Canadian Hemophilia Society: (514) 848-0503,
1-800-668-2686
Web site: www.hemophilia.ca

HIV-AIDS: Canadian AIDS Society: 1-800-499-1986
Web site: www.cdnaids.ca
Canadian AIDS Treatment Information Exchange: 1-800-263-1638
Web site: www.catie.ca

Hypertension: Canadian Hypertension Society
Web site: www.hypertension.ca

Inflammatory Bowel Disease:
Crohn's and Colitis Foundation of Canada: 1-800-387-1479
Web site: www.fcmii.ca

Kidney: The Kidney Foundation of Canada: (514) 369-4806, 1-800-361-7494
Web site: www.kidney.ca

Liver disease: Canadian Liver Foundation: 1-800-563-5483
Web site: www.liver.ca

Lung disease: Canadian Lung Association: 1-800-972-2636
Web site: www.lung.ca
Québec Lung Association:
Web site: www.pq.poumon.ca

Lupus: Lupus Canada: 1-800-661-1468
Web site: www.lupuscanada.org

Multiple sclerosis: Multiple Sclerosis Society of Canada: 1-800-268-7582
Web site: www.mssociety.ca

Osteoporosis: Osteoporosis Canada: 1-800-463-6842
Web site: www.osteoporosis.ca

Parkinson's disease: Parkinson Society Canada: (514) 861-4422,
1-800-565-3000
Web site: www.parkinson.ca

Sjögren's syndrome: The Sjögren's Society of Canada: 1-888-558-0950
Web site: www.sjogrenscanada.org

Thyroid: Thyroid Foundation of Canada: 1-800-267-8822
Web site: www.thyroid.ca

Abbreviations

Abbreviations

A

AAA : abdominal aortic aneurysms
ABI : ankle-brachial index
ABVD : doxorubicin, bleomycin, vinblastine, dacarbazine
AC : before meals
ACCP : American College of Chest Physicians
ACEI : angiotensin-converting enzyme inhibitor
ACS : acute coronary syndrome
ACTH : adrenocorticotropin
ad : up to or until
AD : Alzheimer's disease
ADH : antidiuretic hormone
AF : atrial fibrillation
AIDS : acquired immunodeficiency syndrome
ALL : acute lymphocytic leukemia
ALT : alanine aminotransferases
AM : *ante meridiem*
AML : acute myelogenous leukemia
ANA : antinuclear antibody
ANCA : antineutrophil cytoplasmic autoantibodies
APS : antiphospholipid syndrome
aPTT : activated partial thromboplastin time
ARB : angiotensin II receptor blocker
ARDS : acute respiratory distress syndrome
AS : aortic stenosis
ASA : acetylsalicylic acid
ASO : antistreptolysines O antibodies
AST : aspartate aminotransferases
AV : atrioventricular

B

BCG : bacillus Calmette-Guérin
bid : twice a day
BMD : bone mineral density
BMI : body mass index
BNP : B-type natriuretic peptide
BOOP : bronchiolitis obliterans organizing pneumonia
BP : blood pressure
BUN : blood urea nitrogen

C

[ ] : concentration
5-FU : 5-fluorouracil
5-HIAA : 5-hydroxyindoleacetic acid
C1 Inh : C1 esterase inhibitor
Ca^{++} : calcium
CABG : coronary artery bypass graft
CAD : coronary artery disease
CBC : complete blood count
CDC : Centers for Disease Control
CEA : carcinoembryonic antigen
CHF : congestive heart failure
CHOP : cyclophosphamide, doxorubicin, vincristine, prednisone
CIDP : chronic inflammatory demyelinating polyneuropathy
CK : creatine kinase
CKD: chronic kidney disease
Cl^{-} : chlorides

ClCr: creatinine clearance
CLL : chronic lymphocytic leukemia
cm : centimeter
CMF: cyclophosphamide, methotrexate, 5-FU
CML : chronic myelogenous leukemia
CMV : cytomegalovirus
CNS: central nervous system
COP: cryptogenic organizing pneumonia
COPD : chronic obstructive pulmonary disease
CRH : corticotropin-releasing hormone
CREST : calcinosis cutis, Raynaud's phenomenon, esophageal dysmotility, sclerodactyly, telangiectasia
CRP : C-reactive protein
CSF : cerebrospinal fluid
CT : computed tomography
CVA : cerebrovascular accident
CVP : central venous pressure or cyclophosphamide, vincristine, prednisone

D

d : day
18-OHB : 18-hydroxyprogesterone
DBP : diastolic blood pressure
DDAVP : desmopressin
DHE : dihydroergotamine
DHEA-S : dehydroepiandrosterone sulfate
DIC : disseminated intravascular coagulation
DLCO : CO_2 diffusion
DNA : deoxyribonucleic acid
DS-DNA : double-stranded DNA
DVT : deep-vein thrombosis

E

EBV : Ebstein-Barr virus
ECG : electrocardiogram
EEG : electroencephalogram
e.g. : for example
ELISA : enzyme-linked immunosorbent assay
EMG : electromyogram
ENT : ear nose throat
EPS : electrophysiologic study
ER : estrogen receptors *or* emergency room
ERCP : endoscopic retrograde cholangiography
ESR : erythrocyte sedimentation rate
ESRD: end stage renal disease
Eth : ethambutol
Ex : example

F

1st : first
FEV1: forced expiratory volume in 1 s
FIO2 : inspired oxygen fraction
FSH : follicle-stimulating hormone
FT4 : free T4
FUO : fever of unknown origin
FVC : forced vital capacity

G

g : gram
GABA : gamma-aminobutyric acid
GBM : glomerular membrane basement
G-CSF : granulocyte colony stimulating factor
gen : generation

Abbreviations

GERD : gastroesophageal reflux disease
GFR : glomerular filtration rate
GGT : gamma glutamyltransferase
GH : growth hormone
GHRH : growth hormone-releasing hormone
GI : gastrointestinal
GM-CSF : granulocyte-macrophage colony
    stimulating factor
GnRH : gonadotropin-releasing hormone
GOLD : Global Initiative for Chronic Obstructive
    Lung Disease
GVHD : graft-versus-host disease

H
h : hour
HAV : hepatitis A virus
Hb : hemoglobin
HbA1c : glycosylated hemoglobin
HBP : high blood pressure
HBV : hepatitis B virus
hCG : human chorionic gonadotropin
HCO3 : bicarbonates
Hct : hematocrit
HCTZ : hydrochlorothiazide
HCV : hepatitis C virus
H2O : water
HDL : high density lipoprotein
HDV : hepatitis D virus
HELLP : hemolysis elevated liver enzymes low
    platelets syndrome
HIT : heparin-induced thrombocytopenia
HIV : human immunodeficiency virus
HS : at bedtime
HSV : herpes simplex virus
HTN : hypertension
Hz : Hertz

I
i.e. : that is
IE : infective endocarditis
Ig : immunoglobulins
IGF-I : insulin-like growth factor 1
IM : intramuscular
inh : inhalation
INH : isoniazid
INR : international normalized ratio
IR : intrarectal
ISA : intrinsic sympathomimetic activity
ITP : immune thrombocytopenic purpura
URTI : upper respiratory tract infection
IU : international unit
IUGR : intrauterine growth retardation
IV : intravenous

J

K
K+ : potassium
KCl : potassium chloride
kg : kilogram

L
L : liter
LA : left atrium
LAFB : left anterior fascicular block
LBBB : left bundle-branch block
LCM : lymphocytic choriomeningitis

LDH : lactic dehydrogenase
LDL : low density lipoprotein
LH : luteinizing hormone
LHRH : luteinizing hormone releasing hormone
LKM : Liver-Kidney microsomes
LLQ : left lower quadrant
LMWH : low molecular weight heparin
LPFB : left posterior fascicular block
LUQ : left upper quadrant
LV : left ventricle
LVEF : left ventricular ejection fraction
LVH : left ventricular hypertrophy

M
MALT : mucosa-associated lymphoid tissue
MAO : monoamine oxidase
MAOI : monoamine oxidase inhibitor
max : maximum
mcg : microgram
MCV: mean corpuscular volume
MDMA : methylenedioxy-methamphetamine
    (*ecstasy*)
MEN : multiple endocrine neoplasia
mEq : milliequivalent
mg : milligram
Mg++ : magnesium
MGUS : monoclonal gammapathy of unknown
    significance
MI : myocardial infarction
MIBG : metaiodobenzylguanidine
MIC : minimum inhibitory concentration
min : minute
mL : milliliter
mm : millimeter
mmHg : millimeter of mercury
mmol : millimole
MMSE : MiniMental State Examination
mo : month
MPV : mean platelet volume
ms : millisecond
MRI : magnetic resonance imaging
MRCP : magnetic resonance
    cholangiopancreatography
MRSA : methicillin-resistant *S. aureus*
MS : mitral stenosis
MTX : methotrexate
MU : millions of units

N
Na+ : sodium
nebu : nebulization
neg. : negative
ng : nannogram
NG : nasogastric
NK : natural killer
nmol : nanomole
NMDA : N-methyl-D-aspartate
NPO : *nil per os*
NSAID : nonsteroidal antiinflammatory
drug

O
1,25-OH2D3 : 1,25-dihydroxycholecalciferol
O2 : oxygen
od : once a day
OHA : oral antihyperglycemic agents

Abbreviations

osm : osmolality

P
PaCO2 : partial pressure of carbon dioxide in arterial blood
PAD : peripheral artery disease
PaO2 : partial pressure of oxygen in arterial blood
PAS : periodic acid-Shiff
PC : after meals
PCI : percutaneous coronary intervention
PCP : phencyclidine
PCR : polymerase chain reaction
PE : pulmonary embolism
PEEP : positive end expiratory pressure
PEF : peak expiratory flow
pmol : picomole
PET : positrons emission tomodensitometry
PFT : pulmonary function tests
PO : *per os* or by mouth
PO4⁻ : phosphorus
post-op : post-operative
PP : *post-partum*
PPD : purified protein derivative
PPI : proton-pump inhibitor
pre-op : pre-operative
PRN : as needed
P.S. : *post scriptum*
PSA : prostate-specific antigen
PSVT : paroxysmal supraventricular tachycardia
Pt:patient
PT : prothrombin time
PTH : parathyroid hormone
PTHrP : PTH related peptide
PTU : propylthiouracil
Pyr : pyrazinamide

Q
q : every ...
qid : four time a day
QTc : corrected QT

R
RA : rheumatoid arthritis
RAST : radioallergosorbent test
RBBB : right bundle-branch block
RBC : red blood cells
RF : risk factor or rheumatoid factor
Rif : rifampin
RLQ : right lower quadrant
RNA : ribonucleic acid
RPR : rapid plasma reagin
RR : relative risk
RSV : respiratory syncytial virus
RUQ : right upper quadrant
RVH : right ventricular hypertrophy

S
s : second
2ⁿᵈ : second or secondary
S1 : first heart sound
S2 : second hearth sound
S2a : aortic component of the second hearth sound
S2p : pulmonic component of the second hearth sound
SaO2 : oxygen arterial saturation
Sat: saturation

SBP : systolic blood pressure
s/c : subcutaneous
SIADH : syndrome of inappropriate ADH secretion
SIRS : systemic inflammatory response syndrome
SLE : systemic lupus erythematosus
SMX : sulfamethoxazole
SSRI : selective serotonin reuptake inhibitors
sp. : species
STD : sexually transmitted diseases
Strepto : streptomycine
STAT : immediately
SvO2 : oxygen venous saturation

T
25-OHD : 25-hydroxycholecalciferol
T3 : triiodothyronine
T4 : thyroxine
TB : tuberculosis
TG : triglycerides
TIA : transient ischemic attack
tid : three times a day
TIPS : transjugular intrahepatic portosystemic shunts
TMP : trimethoprim
TNF : tumor necrosis factor
TNM : tumor node metastasis
TO : topical
tPA : alteplase
TPN : total parenteral nutrition
TRH : thyrotropin-releasing hormone
TSH : thyroid-stimulating hormone
TTKG : transtubular K⁺ gradient
TTP : thrombotic thrombocytopenic purpura
TTP-HUS : thrombotic thrombocytopenic purpura-hemolytic uremic syndrome
Tx : treatment

U
U : unit
UF : unfractioned
URTI : upper respiratory tract infection
U/S : ultrasound
UTI : urinary tract infection

V
VAD : vincristine, doxorubicin, dexamethasone
VDRL : venereal disease research laboratory
VIP : vasoactive intestinal peptide
VRE : vancomycin-resistant enterococci
VT : ventricular tachycardia
vWF : von Willebrand factor
Vx : vessel
VZV : varicella zoster virus

W
WBC: White blood cells
WHO : World Health Organization

Y
y.o. : year old

INDEX

Index

Index